中文翻译版

妊娠糖尿病实战手册
A Practical Manual of Diabetes in Pregnancy

原书第 2 版

主　编　David R. McCance
　　　　Michael Maresh
　　　　David A. Sacks
主　译　李洪梅

科学出版社

北　京

图字：01-2018-5232 号

内 容 简 介

本书延续了第 1 版说明性病例的章节格式特点，提出一些问题，在文中给出回答，并配有说明性图表和相关文献，全面介绍了妊娠糖尿病的知识，包括筛查、诊断和治疗。同时阐述了妊娠糖尿病领域已经取得的成就、目前的研究进展和未来的前景。

本书内容简洁、实用，符合妊娠糖尿病管理的需要，可作为内分泌科、产科临床医师及护理人员的参考用书，也可供社区卫生服务机构从业人员及孕产妇阅读和参考。

图书在版编目（CIP）数据

妊娠糖尿病实战手册：原书第2版/（英）D. R. 麦坎斯（David R. McCance）等主编；李洪梅主译.—北京：科学出版社，2020.5
书名原文：A Practical Manual of Diabetes in Pregnancy
ISBN 978-7-03-064654-5

Ⅰ. ①妊⋯ Ⅱ. ①D⋯ ②李⋯ Ⅲ. ①妊娠合并症-糖尿病-诊疗-手册 Ⅳ. ①R714.256-62

中国版本图书馆 CIP 数据核字（2020）第 038786 号

责任编辑：康丽涛 ／ 责任校对：张小霞
责任印制：赵 博 ／ 封面设计：吴朝洪

All rights reserved. This Translation publish under license. Authorized translation from the English language edition, entitled *A Practical Manual of Diabetes in Pregnancy* ISBN 978-1-119-04379-9, by David R. McCance.Published by John Wiley Sons. Responsibility for the accuracy of the translation rests solely with China Science Publishing & Media Ltd(Science Press). No part of this publication may be reproduced, stored in a retrieval system, or transmitted, in any form or by any means, electronic, mechanical, photocopying, recording or otherwise, except as permitted by law.
Copies of this book sold without a Wiley sticker on the cover are unauthorized and illegal.

科学出版社 出版
北京东黄城根北街 16 号
邮政编码：100717
http://www.sciencep.com

天津市新科印刷有限公司 印刷
科学出版社发行 各地新华书店经销
*
2020 年 5 月第 一 版 开本：890×1240 1/32
2020 年 5 月第一次印刷 印张：14 1/2
字数：441 000
定价：78.00 元

（如有印装质量问题，我社负责调换）

《妊娠糖尿病实战手册》（原书第 2 版）翻译人员

主　译　李洪梅
副主译　朱海清　王　冰
译　者　（按姓氏笔画排序）

王　冰　王凯亮　王诗淇　朱海清
任　歆　刘长春　刘雅静　孙　焱
李晶晶　杨　芳　杨　蓉　汪　琦
张　焱　张雪冰　侯淑敏　韩　旸
赖　杰

Contributors

Juan María Adelantado MD
Department of Obstetrics and Gynaecology
Hospital de la Santa Creu i Sant Pau
Barcelona, Spain

Montserrat Balsells
Department of Endocrinology and Nutrition
Hospital Universitari Mútua de Terrassa
Terrassa, Spain

Helen L. Barrett MBBS, PhD
UQ Centre for Clinical Research
Faculty of Medicine
The University of Queensland
Brisbane, Queensland, Australia

Leonie K. Callaway MBBS, PhD
UQ Centre for Clinical Research
Faculty of Medicine
The University of Queensland
Brisbane, Queensland, Australia

Gioia N. Canciani MBBS
Elsie Bertram Diabetes Centre
Norfolk and Norwich University Hospitals
Norwich, UK

Lisa Chasan-Taber ScD
Department of Biostatistics & Epidemiology
University of Massachusetts
Amherst, Massachusetts, USA

Emily Y. Chew MD
National Eye Institute of National
Institutes of Health, Bethesda
Maryland, USA

Rosa Corcoy MD
Department of Endocrinology and Nutrition
Hospital de la Santa Creu i Sant Pau
Barcelona; CIBER Bioengineering,
Biomaterials and Nanotechnology
(CIBER-BBN)
Instituto de Salud Carlos III
Zaragoza; Department of Medicine
Universitat Autònoma de Barcelona
Bellaterra, Spain

Susan Curtis
Manchester Diabetes Centre
Central Manchester University Hospitals
NHS Foundation Trust
Manchester Academic Health
Sciences Centre, Manchester, UK

Dana Dabalea MD, PhD
Department of Epidemiology
University of Colorado School of
Public Health
Aurora, Colorado, USA

Peter Damm MD, DMSc
Center of Pregnant Women with Diabetes
Department of Obstetrics
Rigshospitalet; and
Faculty of Health Sciences
University of Copenhagen
Copenhagen, Denmark

Gernot Desoye PhD
Department of Obstetrics and Gynecology
Medical University of Graz
Graz, Austria

Francine Hughes Einstein MD
Departments of Obstetrics & Gynecology
and Women's Health
Division of Maternal Fetal Medicine
Montefiore Medical Center
The University Hospital for the Albert
Einstein College of Medicine
Bronx, New York, USA

Denice S. Feig MD, MSc
University of Toronto
Diabetes & Endocrinology in Pregnancy
Program; and
Mount Sinai Hospital
Toronto, Canada

Apolonia García-Patterson MD
Department of Endocrinology
and Nutrition
Hospital de la Santa Creu i Sant Pau
Barcelona, Spain

Una M. Graham MD
Regional Centre for Endocrinology
and Diabetes
Royal Victoria Hospital
Belfast,
Northern Ireland, UK

Peter Hammond MD
Harrogate District Hospital
Harrogate, UK

Lorie M. Harper MD, MSCI
Department of Obstetrics
and Gynecology
University of Alabama at Birmingham
Birmingham, Alabama, USA

Jesia Hasan MD
Department of Ophthalmology
University of Montreal
Montreal, Canada

Jane M. Hawdon MD
Women's and Children's Health
Clinical Academic Group
Barts Health NHS Trust
London, UK

Ursula Hiden PhD
Department of Obstetrics and Gynecology
Medical University of Graz
Graz, Austria

David J. Hill D.Phil.
Lawson Health Research Institute
St. Joseph's Health Care
London, Ontario, Canada

Dorte Møller Jensen MD
Department of Endocrinology
Department of Gynecology and Obstetrics
Odense University Hospital; and
Department of Clinical Research
Faculty of Health Sciences
University of Southern Denmark
Odense, Denmark

Nia Jones MD
Department of Obstetrics
and Gynaecology
Nottingham University Hospitals NHS
Trust; and
School of Medicine
University of Nottingham
Nottingham, UK

Dipanwita Kapoor MBBS
Department of Obstetrics and Gynaecology
Nottingham University Hospitals NHS Trust
Nottingham, UK

Gretta Kearney
St Mary's Hospital
Central Manchester University Hospitals
NHS Foundation Trust
Manchester Academic Health Sciences Centre
Manchester, UK

Catherine Kim MD, MPH
Departments of Medicine and
Obstetrics & Gynecology
University of Michigan
Ann Arbor, Michigan, USA

Jacques Lepercq MD
Maternité Port Royal
Université Paris Descartes
Paris, France

Robert S. Lindsay MD
Institute of Cardiovascular
and Medical Sciences
University of Glasgow
Scotland, UK

Michael Maresh MD
St Mary's Hospital
Central Manchester University Hospitals
NHS Foundation Trust
Manchester Academic Health
Sciences Centre
Manchester, UK

Elisabeth R. Mathiesen MD
Center of Pregnant Women with Diabetes
Department of Endocrinology
Rigshospitalet; and
Faculty of Health Sciences
University of Copenhagen
Copenhagen, Denmark

David R. McCance MD
Regional Centre for Endocrinology and
Diabetes
Royal Victoria Hospital
Belfast, Northern Ireland, UK

H. David McIntyre MD
Department of Obstetric Medicine
Mater Health Services
and Mater Research
Faculty of Medicine
The University of Queensland
Brisbane, Queensland, Australia

Geetha Mukerji MD, MSc
University of Toronto;
Women's College Hospital; and
Mount Sinai Hospital (cross-appointed)
Toronto, Canada

Helen R. Murphy MD
University of Cambridge Metabolic
Research Laboratories and NIHR
Cambridge Biomedical Research Centre
Institute of Metabolic Science
Addenbrooke's Hospital
Cambridge, UK

Jenny Myers MD
St Mary's Hospital
Central Manchester University Hospitals
NHS Foundation Trust
Manchester Academic
Health Sciences Centre
Maternal & Fetal Health Research Centre
University of Manchester
Manchester, UK

Anita L. Nelson MD
David Geffen School of Medicine at UCLA
University of California
Los Angeles, California, USA

Marloes Dekker Nitert PhD
School of Chemistry
and Molecular Biosciences
The University of Queensland
Brisbane, Queensland, Australia

Susan Quinn
St Mary's Hospital
Central Manchester University Hospitals
NHS Foundation Trust
Manchester Academic Health
Sciences Centre
Manchester, UK

Aubrey R. Raimondi MD, MPH
Ben-Gurion University of the Negev
Beer-Sheva, Israel

Prasanna Rao-Balakrishna MD
Manchester Diabetes Centre
Central Manchester University Hospitals
NHS Foundation Trust
Manchester Academic Health
Sciences Centre
Manchester, UK

Ravi Retnakaran MD, FRCPC
Leadership Sinai Centre for Diabetes
Mount Sinai Hospital;
Division of Endocrinology
University of Toronto; and
Lunenfeld-Tanenbaum Research Institute
Mount Sinai Hospital, Canada

Lene Ringholm MD, PhD
Center for Pregnant Women with Diabetes;
Department of Endocrinology, Rigshospitalet
Faculty of Health Sciences
University of Copenhagen
Copenhagen; and
Steno Diabetes Center Copenhagen
Gentofte, Denmark

David A. Sacks MD
Associate Investigator
Department of Research and Evaluation
Kaiser Permanente Southern California
Pasadena, California; and
Adjunct Clinical Professor
Division of Maternal-Fetal Medicine
Department of Obstetrics and Gynecology
Keck School of Medicine
University of Southern California
Los Angeles, California, USA

Eyal Sheiner MD, PhD
Department of Obstetrics
and Gynecology
Faculty of Health Sciences
Soroka University Medical Center
Ben-Gurion; and
University of the Negev
Beer-Sheva, Israel

David Simmons MD
School of Medicine
Western Sydney University
Campbelltown, New South Wales
Australia

Katharine P. Stanley
Department of Obstetrics
Norfolk and Norwich University
Hospital NHS Trust
Norwich, UK

Anne P. Starling PhD
Department of Epidemiology
University of Colorado School of
Public Health
Aurora, Colorado
USA

Elizabeth Stenhouse PhD
School of Nursing and Midwifery
Faculty of Health and Human Sciences
Plymouth University
Plymouth, UK

Zoe A. Stewart
University of Cambridge Metabolic
Research Laboratories and NIHR
Cambridge Biomedical Research Centre
Institute of Metabolic Science
Addenbrooke's Hospital
Cambridge, UK

Rosemary C. Temple
Elsie Bertram Diabetes Centre
Norfolk and Norwich University
Hospital NHS Trust
Norwich, UK

Christina Anne Vinter
Department of Gynecology and Obstetrics
Odense University Hospital; and
Department of Clinical Research
Faculty of Health Sciences
University of Southern Denmark
Odense, Denmark

Ewa Wender-Ozegowska MD
Department of Obstetrics
and Women's Diseases
Poznań University of Medical Sciences
Poznań, Poland

原 书 序

我很高兴并且非常荣幸能为第 2 版 *A Practical Manual of Diabetes in Pregnancy* 撰写序言。

第 1 版序言是 David Hadden 教授所写,他是欧洲糖尿病妊娠研究组(DPSG)的创始成员。David 是个有魅力、有个性的人,而且很有激情。他受到很多临床医师、研究人员、卫生机构行政人员的尊敬,当然还受到糖尿病患者的尊敬。

第 2 版是由 David R. McCance、Michael Maresh 和 David A. Sacks 编写的,这三位都是 DPSG 的成员。当然,自 100 年前胰岛素被发现以来,在妊娠糖尿病的认识和治疗方面已经取得了重要的进展,但主要问题尚未得到充分了解,也尚未得到有效解决。因此,该书的观点依旧很受欢迎。

第 2 版强调了妊娠糖尿病的全面治疗,阐述了已取得的成就、目前的进展和未来的前景。对妊娠糖尿病的有效筛查是一个重要的问题,必须在欧洲乃至全世界取得妊娠糖尿病筛查的共识,该书强调了普遍和统一的筛选方法。DPSG 和欧洲妇产科学会(EBCOG)正在合作,将在欧洲达成这一共识,国际妇产科联合会正在制定全球共识。肥胖的流行对妊娠糖尿病的发生和表现也有明显的影响,第 2 版中对此有明确的表述。最重要的是,妊娠糖尿病对母亲、胎儿和新生儿及子代将来来说,依旧是一个高风险的因素,应在这一领域继续努力。一个包括研究人员及患者本人的多学科团队要以患者为中心并应用新的知识和技术一起协同作战。

Andre Van Assche,MD,PhD,
FRCOG,FEBCOG

(王诗淇 译)

译者前言

作为一名内分泌科的医务工作者，在临床工作中遇见最多的就是糖尿病患者，这其中包括大量妊娠糖尿病患者。妊娠原本是件愉快的事情，但是很多女性却因为患有糖尿病而给自身及婴儿带来很高的风险。

现代社会飞速发展，女性面临工作及家庭的双重压力，身体长期处于紧张状态，甚至亚健康状态。而且，随着二孩政策的开放，很多女性生育的年龄偏大，导致糖尿病及代谢综合征的患病率增加。

A Practical Manual of Diabetes in Pregnancy 第 2 版由 David R. McCance、Michael Maresh 和 David A. Sacks 主编，全面介绍了妊娠糖尿病的知识，包括筛查、诊断和治疗。同时阐述了妊娠糖尿病相关研究已取得的成就、目前的进展和未来的前景。

希望本书对内分泌科医师、产科医师的临床工作有所裨益，同时也希望本书对患有妊娠糖尿病的准妈妈有一定的指导作用，但是它不能取代您的医师，如果您对自己的问题有疑问，建议咨询医师。

希望本书能帮助成千上万的妊娠糖尿病女性，使她们孕育出健康的宝宝，并保持自己的健康。

李洪梅
2019 年 5 月

原书前言

任何一本书的再版都会带来新的挑战。编者们可能会感到欣慰的是，他们之前的工作受到好评，出版商已经对第 2 版有足够的信心。编者的困境和责任是确保新版书能包含足够的新资料并采用最合适的形式，以便适应学习和交流方式的迅速变化。我们的结论是，在妊娠期间，糖尿病的管理仍然需要一个简洁、便捷、循证、实用的指导。我们对新的版本进行了广泛的修订并增加了许多新的章节，但它依旧特意保留了简短的说明性病例的章节格式，提出了一些问题，并在正文中做出回答。另外，还有实践要点、说明性图表和相关文献。

自 2010 年第 1 版问世以来，全球妊娠糖尿病和肥胖症的增长趋势更加显著，随之预防和后续影响也显露出来。妊娠前规划，持续避孕直到血糖最优控制已经实现，显然降低了妊娠前糖尿病的不利影响，但更多的女性需要接受这些观点，并思考如何做到这一点。长效可行的避孕方法有助于降低意外妊娠率，医疗保健专业人士需要为这些器具和药物提供及时指导。关于计划生育的相关内容强调了上面这些问题，并讨论了目前可用的避孕方法。现在有更多的 1 型糖尿病患者会使用碳水化合物计量，还有一些会使用胰岛素泵持续皮下胰岛素输注/连续血糖监测系统（CGMS/CSII）。这需要从孕前计划诊所到分娩机构的整个糖尿病团队的支持，现在患者每次咨询都需要更多的时间。

确凿的证据表明，妊娠期间患有 2 型糖尿病与患有 1 型糖尿病者预后相似，急需进行创新，为那些经常照顾这些妇女的初级保健者提供这些知识。继世界卫生组织（WHO）于 2013 年批准国际糖尿病与妊娠研究组（IADPSG）诊断妊娠糖尿病的标准后，我们正在努力就这些诊断标准达成全球共识，但需要更多的不同种族人群和卫生经济学的数据。一个不断演变的问题是，我们是否应该在妊娠早期诊断糖尿病，而不是妊娠晚期。本书最后一章展望了微生物组学、蛋白质组学和代谢组学的作用——这些进展现在都近在咫尺。

在所有这些活动中，必须保持以患者为中心的地位。然而，糖尿病和妊娠的结合仍然是一种高风险的情况，妊娠应该是一种愉快的经历，而作为医疗保健专业人员，我们很容易忘记这一点。多学科小组对于沟通、协调护理和评估风险至关重要。应用技术可以提供很多帮助，远程传送血糖监测结果（甚至是带有移动电话的日记页面的截图）现在已经司空见惯，这有助于减少复诊的频率，特别是对于患有妊娠糖尿病的妇女。

自从第1版出版以来，我们作为主创人员，为David Hadden先生的逝世感到悲伤，他不仅是我们尊敬的同事、导师，更是朋友。他的兴趣和热情使其成为这一领域的传奇，他留下的精神财富还在继续激励后人。在撰写第1版的前言时，他强调这本书是为整个糖尿病小组写的。我们赞同他的看法，并将本书献给他。我们希望本书的临床案例和实践要点能够对临床工作有所裨益。

David R. McCance
Michael Maresh
David A. Sacks
（王诗淇 译）

目 录

第一篇 概 述

第一章 妊娠糖尿病流行病学研究 ……………………………………… 1
第二章 妊娠糖尿病的病理生理学 ………………………………………… 19
第三章 糖尿病合并妊娠期间的胎盘 ……………………………………… 34

第二篇 妊娠糖尿病

第四章 妊娠糖尿病的筛查 …………………………………………………… 51
第五章 妊娠高血糖诊断标准 ………………………………………………… 65
第六章 生活方式的干预 ……………………………………………………… 79
第七章 妊娠期肥胖和糖尿病 ………………………………………………… 94
第八章 妊娠糖尿病的代谢异常 …………………………………………… 114
第九章 妊娠糖尿病母亲的风险 …………………………………………… 125

第三篇 妊娠糖尿病相关问题

第十章 1 型和 2 型糖尿病患者的妊娠前护理 ………………………… 139
第十一章 先天畸形 ……………………………………………………………… 153
第十二章 妊娠期护理 …………………………………………………………… 168
第十三章 1 型糖尿病女性更常遇到的问题 ……………………………… 186
第十四章 2 型糖尿病女性更常遇到的问题 ……………………………… 200
第十五章 妊娠期口服降糖药的研究进展 ………………………………… 210
第十六章 胰岛素治疗的进展 ………………………………………………… 227
第十七章 糖尿病合并妊娠的胰岛素泵治疗 ……………………………… 241
第十八章 减肥手术后的妊娠、围产期和生育结局 …………………… 255
第十九章 胎儿监护 ……………………………………………………………… 274

第二十章 妊娠并发症：高血压和糖尿病肾病 …………………… 290
第二十一章 妊娠糖尿病视网膜病变 …………………………………… 305

第四篇 分娩与产后护理

第二十二章 分娩和产后护理：1型、2型或妊娠期糖尿病妇女的
分娩及分娩和产后的产科管理 …………………………… 324
第二十三章 临产后、产时和产后的饮食管理 ……………………… 336
第二十四章 分娩和分娩后护理：新生儿护理 ……………………… 352
第二十五章 女性糖尿病患者的产后避孕 …………………………… 370
第二十六章 母乳喂养与糖尿病 ……………………………………… 388

第五篇 对未来的影响

第二十七章 妊娠对糖尿病母亲的影响 ……………………………… 401
第二十八章 妊娠糖尿病：对子代的影响 …………………………… 416
第二十九章 从试验到临床：潜在的未来治疗妊娠糖尿病的方法——
改善妊娠期间 B 细胞的质量和功能 …………………… 428

第一篇 概 述

第一章 妊娠糖尿病流行病学研究

David Simmons

School of Medicine, Western Sydney University, Campbelltown, New South Wales, Australia

实践要点

- 世界卫生组织（World Health Organization，WHO）建议在妊娠期任何时间第一次监测到高血糖时应当归为以下任何一种情况：糖尿病合并妊娠或妊娠期糖尿病。
- 妊娠前糖尿病是妊娠前确诊的糖尿病。
- 近40年的时间里全球妊娠前糖尿病的患病率一直在增加，患病率为1%～5%。0.3%～0.8%的妊娠并发1型糖尿病；其余大部分是2型糖尿病，一小部分为罕见类型糖尿病。
- DIP的患病率为0.2%～0.4%，主要为产后2型糖尿病。
- WHO的妊娠糖尿病（GDM）诊断标准现已发生变化，空腹血糖标准更低（≥5.1mmol/L），并且增加了在75g葡萄糖负荷后1h血糖值（≥10.0mmol/L），2h后血糖值切点升高（≥8.5mmol/L）。这些标准的更改增加了GDM的患病率，在某些人群中超过35%。
- 非欧洲种族和肥胖是妊娠高血糖的主要危险因素；其他如糖尿病家族史、既往GDM、多囊卵巢综合征、高龄和既往死产史及巨大儿史等也是重要危险因素。
- 妊娠前糖尿病和妊娠期糖尿病对胎儿畸形有显著影响。
- 妊娠高血糖导致不良妊娠结局，尤其是肩难产。
- GDM是超过34%的女性2型糖尿病的前兆表现。
- 妊娠高血糖与后代发生肥胖、糖尿病及代谢综合征存在关系。

> **病　例**
>
> 　　患者是一名 32 岁的女性，孕 3 产 2，没有明确的糖尿病既往病史，也没有糖尿病家族史。
>
> 　　妊娠 8 周时随机血糖为 7.8mmol/L，11 周时口服葡萄糖耐量试验（OGTT）血糖为 4.3mmol/L、7.6mmol/L 和 7.4mmol/L[1]。妊娠前的体质指数（BMI）为 19.9kg/m^2。在 28 周时，出现了极其严重的全身疲劳，但是无发热。测随机血糖为 27.2mmol/L，血压为 110/84mmHg，心率为 106 次/分。尿酮体为+++，动脉血 pH 为 7.45，碳酸氢盐为 12.1mmol/L，碱剩余-9.8mmol/L（即代偿性代谢性酸中毒）。HbA1c 为 125mmol/mol（13.6%）。抗谷氨酸脱羧酶（GAD）抗体为 25.0（参考范围为 1~5）。她被诊断出患有 1 型糖尿病并开始接受胰岛素治疗。在接下来的妊娠期平安无事，虽然总体重增加仅为 3kg，但孩子出生体重为 3.06kg。
>
> **本章要回答的问题：**
>
> 　　1. 1 型糖尿病、2 型糖尿病、单基因型糖尿病或其他罕见类型的糖尿病合并妊娠的比例是多少？
>
> 　　2. GDM 的比例是多少？
>
> 　　3. 哪种类型的患者在妊娠期首次发现糖尿病？
>
> 　　4. 妊娠高血糖对公众健康的影响是什么？

妊娠高血糖的总患病率

　　糖尿病合并妊娠和妊娠糖尿病这两个术语在临床医学方面应用至今已超过 100 年。在 2010 年和 2013 年，国际糖尿病与妊娠研究组（IADPSG）[2]和 WHO[3]分别将妊娠期的高血糖重新划分为三组，包含可增加妊娠并发症的所有高血糖情况。

已知妊娠前糖尿病	（显性）糖尿病	妊娠糖尿病
已知糖尿病	糖尿病合并妊娠	
例如：1 型糖尿病、2 型糖尿病、罕见类型糖尿病（如单基因型糖尿病）	妊娠期第一次诊断并预计在产后继续存在 通常为 2 型糖尿病；偶有罕见类型或 1 型糖尿病	妊娠期第一次诊断，产后预计没有永久性糖尿病

　　2013 年，全世界在 20~49 岁年龄生出活产婴儿的妊娠妇女中，妊娠高血糖的患病率估计为 16.9%，约 2140 万人[4]。最高患病率发生在

东南亚地区，为 25.0%，北美和加勒比地区占 10.4%。低收入和中等收入国家病例估计占病例数的 90%。

妊娠期已知妊娠糖尿病的患病率

流行病学研究显示，患有 1 型糖尿病和 2 型糖尿病的育龄妇女在全球范围内的数量正在不断增加[5]。在美国，预计到 2050 年 1 型糖尿病和 2 型糖尿病在 20 岁以下人群中的发病率将分别增加 3 倍和 4 倍[5]。图 1.1 是南加利福尼亚州 1999～2005 年妊娠合并妊娠前糖尿病（按年龄组）的数据，年龄和种族调整后的比率由 1999 年的 8.1/1000 增加到了 2005 年的 18.2/1000[6]。

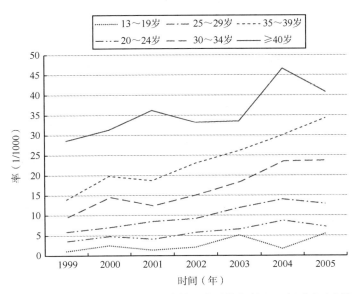

图 1.1 1999～2005 年妊娠合并妊娠前糖尿病（按年龄组，每千人比例）数据

流行病学显示，糖尿病发病率的种族差异很大。例如，2007～2010 年美国各地年龄在 20～44 岁的女性，非西班牙裔白种人患病率为 2.7%（1.8%～4.1%）；西班牙裔女性为 3.7%（2.2%～6.2%）；非西班牙裔黑种人患病率为 4.6%（3.3%～6.4%）[7]。这些群体的发病率高于其他人群[4]。

妊娠期 1 型糖尿病的患病率

鉴于较低的标化生育率（SFR）（生育率与更广泛的人群相比），妊娠期 1 型糖尿病的患病率低于非妊娠人群。1 型糖尿病的 SFR 为 0.80（95%CI：0.77~0.82），在患有视网膜病变、肾病、神经疾病或心血管疾病并发症的女性中分别为 0.63、0.54、0.50 和 0.34[8]。随着时间的推移，患有和未患 1 型糖尿病女性之间的生育率的差距已经明显缩小，儿童期患病者与成人期患病者之间生育率的差距是最大的[9]。

妊娠期 1 型糖尿病的患病率如表 1.1 所示，其为挪威（1999~2004 年）[10]和加拿大安大略省（2005~2006 年）[11]的数据。数据显示，妊娠期 1 型糖尿病患病率随年龄的增长而增加。

除了先前存在 1 型糖尿病的女性，少数患有此类糖尿病的女性是在妊娠期间被首次诊断出来的（参见本章的病例）。在 1986~2005 年的新西兰，有 11/325（3.4%）的女性在产后被诊断为新发的 1 型糖尿病[12]。其他患有 GDM 的女性检测出有自身免疫标志物[胰岛细胞抗体（ICA）、GAD 抗体（GADA）或酪氨酸磷酸酶抗体（IA-2A）]，没有明显的 DIP。总体而言，此类自身免疫标志物阳性率为 1%~10%，而且在 1 型糖尿病患病率较高的人群中，这一比例最高[13]。在瑞典的一项研究中，50%具有抗体阳性的女性患有 1 型糖尿病，而在 GDM 对照受试者中则没有[14]。

表 1.1　妊娠期 1 型、2 型糖尿病患病率按年龄组分布（每千人）

挪威 1999~2004 年	1 型糖尿病患病率	安大略省，加拿大 2005~2006 年	患病率	
			1 型糖尿病	2 型糖尿病
整体	4.5	整体	7.5	4.3
按年龄分组		按年龄分组		
≤20 岁	2.9	≤20 岁	2.0	0.2
21~34 岁	4.5	21~34 岁	5.7	2.9
35~39 岁	5.0	35~39 岁	8.3	4.9
≥40 岁	4.7	≥40 岁	11.5	7.3

妊娠期 2 型糖尿病的患病率

虽然目前还没有明确的关于 2 型糖尿病患者的生育率报道，但预计这一比率会较低（特别是考虑到相关的肥胖、多囊卵巢综合征和血管疾病等）[15]。不过，2 型糖尿病患者妊娠的发病率比妊娠期 1 型糖尿病的发病率增加得更快[16]。

除了年龄标准的提高，2 型糖尿病的发病（受肥胖流行的影响），人口结构（如种族）的变化可以部分解释个别地区流行率随时间的变化。例如，在 1990～1998 年的英国伯明翰，1 型与 2 型糖尿病的比例在南亚人中为 1：2，在欧洲人中为 11：1[17]。在 1996～2008 年的英格兰北部，妊娠期 1 型和 2 型糖尿病的患病率分别为 0.3%和 0.1%[18]，而 97%的女性 1 型糖尿病患者为欧洲人，21%的 2 型糖尿病患者为非欧洲人。表 1.1 还显示，随着年龄的增长，安大略省的 2 型糖尿病妇女的比例越来越高[11]。

妊娠期其他形式的妊娠糖尿病患病率

目前，关于妊娠糖尿病或继发性糖尿病的单基因形式的相关报道很少。葡萄糖激酶突变在高达 5%～6%的 GDM 女性中存在，高达 80%的女性在妊娠期间持续空腹高血糖，并且在 OGTT 期间伴有小幅度的葡萄糖增加，且有糖尿病家族史[19]。囊性纤维化非妊娠患者的糖尿病患病率增加 1 倍，在妊娠期间进一步增加（如从基线时的 9.3%到妊娠期间的 20.6%，以及随访时的 14.4%）[20]。

> **注意**：糖尿病合并妊娠的年轻女性中有相当一部分为未被诊断的罕见类型糖尿病。

妊娠期首次发现高血糖的患病率

1998 年，King 等对全球首次在妊娠期发现的高血糖的患病率进行了调查[21]。然而，如图 1.2 所示，这项研究的流行病学难以解释其中的原因，对此会在第四章和第五章中进行更全面的讨论。关键的问题是使

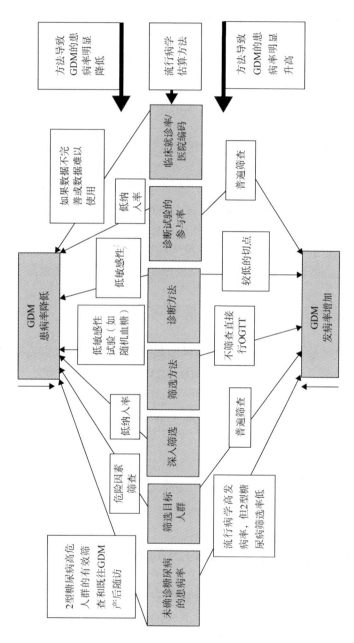

图1.2 不同筛查方式观察到的妊娠糖尿病发病率
OGTT，口服葡萄糖耐量试验

用的诊断标准和筛查方法。此外，筛查时间过早（24周之前）也可能会导致检测到妊娠高血糖的病例减少。在一些女性人群中，GDM的诊断仅在妊娠后期进行，且于24~28周做常规筛选。

超重、肥胖和极度肥胖（BMI≥35kg/m²）是引发GDM和DIP的重要因素。最近，美国南卡罗来纳州的相应人口归因分数（PAF）计算为9.1%、11.8%和15.5%（即GDM的36.4%可归因于超重）[22]。不同民族之间的差别很小[如美国黑种人18.1%（16.0%~20.2%）vs.非西班牙裔白种人14.0%（12.8%~15.3%）vs. 西班牙裔人9.6%（7.3%~12.0%）的所有GDM都归因于极度肥胖]。

糖尿病合并妊娠和妊娠糖尿病的诊断

第五章详细讨论了DIP和GDM的诊断。很少有其他的医学领域涉及这种混乱和争议。而直到最近，诊断标准的不同使流行病学比较存在问题。2013年采用的新的WHO标准[2, 3]首次为这一混乱领域带来了统一性，尽管它们尚未被普遍接受。这些标准基于高血糖与不良妊娠结局（HAPO）研究[23]产生的流行病学数据，而不是未来孕产妇糖尿病的共识或风险。HAPO研究还强调了高血糖和母体内胎儿结局的相关性与母亲的肥胖无关。另一个重要的观察结果是，所有参与种族群体之间高血糖与母体/胎儿结局之间的可比较关系。有一点需要注意的是，一些民族，如波利尼西亚人，没有被纳入HAPO研究。来自新西兰的证据表明，在调整了孕妇体重后，高血糖可能会导致欧洲人群的出生体重增加[24]。

虽然肥胖、种族、母亲年龄和糖尿病家族史是GDM/DIP的主要危险因素，但其他情况也存在（如巨大儿、死产史、多胎妊娠和缺乏身体活动），这些构成了筛选策略的基础[25]（参见第四章）。还有明确的证据表明多囊卵巢综合征作为GDM/DIP危险因素的重要性[26]。GDM患病风险增加的另一个重要人群是那些既往有GDM病史的女性[27]，尤其是与体重超标相关的早期GDM在妊娠早期诊断并需要胰岛素治疗的患者[28]。

糖尿病合并妊娠患病率

很少有研究报道按照WHO 2013年标准[3]所定义的DIP患病率：空腹

血糖≥7.0mmol/L，HbA1c≥6.5%（47mmol/mol），随机血糖≥11.1mmol/L并被其他测试确诊。之前有很多关于妊娠合并 GDM 后立即出现糖尿病的报道，如在新西兰，21%的波利尼西亚人和4%的欧洲孕妇产后患有糖尿病[29]。然而，这些研究是在 IADPSG/WHO 确定 DIP 和 DIP 标准通常与产后糖尿病无关之前进行的。例如，在一项澳大利亚队列研究中，只有 21%的妊娠糖尿病女性产后患有糖尿病（41%的恢复正常）[30]。

> **实践要点**
>
> DIP 并不总是意味着产后出现永久性糖尿病。

在一项关于 133 名妊娠糖尿病患者在产后 6～8 周接受后续 OGTT 的研究中，21%的患者患上了糖尿病，37.6%的患者空腹血糖受损或葡萄糖耐量受损，41.4%的患者最后恢复了正常的葡萄糖耐量。

迄今为止，很少有文献描述 DIP 女性的特征。日本糖尿病和妊娠研究小组的报道指出，与患有 GDM 的女性相比，DIP 女性的妊娠前 BMI 更高[（24.9±5.7）kg/m^2 vs.（26.2±6.1）kg/m^2，$P<0.05$]，分娩孕周更早[（38.19±2.1）周 vs.（37.89±2.5）周，$P<0.05$]，视网膜病变更多（0 vs. 1.2%，$P<0.05$）和妊娠高血压更多（6.1% vs. 10.1%，$P<0.05$）[31]。其他人也发现患有 DIP 的女性 BMI 较高且妊娠结局不良[30]。

妊娠糖尿病的患病率

不同族群之间的 GDM 患病率存在显著差异，同时，2 型糖尿病的整体患病率受发病年龄的影响[32]。现在认为，除欧洲人后裔（甚至包括一些欧洲人口）以外的所有人口都处于高风险之中。流行率也随着时间的推移而普遍增加[33, 34]。虽然这很可能反映了非妊娠状态下肥胖和 2 型糖尿病的流行情况，但另一个特征可能是妊娠的年龄增大，高危民族的移民增加了总人口。流行率在不同地区的同一民族中有所不同，流动人口的流行率通常高于传统农村地区的流行率，可能与生活方式的改变（高能量饮食和身体活动减少）和更严重的肥胖有关。这些数据需要仔细审查以识别这些因素并确认有无发生筛选方法或诊断标准的变化。

> 许多描述 GDM 患病率的研究采用不同的筛查方法，这些方法低估了真实患病率。

目前，使用 WHO 2013 年标准的 GDM 患病率的报道正在不断增加。如表 1.2 所示，原始 HAPO 网址可以获得更全面的图片。患病率较使用旧标准时明显提高，第五章将对此进行更多讨论。

非洲尚未公布使用 WHO 2013 年标准的数据，虽然非洲裔女性的 GDM 患病率很高，如奥斯陆[33]，IDF 糖尿病版图[4]引用非洲妊娠高血糖患病率为 16.0%（2013 年有 460 万的新生儿受到影响），该地区高血糖病例数最多。患病率高于欧洲（15.2%）、北美洲（13.2%）、南美洲/中美洲（13.2%）或西太平洋（11.8%），但低于中东/北非（22.3%）或南/东亚（23.1%）。

表 1.2 在全部人群和 HAPO 研究中使用 WHO（2013）/IADPSG 标准与使用其他标准 GDM 患病率比较

地区	年份	使用 WHO(2013)/IADPSG 标准的患病率（%）	使用其他标准	使用其他标准的患病率（%）
欧洲				
比利时[35]	2014	23	NDDG	8
挪威-西欧[36]	2012	24	WHO（1999）	11
挪威少数民族[36]	2012	37	WHO（1999）	15
西班牙[37]	2010	35.5	NDDG	10.6
英国贝尔法斯特（HAPO）[2]	2010	17.05	WHO（1999）	1.5
英国曼彻斯特（HAPO）[38]	2010	24.28		
爱尔兰[39]	2011	12.4	WHO（1999）	9.4
匈牙利[40]	2011	16.6	WHO（1999）	8.7
中东				
以色列 Petah-Tiqva（HAPO）[38]	2010	10.06		
以色列 Beersheba（HAPO）[38]	2010	9.25		
阿联酋[41]	2010	37.7	ADA	12.9
北美洲				
巴巴多斯（HAPO）[38]	2010	11.9		
加拿大[42]	2014	10.3	CDA（2008）	7.3
加拿大多伦多（HAPO）[38]	2010	15.53		
美国加利福尼亚（HAPO）[38]	2012	25.5		

续表

地区	年份	使用 WHO(2013)/IADPSG 标准的患病率(%)	使用其他标准	使用其他标准的患病率(%)
美国俄亥俄(HAPO)[38]	2012	25.0		
美国芝加哥(HAPO)[38]	2012	17.3		
美国罗德岛(HAPO)[38]	2012	15.5		
南美洲/中美洲				
墨西哥[43]	2011	30.1	NDDG	10.3
亚洲				
印度[44]	2012	14.6	DIPSI	13.4
中国香港(HAPO)[38]	2010	14.39		
新加坡(HAPO)[38]	2010	25.13		
泰国(HAPO)[38]	2010	22.97		
日本[45]	2011	6.6	JSOG	2.4
中国内地[46]	2014	18.9	NDDG	8.4
越南[47]	2012	20.36	ADA	6.07
太平洋地区				
澳大利亚纽卡斯尔(HAPO)[38]	2012	15.3		
澳大利亚布里斯班(HAPO)[38]	2012	12.4		
澳大利亚伍伦贡[48]	2011	13.0	ADIPS	9.6

注：NDDG，美国国家糖尿病数据组；JSOG，日本妇产科医学会；ADA，美国糖尿病协会；DIPSI，印度妊娠糖尿病研究小组；ADIPS，澳大利亚妊娠糖尿病协会。

妊娠高血糖的风险与人口较低的社会经济状况有关。在澳大利亚的一项研究中，生活在社会经济地位最低的 3 个四分位数的女性与生活在社会经济地位最高的四分位数的女性相比，患 GDM 的优势比(OR)更高，OR 为 1.54∶1(1.50~1.59)、1.74∶1(1.69~1.8)、1.65∶1(1.60~1.70)[49]。

HAPO 研究的另一个重要发现是不同种族的不同高血糖模式，55%的女性在空腹血糖检测时诊断，33%在餐后 1h 血糖检测时诊断，12%在餐后 2h 血糖检测时诊断。这对于在 OGTT 选择空腹、餐后 1h 或餐后 2h 时间点的决定上具有重要意义。空腹血糖诊断 GDM 的比例从巴巴多斯的 74%到中国香港的 26%，而泰国仅占 24%[38]。这自然地改变了诊断"时间点"，因此在泰国和巴巴多斯，餐后 1h 时间点诊出率为 64%和 9%，而在中国香港餐后 2h 时间点诊出率为 29%。从妊娠期以外的研究中也可以预测出亚洲人餐后 2h 血糖诊断的可能性更大[50]。

妊娠高血糖对公共健康的影响

妊娠高血糖对公共健康的影响与受影响的人数、对生活质量的影响、额外的资源利用及可能的代际传播有关。表 1.3 显示了减轻妊娠高血糖危害所需的额外资源及干预可能带来的潜在益处。

表 1.3　妊娠高血糖的干预和干预可能减少的风险

项目	干预	干预可能减少的风险
1 型和 2 型糖尿病		
妊娠前	优化代谢控制，补充叶酸，优化药物治疗	畸形、流产
产前管理	优化代谢控制，包括血压控制 优化产科管理	新生儿，产妇分娩并发症 后代患糖尿病及肥胖症的风险
视网膜病变管理	眼底筛查，必要时激光治疗	玻璃体手术，剖宫产
其他并发症管理	肾脏替代治疗，心脏事件住院，自主神经病变	
妊娠糖尿病和妊娠期显性糖尿病		
妊娠糖尿病的诊断	筛查和诊断项目	
产前管理	优化代谢控制，包括血压控制 优化产科管理	新生儿及产妇分娩并发症 后代患糖尿病及肥胖症的风险
视网膜病变管理	眼底筛查，必要时激光治疗	剖宫产（罕见）
产后筛查和干预	筛查 初级预防（生活方式、药物）	预防永久性糖尿病 预防妊娠期显性糖尿病

妊娠前糖尿病患者的妊娠对公共健康的影响

妊娠前糖尿病是胎儿先天畸形的主要危险因素，尤其是先天性心脏缺陷[51]。1 型和 2 型糖尿病可能具有相当的致畸作用[52]。相对于 1 型糖尿病，妊娠期 2 型糖尿病在围产期的死亡率较高（OR：1.50；95%CI：

1.15~1.96)和剖宫产率较低(OR：0.80；95%CI：0.59~0.94)，但在死胎、新生儿死亡率、流产、早产和过期产、新生儿低血糖、黄疸和呼吸困难症等方面两者相似[53]。

在美国，先天性心脏缺陷的 PAF 在妊娠前糖尿病中估计为 8%[7]，但房室隔缺损的 PAF 上升到约 1/4（表 1.4）[7]。除 2%~3%的患者死亡外，其他患者都需要手术和再次手术，此增加了心律失常、心内膜炎、心力衰竭和肺动脉高压的患病风险。人口影响的程度取决于妊娠前护理的实施，对于先天畸形，其风险比（RR）为 0.25（95%CI：0.16~0.37），减少一个事件需治疗的患者数（NNT）为 19（95%CI：14~24），围产期死亡率的 RR 为 0.34（95%CI：0.15~0.75），NNT 为 46（95%CI：28~115）[54]。

表 1.4 妊娠前糖尿病患者先天性心脏病的人群归因分数[7]

先天性心脏病种类	OR（95%CI）	人口归因分数（%）（95%CI）
所有先天性心脏缺陷	3.8（3.0~4.9）	8.3（6.6~11.8）
房室缺陷	10.6（4.7~20.9）	23.4（10.6~40.0）
主动脉缩窄	3.7（1.7~7.4）	7.9（2.1~17.6）
左心发育不良综合征	3.7（1.5~8.9）	8.0（1.6~20.4）
法洛四联症	6.5（3.3~11.8）	14.8（6.6~26.3）
变异大动脉	4.8（2.7~8.5）	10.9（5.1~19.8）

资料来源：Simeone et al.（2015）[7]。

GDM/DIP 对公共卫生的影响

虽然世界各地的标准差异很大，导致 GDM/DIP 的成本难以估计，但 WHO 2013 年标准的日益普及使得卫生经济分析更加可行。之前对 GDM/DIP 人口影响的估计表明，糖尿病妇女在妊娠期发生围产期死亡的比例为 2.8%，胎儿畸形率为 2.5%，5.9%的患者需要剖宫产，9.9%的婴儿≥4.5kg 及 23.5%的为肩难产病例[55]。

然而，这些估计是在新标准和新的筛查方法之前，因此许多具有潜在可预防不良后果的女性在没有 GDM/DIP 治疗机会的情况下被认为是"正常的"。

当然，确诊的程度和从治疗 GDM/DIP 中的获益取决于采用哪种鉴定方法（如普遍筛查与基于风险因素的筛选）。其他重要决定因素还包括实施治疗的程度，以及达到治疗目标的程度。例如，在一项研究中，空腹血糖≤5.3mmol/L 的女性中有 24.8%经历了不良妊娠结局，而 30%的时间空腹血糖＞5.3mmol/L 的女性中有 57.9%经历了不良妊娠结局[56]。

健康经济分析往往会忽略生活质量（QoL）改善带来的好处及预防母亲和后代糖尿病的潜在获益。在澳大利亚孕妇糖类不耐受试验（ACHOIS）研究中（根据 WHO 1999 年较早的标准），随着 GDM 的诊断和治疗，QoL 可显著改善卫生经济模型，这与人口明显增长的基础有关[57]。

从萨斯喀彻温省数据库中首次尝试模拟 GDM 对 2 型糖尿病的代际和代内作用，发现在高风险的原住民人口中，先前的 GDM 病史可能导致 2 型糖尿病的患病者从 19%增加至 30%。而在其他人群中，这一影响的比例为 6%[58]。

目前的卫生经济分析并不包括前次妊娠期合并 GDM 对下次妊娠前糖尿病的影响。有证据表明，妊娠期并发 GDM 的母亲患永久性糖尿病的风险更高[59]。GDM 的识别还提供了通过及时使用可靠避孕措施来管理这种风险的机会。即使有上面提到的不足，许多模型研究已经显示了 GDM 的成本和治疗的成本效益。来自一些国家的报道显示，GDM 有很高的花费（如 2011 年，美国每 10 万名妇女的治疗成本为 831 622 028 美元）和治疗的成本效益（如美国、以色列和印度[60, 61]）。

> 卫生经济分析应包括对其益处的估计和识别，并干预有发展为 2 型糖尿病风险的妇女。

未来的需求

1. 更多的研究使用 WHO 的 GDM 和 DIP 标准进行普遍筛查。
2. 研究了更多人群之间的相互作用和独立影响。
3. 肥胖和 GDM。
4. 关于妊娠早期 GDM 所需标准的研究。
5. 更多关于单基因型糖尿病和其他罕见糖尿病的研究。
6. 来自非洲的更多研究。
7. 更多研究关注人口对母体代际的影响。

8. 糖尿病，包括 GDM，更多关于 GDM 流行病学的研究。
9. 更多关于不同经济体的妊娠高血糖对健康经济影响的总体研究。

选择题

一个或多个答案是正确的。

1. WHO 2013 年妊娠糖尿病标准基于（　　）
   A. 母亲患糖尿病的长期风险
   B. 后代肥胖的长期风险
   C. 与"正常"女性相比，妊娠并发症的风险增加 100%
   D. 与"正常"女性相比，妊娠并发症的风险增加 75%
   E. 与"正常"女性相比，妊娠并发症的风险增加 50%
正确答案是 D。

2. 如果出现以下情况，GDM 的风险会更大的是（　　）
   A. 一个女性体重正常
   B. 女性患有多囊卵巢综合征
   C. 女性有死产史
   D. 女性过去曾出现过产前大出血
   E. 女性在妊娠前和妊娠期间都处于缺少活动状态
正确答案是 B、C、E。

（杨　芳　译，朱海清　校）

参 考 文 献

1 Himuro H, Sugiyama T, Nishigori H, Saito M, Nagase S, Sugawara J, Yaegashi N. A case of a woman with late-pregnancy-onset DKA who had normal glucose tolerance in the first trimester. Endocrinol Diabetes Metab Case Rep 2014;2014:130085. doi:10.1530/EDM-13-0085

2 IADPSG Consensus Panel. International Association of Diabetes and Pregnancy Study Groups (IADPSG) Recommendations on the Diagnosis and Classification of Hyperglycemia in Pregnancy. Diabetes Care 2010;33:676–682.

3 World Health Organization. Diagnostic Criteria and Classification of Hyperglycaemia First Detected in Pregnancy WHO/NMH/MND/13.2. WHO: Geneva, 2013. http://apps.who.int/iris/bitstream/10665/85975/1/WHO_NMH_

MND_13.2_eng.pdf
4. Guariguata L, Linnenkamp U, Beagley J, Whiting DR, Cho NH. Global estimates of the prevalence of hyperglycaemia in pregnancy. Diabetes Res Clin Pract 2014;103(2):176–185.
5. Imperatore G, Boyle JP, Thompson TJ, et al. Projections of type 1 and type 2 diabetes burden in the U.S. population aged <20 years through 2050: dynamic modeling of incidence, mortality, and population growth. Diabetes Care 2012;35(12):2515–2520.
6. Lawrence JM, Contreras R, Chen WS, Sacks DA. Trends in the prevalence of preexisting diabetes and gestational diabetes mellitus among a racially/ethnically diverse population of pregnant women, 1999–2005. Diabetes Care 2008;31(5):899–904.
7. Simeone RM, Devine OJ, Marcinkevage JA, Gilboa SM, Razzaghi H, Bardenheier BH, Sharma AJ, Honein MA. Diabetes and congenital heart defects: a systematic review, meta-analysis and modelling project. Am J Prev Med 2015;48(2):195–204.
8. Jonasson JM, Brismar K, Sparen P et al. Fertility in women with Type 1 diabetes. Diabetes Care 2007;30:2271–2276.
9. Wiebe JC, Santana A, Medina-Rodríguez N, Hernández M, Nóvoa J, Mauricio D, Wägner AM on behalf of the T1DGC. Fertility is reduced in women and in men with type 1 diabetes: results from the Type 1 Diabetes Genetics Consortium (T1DGC). Diabetologia 2014;57:2501–2504.
10. Eidem I, Stene LC, Henriksen T, Hanssen KF, Vangen S, Vollset SE, Joner G. Congenital anomalies in newborns of women with type 1 diabetes: nationwide population-based study in Norway, 1999–2004. Acta Obstetric Gynecolog Scandinav 2010;89:1403–1411.
11. Peticca P, Keely E, Walker M, Yang Q, Bottomley J. Pregnancy outcomes in diabetes subtypes: how do they compare? A province-based study of Ontario, 2005–2006. J Obstetr Gynaecol Canada 2009;31:487–496.
12. Cundy T, Gamble G, Neale L, Henley PG, MacPherson P, Roberts AB, Rowan J. Differing causes of pregnancy loss in type 1 and type 2 diabetes. Diabetes Care 2007;30:2603–2607.
13. Wucher H, Lepercq J, Timsit J. Onset of autoimmune type 1 diabetes during pregnancy: prevalence and outcomes. Best Pract Clin Endo Metab 2010;24:617–624.
14. Nilsson C, Ursing D, Törn C, Aberg A, Landin-Olsson M. Presence of GAD antibodies during gestational diabetes mellitus predicts type 1 diabetes. Diabetes Care [serial online]. August 2007;30(8):1968–1971.
15. Livshits A, Seidman D. Fertility issues in women with diabetes. Women's Health (London, England) 2009;5:701–707.
16. Engelgau MM, Herman WH, Smith PJ, German RR, Aubert RE. The epidemiology of diabetes and pregnancy in the U.S., 1988. Diabetes Care 1995;18:1029–1033.
17. Dunne FP, Brydon PA, Proffit M, Smith T, Gee H, Holder RL. Fetal and maternal outcomes in Indo-Asian compared to Caucasian women with diabetes in pregnancy. Q J Med 2000;93:813–818.
18. Bell R, Glinianaia S, Tennant PWG, Bilous R, Rankin J. Peri-conception hyperglycaemia and nephropathy are associated with risk of congenital anomaly in women with pre-existing diabetes: a population-based cohort study. Diabetologia 2012;55:936–947.
19. Ellard S, Beards F, Allen LIS, et al. A high prevalence of glucokinase mutations in gestational diabetic subjects selected by clinical criteria. Diabetologia 2000;43:250.
20. McMullen AH, Pasta D, Frederick P, et al. Impact of pregnancy on women with cystic fibrosis. Chest 2006;129:706–711.
21. King H. Epidemiology of glucose intolerance and gestational diabetes in women of childbearing age. Diabetes Care 1998;21:B9–B13.
22. Cavicchia PP, Liu J, Adams SA, Steck SE, Hussey JR, Daguisé VG, Hebert JR. Proportion of gestational diabetes mellitus attributable to overweight and obesity among non-Hispanic black, non-Hispanic

white, and Hispanic women in South Carolina. Matern Child Health J 2014;18:1919-1926.
23 The HAPO Study Cooperative Research Group. Hyperglycemia and adverse pregnancy outcomes. N Engl J Med 2008;358:1999-2002.
24 Simmons D. Relationship between maternal glycaemia and birthweight among women without diabetes from difference ethnic groups in New Zealand. Diabet Med 2007;24:240-244.
25 Ben Haroush A, Yogev Y, Hod M. Epidemiology of gestational diabetes mellitus and its association with Type 2 diabetes. Diabet Med 2004;21:103-113.
26 Simmons D, Walters BNJ, Rowan JA, McIntyre HD. Metformin therapy and diabetes in pregnancy. Med J Aust 2004;180:462-464.
27 Kim, C, Berger DK, Chamany S. Recurrence of gestational diabetes mellitus: a systematic review. Diabetes Care 2007;30:1314-1319.
28 Major CA, de Veciana M, Weeks J, Morgan MA. Recurrence of gestational diabetes mellitus: who is at risk? Am J Obstet Gynecol 1998;179:1038-1042.
29 Simmons D, Thompson CF, Conroy C. Incidence and risk factors for neonatal hypoglycaemia among women with gestational diabetes mellitus in South Auckland. Diabet Med. 2000;17:830-834.
30 Wong T, Ross GP, Jalaludin BB, Flack JR. The clinical significance of overt diabetes in pregnancy. Diabet Med 2013;30:468-474.
31 Sugiyama T, Saito M, Nishigori H, Nagase S, Yaegashi N, Sagawa N, Kawano R, Ichihara K, Sanaka M, Akazawa S, Anazawa S, Waguri M, Sameshima H, Hiramatsu Y, Toyoda N, Japan Diabetes and Pregnancy Study Group. Comparison of pregnancy outcomes between women with gestational diabetes and overt diabetes first diagnosed in pregnancy: A retrospective multi-institutional study in Japan. Diab Res Clin Pract 2014;103:20-25.
32 Yue DK, Molyneaux LM, Ross GP, Constantino MI, Child AG, Turtle JR. Why does ethnicity affect prevalence of gestational diabetes? The underwater volcano theory. Diabet Med 1996;13:748-752.
33 Ferrara A. Increasing prevalence of gestational diabetes: a public health perspective. Diabetes Care 2007;30 (Suppl 2): S141-S146.
34 Beischer NA, Oats JN, Henry OA, Sheedy MT, Walstab JE. Incidence and severity of gestational diabetes mellitus according to country of birth in women living in Australia. Diabetes 1991;40 (Suppl 2):35-38.
35 Oriot P, Selvais P, Radikov J, Jacobs JL, Gilleman U, Loumaye R, Fernandez C. Assessing the incidence of gestational diabetes and neonatal outcomes using the IADPSG guidelines in comparison with the Carpenter and Coustan criteria in a Belgian general hospital. Acta Clinica Belgica 2014;69. doi:10.1179/0001551213Z
36 Jenum AK, Mørkrid K, Sletner L, Vange S, Torper JL, Nakstad B, Voldner N, Rognerud-Jensen OH, Berntsen S, Mosdøl A, Skrivarhaug T, Va°rdal MH, Holme I, Yajnik CS, Birkeland KI. Impact of ethnicity on gestational diabetes identified with the WHO and the modified International Association of Diabetes and Pregnancy Study Groups criteria: a population-based cohort study. Euro J Endocrinol 2012;166:317-324.
37 Duran A, Sáenz S, Torrejón MJ, Bordiú E, Del Valle L, Galindo M, Perez N, Herraiz MA, Izquierdo N, Rubio MA, Runkle I, Pérez-Ferre N, Cusihuallpa I, Jiménez S, García de la Torre N, Fernández MD, Montañez C, Familiar C, Calle-Pascual AL. Introduction of IADPSG criteria for the screening and diagnosis of gestational diabetes mellitus results in improved pregnancy outcomes at a lower cost in a large cohort of pregnant women: the St. Carlos Gestational Diabetes Study. Diabetes Care 2014;37:2442-2450.
38 Sacks DA, Hadden DR, Maresh M, et al.,

for the HAPO Study Cooperative Research Group. Frequency of Gestational Diabetes Mellitus at Collaborating Centers Based on IADPSG Consensus Panel-Recommended Criteria: The Hyperglycemia and Adverse Pregnancy Outcome (HAPO) Study. Diabetes Care 2012;35:526-528.
39. O'Sullivan EP, Avalos G, O'Reilly M, Dennedy MC, Gaffney G, Dunne F, on behalf of the Atlantic DIP collaborators. Atlantic Diabetes in Pregnancy (DIP): the prevalence and outcomes of gestational diabetes mellitus using new diagnostic criteria. Diabetologia 2011;54:1670-1675.
40. Kun A, Tornóczky J, Tabák AG. The prevalence and predictors of gestational diabetes mellitus in Hungary. Horm Metab Res 2011;43:788-793.
41. Agarwal MM, Dhatt GS, Shah SM. Gestational diabetes mellitus: simplifying the International Association of Diabetes and Pregnancy diagnostic algorithm using fasting plasma glucose. Diabetes Care 2010;33(9):2018-2020.
42. Mayo K, Melamed N, Vandenberghe H, Berger H. The impact of adoption of the International Association of Diabetes in Pregnancy Study Group criteria for the screening and diagnosis of gestational diabetes. Am J Obstet Gynecol 2015;211:e1-9.
43. Reyes-Muñoz E, Parra A, Castillo-Mora A, Ortega-González C. Impact of the international association of diabetes and pregnancy study groups diagnostic criteria on the prevalence of gestational diabetes mellitus in urban Mexican women: a cross sectional study. Endocr Pract 2011;19:1-17.
44. Seshiaha V, Balaji V, Shah SN, Joshi S, Das AK, Sahay BK, Banerjee S, Zargar AH, Balaji M. Diagnosis of gestational diabetes mellitus in the community. JAPI 2012;60:15-17.
45. Morikawa M, Yamada T, Yamada T, Akaishi R, Nishida R, Cho K, Minakami H. Change in the number of patients after the adoption of IADPSG criteria for hyperglycemia during pregnancy in Japanese women. Diabetes Res Clin Prac 2010;90:339-342.
46. Yumei W, Huixia Y, Weiwei Z, Hongyun Y, Haixia L, Jie Y, Cuilin Z. International Association of Diabetes and Pregnancy Study Group criteria is suitable for gestational diabetes mellitus diagnosis: further evidence from China. Chin Med J 2014;127:3553-3556.
47. Hirst JE, Tran TS, Do MAT, Morris JM, Jeffery HE. Consequences of gestational diabetes in an urban hospital in Viet Nam: a prospective cohort study. PLoS Med 2012;9:e1001272. doi:10.1371/journal.pmed.1001272
48. Moses RG, Morris GJ, Petocz P, Gil FS, Garg D. The impact of potential new diagnostic criteria on the prevalence of gestational diabetes mellitus in Australia. MJA 2011;194:338-340.
49. Vibeke A, Huxley RR, Van der Ploeg HP, Bauman AE, Cheung NW. Sociodemographic correlates of the increasing trend in prevalence of gestational diabetes mellitus in a large population of women between 1995 and 2005. Diabetes Care 2008;31:2288-2293.
50. Qiao Q, Hu G, Tuomilehto J et al. Age- and sex-specific prevalence of diabetes and impaired glucose regulation in 11 Asian cohorts. Diabetes Care 2003;26:1770-1780.
51. Garne E, Loane M, Dolk H et al. Spectrum of congenital anomalies in pregnancies with pregestational diabetes. Birth Defects Res A Clin Mol Teratol 2012;94:134-140.
52. Inkster ME, Fahey TP, Donnan PT, Leese GP, Mired GJ, Murphy DJ. Poor glycated haemoglobin control and adverse pregnancy outcomes in type 1 and type 2 diabetes mellitus: systematic review of observational studies. BMC Pregnancy Childbirth 2006;6:30.
53. Balsells M, Garcia-Patterson A, Gich I, Corcoy R. Maternal and fetal outcome in women with type 2 versus type 1 diabetes mellitus: a systematic review and meta-analysis. J Clin Endocrinol Metab 2009;94(11):4284-4291.
54. Wahabi HA, Alzeidan RA, Bawazeer GA, Alansari LA, Esmaeil SA. Preconception care for diabetic women for improving

maternal and fetal outcomes: a systematic review and meta-analysis. BMC Pregnancy Childbirth 2010;10:63.

55 Simmons D. Epidemiology of diabetes in pregnancy. In: Practical Management of Diabetes in Pregnancy (ed. McCance D, Maresh M). Blackwell: London, 2010.

56 Gonzalez-Quintero VH, Istwan NB, Rhea DJ, Rodriguez LI, Cotter A, Carter J, Mueller A, Stanziano GJ. The impact of glycaemic control on neonatal outcomes in singleton pregnancies complicated by gestational diabetes. Diabet Care 2007;30:467–470.

57 Moss JR, Crowther CA, Hiller JE, Willson KJ, Robinson JS. Costs and consequences of treatment for mild gestational diabetes mellitus – evaluation from the ACHOIS randomised trial. BMC Pregnancy Childbirth 2007;7:27.

58 Osgood ND, Dyck RF, Grassmann WK. The inter- and intragenerational impact of gestational diabetes on the epidemic of type 2 diabetes. American Journal of Public Health 2011;101:173–179.

59 Peters RK, Kjos SL, Xiang A, Buchanan TA. Long-term diabetogenic effect of a single pregnancy in women with prior gestational diabetes mellitus. Lancet 1996;347:227–230.

60 Werner EF, Pettker CM, Zuckerwise L, Reel M, Funai EF, Henderson J, Thung SF. Screening for gestational diabetes mellitus: are the criteria proposed by the international association of the Diabetes and Pregnancy Study Groups cost-effective? Diabetes Care 2012;35:529–535.

61 Marseille E, Lohse N, Jiwani A, *et al.* The cost-effectiveness of gestational diabetes screening including prevention of type 2 diabetes: application of a new model in India and Israel. J Matern Fetal Neonatal Med 2013;26:802–810.

第二章 妊娠糖尿病的病理生理学

Francine Hughes Einstein

Departments of Obstetrics & Gynecology and Women's Health, Division of Maternal Fetal Medicine, Montefiore Medical Center, The University Hospital for the Albert Einstein College of Medicine, Bronx, New York, USA

实践要点

- 胰岛素抵抗和代偿性高胰岛素血症对正常妊娠的适应。
- 妊娠期胰岛素抵抗的病因学是多方面的，可能包括胎盘因子等，如人胎盘生长激素和肿瘤坏死因子-α（TNF-α），同时也包括身体成分变化和营养过剩等因素。
- 当胰岛 B 细胞功能不能充分补偿妊娠期胰岛素抵抗的程度时，会导致葡萄糖耐量不足和妊娠糖尿病。
- 妊娠期间的代谢可塑性可在有限的母体资源期间保护胎儿。

妊娠期母体代谢适应

妊娠期是一个重要的母体代谢适应期。从目的上看，孕妇解剖和生理上的改变是为了支持胎儿的生长发育，并为母亲的妊娠和哺乳期的生理需求做准备。变化的整体是动态的，并且在整个妊娠过程中发展。

正常的代谢平衡

代谢能量来源于饮食中的糖类、脂肪和蛋白质。所有的细胞都需要稳定的能量供应，为生产腺苷三磷酸（ATP）和细胞维持提供能量。餐后，膳食成分（葡萄糖、游离脂肪酸和氨基酸）被运送到组织中，被细胞吸收、氧化产生能量。任何多余的（超出身体直接需要的）膳食能量都会以脂肪的形式储存在体内，主要是三酰甘油，如肝、肌肉和其他细胞中的糖原，或者在较小程度上是肌肉中的蛋白质。在两餐之间，机体会调动内源性能量储备，并根据需要提供能量。身体代谢能量的调节是营养和激素之间的一种复杂相互作用，确保能量的连续供给、间歇性添加或提供底物。

胰岛素和胰高血糖素是调节能量动员与储存的两种主要激素。胰岛素是胰岛 B 细胞中胰岛素原合成的多肽，裂解成胰岛素和 C 肽。胰岛素的主要作用是协调葡萄糖、脂类和氨基酸的代谢。胰岛素具有合成代谢和抗分解代谢的特性。在肝脏中，胰岛素能够促进糖原和脂肪合成，同时抑制糖原分解和酮体生成。在脂肪组织中，胰岛素可促进脂肪储存和甘油合成，并抑制脂质分解。在肌肉组织中，胰岛素促进糖酵解及糖原和蛋白质的合成，并抑制蛋白质水解。胰高血糖素在胰岛 A 细胞中合成，是胰岛素的主要拮抗激素。当血糖水平较低时，胰高血糖素分泌增多，通过促进糖原分解和糖异生过程使葡萄糖生成增多。

吸收后期

在吸收后或禁食状态下，葡萄糖依赖的组织，如脑、肾髓质和某些血细胞，以葡萄糖作为主要的能量源。因为葡萄糖是脑的首选底物，所以维持血浆葡萄糖的恰当水平是一种生理优先选择。低胰岛素水平会使组织对外周葡萄糖的吸收减少，如脂肪组织和肌肉。最初，肝糖原被降解并为葡萄糖依赖组织提供葡萄糖。约 70g 糖原被储存在肝脏中[1]，而总的基础葡萄糖消耗量是 200~250g/d[2]，这远远超过储存的肝糖原。当糖原的有限储备被耗尽时，肝脏利用来自乳酸、甘油和氨基酸的碳通过糖异生合成葡萄糖。胰岛素水平降低会促进糖皮质激素的生成，而胰高血糖素在维持持续的内源性葡萄糖供应中起着补充作用。在禁食期间，糖原分解和葡萄糖生成的增加要与葡萄糖依赖组织对葡萄糖的基本需求量相匹配（图 2.1A）。

在禁食期间，胰岛素水平会影响所有营养素的供应，包括氨基酸和脂肪酸。低胰岛素水平会使蛋白水解增加和骨骼肌释放氨基酸增加，两者均为体内主要的蛋白质储备。氨基酸的净通量是从肌肉组织到肝脏，其中葡萄糖异生前体丙氨酸和谷氨酰胺占所释放氨基酸的最大比例[3]。在脂肪组织中，胰岛素抑制激素敏感脂肪酶，该酶催化储存的三酰甘油水解成游离甘油和游离脂肪酸。骨骼肌中游离脂肪酸的消耗是限制肌肉糖酵解和葡萄糖氧化的重要因素。

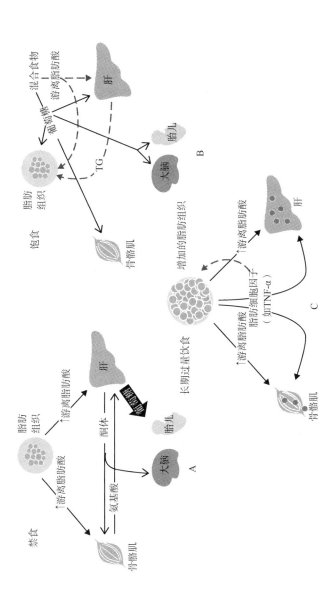

图2.1 A. 在禁食状态下,依赖葡萄糖的组织如大脑和胎儿,所需的葡萄糖来源于肝糖原储存的分解。一旦肝糖原储备被耗尽,葡萄糖从肌肉中的蛋白质释放释放的氨基酸会重新产生。游离脂肪酸(FFA)从脂肪组织中释放出来,转化为肝脏中的酮体,并用于防止非葡萄糖依赖性组织中葡萄糖的过度糖酵解。糖类混合物,糖类被分解成葡萄糖和其他酮体,并被组织吸收以后使用。将脂质水解成脂肪酸,再合成三酰甘油(TG),并储存在脂肪组织中。C. 长期过量进食,肌肉和肝脂肪组织中供应单糖。将脂质水解成脂肪酸,再合成三酰甘油(TG),并储存在脂肪组织中。C. 长期过量进食,肌肉和肝脏营养过剩和肥胖可导致脂肪细胞功能障碍与细胞炎症。各种脂肪因子包括TNF-α的释放会使脂肪组织和肝脏释放FFA抵抗也会导致胰岛素抵抗增加,慢性营养过剩和胰岛素抵抗发生。即使已有相对增加的胰岛素水平,但是脂肪组织中的胰岛素抵抗也会导致FFA释放增加,使胰岛素抵抗加剧随着营养物质的持续过量,通过脂肪细胞的储存能力,脂质"溢出"到其他组织(如肌肉和肝脏),并导致脂毒性和代谢重置化

· 21 ·

妊娠后的吸收状态

在禁食期间，孕妇有额外的负担，因为孕妇要为正在生长的胎儿提供能量底物。葡萄糖是胎儿的主要能量来源，因为胎儿无法进行糖异生[4]，所以要从母体的血浆中获得大部分葡萄糖。胎盘中载体介导的转运系统（GLUT1）[5]可满足胎儿对葡萄糖的高需求，该转运系统可以将葡萄糖从母体快速转移到胎儿。母体血浆葡萄糖浓度和子宫/胎盘血流量决定了葡萄糖的供应，这使胎盘屏障的转运过程相对快速，被称为流动受限过程[6]。

由于胎儿对能量底物葡萄糖的需求不断增加，妊娠期禁食对母体来说更具挑战性。妊娠早期以后，空腹血糖水平会随着孕龄的增加而逐渐降低[7]。通过短时间的禁食，人类妊娠期的特点是与非妊娠期相比空腹血浆胰岛素水平升高，基础肝葡萄糖产量增加[8, 9]。胰岛素诱导抑制肝葡萄糖的产生可以增加内源性葡萄糖的产生，从而增加母体和胎儿在两餐之间的葡萄糖供给。1970年Felig等[3]进行了研究，该研究为计划妊娠中期终止妊娠的健康妇女和未妊娠的健康妇女均预期持续禁食84h。与未妊娠的妇女相比，禁食的妊娠妇女的血浆葡萄糖和胰岛素浓度较低，酮体浓度较高。菲利格的研究提出了妊娠期间"加速饥饿"的概念。在禁食的妊娠妇女中发现较高的血浆酮体水平仅在胰岛素水平降低的情况下出现，并且推测是由脂解增多引起的。

为什么在妊娠期虽然内源性葡萄糖生成增加但妊娠妇女空腹血糖水平较低？发生机制目前尚不清楚。与未妊娠妇女相比，妊娠妇女空腹血糖降低似乎不是因为以妊娠妇女的尿氮排泄为依据所得出的母体蛋白分解减少。与未妊娠妇女相比，禁食妊娠妇女的血浆丙氨酸水平降低，并且可能代表胎儿对生糖前体的吸收。虽然妊娠期蛋白质分解代谢增加，但胎盘和胎儿对其利用率的增加可能导致循环糖异生前体的减少[10]。有些学者认为，对肝脏产生葡萄糖的抑制作用在妊娠晚期并没有降低，而是降低了血浆葡萄糖水平的调定点[11]。

未妊娠女性的餐后状态

对混合营养膳食的反应变化是建立在平衡的机制上的，这种机制允许在预期的禁食期间使用或储存能量（图 2.1B）。肠泌素肽，如葡萄糖依赖性胰岛素促性腺激素多肽（GIP）和胰高血糖素样肽-1（GLP-1），进食后会在胃肠道中分泌出来，从而增强葡萄糖刺激胰岛素分泌的作用。初期，胰岛素释放在肝脏中占主导地位，以降低或终止肝葡萄糖生成[12]。内脏的葡萄糖摄取在很大程度上是葡萄糖可用性增加的结果，其中大部分将由肝脏摄取[13]。随后，胰岛素水平升高介导周围的葡萄糖摄取，主要集中于肌肉和脂肪组织[14]。此时需要大量的胰岛素来调节周围的葡萄糖摄取，而不是抑制肝葡萄糖的产生[12]。肌肉组织氮的含量依赖于餐后肌肉中氨基酸的净摄取量。除了其他功能外，胰岛素还能抑制蛋白水解，加速游离脂肪酸的摄取，促进脂肪组织和肝脏的脂肪合成及三酰甘油的储存。餐后胰岛素水平升高促进了所有营养素（葡萄糖、氨基酸和脂质）的储存，供以后使用。

妊娠期女性的餐后状态

除了短期的能量管理之外，妊娠妇女还必须调节长期的能量平衡，这种动态平衡随着母亲和胎儿在妊娠期和哺乳期的新陈代谢需求的变化而变化。早期妊娠的标志是储存营养物质（合成代谢状态），为能量需求增加（分解代谢状态）的妊娠晚期和哺乳期做准备。妊娠早期至中期的能量平衡适应可能是由于雌激素、孕激素和泌乳素的大量增加（Freemark的评论观点[15]）。催乳素和孕激素能够增强食欲并引起食欲亢进，可致孕妇的食物摄入量增加 10%～15%。一方面孕激素有助于脂肪的储存；另一方面垂体生长激素水平的下降对体内脂肪沉积也存在促进作用。催乳素和雌激素在脂肪生成中的作用目前尚不清楚，且相关研究存在相互矛盾的地方[15]。人胎盘催乳素刺激胰岛 B 细胞的增生和肥大，这会导致在妊娠早期，胰岛素分泌增多的同时，正常的外周胰岛素和肝胰岛素敏感性也会增强，从而通过抑制脂多糖、蛋白质水解和糖原分解来促进能量底物的储存。

总体而言，在妊娠早期，胰岛素敏感性会随着妊娠期的延长而逐渐降低。妊娠早期和晚期的变化差异显著。尽管存在一些关于在妊娠早期胰岛素作用的争论，Catalano 等使用高胰岛素-正葡萄糖钳夹技术和葡萄糖示踪剂发现了妊娠早期外周和肝胰岛素敏感性并无变化，但葡萄糖耐量却得到改善[7, 8, 16]。在妊娠早期，胰岛素分泌增加，而胰岛素的作用却是可变的，因此一些妇女的葡萄糖耐量可能增加。胰岛素抵抗和代偿性高胰岛素血症是妊娠晚期的特征。与妊娠前相比，妊娠晚期胰岛素诱导的外周血糖摄取减少56%，胰岛素分泌则增加3～3.5倍[8]。某些动物[17, 18]和人类[19, 20]研究表明，妊娠期胰岛素抑制肝葡萄糖生成，而其他动物则没有[11, 21]。胰岛素钳夹过程中的方法学差异可能是解释差异的原因，但有力的证据表明，在妊娠晚期胰岛素抑制肝葡萄糖生成的能力下降。糖耐量正常的肥胖女性与偏瘦女性相比，胰岛素诱导的肝葡萄糖生成减少[20]。在妊娠的啮齿类动物中，内脏脂肪的积累有助于肝胰岛素抵抗的发展，其作用可能是通过肝脏三酰甘油的积累介导的[22]。

妊娠期胰岛素抵抗

妊娠期胰岛素抵抗的病因尚不完全清楚，很可能是多因素造成的。一直以来，胎盘激素受到牵连的原因有很多。妊娠期胰岛素抵抗的程度与胎盘的生长相符，许多胎盘激素对非妊娠个体而言会诱导胰岛素抵抗，包括人胎盘催乳素（HPL）[23, 24]、人胎盘生长激素（HPGH）[25]和孕酮[26, 27]。HPGH通过抑制脂肪组织中胰岛素信号级联的关键调节因子诱导胰岛素抵抗[28]。胎盘因素在妊娠期胰岛素抵抗的发生中起重要作用。一些激素，如HPGH可能直接影响胰岛素的作用；其他因素可能通过增加食物摄取和促进脂肪生成间接影响胰岛素抵抗。

正常妊娠与代谢综合征有许多共同特征，包括肥胖、胰岛素抵抗、高胰岛素血症和高脂血症。在相对较短的时间间隔内，妊娠妇女体内脂肪平均增加超过3kg[29]。虽然流行病学[30, 31]和动物[22]研究表明，内脏脂肪在妊娠期间显著增加。但是对人体组成成分的描述因体内水分的增加和妊娠期间可使用的测量方式的限制而受到限制[32-35]，脂肪组织在调节食物摄取、能量平衡和代谢平衡的过程中发挥作用。有几种生物活性肽（adipokines）会影响能量平衡，如瘦素，它主要由脂肪细胞表达和分泌。脂肪细胞在下丘脑储存了充足的瘦素信号，供给动态平衡中的传入支[36, 37]。除了母体脂肪作为瘦素的来源外，人胎盘会产生和分泌瘦素到母体和胎儿的循环中[38]，而且在不考虑体重指数的情况下[39]，妊娠时的瘦素浓度与非妊娠状态相比升高。因为食物摄入量增加了，所以这看上去有些矛盾。这种现象被称为瘦素抵抗，妊娠时处于瘦素抵抗状态。最新的实验证据表明在妊娠期存在针对瘦素的中枢细胞阻力[40-42]。与肥胖一样，细胞瘦素抵抗可以通过有限的瘦素作用和更强地抑制食物摄入需求，使食物摄入达到新的平衡。

虽然脂肪细胞产生的脂肪因子在代谢过程中发挥着重要的作用，但一些脂肪因子可能会介导肥胖症增加的有害生物效应。例如，在除妊娠外的许多情况下，TNF-α 与胰岛素敏感性降低有关，包括肥胖[43]和衰老[44]。在妊娠期间，与皮质醇、人绒毛膜促性腺激素（HCG）、雌二醇、人胎盘催乳素和泌乳素[45]相比，TNF-α 血浆浓度更能预判胰岛素抵抗。其他的脂肪因子（抵抗素、IL-1 和 IL-6）也被认为是胰岛素抵抗的介质[46]。

营养过剩和代谢功能障碍

慢性营养过剩、肥胖及脂肪组织的扩张可能导致脂肪细胞功能紊乱、细胞炎症和胰岛素抵抗（图2.1C）。除了脂肪组织过多引起的代谢功能障碍外，过量脂肪组织的积累过程也会导致代谢失调。Gregor 和 Hotamisligil[47]提出，脂肪细胞中营养物质和脂质储存过量会导致线粒体功能丧失、内质网应激增加和脂肪细胞功能障碍，所有这些都会产生胰岛素抵抗。另外，当持续的营养过剩超过脂肪细胞的储存能力时，脂质就会"溢出"到其他组织中[48]。大量脂肪进入肝脏、骨骼肌和胰岛会导致组织特异性胰岛素抵抗及胰岛素分泌受损，通常被称为脂毒性[48]。1963年，Randle 等[49]提出了增加脂肪酸氧化来抑制葡萄糖氧化的观点。后来，McGarry 等的研究[50]表明，高血糖会抑制脂肪酸氧化。因为这两种观点的提出出现了代谢僵化的概念，它是指在慢性营养过剩的环境下，肌肉组织无法针对当前的营养供应情况而选择合适的氧化底物（葡萄糖与脂肪酸）[51]，从而导致骨骼肌代谢失调，骨骼肌是未妊娠状态下周围葡萄糖摄取的主要组织。这一理论适用于妊娠期、多食症和孕妇体内脂肪快速增加的患者，其对代谢功能有重要的影响，这些影响包括更强的外周胰岛素抵抗。

胰岛素抵抗与糖耐量异常

人们经常误用胰岛素抵抗和葡萄糖耐受这两个概念，其实两者应该被区分开来。胰岛素抵抗是指胰岛素作用于靶组织的能力降低。在一般情况下，胰岛素在抑制肝糖原产生方面效果较差，并且需要更多的胰岛素来诱导肌肉和脂肪组织中的外周葡萄糖摄取。在胰岛素抵抗的状态下，需要更多的胰岛素来维持葡萄糖稳态。糖耐量异常通常包括一定程度的胰岛素抵抗和高胰岛素血症，但是对胰岛素抵抗的程度而言，胰岛素的分泌相对不足，结果导致空腹和（或）餐后血糖水平升高。

在正常妊娠中，尽管有明显的胰岛素抵抗，但在正常体重的女性中，胰岛素分泌量补偿性增加会使妊娠妇女血浆葡萄糖水平保持在相对较窄的范围内[19]。血糖监测显示，妊娠29周左右的正常体重的女性平均空腹血糖水平为（4.0±0.7）mmol/L，餐后高峰水平为（5.9±0.9）mmol/L[52]。胰岛素分泌量无法补偿性增加的女性会变得葡萄糖不耐受。虽然测得的糖耐量是持续分布的，但妊娠妇女依旧被归类为葡萄糖耐受或不耐受。妊娠糖尿病的检测旨在确定可能出现不良母婴妊娠结果的风险，并在某种程度上确定未来可能患2型糖尿病风险的女性。目前有关胎儿风险增高的母体血糖阈值，学者们还在讨论（参见第六章和第七章）。

胰岛素敏感性和胰岛素分泌之间的关系本质上是呈倒数和非线性的（图2.2）。为了维持正常的糖耐量，胰岛素敏感性的变化必须与循环胰岛素水平的相对变化相匹配。如在妊娠期，随着胰岛素敏感性的降低，胰岛素分泌必须增加，而葡萄糖浓度则保持不变。因为胰岛素抵抗程度而分泌足够量的胰岛素会导致曲线向左偏移并且糖耐量降低。这个过程是糖尿病发生的基础。

在整个妊娠期间，增加胰岛素抵抗和高胰岛素血症都是渐进的。如果胰岛素分泌不能补偿胰岛素抵抗的增加，就会发生葡萄糖耐受不良。目前对妊娠期胰岛素敏感性和分泌的了解大部分来自Catalano教授及其同事在20世纪80年代[53]和90年代[54,55]的发现。基于高胰岛素-正葡萄糖钳夹的研究发现，有妊娠糖尿病病史的非妊娠妇女与正常糖耐量的妇女相比，胰岛素敏感性降低[53]。所有妊娠妇女在妊娠晚期的胰岛素敏感性与

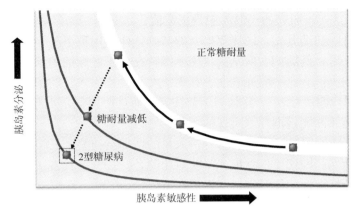

图 2.2 为了维持正常的葡萄糖耐量，胰岛素分泌必须增加以补偿妊娠期间胰岛素敏感性降低（实线箭头）。未能分泌足够量的胰岛素以达到胰岛素抵抗的程度会导致曲线向左移位并且葡萄糖耐量降低（虚线箭头）。这个过程是糖尿病（妊娠期糖尿病和 2 型糖尿病）发展的基础[经许可引自 Kahn 等 Nature 2006；444：840-846（63）]

妊娠前相比，似乎都有 50%～60%的下降，妊娠晚期胰岛素敏感性差异在很大程度上代表了妊娠前差异。妊娠早期胰岛素敏感性的变化与母体脂肪质量的变化呈负相关。为了补偿妊娠期间的胰岛素抵抗，胰岛素分泌增加。正常糖耐量的体重偏瘦型妇女在第一阶段胰岛素反应中，胰岛素分泌量会显著增加，而妊娠糖尿病妇女在第二阶段胰岛素反应中增加得更多。肥胖女性在第一和第二阶段的反应都有所增加[54, 55]。这些研究结果表明，妊娠糖尿病的肥胖女性胰岛 B 细胞受损和患 2 型糖尿病的风险最高。

妊娠期的代谢可塑性

妊娠期母体的代谢可塑性可以在有限的资源内保护胎儿。虽然科学家们对影响母亲和胎儿竞争需求平衡的复杂因素尚未完全解释清楚，但资源贫乏的冈比亚国家对特殊女性人口的研究结果提供了一些见解。Poppitt 教授和他的同事[56]在资源贫乏的冈比亚女性群体中进行了全身热量测量的纵向研究。这些女性虽然瘦但体重正常，她们在妊娠期间的体重增加量低于美国医学研究所的建议，而胎儿的平均出生体重是

3.02kg，这在该研究的小群体中是正常值。

从妊娠初期开始，冈比亚妇女的基础代谢率出现下降，当偏瘦体重得到纠正后，妊娠妇女的基础代谢率维持在低于妊娠前的水平，甚至在妊娠末期更低。这项研究表明，在无法增加食物摄入量的情况下，妊娠妇女有"代谢可塑性"，并且为了节约能量而进行调整，可能是通过改变发育中胎儿的能量消耗来实现的。

在资源充足的环境中，营养摄入量的增加会使整个妊娠期间产生正能量平衡。与冈比亚妇女形成鲜明对比的是，在资源较富裕的国家，女性在整个妊娠期间的基础代谢率都在持续增高[57]。

上述这些发现表明，妊娠期能量需求的增加可以通过许多方式来满足，如摄入量增加、活动减少和妊娠妇女脂肪储存量减少。此外，来自资源富裕国家和贫乏国家妇女的妊娠期总能量消耗（胎儿、脂肪沉积和维持）与妊娠前的脂肪和体重的增加密切相关[57]。没有条件增加食物摄入量的妊娠妇女的代谢可塑性可能对胎儿起到保护作用。因此，关于能量摄入量是否要充足的建议是因情况而变的，并且在很大程度上取决于母亲在妊娠初期可获得的资源和营养状况。

妊娠前糖尿病

1型糖尿病是一种免疫介导的胰岛B细胞破坏过程。随着时间的推移，胰岛B细胞功能下降导致分泌胰岛素的能力受损，并且在临床发病之前就已开始。有学者认为，1型糖尿病的病因包括遗传易感性和暴露于尚未确定的环境诱因[58]。风险等位基因与HLA-DQ有关，但易感性与40多种遗传因素有关[59]。胰岛素、谷氨酸脱羧酶-65（GAD65）、IA2和ZNT8转运蛋白的存在是自身免疫的临床标志[60]，疾病临床检测的风险水平和间隔时间与存在的胰岛B细胞蛋白抗体的数量有关[61]。

胰岛素抵抗和胰岛B细胞功能障碍是导致2型糖尿病的两个关键性病理生理因素。营养过剩（如高血糖症和高脂血症）和肥胖导致高代谢负荷、胰岛素抵抗和慢性炎症。胰岛B细胞对这些环境变化和长期应激状态的细胞反应根据个体的遗传易感性而变化。不同的基因-环境相互作用导致不同时期的情况和临床表现[62]。

总结和未来研究方向

妊娠期间发生的生理适应为胎儿生长提供了充足的能量和基础，并使母亲为妊娠和哺乳期负担增加做好了准备。胰岛素抵抗在整个妊娠期是渐进的，并且胰岛素分泌的代偿性增加将血浆葡萄糖水平维持在相对稳定的范围内。胎盘因素直接导致胰岛素抵抗（如 HPGH 和 TNF-α），并通过食欲和体重的增加而间接增强胰岛素抵抗。长期的正能量平衡会导致脂肪组织增生，这可能会用于在妊娠晚期和哺乳期胎儿对能量需求的增加。然而，妊娠前单纯性肥胖及妊娠期间体重过度增加可能会对胰岛素的作用和糖耐量产生不良影响。我们尚不清楚可以满足胎儿正常生长所需要的未妊娠女性健康的脂肪量、妊娠期体重增加的理想指数或胰岛素抵抗的必要程度，这应该是未来研究的重点。

选择题

1. 胰岛素具有以下哪些代谢调节特征（　　）
   A. 糖原合成　　　　　　B. 抑制脂类分解
   C. 糖蛋白水解　　　　　D. 蛋白的合成

正确答案是 C。胰岛素可促进肝脏中的糖原合成和肌肉中的蛋白质合成，并抑制脂肪分解。反调节激素——胰高血糖素促进空腹状态下的糖原分解。

2. 下列正确的是（　　）
   A. 妊娠晚期胰岛素抵抗与妊娠早期相比减少
   B. 妊娠早期葡萄糖耐量可能是变化的
   C. 胰岛素分泌不足会导致妊娠期胰岛素抵抗
   D. 胰岛素分泌与胰岛素敏感性之间的关系呈线性关系

正确答案是 B。妊娠早期胰岛素分泌增加，但不同妇女的胰岛素敏感性可能不同，使得妊娠早期糖耐量发生变化。

3. 以下不会影响妊娠期胰岛素抵抗的是（　　）

A. 人胎盘生长因子　　B. TNF-α（肿瘤坏死因子）
C. 过量的营养素　　　D. GLP-1（胰高血糖素样肽-1）

正确答案是 D。胎盘激素、脂肪因子和过量营养素都可能导致妊娠期胰岛素抵抗的发生。GLP-1 在餐后由胃肠道分泌并促进胰腺分泌胰岛素。

（王诗淇　译，朱海清　校）

参 考 文 献

1. Hultman E. [Carbohydrate metabolism normally and under trauma]. Nord Med 1971;85(11):330-346.
2. Rothman DL, Shulman RG, Shulman GI. 31P nuclear magnetic resonance measurements of muscle glucose-6-phosphate. Evidence for reduced insulin-dependent muscle glucose transport or phosphorylation activity in non-insulin-dependent diabetes mellitus. J Clin Invest 1992;89(4):1069-1075.
3. Felig P, Lynch V. [Starvation in human pregnancy: hypoglycemia, hypoinsulinemia, and hyperketonemia]. Science 1970;170(961):990-992.
4. Baumann MU, Deborde S, Illsley NP. Placental glucose transfer and fetal growth. Endocrine 2002;19(1):13-22.
5. Teasdale F, Jean-Jacques G. Morphometric evaluation of the microvillous surface enlargement factor in the human placenta from mid-gestation to term. Placenta 1985;6(5):375-381.
6. Illsley NP, Lin HY, Verkman AS. Lipid domain structure correlated with membrane protein function in placental microvillus vesicles. Biochemistry 1987;26(2):446-454.
7. Catalano PM, Tyzbir ED, Roman NM, Amini SB, Sims EA. Longitudinal changes in insulin release and insulin resistance in nonobese pregnant women. Am J Obstet Gynecol 1991;165(6 Pt 1):1667-1672.
8. Catalano PM, Tyzbir ED, Wolfe RR, Roman NM, Amini SB, Sims EA. Longitudinal changes in basal hepatic glucose production and suppression during insulin infusion in normal pregnant women. Am J Obstet Gynecol 1992;167(4 Pt 1):913-919.
9. Cowett RM, Susa JB, Kahn CB, Giletti B, Oh W, Schwartz R. Glucose kinetics in nondiabetic and diabetic women during the third trimester of pregnancy. Am J Obstet Gynecol 1983;146(7):773-780.
10. Felig P. Maternal and fetal fuel homeostasis in human pregnancy. Am J Clin Nutr 1973;26(9):998-1005.
11. Nolan CJ, Proietto J. The set point for maternal glucose homeostasis is lowered during late pregnancy in the rat: the role of the islet beta-cell and liver. Diabetologia 1996;39(7):785-792.
12. Rizza RA, Mandarino LJ, Gerich JE. Dose-response characteristics for effects of insulin on production and utilization of glucose in man. Am J Physiol 1981;240(6):E630-E639.
13. Sherwin RS, Hendler R, DeFronzo R, Wahren J, Felic P. Glucose homeostasis during prolonged suppression of glucagon and insulin secretion by somatostatin. Proc Natl Acad Sci USA 1977;74(1):348-352.
14. Sacca L, Cicala M, Trimarco B, Ungaro B, Vigorito C. Differential effects of insulin on splanchnic and peripheral glucose disposal after an intravenous glucose load in man. J Clin Invest 1982;70(1):117-126.
15. Freemark M. Regulation of maternal metabolism by pituitary and placental hormones: roles in fetal development and

metabolic programming. Horm Res 2006;65(Suppl 3):41–49.
16 Catalano PM, Tyzbir ED, Wolfe RR, Calles J, Roman NM, Amini SB, et al. Carbohydrate metabolism during pregnancy in control subjects and women with gestational diabetes. Am J Physiol 1993;264(1 Pt 1):E60–E67.
17 Hauguel S, Gilbert M, Girard J. Pregnancy-induced insulin resistance in liver and skeletal muscles of the conscious rabbit. Am J Physiol 1987;252(2 Pt 1):E165–E169.
18 Rossi G, Sherwin RS, Penzias AS, Lapaczewski P, Jacob RJ, Shulman GI, et al. Temporal changes in insulin resistance and secretion in 24-h-fasted conscious pregnant rats. Am J Physiol 1993;265(6 Pt 1): E845–E851.
19 Catalano PM, Huston L, Amini SB, Kalhan SC. Longitudinal changes in glucose metabolism during pregnancy in obese women with normal glucose tolerance and gestational diabetes mellitus. Am J Obstet Gynecol 1999;180(4):903–916.
20 Sivan E, Chen X, Homko CJ, Reece EA, Boden G. Longitudinal study of carbohydrate metabolism in healthy obese pregnant women. Diabetes Care 1997;20(9):1470–1475.
21 Connolly CC, Papa T, Smith MS, Lacy DB, Williams PE, Moore MC. Hepatic and muscle insulin action during late pregnancy in the dog. Am J Physiol Reg Integ Comp Physiol 2007;292(1): R447–R452.
22 Einstein FH, Fishman S, Muzumdar RH, Yang XM, Atzmon G, Barzilai N. Accretion of visceral fat and hepatic insulin resistance in pregnant rats. Am J Physiol Endocrinol Metab 2008;294(2):E451–E455.
23 Kalkhoff RK, Richardson BL, Beck P. Relative effects of pregnancy, human placental lactogen and prednisolone on carbohydrate tolerance in normal and subclinical diabetic subjects. Diabetes 1969;18(3):153–163.
24 Samaan N, Yen SC, Gonzalez D, Pearson OH. Metabolic effects of placental lactogen (HPL) in man. J Clin Endocrinol Metab 1968;28(4):485–491.

25 Barbour LA, Shao J, Qiao L, Pulawa LK, Jensen DR, Bartke A, et al. Human placental growth hormone causes severe insulin resistance in transgenic mice. Am J Obstet Gynecol 2002;186(3):512–517.
26 Beck P. Progestin enhancement of the plasma insulin response to glucose in Rhesus monkeys. Diabetes 1969;18(3):146–152.
27 Kalkhoff RK, Jacobson M, Lemper D. Progesterone, pregnancy and the augmented plasma insulin response. J Clin Endocrinol Metab 1970;31(1):24–28.
28 Barbour LA, Shao J, Qiao L, Leitner W, Anderson M, Friedman JE, et al. Human placental growth hormone increases expression of the p85 regulatory unit of phosphatidylinositol 3-kinase and triggers severe insulin resistance in skeletal muscle. Endocrinology 2004;145(3):1144–1150.
29 Hytten FE. Weight gain in pregnancy: 30 year of research. S Afr Med J 1981;60(1):15–19.
30 Blaudeau TE, Hunter GR, Sirikul B. Intra-abdominal adipose tissue deposition and parity. Int J Obes (Lond) 2006;30(7):1119–1124.
31 Kinoshita T, Itoh M. Longitudinal variance of fat mass deposition during pregnancy evaluated by ultrasonography: the ratio of visceral fat to subcutaneous fat in the abdomen. Gynecol Obstet Invest 2006;61(2):115–118.
32 Hopkinson JM, Butte NF, Ellis KJ, Wong WW, Puyau MR, Smith EO. Body fat estimation in late pregnancy and early postpartum: comparison of two-, three-, and four-component models. Am J Clin Nutr 1997;65(2):432–438.
33 McManus RM, Cunningham I, Watson A, Harker L, Finegood DT. Beta-cell function and visceral fat in lactating women with a history of gestational diabetes. Metab Clin Exper 2001;50(6):715–719.
34 Sidebottom AC, Brown JE, Jacobs DR, Jr. Pregnancy-related changes in body fat. Eur J Obstet Gynecol Reprod Biol 2001;94(2):216–223.
35 Sohlstrom A, Forsum E. Changes in total body fat during the human reproductive

cycle as assessed by magnetic resonance imaging, body water dilution, and skinfold thickness: a comparison of methods. Am J Clin Nutr 1997;66(6):1315-1322.
36. Campfield LA, Smith FJ, Guisez Y, Devos R, Burn P. Recombinant mouse OB protein: evidence for a peripheral signal linking adiposity and central neural networks. Science 1995;269(5223):546-549.
37. Zhang F, Basinski MB, Beals JM, Briggs SL, Churgay LM, Clawson DK, et al. Crystal structure of the obese protein leptin-E100. Nature 1997;387(6629):206-209.
38. Masuzaki H, Ogawa Y, Sagawa N, Hosoda K, Matsumoto T, Mise H, et al. Nonadipose tissue production of leptin: leptin as a novel placenta-derived hormone in humans. Nature Med 1997;3(9):1029-1033.
39. Finn PD, Cunningham MJ, Pau KY, Spies HG, Clifton DK, Steiner RA. The stimulatory effect of leptin on the neuroendocrine reproductive axis of the monkey. Endocrinology 1998;139(11):4652-4662.
40. Peters A, Schweiger U, Pellerin L, Hubold C, Oltmanns KM, Conrad M, et al. The selfish brain: competition for energy resources. Neurosci Biobehav Rev 2004;28(2):143-180.
41. Ladyman SR, Grattan DR. Region-specific reduction in leptin-induced phosphorylation of signal transducer and activator of transcription-3 (STAT3) in the rat hypothalamus is associated with leptin resistance during pregnancy. Endocrinology 2004;145(8):3704-3711.
42. Ladyman SR, Grattan DR. Suppression of leptin receptor messenger ribonucleic acid and leptin responsiveness in the ventromedial nucleus of the hypothalamus during pregnancy in the rat. Endocrinology 2005;146(9):3868-3874.
43. Hotamisligil GS, Peraldi P, Budavari A, Ellis R, White MF, Spiegelman BM. IRS-1-mediated inhibition of insulin receptor tyrosine kinase activity in TNF-alpha- and obesity-induced insulin resistance. Science 1996;271(5249):665-668.
44. Kirwan JP, Krishnan RK, Weaver JA, Del Aguila LF, Evans WJ. Human aging is associated with altered TNF-alpha production during hyperglycemia and hyperinsulinemia. Am J Physiol Endocrinol Metab 2001;281(6):E1137-E1143.
45. Kirwan JP, Hauguel-De Mouzon S, Lepercq J, Challier JC, Huston-Presley L, Friedman JE, et al. TNF-alpha is a predictor of insulin resistance in human pregnancy. Diabetes 2002;51(7):2207-2213.
46. Hotamisligil GS, Murray DL, Choy LN, Spiegelman BM. Tumor necrosis factor alpha inhibits signaling from the insulin receptor. Proc Natl Acad Sci USA 1994;91(11):4854-4858.
47. Gregor MG, Hotamisligil GS. Adipocyte stress: the endoplasmic reticulum and metabolic disease. J Lipid Res 2007;48(9):1905-1914.
48. Muoio DM, Newgard CB. Obesity-related derangements in metabolic regulation. Ann Rev Biochem 2006;75:367-401.
49. Randle PJ, Garland PB, Hales CN, Newsholme EA. The glucose fatty-acid cycle. Its role in insulin sensitivity and the metabolic disturbances of diabetes mellitus. Lancet 1963;1(7285):785-789.
50. McGarry JD, Mannaerts GP, Foster DW. A possible role for malonyl-CoA in the regulation of hepatic fatty acid oxidation and ketogenesis. J Clin Invest 1977;60(1):265-270.
51. Kelley DE, Mandarino LJ. Fuel selection in human skeletal muscle in insulin resistance: a reexamination. Diabetes 2000;49(5):677-683.
52. Yogev Y, Ben-Haroush A, Chen R, Rosenn B, Hod M, Langer O. Diurnal glycemic profile in obese and normal weight nondiabetic pregnant women. Am J Obstet Gynecol 2004;191(3):949-953.
53. Catalano PM, Bernstein IM, Wolfe RR, Srikanta S, Tyzbir E, Sims EA. Subclinical abnormalities of glucose metabolism in subjects with previous gestational diabetes. Am J Obstet Gynecol 1986; 155 (6): 1255-1262.
54. Catalano PM, Roman-Drago NM, Amini SB, Sims EA. Longitudinal c hanges in body composition and energy balance in

lean women with normal and abnormal glucose tolerance during pregnancy. Am J Obstet Gynecol 1998; 179 (1): 156–165.
55 Catalano PM, Huston L, Amini SB, Kalhan SC. Longitudinal changes in glucose metabolism during pregnancy in obese women with normal glucose tolerance and gestational diabetes mellitus. Am J Obstet Gynecol 1999; 180(4): 903–916.
56 Poppitt SD, Prentice AM, Jequier E, Schutz Y, Whitehead RG. Evidence of energy sparing in Gambian women during pregnancy: a longitudinal study using whole-body calorimetry. Am J Clin Nutr 1993;57(3):353–364.
57 Prentice AM, Goldberg GR. Energy adaptations in human pregnancy: limits and long-term consequences. Am J Clin Nutr 2000;71(5 Suppl):1226S–1232S.
58 Steenkiste A, Valdes AM, Feolo M, Hoffman D, Concannon P, Noble J, et al. 14th International HLA and Immunogenetics Workshop: report on the HLA component of type 1 diabetes. Tissue Antigens 2007;69(Suppl 1):214–225.
59 Concannon P, Rich SS, Nepom GT. Genetics of type 1A diabetes. N Engl J Med 2009;360(16):1646–1654.
60 Pihoker C, Gilliam LK, Hampe CS, Lernmark A. Autoantibodies in diabetes. Diabetes 2005;54(Suppl 2):S52–S61.
61 Lernmark A, Larsson HE. Immune therapy in type 1 diabetes mellitus. Nat Rev Endocrinol 2013;9(2):92–103.
62 Halban PA, Polonsky KS, Bowden DW, Hawkins MA, Ling C, Mather KJ, et al. Beta-cell failure in type 2 diabetes: postulated mechanisms and prospects for prevention and treatment. Diabetes Care 2014;37(6):1751–1758.

其他可参阅文献

63 Kahn SE, Hull RL, Utzschneider KM. Mechanisms linking obesity to insulin resistance and type 2 diabetes. Nature 2006;444(7121):840–846.

第三章 糖尿病合并妊娠期间的胎盘

Ursula Hiden and Gernot Desoye

Department of Obstetrics and Gynecology, Medical University of Graz, Graz, Austria

实践要点

- 与糖尿病相关的不同胎盘变化取决于妊娠糖尿病的发生时间及糖尿病的类型。
- 早期胎盘发育可能随胰岛素和肿瘤坏死因子-α（TNF-α）诱导的基质金属蛋白酶降解细胞外基质的变化而改变。
- 糖尿病妇女通常胎盘较重，母体（即合体滋养细胞）和胎儿（即内皮）表面积增多。
- 滋养层细胞增殖受母体胰岛素调节，血管过度形成是胎儿缺氧的结果。
- GDM 母体葡萄糖对胎儿循环的影响无明显变化。高通量来自更明显的母体胎儿浓度梯度。氨基酸转运可能发生改变。
- 胎儿胰岛素和类胰岛素生长因子可直接影响胎儿的生长，但同时也可促进母体对胎儿氨基酸的转运，从而维持胎儿的生长。
- 瘦素与胰岛素共有部分信号通路，通过胎盘高表达，且分泌到母体和胎儿的血液循环中，可能有助于糖尿病的发展变化。
- 胎儿性别可能调节 GDM 对胎盘和胎儿发育及功能的影响。
- GDM 的糖尿病环境改变了 DNA 甲基化谱，因此长期影响子代。

正常发展

胎盘是促进胎儿生长发育必不可少的复杂器官。它具有广泛的功能，最重要的就是将母体的营养物质传输给胎儿及合成各种激素和生长因子。它的发育和功能受到一系列激素、细胞因子、生长因子和存在于母体及胎儿循环中基质的严格调节。胎盘因素影响母体对妊娠的适应及胎儿的生长发育。

在胚囊植入蜕膜表面后，胎盘通过滋养细胞的分裂和增殖而持续发育，最终形成不同成熟程度的胎盘绒毛[1]，其中大部分自由地漂浮在绒毛间隙（即区域）中（图3.1）。高度增殖的绒毛滋养细胞融合形成合体滋养细胞，代表胎盘与母体循环接触的最外层界面。该合胞体的微绒毛膜与母血接触，具有丰富的受体[2]、酶[3]和转运体[4]。母体血液由重塑和开放的螺旋动脉滋润绒毛。

一些绒毛将胎盘完全地固定在子宫上，从而在胎儿和母体蜕膜之间建立连接（图3.1）。这些固定绒毛由蜕膜腔内层的滋养细胞增殖、分化和侵入形成。绒毛外滋养层细胞也侵入蜕膜螺旋动脉，并将其转化为低阻力动脉。由此产生的流入间隙空间的母体血流的增加确保了向胎儿提供足够的母体营养[1]。滋养层细胞的侵袭在时间和空间上受到母体来源的促侵袭因子和抑制因子的严格调控。蜕膜来源于胚胎植入前蜕膜化后的母体子宫内膜。蜕膜化产生致密的细胞外基质和细胞因子环境，减少滋养细胞侵入[5]。这些因素的水平在出现妊娠相关疾病与糖尿病时会发生变化（表3.1）。

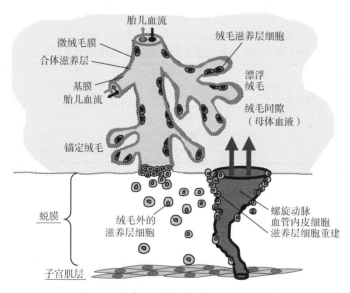

图3.1 妊娠20周后的胎盘绒毛组织

合体滋养细胞代表胎盘的最外层，并通过其微绒毛膜与母体血液接触，该微绒毛膜富含受体、酶和转运体。合体细胞通过位于下方的细胞滋养细胞的增殖和融合而再生与扩展。漂浮绒毛顶端的一些细胞滋养层侵入蜕膜，从而固定绒毛。部分绒毛外细胞滋养细胞进一步侵入子宫螺旋动脉，导致其重塑为低阻力血管。为了区分母体和胎盘细胞及组织，图中母体结构加下划线标记

表 3.1　GDM 和 T_1DM 患者滋养细胞浸润抑制及侵袭促进因子水平的变化

抑制浸润	促进浸润				
TNF-α	VEGF	Leptin	IGF1	IGF2	胰岛素
GDM ↑(84)	↑(38)	↑(85)	↑(86) NC(87)	↑(87) NC(37,86)	↑(45)胰岛素治疗 ↑(88)
T_1DM ↑(36)		NC(89)	↓(37) NC(87)	↑(87) NC(37)	↑(45)

注：肿瘤坏死因子-α（TNF-α）抑制滋养层浸润，而 VEGF（血管内皮生长因子）、Leptin（瘦素）、胰岛素样生长因子-1（IGF1）和胰岛素样生长因子-2（IGF2）促进滋养层浸润。
GDM，妊娠糖尿病；NC，无变化；T_1DM，1 型糖尿病；TNF-α，肿瘤坏死因-α；VEGF，血管内皮生长因子。

在绒毛发育期间，血管生成导致胎盘血管的形成，这一过程再次受到各种生长因子、细胞因子和氧气的控制（表 3.2），因此在罹患糖尿病时可能会出现失调。

表 3.2　GDM 和 T_1DM 胎儿的促血管生成因子或抗血管生成因子的变化

抗血管生成	促血管生成							其他
TNF-α	VEGF	FGF2	PGF	Leptin	IGF1	IGF2	缺氧	胰岛素
GDM ↓(84)	NC(90)	↑(38)	↓(90) NC(91)	↑(92) NC(93,94)	↑(90)	↑(87) NC(90)	↑(95)	↑(96)
T_1DM	↓(97)	↑(98)	↓(90)	↑(92)	↑(37,52)	↑(52,87)	↑(99)	↑(45)

注：两种类型的糖尿病都以血管化增强为特征。PGF，胎盘生长因子。

糖尿病期间的胎盘

由于受体和酶在胎盘表面（即微绒毛合体滋养细胞膜及合体滋养细胞和胎盘内皮细胞的基膜）的存在，糖尿病可能对胎盘发育和功能产生深远的影响。这些具体影响及其严重性取决于妊娠糖尿病环境的损害作用于胎盘的时间[6]。

由于葡萄糖可以刺激和抑制基因表达[7]，母体和胎儿的高血糖可能影响各种胎盘蛋白的生成，但具体研究尚待进行。此外，母体和胎儿高胰岛素血症也影响胎盘代谢、生长和发育[3,8,9]。然而，糖尿病环境的变化并不局限于葡萄糖和胰岛素（表 3.1 和表 3.2）。母亲体内的这些细胞可诱导胎盘发生改变，包括细胞因子和生长因子的合成发生改变，而细胞因子和生长因子又可能以自分泌或旁分泌的方式局部起作用。改变的细胞因子和生长因子及代谢物可被分泌到母体循环和胎儿循环中，从而影响母体和胎儿（图 3.2）。

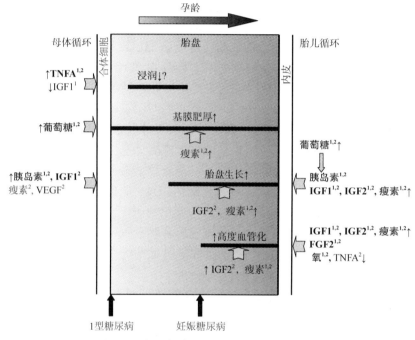

图 3.2 糖尿病诱导人胎盘改变的假设模型

1 型糖尿病妊娠妇女中 TNF-α 的升高和胰岛素样生长因子-1 水平的降低可能抑制胎盘浸润，同时糖尿病早期妊娠流产的发生率也较高。母体高血糖症导致胎盘基膜增厚，从而减少氧转运。胎盘瘦素水平的升高甚至可能进一步促进细胞外基质（ECM）的过度合成。糖尿病患者胎盘（IGF2、瘦素）、母体（胰岛素、VEGF）或胎儿（胰岛素、IGF1、IGF2、瘦素）循环中升高的各种因子可促进增殖和胎盘生长。胎盘 IGF2 和瘦素水平升高，胎儿 IGF1、IGF2、瘦素和 FGF2 水平升高，胎儿 TNF-α 水平降低及胎儿缺氧导致胎盘高度血管化。胎儿胎盘的这些结构紊乱是妊娠糖尿病、显性糖尿病或两者的特征（粗体表示 1 型糖尿病和妊娠糖尿病有类似的失调）

1 为 T_1DM 中的变化；2 为 GDM 中的变化

尽管在过去的几十年[10]中，母亲血糖控制有所改善，但足月时糖尿病胎盘的结构和功能变化可能独立于糖尿病类型而发生[11]。与胎儿体重相似，糖尿病妊娠妇女的胎盘重量也趋向于较重，但胎盘的重量增加比胎儿更为明显，这反映出胎盘与胎儿重量比高于正常妊娠者[12, 13]。胎盘超重是否是糖尿病中胎儿过度生长的原因或结果一直是一个尚未解决的问题。

直观地说，糖尿病可能导致胎盘运输系统发生变化。在 GDM 患者中，母体对胎儿的葡萄糖转运目前已被广泛研究。GLUT1 是人胎盘中主要的葡萄糖转运体（GLUT），在妊娠的所有阶段的所有细胞类型中都有所发现[14]。此外，高亲和力葡萄糖转运蛋白 GLUT3 主要存在于胎儿胎盘内皮细胞上。在早期人类妊娠中[15]，胰岛素调节的 GLUT4 位于合体滋养细胞上，而在妊娠结束时，它主要位于胎盘绒毛基质中[16]。这些胎盘葡萄糖转运体之间的相互作用，以及它们对胎盘葡萄糖代谢和胎盘葡萄糖流量的作用尚不清楚。这些转运体可由多种激素和代谢刺激物调节，包括环境葡萄糖水平[17-19]。结果是 GDM 患者胎盘中葡萄糖转运体水平的改变及显性糖尿病母体的变化[20, 21]。尽管这些分子发生了变化，灌注实验已经证实即使以胎盘总重量为基础，GDM 的葡萄糖经胎盘转运没有减少，也没有改变[22]。整合潜在结构变化的研究清晰地显示，母体到胎儿葡萄糖浓度梯度越明显，是糖尿病患者胎盘葡萄糖流量增加的主要原因，也是重要原因。GDM 脐动脉和静脉葡萄糖浓度的变化也证实了这一结论[23]。

合胞滋养层氨基酸转运系统可能在糖尿病时发生改变[4, 24]。然而，即使对于未改变的运输系统，当单位蛋白或组织重量表达时，胎盘总重量的增加将导致营养运输的增加。目前尚不清楚这是否会刺激胎儿的生长，或只是用来弥补胎儿营养需求增加，其过度增长是由其他因素驱动的。

无论是哪种类型的糖尿病，胎盘结构都可能被改变。要注意的是，由于血管过度增生，表面和交换区域增大[25]，绒毛表面增加的潜在机制尚不清楚。妊娠早期母体高胰岛素血症是一个因素[8]，但其他母体生长因子也可能起作用。

胎盘毛细血管表面较大可能由胎儿胎盘缺氧调节机制所致。从妊娠糖尿病的患者中经常能观察到体内的胎儿促红细胞生成素水平升高、红细胞增多和有核红细胞增多[26]。妊娠糖尿病患者的胎盘氧供应减少的原因可能是：

（1）母体动脉血氧饱和度降低，糖化血红蛋白比例增加，对氧的亲和力高于非糖化血红蛋白[27]。

（2）滋养层基膜增厚[28]，但没有一致的发现[29]。

（3）在某些情况下，由于子宫动脉和脐动脉血流阻抗增加，子宫胎盘血流减少[30-32]。

除了氧气供应受损外，胎儿对氧气的需求也因胎儿高胰岛素血症刺激有氧代谢而增加。由此产生的胎儿低氧水平最终上调胎盘促血管生成因子的转录合成。已有的研究包括成纤维细胞生长因子-2（FGF2）、血管内皮生长因子（VEGF）和瘦素[33-35]，更高水平的这些因素可促进胎盘血管内皮细胞增殖，这是血管生成的关键过程。在母体营养过剩的情况下，胎儿缺氧背景下胎盘血管交换面积的增加似乎是矛盾的，并且可能强调了对胎儿有足够的氧气输送的重要性。

在妊娠早期，当发育中的胎盘暴露于母体糖尿病环境，如高血糖、高胰岛素血症时，由于维持严格的代谢控制所需的相对过量的胰岛素剂量，使 TNF-α 的分泌增加[36]，胰岛素样生长因子-1（IGF1）减少[37]，FGF2 增加[38]。在形成胎盘结构的关键时期，糖尿病环境将对胎盘的发育和功能产生影响，并且胎盘可能对环境紊乱最敏感，这似乎是合理的。胎盘的生长和发育有时似乎在第一个妊娠周被阻塞，可能由高血糖引起的滋养细胞增殖减少导致[39, 40]。自然流产[41]和妊娠病理[如子痫前期和宫内生长受限（IUGR）]的更高发病率提示滋养细胞侵入受损，这将导致胎盘固定不足和母体螺旋动脉开放[42]。这进一步由偶尔观察到的子宫胎盘血流减少所支持[30]，尽管不是统一的[43, 44]。

基质金属蛋白酶 MMP14 和 MMP15 参与了与侵入、血管生成和增殖相关的组织重塑过程。基质金属蛋白酶在 1 型糖尿病[3]中的升高是由母体胰岛素和 TNF-α[36, 45]引起的。MMP14 和 MMP15 具有非常宽的底物谱，包括细胞外基质成分[46]。此外，成熟和不成熟的细胞因子可能被激活或失活，从而有助于糖尿病的进一步改变。特别是由弗林蛋白酶裂解产生的胎盘 MMP14 的活性在糖尿病时增加。弗林蛋白酶含有低氧诱导因子 1α（HIF1α）启动子结合位点。这使得人们倾向于假设糖尿病绒毛状胎盘结构中的缺氧状况可能与 MMP14 活性增加有关。这些结果表明，早期胎盘发育对生长因子和细胞因子水平变化的敏感性。然而，在母体糖尿病中减少滋养层细胞的侵入仍然是推测性的。

胰岛素/胰岛素样生长因子系统和瘦素在糖尿病胎盘中的作用

母亲和胎儿高瘦素血症,以及胎盘瘦素合成增加,在糖尿病和肥胖症中得到证实。然而,最近的报道并没有支持 GDM 中更高的胎儿瘦素水平(表 3.1 和表 3.2)。胰岛素和瘦素发挥的作用超出了新陈代谢调节的功能,包括刺激生长因子活性和效力,这反过来又刺激各种靶基因的表达[9, 47]。在人类肥胖症中,由于胰岛素和瘦素的信号通路之间有相当大的重叠,因此常巧合地发生对胰岛素和瘦素的耐药性[48]。这些信号级联之间的广泛交叉交流可能是糖尿病引起胎盘改变的主要原因,特别是在肥胖妊娠的前 3 个月。

胰岛素、胰岛素样生长因子 1 和胰岛素样生长因子 2

胰岛素/胰岛素样生长因子(LGF)系统在控制胎儿和胎盘生长发育方面被认为具有中心地位[49]。胰岛素受体和高度相关的 IGF1 受体(IGF1R)均主要通过两条细胞内途径[50]发出信号:ERK1/2 途径刺激细胞增殖,PI3K-AKT 途径主要调节代谢功能。

胎儿胎盘胰岛素、IGF1、IGF2 及其受体的表达在发育过程中以组织特异性的方式调节,并可受营养和内分泌条件的影响[49]。胰岛素受体的胎盘表达经历了从妊娠早期滋养细胞到妊娠晚期胎盘内皮细胞[9, 51]的发展转变。胎盘 IGF1R 主要表达于合体滋养细胞的基膜上。因此,它主要可用于胎儿 IGF1 和 IGF2[2]。这些生长因子对人类胎盘的具体作用还没有被详细研究。小鼠胚胎 IGF1、IGF2 或 IGF1R 基因的靶向性破坏导致胎儿生长迟缓,而 IGF2 过度合成则促进胎儿生长。IGF1 依赖于营养供应刺激胎儿生长,而胎盘 IGF2 是胎盘生长和营养转运的关键调节因子,可促进胎儿生长发育[49]。

IGF1 和 IGF2 效应可通过影响其生物利用度的可溶性胰岛素样生长因子结合蛋白(IGFBP)来减弱或增加。在人类中,胎儿血浆和组织中最普遍的 IGFBP 是 IGFBP1~IGFBP4。胎儿脐带血分析表明,这些结合蛋白可能在糖尿病妊娠中失调[52]。IGFBP 的减少将导致 IGF 更高的生物利用度，从而可能间接地导致胎儿的过度生长。

母体、胎儿和胎盘之间的内分泌系统相互作用，通过母体胰岛素和胎儿胰岛素对胎盘的作用来体现。母体胰岛素通过合体滋养细胞微绒毛膜上表达的受体影响胎盘发育[3]。反过来，胎盘通过分泌激素、细胞因子和代谢产物来影响母亲。例如，母体胰岛素上调滋养层细胞[53]中的瘦素生成，并且在母体循环后分泌增加的瘦素水平可增强母体胰岛素抵抗。瘦素和胰岛素均抑制滋养层细胞中胎盘生长激素（PGH）的分泌[54]。PGH 可引起母体胰岛素抵抗[55]。因此，作为推测，胰岛素和瘦素减少 PGH 分泌可能代表母体胎盘前向反馈机制最终减轻母体胰岛素抵抗。

胎儿胰岛素影响胎盘动脉和静脉内皮细胞的基因表达[9]，这直接或间接影响胎盘和胎儿的发育。胰岛素受体表达从妊娠早期滋养细胞到足月期内皮的变化，使母亲体内的胰岛素能够在妊娠初期调节胎盘功能，而随着妊娠的进展，胎儿控制了胎盘胰岛素的作用（图 3.3）[9]。IGF1 和 IGF2

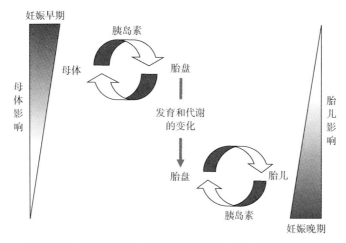

图 3.3　胎盘胰岛素受体表达的时空变化允许胰岛素调控从母体到胎儿的转变

胰岛素受体表达从妊娠早期滋养细胞向妊娠晚期内皮细胞转移。在妊娠早期，母体胰岛素通过与滋养层胰岛素受体的相互作用而影响胎盘。这些可能反过来影响母体分泌细胞因子、激素或代谢产物。在妊娠后期，胎儿通过与胎盘内皮细胞相互作用，控制胰岛素依赖胎盘的过程。妊娠早期母体胰岛素对胎盘发育和代谢的影响及妊娠后期胎儿胰岛素对胎盘的影响可能对胎儿发育和代谢产生影响

（版权所有归美国糖尿病协会[6]。转载经美国糖尿病协会许可）

通过上调基质金属蛋白酶 MMP2 和 MMP9 刺激滋养层细胞侵入[56]，从而降解明胶和胶原，影响细胞外基质的组分。1 型糖尿病患者母体 IGF1 水平较低，这可能会导致滋养细胞侵入异常。胰岛素和 IGF 刺激营养物质通过合体滋养层转运，特别是通过上调氨基酸转运系统 A[57-59]来转运大量中性氨基酸。因此，在妊娠糖尿病患者中，母体生长因子浓度的增加可能促进胎盘氨基酸转运，从而促进胎儿生长（表 3.1）。

在胎儿循环中也可以看到变化（表 3.2）。然而，除了众所周知的胰岛素刺激脂肪增生外，这些变化对胎儿的影响目前还不清楚。

瘦素

瘦素是通过代谢控制间接促进胰岛素抵抗的中枢激素[60]。在人类中，瘦素水平与肥胖密切相关。然而，激素除了代谢控制外，还具有多种功能，如刺激血管生成、调节造血和炎症反应[61]。瘦素的主要来源是脂肪组织，但也可在胎儿胎盘单位的各种器官中合成。妊娠期间，孕妇体内的瘦素浓度上升 30%，胎盘成为瘦素的另一来源。

胎盘中瘦素受体的主要合成部位是合体滋养细胞。瘦素诱导人绒毛膜促性腺激素（HCG）产生，促进有丝分裂发生，刺激氨基酸摄取，并增加细胞外基质蛋白和金属蛋白酶[61]的合成，后者意味着激素在胎盘生长调节中的作用。此外，高瘦素血症能够改变胶原合成，因此可以进一步假设高瘦素血症对糖尿病胎盘其他改变（如基底膜增厚）的贡献[62]。此外，瘦素的促血管生成作用提示糖尿病相关胎盘血管过多（图 3.2）。

胎儿性别对妊娠糖尿病患者胎盘功能的影响

人们早已认识到胎儿性别对于妊娠结局的影响是不同的[63]，甚至 GDM 作为母体疾病的发病率也受到胎儿性别的影响：怀有男性胎儿的母亲患 GDM 的风险更高[63, 64]。胎盘是母体代谢适应妊娠的主要驱动力之一，因此可能与妊娠疾病的性别依赖有关。事实上，男性和女性胎儿胎盘在分子上和功能上是不同的。它表达了不同水平的转录本[65, 66]，这些差异不仅存在于胎盘组织中,而且胎盘中不同的细胞类型[66]基因表达也是不同的。到目前为止,功能性的后果尚不清楚,但可能与男性和女性胎儿的不同的生长能力有关[67]。

除了这些性别依赖性的分子差异外,男性和女性胎盘对环境因素的反应也是不同的:妊娠期饮食干预导致胎盘转录本的性别特异性改变,这在女性胎儿中更为明显。此外,女性胎儿似乎对与 GDM 相关的宫内变化(如高胰岛素血症)也有更强的反应,因为她们在出生时具有胰岛素抵抗[68, 69]。这些数据可能反映女性胎儿比男性更易受到环境挑战的影响[70]。到目前为止,没有性别差异在胎盘适应 GDM 中的描述。然而,考虑到女性胎盘和胎儿的可塑性,可以预料到这样的变化[71, 72]。

胎盘甲基化

胎儿宫内环境对后代健康的长期影响导致了这样一种概念,即在早期生命暴露于"程序化"的胎儿组织,以便他们在生命后期记住这些宫内事件。表观遗传改变,主要是富含胞嘧啶鸟苷二核苷酸(CpG)的 DNA 区域的甲基化,已经被建立作为这种记忆效应的分子表征。由于胎盘是一种容易获得的胎儿组织,它与 GDM 相关的甲基化改变最近成为一些研究的焦点。

在胎盘[73-77]中发现了一些与 GDM 相关的甲基化改变,这些改变不同于其他妊娠病理学,如子痫前期[75]引起的改变。有趣的是,GDM 中分别参与调节胰岛素敏感性和胰岛素抵抗的脂联素与瘦素编码基因的胎盘甲基化,以与妊娠前和妊娠期间的母体代谢状态有关的方式改变[78]。母体印迹 MEST 基因甲基化降低,是 α/β 水解酶超家族的成员,不仅在 GDM 出生时的胎盘中发现,而且在病态肥胖的成年人的血细胞中也被发现[73]。此外,GDM 后代脐血中的循环细胞显示其 DNA 甲基化变化[73, 74, 77]。在这些变化中,维甲酸受体启动子中一个独特的 CpG 位点的甲基化与两个独立队列中的儿童 9 岁时的脂肪量有关[79, 80]。总之,这些结果表明,宫内暴露于 GDM 环境的后代的长期后果部分通过甲基化改变(即后代表观基因组的改变)介导。

DNA 甲基化是高度细胞特异性的。这里所描述的研究已经在全胎盘组织中进行。因此，不能排除甲基化变化仅仅是细胞组成变化与 GDM 相关的反映。因此，这类研究可能导致后代晚年疾病风险的生物标志物识别，而不是提供对子宫内 GDM 环境如何影响疾病风险的机制见解。

总结

胎盘结构和功能可因母体糖尿病而改变。这些变化的具体性质和程度取决于妊娠糖尿病的损害，以及糖尿病的类型。尽管近几十年母体血糖控制有所改善，但仍继续发生一些变化[81,82]，这表明高血糖不是唯一的病因。然而，如果糖尿病得到很好的控制[11,83]，绒毛形态的各种变化也可能会随之改善。母亲和胎儿中几种生长因子、细胞因子和激素的浓度在糖尿病中也发生变化，并可能影响胎儿与胎盘的生长与发育。最近发现胎儿性别可以调节母体的代谢状况，因此 GDM 也可能影响胎盘功能。GDM 的宫内环境改变不仅影响胎盘和胎儿的发育，而且通过改变 DNA 甲基化谱引起持续变化。目前在这方面的研究是试图确定具体的生物效应和详细的机制。

问题

1. 胰岛素如何改变早期胎盘发育？

答：至少通过改变基质金属蛋白酶的表达，如 MMP14，它可以调节胎盘生长和发育，如在侵袭和血管生成中发挥多种作用。

2. 糖尿病患者胎盘葡萄糖流量增加的主要驱动力是什么？

答：妊娠后期母胎浓度梯度是调节葡萄糖流量的主要驱动因素。子宫胎盘和胎儿胎盘血流量也有助于调节葡萄糖流量。糖尿病早期血糖调节因子尚不清楚。

3. 胎盘分泌瘦素吗？如果分泌，进入哪个循环？

答：是的，瘦素被分泌到母体和胎儿的血液循环中。

4. 胎盘功能取决于胎儿性别吗？

答：是的，虽然还没有很多证据，但总的来说，男性和女性胎盘的基因表达在细胞类型上有所不同。这很可能也会导致胎盘功能的性别差异。

5. GDM 是否改变了胎盘基因的甲基化谱？

答：是的，有很好的证据表明 GDM 基因改变了胎盘基因的甲基化谱。然而，由于缺乏数据，且甲基化是非常细胞特异性的，目前尚不清楚这是否是 GDM 患者胎盘细胞成分真正的改变，或仅是对照组胎盘细胞成分改变的反映。

（刘雅静 译，王 冰 校）

参 考 文 献

1. Aplin JD. Implantation, trophoblast differentiation and haemochorial placentation: mechanistic evidence in vivo and in vitro. J Cell Sci 1991;99(Pt 4):681–692.
2. Hayati AR, Cheah FC, Tan AE, & Tan GC. Insulin-like growth factor-1 receptor expression in the placentae of diabetic and normal pregnancies. Early Hum Dev 2007;83(1):414–416.
3. Hiden U, Glitzner E, Ivanisevic M, Djelmis J, Wadsack C, Lang U, et al. MT1-MMP expression in first-trimester placental tissue is upregulated in type 1 diabetes as a result of elevated insulin and tumor necrosis factor-alpha levels. Diabetes 2008;57(1):150–157.
4. Jansson T, Ekstrand Y, Bjorn C, Wennergren M, & Powell TL. Alterations in the activity of placental amino acid transporters in pregnancies complicated by diabetes. Diabetes 2002;51(7):2214–2219.
5. Kliman HJ. Uteroplacental blood flow. The story of decidualization, menstruation, and trophoblast invasion. Am J Pathol 2000;157(6):1759–1768.
6. Desoye G & Hauguel-de Mouzon S. The human placenta in gestational diabetes mellitus. The insulin and cytokine network. Diabetes Care 2007;30(Suppl 2):S120–S126.
7. Foufelle F, Girard J, & Ferre P. Regulation of lipogenic enzyme expression by glucose in liver and adipose tissue: a review of the potential cellular and molecular mechanisms. Adv Enzyme Regul 1996;36:199–226.
8. Mandl M, Haas J, Bischof P, Nohammer G, & Desoye G. Serum-dependent effects of IGF-I and insulin on proliferation and invasion of human first trimester trophoblast cell models. Histochem Cell Biol 2002;117(5):391–399.
9. Hiden U, Maier A, Bilban M, Ghaffari-Tabrizi N, Wadsack C, Lang I, et al. Insulin control of placental gene expression shifts from mother to foetus over the course of pregnancy. Diabetologia 2006;49(1):123–131.
10. Younes B, Baez-Giangreco A, al-Nuaim L, al-Hakeem A, & Abu Talib Z. Basement membrane thickening in the placentae from diabetic women. Pathol Intl 1996;46(2):100–104.
11. Calderon IM, Damasceno DC, Amorin RL, Costa RA, Brasil MA, & Rudge MV. Morphometric study of placental villi and vessels in women with mild hyperglycemia or gestational or overt diabetes. Diabetes Res Clin Pract 2007;78(1):65–71.
12. Taricco E, Radaelli T, Nobile de Santis MS, & Cetin I. Foetal and placental weights in relation to maternal characteristics in gestational diabetes. Placenta 2003;24(4):343–347.
13. Lao TT, Lee CP, & Wong WM. Placental weight to birthweight ratio is increased in mild gestational glucose intolerance. Placenta 1997;18(2–3):227–230.
14. Hahn T & Desoye G. Ontogeny of glucose transport systems in the placenta and its progenitor tissues. Early Pregnancy 1996;2(3):168–182.
15. Ericsson A, Hamark B, Powell TL, & Jansson T. Glucose transporter isoform 4 is

expressed in the syncytiotrophoblast of first trimester human placenta. Hum Reprod 2005;20(2):521–530.
16. Xing AY, Challier JC, Lepercq J, Cauzac M, Charron MJ, Girard J, et al. Unexpected expression of glucose transporter 4 in villous stromal cells of human placenta. J Clin Endocrinol Metab 1998;83(11):4097–4101.
17. Ericsson A, Hamark B, Jansson N, Johansson BR, Powell TL, & Jansson T. Hormonal regulation of glucose and system A amino acid transport in first trimester placental villous fragments. Am J Physiol Regul Integr Comp Physiol 2005;288(3):R656–R662.
18. Hahn T, Barth S, Graf R, Engelmann M, Beslagic D, Reul JM, et al. Placental glucose transporter expression is regulated by glucocorticoids. J Clin Endocrinol Metab 1999;84(4):1445–1452.
19. Hahn T, Barth S, Weiss U, Mosgoeller W, & Desoye G. Sustained hyperglycemia in vitro down-regulates the GLUT1 glucose transport system of cultured human term placental trophoblast: a mechanism to protect fetal development? FASEB J 1998;12(12):1221–1231.
20. Colomiere M, Permezel M, Riley C, Desoye G, & Lappas M. Defective insulin signaling in placenta from pregnancies complicated by gestational diabetes mellitus. Eur J Endocrinol 2009;160(4):567–578.
21. Gaither K, Quraishi AN, & Illsley NP. Diabetes alters the expression and activity of the human placental GLUT1 glucose transporter. J Clin Endocrinol Metab 1999;84(2):695–701.
22. Osmond DT, King RG, Brennecke SP, & Gude NM. Placental glucose transport and utilisation is altered at term in insulin-treated, gestational-diabetic patients. Diabetologia 2001;44(9):1133–1139.
23. Radaelli T, Taricco E, Rossi G, Antonazzo P, Ciappina N, Pileri P, et al. Oxygenation, acid-base balance and glucose levels in fetuses from gestational diabetic pregnancies. JSGI 2005;2(Suppl):221A.
24. Kuruvilla AG, D'Souza SW, Glazier JD, Mahendran D, Maresh MJ, & Sibley CP. Altered activity of the system A amino acid transporter in microvillous membrane

vesicles from placentas of macrosomic babies born to diabetic women. J Clin Invest 1994;94(2):689–695.
25. Mayhew TM, Sorensen FB, Klebe JG, & Jackson MR. Growth and maturation of villi in placentae from well–controlled diabetic women. Placenta 1994;15(1):57–65.
26. Mimouni F, Miodovnik M, Siddiqi TA, Butler JB, Holroyde J, & Tsang RC. Neonatal polycythemia in infants of insulin-dependent diabetic mothers. Obstet Gynecol 1986;68(3):370–372.
27. Madsen H & Ditzel J. Red cell 2,3-diphosphoglycerate and hemoglobin-oxygen affinity during diabetic pregnancy. Acta Obstet Gynecol Scand 1984;63(5):403–406.
28. al-Okail MS & al-Attas OS. Histological changes in placental syncytiotrophoblasts of poorly controlled gestational diabetic patients. Endocr J 1994;41(4):355–360.
29. Jirkovska M. Comparison of the thickness of the capillary basement membrane of the human placenta under normal conditions and in type 1 diabetes. Funct Dev Morphol 1991;1(3):9–16.
30. Nylund L, Lunell NO, Lewander R, Persson B, & Sarby B. Uteroplacental blood flow in diabetic pregnancy: measurements with indium 113 m and a computer-linked gamma camera. Am J Obstet Gynecol 1982;144(3):298–302.
31. Bracero LA, Jovanovic L, Rochelson B, Bauman W, & Farmakides G. Significance of umbilical and uterine artery velocimetry in the well-controlled pregnant diabetic. J Reprod Med 1989;34(4):273–276.
32. Bracero LA & Schulman H. Doppler studies of the uteroplacental circulation in pregnancies complicated by diabetes. Ultrasound Obstet Gynecol 1991;1(6):391–394.
33. Black SM, Devol JM, & Wedgwood S. Regulation of fibroblast growth factor-2 expression in pulmonary arterial smooth muscle cells involves increased reactive oxygen species generation. Am J Physiol Cell Physiol 2008;294(1):C345–C354.
34. Grosfeld A, Andre J, Hauguel-De Mouzon

S, Berra E, Pouyssegur J, & Guerre-Millo M. Hypoxia-inducible factor 1 transactivates the human leptin gene promoter. J Biol Chem 2002;277(45):42953–42957.

35 Josko J & Mazurek M. Transcription factors having impact on vascular endothelial growth factor (VEGF) gene expression in angiogenesis. Med Sci Monit 2004;10(4):RA89–R!98.

36 Abdel Aziz MT, Fouad HH, Mohsen GA, Mansour M, & Abdel Ghaffar S. TNF-alpha and homocysteine levels in type 1 diabetes mellitus. East Mediterr Health J 2001;7(4–5):679–688.

37 Bhaumick B, Danilkewich AD, & Bala RM. Insulin-like growth factors (IGF) I and II in diabetic pregnancy: suppression of normal pregnancy-induced rise of IGF-I. Diabetologia 1986;29(11):792–797.

38 Lygnos MC, Pappa KI, Papadaki HA, Relakis C, Koumantakis E, Anagnou NP, et al. Changes in maternal plasma levels of VEGF, bFGF, TGF-beta1, ET-1 and sKL during uncomplicated pregnancy, hypertensive pregnancy and gestational diabetes. In Vivo 2006;20(1):157–163.

39 Brown ZA, Mills JL, Metzger BE, Knopp RH, Simpson JL, Jovanovic-Peterson L, et al. Early sonographic evaluation for fetal growth delay and congenital malformations in pregnancies complicated by insulin-requiring diabetes. National Institute of Child Health and Human Development Diabetes in Early Pregnancy Study. Diabetes Care 1992;15(5):613–619.

40 Weiss U, Cervar M, Puerstner P, Schmut O, Haas J, Mauschitz R, et al. Hyperglycaemia in vitro alters the proliferation and mitochondrial activity of the choriocarcinoma cell lines BeWo, JAR and JEG-3 as models for human first-trimester trophoblast. Diabetologia 2001;44(2):209–219.

41 Galindo A, Burguillo AG, Azriel S, & Fuente Pde L. Outcome of fetuses in women with pregestational diabetes mellitus. J Perinat Med 2006;34(4):323–331.

42 Desoye G & Shafrir E. The human placenta in diabetic pregnancy. Diabetes Rev 1996;4:70–89.

43 Salvesen DR, Higueras MT, Mansur CA, Freeman J, Brudenell JM, & Nicolaides KH. Placental and fetal Doppler velocimetry in pregnancies complicated by maternal diabetes mellitus. Am J Obstet Gynecol 1993;168(2):645–652.

44 Johnstone FD, Steel JM, Haddad NG, Hoskins PR, Greer IA, & Chambers S. Doppler umbilical artery flow velocity waveforms in diabetic pregnancy. Br J Obstet Gynaecol 1992;99(2):135–140.

45 Desoye G, Hofmann HH, & Weiss PA. Insulin binding to trophoblast plasma membranes and placental glycogen content in well-controlled gestational diabetic women treated with diet or insulin, in well-controlled overt diabetic patients and in healthy control subjects. Diabetologia 1992;35(1):45–55.

46 d'Ortho MP, Will H, Atkinson S, Butler G, Messent A, Gavrilovic J, et al. Membrane-type matrix metalloproteinases 1 and 2 exhibit broad-spectrum proteolytic capacities comparable to many matrix metalloproteinases. Eur J Biochem 1997;250(3):751–757.

47 Taleb S, Van Haaften R, Henegar C, Hukshorn C, Cancello R, Pelloux V, et al. Microarray profiling of human white adipose tissue after exogenous leptin injection. Eur J Clin Invest 2006;36(3):153–163.

48 Myers MG Jr. Leptin receptor signaling and the regulation of mammalian physiology. Recent Prog Horm Res 2004;59:287–304.

49 Gicquel C & Le Bouc Y. Hormonal regulation of fetal growth. Horm Res 2006;65(Suppl 3):28–33.

50 Pirola L, Johnston AM, & Van Obberghen E. Modulation of insulin action. Diabetologia 2004;47(2):170–184.

51 Desoye G, Hartmann M, Jones CJ, Wolf HJ, Kohnen G, Kosanke G, et al. Location of insulin receptors in the placenta and its progenitor tissues. Microsc Res Tech 1997;38(1–2):63–75.

52 Yan-Jun L, Tsushima T, Minei S, Sanaka M, Nagashima T, Yanagisawa K, et al. Insulin-like growth factors (IGFs) and IGF-binding proteins (IGFBP-1, -2 and -3) in diabetic pregnancy: relationship to macrosomia. Endocr J 1996;43(2):221–231.

53 Coya R, Gualillo O, Pineda J, Garcia MC, Busturia MA, Aniel-Quiroga A, et al. Effect of cyclic 3′,5′-adenosine monophosphate, glucocorticoids, and insulin on leptin messenger RNA levels and leptin secretion in cultured human trophoblast. Biol Reprod 2001;65(3):814–819.

54 Zeck W, Widberg C, Maylin E, Desoye G, Lang U, McIntyre D, et al. Regulation of placental growth hormone secretion in a human trophoblast model – the effects of hormones and adipokines. Pediatr Res 2008;63(4):353–357.

55 Barbour LA, Shao J, Qiao L, Pulawa LK, Jensen DR, Bartke A, et al. Human placental growth hormone causes severe insulin resistance in transgenic mice. Am J Obstet Gynecol 2002;186(3):512–517.

56 Chakraborty C, Gleeson LM, McKinnon T & Lala PK. Regulation of human trophoblast migration and invasiveness. Can J Physiol Pharmacol 2002;80(2):116–124.

57 Constancia M, Hemberger M, Hughes J, Dean W, Ferguson-Smith A, Fundele R, et al. Placental-specific IGF-II is a major modulator of placental and fetal growth. Nature 2002;417(6892):945–948.

58 Karl PI. Insulin-like growth factor-1 stimulates amino acid uptake by the cultured human placental trophoblast. J Cell Physiol 1995;165(1):83–88.

59 Karl PI, Alpy KL, & Fisher SE. Amino acid transport by the cultured human placental trophoblast: effect of insulin on AIB transport. Am J Physiol 1992;262(4 Pt 1):C834–C839.

60 Webber J. Energy balance in obesity. Proc Nutr Soc 2003;62(2):539–543.

61 Hauguel-de Mouzon S, Lepercq J, & Catalano P. The known and unknown of leptin in pregnancy. Am J Obstet Gynecol 2006;194(6):1537–1545.

62 Madani S, De Girolamo S, Munoz DM, Li RK, & Sweeney G. Direct effects of leptin on size and extracellular matrix components of human pediatric ventricular myocytes. Cardiovasc Res 2006;69(3):716–725.

63 Sheiner E, Levy A, Katz M, Hershkovitz R, Leron E, & Mazor M. Gender does matter in perinatal medicine. Fetal Diag Ther 2004;19(4):366–369.

64 Retnakaran R, Kramer CK, Ye C, Kew S, Hanley AJ, Connelly PW, et al. Fetal sex and maternal risk of gestational diabetes mellitus: the impact of having a boy. Diabetes Care 2015.

65 Buckberry S, Bianco-Miotto T, Bent SJ, Dekker GA, & Roberts CT. Integrative transcriptome meta-analysis reveals widespread sex-biased gene expression at the human fetal-maternal interface. Mol Hum Reprod 2014;20(8):810–819.

66 Cvitic S, Longtine MS, Hackl H, Wagner K, Nelson MD, Desoye G, et al. The human placental sexome differs between trophoblast epithelium and villous vessel endothelium. PLoS One 2013;8(10):e79233.

67 Lampl M & Jeanty P. Timing is everything: a reconsideration of fetal growth velocity patterns identifies the importance of individual and sex differences. Am J Human Biol 2003;15(5):667–680.

68 Wilkin TJ & Murphy MJ. The gender insulin hypothesis: why girls are born lighter than boys, and the implications for insulin resistance. Int J Obes (Lond) 2006;30(7):1056–1061.

69 Basu S, Laffineuse L, Presley L, Minium J, Catalano PM, & Hauguel-de Mouzon S. In utero gender dimorphism of adiponectin reflects insulin sensitivity and adiposity of the fetus. Obesity 2009;17(6):1144–1149.

70 Sedlmeier EM, Brunner S, Much D, Pagel P, Ulbrich SE, Meyer HH, et al. Human placental transcriptome shows sexually dimorphic gene expression and responsiveness to maternal dietary n-3 long-chain polyunsaturated fatty acid intervention during pregnancy. BMC

Genomics 2014;15:941.
71. Gabory A, Attig L, & Junien C. Sexual dimorphism in environmental epigenetic programming. Mol Cell Endocrinol 2009;304(1–2):8–18.
72. Tarrade A, Panchenko P, Junien C, & Gabory A. Placental contribution to nutritional programming of health and diseases: epigenetics and sexual dimorphism. J Exper Biol 2015;218(Pt 1):50–58.
73. El Hajj N, Pliushch G, Schneider E, Dittrich M, Muller T, Korenkov M, et al. Metabolic programming of MEST DNA methylation by intrauterine exposure to gestational diabetes mellitus. Diabetes 2013;62(4):1320–1328.
74. Nomura Y, Lambertini L, Rialdi A, Lee M, Mystal EY, Grabie M, et al. Global methylation in the placenta and umbilical cord blood from pregnancies with maternal gestational diabetes, preeclampsia, and obesity. Reprod Sci 2014;21(1):131–137.
75. Liu L, Zhang X, Rong C, Rui C, Ji H, Qian YJ, et al. Distinct DNA methylomes of human placentas between pre-eclampsia and gestational diabetes mellitus. Cell Physiol Biochem 2014;34(6):1877–1889.
76. Petropoulos S, Guillemin C, Ergaz Z, Dimov S, Suderman M, Weinstein-Fudim L, et al. Gestational diabetes alters offspring DNA methylation profiles in human and rat: identification of key pathways involved in endocrine system disorders, insulin signaling, diabetes signaling and IL-K signaling. Endocrinology 2014:en20141643.
77. Finer S, Mathews C, Lowe R, Smart M, Hillman S, Foo L, et al. Maternal gestational diabetes is associated with genome-wide DNA methylation variation in placenta and cord blood of exposed offspring. Hum Mol Genet 2015;24(11):3021–3029.
78. Lesseur C, Armstrong DA, Paquette AG, Li Z, Padbury JF, & Marsit CJ. Maternal obesity and gestational diabetes are associated with placental leptin DNA methylation. Am J Obstet Gynecol 2014;211(6):654 e1–e9.
79. Godfrey KM, Hales CN, Osmond C, Barker DJ, & Taylor KP. Relation of cord plasma concentrations of proinsulin, 32-33 split proinsulin, insulin and C-peptide to placental weight and the baby's size and proportions at birth. Early Hum Dev 1996;46(1–2):129–140.
80. Godfrey KM, Sheppard A, Gluckman PD, Lillycrop KA, Burdge GC, McLean C, et al. Epigenetic gene promoter methylation at birth is associated with child's later adiposity. Diabetes 2011;60(5):1528–1534.
81. Evers IM, de Valk HW, Mol BW, ter Braak EW, & Visser GH. Macrosomia despite good glycaemic control in Type I diabetic pregnancy; results of a nationwide study in The Netherlands. Diabetologia 2002;45(11):1484–1489.
82. Pietryga M, Brazert J, Wender-Ozegowska E, Dubiel M, & Gudmundsson S. Placental Doppler velocimetry in gestational diabetes mellitus. J Perinat Med 2006;34(2):108–110.
83. Mayhew TM & Jairam IC. Stereological comparison of 3D spatial relationships involving villi and intervillous pores in human placentas from control and diabetic pregnancies. J Anat 2000;197(Pt 2):263–274.

其他可参阅文献

84. Ategbo JM, Grissa O, Yessoufou A, Hichami A, Dramane KL, Moutairou K, et al. Modulation of adipokines and cytokines in gestational diabetes and macrosomia. J Clin Endocrinol Metab 2006;91(10):4137–4143.
85. Vitoratos N, Salamalekis E, Kassanos D, Loghis C, Panayotopoulos N, Kouskouni E, et al. Maternal plasma leptin levels and their relationship to insulin and glucose in gestational-onset diabetes. Gynecol Obstet Invest 2001;51(1):17–21.
86. Hughes SC, Johnson MR, Heinrich G, & Holly JM. Could abnormalities in insulin-like growth factors and their binding proteins during pregnancy result in gestational diabetes? J Endocrinol 1995;147(3):517–524.
87. Gelato MC, Rutherford C, San-Roman G, Shmoys S, & Monheit A. The serum

insulin-like growth factor-II/mannose-6-phosphate receptor in normal and diabetic pregnancy. Metabolism 1993;42(8):1031–1038.
88 Homko C, Sivan E, Chen X, Reece EA, & Boden G. Insulin secretion during and after pregnancy in patients with gestational diabetes mellitus. J Clin Endocrinol Metab 2001;86(2):568–573.
89 Higgins MF, Russell NM, Brazil DP, Firth RG, & McAuliffe FM. Fetal and maternal leptin in pre-gestational diabetic pregnancy. Int J Gynaecol Obstet 2013;120(2):169–172.
90 Cvitic S, Desoye G, & Hiden U. Glucose, insulin, and oxygen interplay in placental hypervascularisation in diabetes mellitus. BioMed Res Intl 2014;2014:145846.
91 Loukovaara M, Leinonen P, Teramo K, & Andersson S. Concentration of cord serum placenta growth factor in normal and diabetic pregnancies. BJOG 2005;112(1):75–79.
92 Lea RG, Howe D, Hannah LT, Bonneau O, Hunter L, & Hoggard N. Placental leptin in normal, diabetic and fetal growth-retarded pregnancies. Mol Hum Reprod 2000;6(8):763–769.
93 Uebel K, Pusch K, Gedrich K, Schneider KT, Hauner H, & Bader BL. Effect of maternal obesity with and without gestational diabetes on offspring subcutaneous and preperitoneal adipose tissue development from birth up to year-1. BMC Preg Childbirth 2014;14:138.
94 Ortega-Senovilla H, Schaefer-Graf U, Meitzner K, Abou-Dakn M, Graf K, Kintscher U, et al. Gestational diabetes mellitus causes changes in the concentrations of adipocyte fatty acid-binding protein and other adipocytokines in cord blood. Diabetes Care 2011;34(9):2061–2066.
95 Salvesen DR, Brudenell JM, Snijders RJ, Ireland RM, & Nicolaides KH. Fetal plasma erythropoietin in pregnancies complicated by maternal diabetes mellitus. Am J Obstet Gynecol 1993;168(1 Pt 1):88–94.
96 Westgate JA, Lindsay RS, Beattie J, Pattison NS, Gamble G, Mildenhall LF, et al. Hyperinsulinemia in cord blood in mothers with type 2 diabetes and gestational diabetes mellitus in New Zealand. Diabetes Care 2006;29(6):1345–1350.
97 Lassus P, Teramo K, Nupponen I, Markkanen H, Cederqvist K, & Andersson S. Vascular endothelial growth factor and angiogenin levels during fetal development and in maternal diabetes. Biol Neonate 2003;84(4):287–292.
98 Hill DJ, Tevaarwerk GJ, Caddell C, Arany E, Kilkenny D, & Gregory M. Fibroblast growth factor 2 is elevated in term maternal and cord serum and amniotic fluid in pregnancies complicated by diabetes: relationship to fetal and placental size. J Clin Endocrinol Metab 1995;80(9):2626–2632.
99 Teramo K, Kari MA, Eronen M, Markkanen H, & Hiilesmaa V. High amniotic fluid erythropoietin levels are associated with an increased frequency of fetal and neonatal morbidity in type 1 diabetic pregnancies. Diabetologia 2004;47(10):1695–1703.

第二篇 妊娠糖尿病

第四章 妊娠糖尿病的筛查

David A. Sacks

Associate Investigator, Department of Research and Evaluation, Kaiser Permanente Southern California, Pasadena, California, USA Adjunct Clinical Professor, Division of Maternal-Fetal Medicine, Department of Obstetrics and Gynecology, Keck School of Medicine, University of Southern California, Los Angeles, California, USA

实践要点

- 在许多人群中,患有 GDM 的女性病史中没有风险因素。因此,仅基于风险因素的存在与否来确定哪些患者应该或不应该针对 GDM 进行筛查可能无法识别出患有该疾病的大量女性。
- 50g 葡萄糖筛查试验(GST)的结果随着上一餐的时间和抽血时间而变化,并且重复性差。
- GST≥11.1mmol/L 无法诊断为妊娠糖尿病,应进行空腹血糖测试。
- 当用作 GDM 筛查试验时,空腹血糖测试的敏感性和特异性较差。
- 由于不同研究中糖化血红蛋白用于诊断的敏感性和特异性差异较大,因此不建议使用血红蛋白 HbA1c 代替传统的妊娠中期或妊娠晚期 GDM 筛查试验。

病 例

一名 26 岁的女性,孕 5 产 2,在妊娠早期曾发生过两次自然流产,在第 2 次妊娠期间被发现患有 GDM,并且在妊娠的第 8 个月开始口服降糖药。她最小的孩子是 5 岁。自上次分娩以来,体重已增加了 6kg,并且自那次分娩后再没有进行任何血糖测试。目前是在第 5 次妊娠时的第 13 周时被发现患有高血压,BMI 为 37kg/m^2。是否应该在 24~28 周之前接受 GDM 测试呢?如果现在进行测试,最好是使用 50g GST、空腹血糖测试、75g 或 100g 葡萄糖耐量试验(GTT)或是糖化血红蛋白检测,还是这些试验的组合?或者,根据经验应该给予糖尿病治疗吗?如果 50g GST 结果还不到需要做 GTT 试验的阈值,是否应该对其血糖状态进行一些验证性抽血检查?

概述

GDM 这一术语最早是在 1957 年对 621 名孕妇进行的一项研究中提出来的,这些孕妇接受了 100g 3h 葡萄糖耐量试验(GTT)[1]。虽然 GDM 这个标签是指葡萄糖不耐受水平最高的女性,但这个术语后来被广泛用于妊娠期间发病或首次识别的葡萄糖耐受不良[2]。在美国,O'Sullivan 等著作推广了筛查 GDM 的概念[3, 4]。在本章中,将讨论筛选 GDM 的定义、方法、风险、益处和成本。希望通过这次讨论,读者可以决定是否应将筛查纳入 GDM 的诊断中,如果是,哪种方法更适合临床实践。

定义

诊断和筛查这两个术语经常在医学术语中互换使用。在 GDM 方面,应使用筛查试验来鉴定疾病风险较高的患者(即在未经选择的人群中,通过诊断试验检测更有可能患 GDM 的人)。进行最终确诊试验之前使用一些筛查程序的主要好处是,会有更少的患者需要进行确诊试验(对于大多数女性,确诊试验是令人不愉快的)和更昂贵的测试。因此,筛查试验的两个重要特征是其阈值设定得足够低,以包括绝大多数患有该疾病的女性(灵敏度),同时阈值又必须足够高,以排除大多数没有患病的女性接受诊断检测(特异度)。确定筛查试验的灵敏度和特异度之间的适当平衡的困境,如图 4.1 所示。

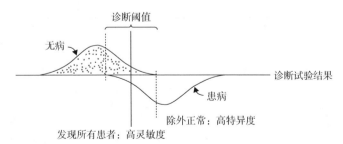

图 4.1 灵敏度、特异度和筛查试验阈值的关系(引自 Carpenter & Coustan 1982。经爱思唯尔许可转载)

我们应该筛查妊娠糖尿病吗?

近几年 GDM 是否值得进行任何类型的筛查试验仍一直存在争议[5]。需要筛查的疾病应具有某些特征:
- 这种疾病应该很普遍。
- 该疾病应与选定的不良后果因果关联。
- 疾病应该有一个无症状的阶段,在这个阶段可以进行检测。
- 应该有治疗方法来改善疾病的影响。

GDM 全球患病率为 1.7%~25%[6, 7],数据显示 GTT 中母体血糖水平与不良妊娠结局之间存在正相关关系[8],GDM 常缺乏特异的症状及来自两个随机对照试验的证据提示治疗将改善一些相关疾病[9, 10],目前可获得的信息表明,GDM 非常适合筛查。

筛查方法

在讨论可用于筛查 GDM 的不同测试和策略之前,重要的是要解决用于评估筛查测试用的参数。如本章所述,理想的筛查试验应当有很高的敏感性,并且具有令人满意的特异性。必须指出的是,为了计算这两项指标,需使用诊断试验和筛查试验对所有研究人群进行测试。大多数研究认为,通常只对有风险因素的孕妇进行筛查试验,然后只对那些在筛查试验中达到选定阈值的人进行诊断试验。虽然这可以计算阳性测试的预测值[阳性预测值(PPV)],但它无法计算测试灵敏度。为了计算后者的统计数据,还必须知道筛查试验结果低于筛查测试阈值但确实患有疾病(假阴性)的女性人数。为了计算筛查试验特异度,还必须知道在筛查试验中检测为阴性且没有患病的女性人数(真阴性)及在筛查试验中检测为阳性但确诊试验为阴性的女性人数(误诊)。同样,对于两种测定,必须同时进行筛查试验和诊断试验,如图 4.1[11] 所示。

筛查风险因素

具有一种或多种历史风险因素的女性通常比没有风险因素的女性患 GDM 的风险更大。这些因素包括超过选定阈值（如 30 岁）的母亲年龄、属于某些种族群体（如来自拉丁美洲、非洲、太平洋岛屿、东南亚和亚洲）、多次生育、超重和肥胖、既往 GDM 的个人史、既往巨大儿史及有糖尿病史的一级亲属[12]。某些风险因素（如既往 GDM）对于 GDM 具有比其他因素更大的 PPV。个体的风险因素越多，GDM 的 PPV 越大[13]。有些因素可能仅在既往妊娠的女性中发现（如既往的 GDM 史、既往巨大儿史），这使得女性患 GDM 风险偏倚增加[13, 14]。最后，无论风险如何定义或存在多少风险因素，每个人群中都会有那些没有风险因素的女性，但如果经过普遍测试，将会发现患有 GDM 的女性[13, 15]。

50g 葡萄糖耐量试验

概述

50g 葡萄糖耐量试验也称为葡萄糖激发试验（GCT）或葡萄糖筛查试验（GST），给妊娠妇女口服 50g 葡萄糖并在 1h 后抽取血糖以确定她们是否具有足够高的风险以便进行确诊试验。GTT 已被用于多个场所，目前被认可为美国权威机构选择的方法[16]或两种有效的 GDM 测试方法之一[17]。因为在 IADPSG 推出针对 GDM[18]的通用一步法测试之前，它已被广泛使用，用二步法还是一步法筛查 GDM 一直存在争议，现在将详细讨论有关其应用的具体信息。

敏感度与特异度

在 O'Sullivan 的原始研究中，对 752 名未经选择的妊娠妇女在建档的当天下午进行了 50g 口服葡萄糖 1h 血糖检测[3]。这些女性中有 3% 的为妊娠早期，45% 的为妊娠中期，52% 的为妊娠晚期。

选择全血葡萄糖 7.2mmol/L 作为 GST 阈值。必须注意的是，

O'Sullivan 的测定方法（Somogyi-Nelson）测定了除葡萄糖外的所有还原物质（如谷胱甘肽、葡糖醛酸）。另外，血浆葡萄糖浓度低于全血。在对血清或血浆中血糖含量使用现代实验室酶活性测定方法，O'Sullivan 的 7.2mmol/L 血糖值粗略相当于 7.8mmol/L。由此发现，GDM 的敏感度和特异度分别为 79% 和 87%。在 GST 阳性的女性中，有 14% 被诊断为 GDM，GDM 诊断试验为 100g 3h GTT。在临床上，如果只有那些 GST≥7.2mmol/L 的女性给予 GTT，79% 的 GDM 女性将被诊断，21% 将被遗漏，但 87% 的没有 GDM 的女性会避免 GTT[4]。

必须指出的是，在 O'Sullivan 研究中仅发现 19 名患有 GDM 的妇女。自该研究发表以来，许多其他研究已经解决了与该筛查测试的灵敏度和特异度有关的问题。一项针对 26 项研究 50g、1h GST 的综述报道称，毫不奇怪，该测试的阈值越低，灵敏度越高，特异度越低。根据危险因素的存在（测试阈值为 7.8mmol/L）选择进行葡萄糖耐量测试的女性对 GDM 的敏感度与在相同测试中普遍筛查的女性无明显差异。但是，在此阈值下，具有危险因素的女性的特异性低于普遍筛查的女性（分别为 77% 和 85%）；也就是说，增加危险因素作为 GDM 明确测试的标准并不能增加对患有 GDM 女性的检查率，但确实可以增加没有接受 GTT 测试的 GDM 女性的比例[19]。

妊娠期筛查时间的选择

妊娠早期到晚期，胰岛素的敏感度逐渐降低，但在给定孕龄时，没有 GDM 的女性对胰岛素的敏感性高于那些患有 GDM 的女性。随着妊娠的进展，患有 GDM 女性的胰岛 B 细胞功能（响应葡萄糖负荷的胰岛素分泌）逐渐成比例地减弱[20]。因此，似乎有理由认为，虽然一些患有 GDM 的女性在妊娠早期会有较高的 GST 结果，但是 GST 升高的女性及患有 GDM 的女性更有可能在妊娠后期被发现。在一项研究中证实了这一假设，其中所有在妊娠早期超过 150mg/dl 阈值的女性在妊娠中期接受了 GTT 检测。未发现患有 GDM 的患者在妊娠后期行 GTT。在妊娠后期进行的测试中发现更多的女性患有 GDM[21]。

在另一项研究中，女性在妊娠 6~14 周时接受了 GST 和 GTT。除了那些在第一组测试中发现有 GDM 的人，同样的女性在 20~30 周再次进行测试。在妊娠晚期进行的检查中，GST 和 GTT 的绝对葡萄糖浓度显著增加。在 85 名被发现患有 GDM 的女性中，68%是在妊娠后期进行的测试中被发现的[22]。虽然尚未确定早期筛查的胎儿益处，但妊娠早期筛查可能对 2 型糖尿病患病率高的人群有价值。筛查 GDM 可以更好地识别那些最近没有接受过检测且有葡萄糖耐受不良可能的妊娠女性。

在 O'Sullivan 的开创性工作中，752 名女性在建档的当天下午进行了 50g 口服葡萄糖 1h 血糖检测。结果没有提及自上次进餐以来的时间与 GST 结果之间的时间关系，也没有提到关于在一天的其他时间进行测试的数据。另一个人群的横断面数据发现，最后一餐和 50g GST 的间隔时间越长，母体血糖结果越高[23]。另外两项研究比较了在不同的日子对相同患者进行 50g 葡萄糖负荷的管理，分别是禁食一晚和早餐后 1h[24, 25]。虽然没有 GDM 女性的测试结果没有差异，但是那些有 GDM 的女性在禁食一晚后测试的葡萄糖浓度明显更高[24]。连续葡萄糖负荷（Staub-Traugott 效应）后这种明显增加的葡萄糖浓度似乎不是由胰岛素分泌增加所介导的[25]。

一天中何时进行筛查

在患有 GDM 的女性中用自身作为对照，早餐后 1h 的葡萄糖浓度与晚餐后 1h 相比前者更高，在 2h 时没有差异，并且在餐后 3~9h 的葡萄糖浓度显著低于后者。GDM 女性的早晨高血糖与早晨皮质醇增加有关[26]。早晨葡萄糖升高也与慢性高血压有关，可能归因于交感神经过度活跃[27]。在另一项研究中，GTT 从早上进行到下午，12 名有 GDM 的女性虽然在空腹葡萄糖结果中没有发现差异，但是在下午 100g 葡萄糖负荷后相应的 1h、2h 和 3h 结果显著高于早晨[28]葡萄糖负荷之后的结果。总结以上，这些研究确实表明 GST 和 GTT 结果的日变化，但差异的方向似乎不一致。

什么是 GST 的理想阈值

任何疾病的理想筛查测试是提供高水平的敏感度和特异度。反过来，敏感度和特异度取决于筛查试验所选择的阈值。在 O'Sullivan 的研究中，19 名 GDM 女性患者中有 15 名血糖≥7.2mmol/L，79%的敏感度，相应的特异度为 87%。鉴于 GDM 女性人数较少，GST 值的微小变化可能导致敏感度和特异度发生较大变化。随后对 704 名妇女进行了一项研究，其中 90 名患有 GDM，使用受试者特征曲线和 Youden 指数[（敏感度+特异度）-1][29]以确定可达到最佳敏感度和特异度的平衡点[30]。GST 阈值定为 7.8mmol/L，该阈值为 90%的敏感度和 74%的特异度。根据这些数据，似乎可以在接近 7.8mmol/L 的 GST 阈值下实现敏感度和特异度的合理平衡。然而，要注意的是，这一阈值将使一部分符合 GDM 标准的妊娠妇女未被发现。

是否经过葡萄糖筛查测试

大多数但不是所有 GST≥11.1mmol/L 的女性都有 GDM（表 4.1）。

尚不清楚 GST≥11.1mmol/L 且 GTT 正常的女性中有多少比例的妊娠妇女表现出 GDM 的不良后果[31-35]。

表 4.1 GDM 患者行 50g GST 血糖≥11.1mmol/L

作者	GTT	GST 血糖≥ 11.1mmol/L 人数	GST 血糖≥ 11.1mmol/L 同时诊断 GDM 人数（比例）	无 GDM GST 血糖最高值
Sacks[31]	2nd IWC	15	8（53%）	12.5mmol/L
Bobrowski[32]	NDDG	27	18（67%）	12.0mmol/L
Landy[33]	NDDG	51	46（90%）	NS
Shivvers[34]	NDDG	59	48（81%）	14.2mmol/L
Wong[35]	ADIPS	528*	465（88%）	12.0mmol/L

*GST≥11.0mmol/L（198mg/dl），检查在中午前进行。
2nd IWC，第二届妊娠糖尿病国际研讨会；ADIPS，澳大利亚妊娠糖尿病协会；GDM，妊娠糖尿病；GST，葡萄糖筛查试验；GTT，葡萄糖耐量试验；NDDG，美国国家糖尿病数据组；NS，未陈述。

对可能有未被发现糖尿病同时 GST 血糖结果明显升高的女性行 GTT。最安全的策略是在 GST 后加测空腹血糖，如果后者的血糖结果低于 GDM 诊断标准，则行 GTT 的必要性减少。如果 GST 血糖结果≥11.1mmol/L，但 GTT 血糖结果正常，随着妊娠进展仍需要密切监测血糖。

50g 1h 葡萄糖筛查试验的重复性

精确度或在重复测试中达到相同测试结果的能力是筛选测试的重要

特征。同一个体的 GST 结果在一天内超过最终测试的阈值，而在另一天低于该阈值可能导致无法诊断该个体患有 GDM。为了测试 GST 的可重复性，必须控制混淆。因此，第二次测试应该在第一次测试的相邻时间进行，在一天的同一时间，在上一餐后的相同时间间隔之后并且通过相同的分析方法在相同的血液成分上进行。有两项针对未诊断 GDM 妇女进行 50g 1h GST 的研究。第一项研究中所有受试者在早晨进行测试，在测试之前采用不同的禁食和进食顺序。一半受试者在 12~24 周进行测试，一半在 24~28 周进行测试。在早期组中，43%在两天均超过 7.8mmol/L 阈值，而在妊娠后期这一数字上升至 83%[36]。在第二项研究中，参加研究的女性在第 1 天进行 50g 1h 葡萄糖耐量试验，然后被要求在第 2 天相似的时间点重复上述检查。在参加研究的 30 名 GDM 女性中，3 名患者的 GST 结果 2 天低于 7.5mmol/L，另有 10 名仅在 2 天检查中有 1 天结果超过正常（也就是说如果仅进行单次 GST，可能有 27%的 GDM 女性不能被筛查出来）[37]，另外两项研究在妊娠期间隔 1 周重复行 100g GTT，旨在研究其可重复性，结果发现 2 次 GTT 中仅有 1 次提示 GDM 的比例分别为 22%[38]和 24%[39]。总结以上两项研究的结果发现，GDM 患者糖负荷后结果的重现性仅为 45%（27%+73%×24%）。

空腹血糖筛查试验

空腹血浆葡萄糖（FPG）浓度在妊娠第 12 周时达到最低点，然后在整个妊娠期间保持相对稳定[40]。FPG 似乎是筛选 GDM 的有吸引力的替代方案，因为它易于操作，耐受性好，可重复性好[41]，价格低廉[42]。用于确定 FPG 的敏感度、特异度及阳性和阴性预测值的理想方案是在接近的时间内行 FPG 和 GTT。不幸的是，FPG 筛查试验的大多数研究通过仅检测具有风险因素（包括升高的 50g GST）的患者而表现出选择偏倚。全部使用 GTT 的 FPG 作为筛选测试值。虽然这种方法可以提高敏感度，但它需假定 FPG 具有 100%的可重复性，且实际情况可能并非如此。评估 FPG 筛查试验的研究在葡萄糖负荷、数值标准和等于或超过的血糖阈值数量方面也有所不同，所有这些都可能影响对试验结果的解释[43]。在两项研究中，一项使用 Carpenter-Coustan，另一项使用 WHO 标准来定义 GDM,在 FPG 阈值为 4.8mmol/L 时发现类似的敏感度(分别为 81%[44]和 88%[45])和特异度(76%[44]和 72%[45])。相反,两项研究均通过 IADPSG 标准[18]定义了 GDM,报道了 FPG 为 4.7mmol/L 时各自的敏感度为 92.5%[46]和 74%[47]。

两项研究分别以妊娠早期 FPG 作为筛查试验,另一项研究在妊娠早期按 IADPSG 标准[18]进行筛查试验。在 FPG 阈值为 5.1mmol/L 时,敏感度分别为 27%[48]和 26%[49],各自的特异度分别为 95%[48]和 90%[49]。也许是由于妊娠早期结束时 FPG 的生理性下降,如果将第一次血浆 FPG 为 5.1mmol/L 定义为患有 GDM,那么妊娠早期 FPG 诊断 GDM 而妊娠晚期 GTT 未诊断 GDM 的假阳性率在两项研究中均超过 50%。特别是当在妊娠早期进行筛查时,不应仅依赖 FPG 来确定是否需要行 GTT。

糖化血红蛋白作为筛选试验

葡萄糖通过非酶促不可逆反应与血红蛋白 β 链中的 N 端缬氨酸结合。红细胞内所得 HbA1c 的浓度直接随着暴露于葡萄糖的持续时间和红细胞的寿命(120 天)而变化。因此,HbA1c 最能反映前 4 个月的平均葡萄糖浓度[50]。在分析其作为 GDM 筛查试验的用途中,很明显,在妊娠期间,无论何时进行试验,HbA1c 越高,GDM 的诊断率也就越高[51-55]。然而,由于 GDM 女性和没有 GDM 的女性的数值存在重叠,HbA1c 作为 GDM 筛查试验的价值非常有限[53]。在四项研究中,所有受试者均使用 HbA1c 5.45%~5.7%的阈值接受 GDM 诊断检测,敏感度从 26%变为 86%,特异度从 21%变为 92%[52-55]。一项大型($n=8497$)HbA1c 作为妊娠早期筛查试验的研究解决了筛查试验阈值和何时进行 GTT 的问题。所有女性在首次产前检查时均接受 HbA1c 筛查(中位数为 47 天),并被要求进行随访 GTT。

在发现有 GDM 的 692 例中,82%的 HbA1c<5.9%。23%是在 20 周之前测试发现了 GDM。剩下的 77%的 GDM 是在 20 周后的初始或重复 GTT 中发现的。值得注意的是,接受 HbA1c 筛查的 8497 名女性中只有 55%接受了 GTT[56]。

筛查的成本

在医疗资源有限的时代，必须关注提供医疗保健的成本。对于 GDM，评估筛查试验的风险和效益时，应考虑到确诊为 GDM 患者的治疗成本和效益，以及因筛查试验结果血糖低而未确诊为 GDM 患者的成本和风险。成本模型因输入变量不同而有差异。例如，仅限于改善孕产妇和围产期结局的成本分析与包括诊断和治疗妊娠后糖尿病的成本分析大不相同。使用质量调整生命年（QALY），一项研究分析发现 GDM 风险小于 1% 的人群不进行筛查是最经济有效的方法，而对于风险大于 4.2% 的人群，使用 GTT 进行普遍检测是最经济有效的方法[57]。另一项研究统一使用 75g GTT，并将减少伤残调整寿命年（DALY）的成本作为终点，确定了 GDM 的普遍筛查经济有效。已经有研究分析了两步测试（GST 和 GTT 对于那些等于或超过选定阈值的妇女）或一步测试方案中哪种更具成本效益。虽然两项研究得出结论，采用新的 IADPSG 标准进行测试成本高，但具有成本效益[58, 59]，而有一项研究报道称，只有在完成产后相关护理后才能证明成本效益[59]。

结论

虽然 ACHOIS[10]和母婴医学协作网（MFMU）[9]试验的结果已经基本上搁置了关于 GDM 治疗益处的争论，但确定 GDM 的最佳检测策略仍然是一个难以实现的目标。目前的筛查策略在短期内可以节省成本，但如果考虑到给 GDM 女性及其后代带来的相关并发症和死亡风险，个人和社会可能会花费更多。由于伦理限制，解决这个问题不能通过随机对照试验而需要通过大型队列研究。

选择题

关于 50g 葡萄糖筛查试验，以下陈述正确的是（　　）

A. 当使用 IADPSG 标准进行 50g 葡萄糖耐量试验的随访测试时，其灵敏度超过 75%

B. 可以在不考虑一天中的时间或最后一餐的时间的情况下使用，基本上不影响测试结果
C. 同一女性连续两天在相同时间行该试验，结果可能会有很大差异
D. 用于表示随访葡萄糖耐量试验的阈值越低，识别患有妊娠糖尿病的女性的可能性越大

正确答案是 C、D。

（王凯亮　译，朱海清　校）

参 考 文 献

1. Carrington ER, Shuman CR, Reardon HS. Evaluation of the prediabetic state during pregnancy. Obstet Gynecol 1957;9:664–669.
2. Metzger BE, Coustan DR. Summary and recommendations of the Fourth International Workshop-Conference on Gestational Diabetes Mellitus. The Organizing Committee. Diabetes Care 1998;21(Suppl 2):B161–167.
3. O'Sullivan JB, Mahan CM. Criteria for the oral glucose tolerance test in pregnancy. Diabetes 1964;13:278–285.
4. O'Sullivan JB, Mahan CM, Charles D, Dandrow RV. Screening criteria for high-risk gestational diabetic patients. Am J Obstet Gynecol 1973;116:895–900.
5. Jarrett RJ, Castro-Soares J, Dornhorst A, Beard RW. Should we screen for gestational diabetes? BMJ 1997;315:736–739.
6. Schneider S, Bock C, Wetzel M, Maul H, Loerbroks A. The prevalence of gestational diabetes in advanced economies. J Perinat Med 2012;0:1–10.
7. Sacks DA, Hadden DR, Maresh M, *et al*. Frequency of gestational diabetes mellitus at collaborating centers based on IADPSG consensus panel-recommended criteria: the Hyperglycemia and Adverse Pregnancy Outcome (HAPO) Study. Diabetes Care 2012;35:526–528.
8. Metzger BE, Lowe LP, Dyer AR, *et al*. Hyperglycemia and adverse pregnancy outcomes. N Engl J Med 2008;358:1991–2002.
9. Landon MB, Spong CY, Thom E, *et al*. A multicenter, randomized trial of treatment for mild gestational diabetes. N Engl J Med 2009;361:1339–1348.
10. Crowther CA, Hiller JE, Moss JR, McPhee AJ, Jeffries WS, Robinson JS. Effect of treatment of gestational diabetes mellitus on pregnancy outcomes. N Engl J Med 2005;352:2477–2486.
11. Carpenter MW, Coustan DR. Criteria for screening tests for gestational diabetes. Am J Obstet Gynecol 1982;144:768–773.
12. American Diabetes Association. Classification and diagnosis of diabetes. Diabetes Care 2015;38(Suppl):S8–S16.
13. Jimenez-Moleon JJ, Bueno-Cavanillas A, Luna-del-Castillo JD, Lardelli-Claret P, Garcia-Martin M, Galvez-Vargas R. Predictive value of a screen for gestational diabetes mellitus: influence of associated risk factors. Acta Obstet Gynecol Scand 2000;79:991–998.
14. McCarthy AD, Curciarello R, Castiglione N, *et al*. Universal versus selective screening for the detection, control and prognosis of gestational diabetes mellitus in Argentina. Acta Diabetol 2010;47:97–103.
15. Arora D, Arora R, Sangthong S, Leelaporn W, Sangratanathongchai J. Universal screening of gestational diabetes mellitus: prevalence and diagnostic value of clinical risk factors. J Med Assoc Thai

2013;96:266-271.
16 American College of Obstetricians and Gynecologists. Practice Bulletin No. 137: Gestational diabetes mellitus. Obstet Gynecol 2013;122:406-416.
17 Standards of medical care in diabetes: 2014. Diabetes Care 2014;37 (Suppl 1): S14-80.
18 Metzger BE, Gabbe SG, Persson B, et al. International association of diabetes and pregnancy study groups recommendations on the diagnosis and classification of hyperglycemia in pregnancy. Diabetes Care 2010;33:676-682.
19 van Leeuwen M, Louwerse MD, Opmeer BC, et al. Glucose challenge test for detecting gestational diabetes mellitus: a systematic review. BJOG 2012;119:393-401.
20 Lain KY, Catalano PM. Metabolic changes in pregnancy. Clin Obstet Gynecol 2007;50:938-948.
21 Benjamin F, Wilson SJ, Deutsch S, Seltzer VL, Droesch K, Droesch J. Effect of advancing pregnancy on the glucose tolerance test and on the 50-g oral glucose load screening test for gestational diabetes. Obstet Gynecol 1986;68:362-365.
22 Plasencia W, Garcia R, Pereira S, Akolekar R, Nicolaides KH. Criteria for screening and diagnosis of gestational diabetes mellitus in the first trimester of pregnancy. Fetal Diagn Ther 2011;30:108-115.
23 Sermer M, Naylor CD, Gare DJ, et al. Impact of time since last meal on the gestational glucose challenge test: the Toronto Tri-Hospital Gestational Diabetes Project. Am J Obstet Gynecol 1994;171:607-616.
24 Coustan DR, Widness JA, Carpenter MW, Rotondo L, Pratt DC, Oh W. Should the fifty-gram, one-hour plasma glucose screening test for gestational diabetes be administered in the fasting or fed state? Am J Obstet Gynecol 1986;154:1031-1035.
25 Lewis GF, McNally C, Blackman JD, Polonsky KS, Barron WM. Prior feeding alters the response to the 50-g glucose challenge test in pregnancy: the Staub-Traugott effect revisited. Diabetes Care 1993;16:1551-1556.
26 Sacks DA, Chen W, Wolde-Tsadik G, Buchanan TA. When is fasting really fasting? The influence of time of day, interval after a meal, and maternal body mass on maternal glycemia in gestational diabetes. Am J Obstet Gynecol 1999;181:904-911.
27 Leinonen A, Hiilesmaa V, Andersen H, Teramo K, Kaaja R. Diurnal blood glucose profiles in women with gestational diabetes with or without hypertension. Diabet Med 2004;21:1181-1184.
28 Aparicio NJ, Joao MA, Cortelezzi M, et al. Pregnant women with impaired tolerance to an oral glucose load in the afternoon: evidence suggesting that they behave metabolically as patients with gestational diabetes. Am J Obstet Gynecol 1998;178:1059-1066.
29 Youden WJ. Index for rating diagnostic tests. Cancer 1950;3:32-35.
30 Bonomo M, Gandini ML, Mastropasqua A, et al. Which cutoff level should be used in screening for glucose intolerance in pregnancy? Definition of Screening Methods for Gestational Diabetes Study Group of the Lombardy Section of the Italian Society of Diabetology. Am J Obstet Gynecol 1998;179:179-185.
31 Sacks DA, Abu-Fadil S, Karten GJ, Forsythe AB, Hackett JR. Screening for gestational diabetes with the one-hour 50-g glucose test. Obstet Gynecol 1987;70:89-93.
32 Bobrowski RA, Bottoms SF, Micallef JA, Dombrowski MP. Is the 50-gram glucose screening test ever diagnostic? J Matern Fetal Med 1996;5:317-320.
33 Landy HJ, Gomez-Marin O, O'Sullivan MJ. Diagnosing gestational diabetes mellitus: use of a glucose screen without administering the glucose tolerance test. Obstet Gynecol 1996;87:395-400.
34 Shivvers SA, Lucas MJ. Gestational diabetes: is a 50-g screening result > or = 200 mg/dL diagnostic? J Reprod Med 1999;44:685-688.
35 Wong VW, Garden F, Jalaludin B.

Hyperglycaemia following glucose challenge test during pregnancy: when can a screening test become diagnostic? Diabetes Res Clin Pract 2009;83:394–396.
36. Espinosa de los Monteros A, Parra A, Carino N, Ramirez A. The reproducibility of the 50-g, 1-hour glucose screen for diabetes in pregnancy. Obstet Gynecol 1993;82:515–518.
37. Sacks DA, Abu-Fadil S, Greenspoon JS, Fotheringham N. How reliable is the fifty-gram, one-hour glucose screening test? Am J Obstet Gynecol 1989;161:642–645.
38. Harlass FE, Brady K, Read JA. Reproducibility of the oral glucose tolerance test in pregnancy. Am J Obstet Gynecol 1991;164:564–568.
39. Catalano PM, Avallone DA, Drago NM, Amini SB. Reproducibility of the oral glucose tolerance test in pregnant women. Am J Obstet Gynecol 1993;169:874–881.
40. Reece EA, Homko C, Wiznitzer A. Metabolic changes in diabetic and nondiabetic subjects during pregnancy. Obstet Gynecol Surv 1994;49:64–71.
41. Mooy JM, Grootenhuis PA, de Vries H, et al. Intra-individual variation of glucose, specific insulin and proinsulin concentrations measured by two oral glucose tolerance tests in a general Caucasian population: the Hoorn Study. Diabetologia 1996;39:298–305.
42. Agarwal MM, Dhatt GS. Fasting plasma glucose as a screening test for gestational diabetes mellitus. Arch Gynecol Obstet 2007;275:81–87.
43. Agarwal MM, Dhatt GS, Punnose J. Gestational diabetes: utility of fasting plasma glucose as a screening test depends on the diagnostic criteria. Diabet Med 2006;23:1319–1326.
44. Perucchini D, Fischer U, Spinas GA, Huch R, Huch A, Lehmann R. Using fasting plasma glucose concentrations to screen for gestational diabetes mellitus: prospective population based study. BMJ 1999;319:812–815.
45. Reichelt AJ, Spichler ER, Branchtein L, Nucci LB, Franco LJ, Schmidt MI. Fasting plasma glucose is a useful test for the detection of gestational diabetes. Brazilian Study of Gestational Diabetes (EBDG) Working Group. Diabetes Care 1998;21:1246–1249.
46. Trujillo J, Vigo A, Reichelt A, Duncan BB, Schmidt MI. Fasting plasma glucose to avoid a full OGTT in the diagnosis of gestational diabetes. Diabetes Res Clin Pract 2014;105(3):322–326.
47. Zhu WW, Fan L, Yang HX, et al. Fasting plasma glucose at 24-28 weeks to screen for gestational diabetes mellitus: new evidence from China. Diabetes Care 2013;36:2038–2040.
48. Corrado F, D'Anna R, Cannata ML, Interdonato ML, Pintaudi B, Di Benedetto A. Correspondence between first-trimester fasting glycaemia, and oral glucose tolerance test in gestational diabetes diagnosis. Diabetes Metab 2012;38:458–461.
49. Zhu WW, Yang HX, Wei YM, et al. Evaluation of the value of fasting plasma glucose in the first prenatal visit to diagnose gestational diabetes mellitus in china. Diabetes Care 2013;36:586–590.
50. Sacks DB, John WG. Interpretation of hemoglobin A1c values. JAMA 2014;311:2271–2.
51. Garner LA, Miller E, Katon J. First-trimester A1C as a tool to predict the development of gestational diabetes in high-risk women. Obstet Gynecol 2014;123(Suppl 1):52S.
52. Fong A, Serra AE, Gabby L, Wing DA, Berkowitz KM. Use of hemoglobin A1c as an early predictor of gestational diabetes mellitus. Am J Obstet Gynecol 2014;211(6):641.e1–7.
53. Agarwal MM, Dhatt GS, Punnose J, Koster G. Gestational diabetes: a reappraisal of HBA1c as a screening test. Acta Obstet Gynecol Scand 2005;84:1159–1163.
54. Rajput R, Yogesh Y, Rajput M, Nanda S. Utility of HbA1c for diagnosis of gestational diabetes mellitus. Diabetes Res Clin Pract 2012;98:104–107.

55 Puavilai G, Chanprasertyotin S, Jirapinyo M. An evaluation of glycosylated hemoglobin measurement by a colorimetric method as a screening test for gestational diabetes mellitus. J Med Assoc Thai 1993;76:549–553.
56 Hughes RC, Moore MP, Gullam JE, Mohamed K, Rowan J. An early pregnancy HbA1c >/=5.9% (41 mmol/mol) Is optimal for detecting diabetes and identifies women at increased risk of adverse pregnancy outcomes. Diabetes Care 2014;37:2953–2959.
57 Round JA, Jacklin P, Fraser RB, Hughes RG, Mugglestone MA, Holt RI. Screening for gestational diabetes mellitus: cost-utility of different screening strategies based on a woman's individual risk of disease. Diabetologia 2011;54:256–263.
58 Mission JF, Ohno MS, Cheng YW, Caughey AB. Gestational diabetes screening with the new IADPSG guidelines: a cost-effectiveness analysis. Am J Obstet Gynecol 2012;207:326.e1–9.
59 Werner EF, Pettker CM, Zuckerwise L, et al. Screening for gestational diabetes mellitus: are the criteria proposed by the international association of the Diabetes and Pregnancy Study Groups cost-effective? Diabetes Care 2012;35:529–535.

其他参考文献

60 Proceedings of the Second International Workshop-Conference on Gestational Diabetes Mellitus. October 25–27, 1984, Chicago, Illinois. Diabetes 1985;34(Suppl 2): 1–130.
61 Classification and diagnosis of diabetes mellitus and other categories of glucose intolerance. National Diabetes Data Group. Diabetes 1979;28:1039–1057.
62 Hoffman L, Nolan C, Wilson JD, Oats JJ, Simmons D. Gestational diabetes mellitus-management guidelines. The Australasian Diabetes in Pregnancy Society. Med J Aust 1998;169:93–97.

第五章 妊娠高血糖诊断标准

Robert S. Lindsay

Institute of Cardiovascular and Medical Sciences, University of Glasgow, Scotland

实践要点

- 围绕 GDM 最合适的诊断标准的争议。

病 例

史密斯女士，28岁，孕1产1。她的祖母在55岁时被诊断出患有2型糖尿病，除此之外，无其他糖尿病家族病史。HbA1c 的测定值为 47mmol/mol（6.4%）[正常值为 20~42mmol/mol（4.0%~6.0%）]。体重指数（32kg/m²）偏高，这是妊娠高血糖的公认危险因素；在妊娠 24 周时进行 75g 口服葡萄糖耐量试验，结果显示空腹血糖为 5.2mmol/L，餐后 1h 血糖为 9.6mmol/L，餐后 2h 血糖为 7.8mmol/L。她被诊断出患有妊娠糖尿病。开始饮食控制和家庭血糖监测。在妊娠 30 周时，她的血糖值超过了标准值，空腹血糖为 5.5mmol/L，餐后 2h 血糖为 7.0mmol/L，开始服用二甲双胍。在妊娠 38 周时，由于胎儿宫内窘迫，进行了紧急剖宫产。

1. GDM 诊断阈值的科学证据是什么？
2. 检测和治疗 GDM 的好处有哪些？

概述

第四章讨论了 GDM 的筛查方法。在本章中，我们考虑目前用于定义 GDM 或妊娠高血糖的诊断标准。这仍然是一个有争议的领域，对于诊断阈值，甚至是否应该以纯临床为基础，仍然没有国际共识，或如最近提出的卫生经济学分析结论。

妊娠糖尿病：历史发展

临床上对妊娠高血糖重要性的认识，早期主要来源于先前患有糖尿病的孕产妇的妊娠结果通常令人担忧[1]。在 1922 年之前，因胰岛素尚未被发现，妊娠结局大多很差，孕产妇和胎儿死亡率高，容易出现酮症酸中毒[1]。对于血糖高的人口，围产期死亡率和死胎率仍成倍地增加，直到胰岛素的出现才显著改善了这种局面[2]。早在 1823 年，就有第一个记录在案的 GDM 病例，一名妊娠期间患有新发口渴和糖尿病的产妇最后分娩了一个巨大的死胎[1]。

直到 20 世纪 50 年代才首次对妊娠期糖代谢进行了前瞻性研究[3,4]。在 1964 年的一项开放性研究中，O'Sullivan 和 Mahan 测量了 752 名孕产妇的葡萄糖耐量，并定义了在 100g 葡萄糖负荷后，空腹状态和餐后 1h、2h、3h 血糖值的正常范围[5]。他们进一步提出，当检测结果出现两项或两项以上的异常时，被认为是不正常的[5]。他们基于对同一家医院的 1013 名老年妇女的跟踪研究，结果显示 2% 的超过这些阈值的妇女在 8 年后患糖尿病的风险增加[5]。在另外的研究中显示，确诊组围产期死亡率增加了 4 倍[6]，孕产妇 16 年后糖尿病的发病率明显增加[7]。

上述这些发现及后来对所用分析技术的各种修改成为 GDM 诊断的基础，至少在美国已经超过了 40 年，在某些情况下直到今天依旧在应用。值得注意的是，标准主要基于这些妊娠妇女在分娩后患 2 型糖尿病的风险。

20 世纪 60 年代末，Pedersen 等使用了 "*gestational diabetes*" 一词，但直到 70 年代末，美国国家糖尿病数据组（NDDG）和世界卫生组织（WHO）才开始正式制定 GDM 诊断标准[8]。

NDDG 的工作也受到 1979 年在芝加哥举行的 GDM 国际研讨会的影响[9]，这是在今后 20 年内断断续续举行的一系列一致性研讨会的第一个会议。人们一致认为，GDM 应定义为"在妊娠期间首次发生的葡萄糖耐受不良"。在 1980 年发表的一致性讨论文件中还指出，妇女在妊娠期间应接受常规筛查，所有妇女（如果尚未发现有糖尿病）在妊娠第 24 周后应测量血糖。至少在会议上，均就使用 100g 葡萄糖负荷和由

O'Sullivan 标准解释的 3h 口服葡萄糖耐量试验（OGTT）达成了共识。然而在国际上，对于要使用的葡萄糖负荷量，妊娠期间的筛查时间或用于筛查的血样类型都没有达成一致意见。

1979 年的美国 NDDG 报告和 1980 年的 WHO 报告对妊娠以外的糖尿病的定义基本一致；然而，在妊娠期并没有达成这种共识。WHO 的标准仅从非糖尿病的背景中推断出来，建议患有糖尿病或糖耐量受损（IGT）的妇女（空腹血糖≥7.8mmol/L 和 OGTT 后 2h 血糖≥7.8mmol/L*）需要接受严格监督。相比之下，美国 NDDG（符合第一次 GDM 协商一致会议的建议）支持首先采用 50g 葡萄糖耐量测试的普遍筛查，其次是基于奥沙利文标准的 100g OGTT[5]。这些不同的诊断方法不仅具有历史意义，同时在这期间，对这两套标准（包括非妊娠糖尿病的诊断）进行了随后的修改，这些不同的 GDM 诊断方法一直沿用至今。事实上，2005 年 Crowther 在澳大利亚[10]和 2009 年 Landon 在美国[11]发表的关于治疗轻度 GDM 诊断的两项有影响力的随机临床试验所使用的标准和方法都来自于这一广泛的分类。

随后在 1984 年、1990 年和 1998 年召开的国际 GDM 研讨会上，对 GDM 的诊断进行了渐进式的改变。第二次会议达成共识，正式采用 50g 口服葡萄糖负荷作为筛选标准，并批准采用 7.8mmol/L 的负荷后静脉血浆值作为进一步行 OGTT 的标准[12]。此外，人们认识到，GDM 的定义包括那些在妊娠前可能患有未被识别的糖尿病的妇女。第三次会议指出了其他可能影响结果的因素，包括产妇肥胖、种族、既往的产科经历和家族病史。

1998 年，WHO 将 GDM 的定义细化为"糖类不耐受导致妊娠开始或第一次识别时出现不同程度的高血糖"[13]。同样，这显然包括了一组重要的女性，她们可能已经患有糖尿病。此时，非妊娠糖尿病的诊断标准在 OGTT 后 2h 被修订为空腹静脉血糖≥7.0mmol/L 或≥11.1mmol/L；对于 IGT 来说，在 OGTT 后 2h 血糖≥7.8mmol/L，但＜11.1mmol/L[13]。WHO 对 GDM 的阈值作为妊娠以外糖尿病和 IGT 的组合被保留。尽管有了新的诊断标准，WHO 还是基于有效风险因素的方法，而不是做普

---

*WHO 的报告实际上建议对这两个值都取 8.0mmol/L，但这只是四舍五入到最近的 mmol。后来在 1985 年的报告中澄清为 7.8mmol/L，与 NDDG 一致。

遍筛查。建议75g OGTT 应限于GDM 高危妇女，即针对那些"有巨大儿生产病史的妇女、来自某些高危族群的妇女及任何空腹或血糖升高的孕妇"。

最后，应该指出的是，其他国家指导小组也对这两种广泛应用的方法进行了修改。例如，在南半球，澳大利亚妊娠糖尿病协会推荐空腹血糖阈值≥5.5mmol/L(99mg/dl)，餐后2h 血糖阈值≥9mmol/L(162mg/dl)，尽管在新西兰使用了较低的餐后2h 阈值[≥8mmol/L（144mg/dl）][14]。这个由不同定义和筛选方法组成的诊断网络造成了很多混乱。几个筛查和产科团体对GDM 的诊断意义持怀疑态度（如加拿大[15]和英国[16]），对筛查和诊断的最佳方法也没有达成共识。一些因素导致了这些早期意见的修订[17]。大规模试验数据开始定义GDM 诊断和治疗的益处[10, 11]。多国观察高血糖和不良妊娠结局（HAPO）的研究涉及9个国家的23 316名妇女，该研究更精确地描绘了孕产妇葡萄糖和不良妊娠结局之间的关系[18]。

这些证据使得 IADPSG 于2010 年公布了商定的诊断阈值[19]。推荐的血糖阈值（本章将进一步讨论）是基于出生体重、脐带血C 肽和新生儿皮肤褶皱概率增加1.75 倍的平均值，高于人口的第90 百分位。自公布以来，IADPSG 的建议继续引起争论，在一些国家得到不同程度的采纳。然而，全球对所建议的标准的反应是对HAPO 数据和IADPSG 倡议的影响及重要性的衡量。美国妇产科医师学会（ACOG）选择保留两阶段过程，包括50g 葡萄糖负荷和100g OGTT[18]。相比之下，美国糖尿病协会[20]允许IADPSG 或两阶段方法。HAPO 合并并发症增加1.75 倍的选择也引起了争议——一些人建议[21, 22]增加1倍更合适，这反过来会导致诊断阈值更接近之前的ACOG 指南。相比之下，2013 年，WHO 普遍接受了IADPSG 的方法[23]。

最近，英国国家卫生和临床技术优化研究所（NICE）推荐了一种单独的诊断方法。该机构几乎完全基于健康经济分析得出阈值，其筛查和治疗费用符合质量调整生命年（QALY）30 000 英镑的标准。首选阈值明显不同于IADPSG 倡导的阈值——禁食空腹血糖≥5.6mmol/L 和餐后2h 血糖≥7.8mmol/L[24]。其他群体的分析基于IADPSG 1.75 倍的风险增加，但建议这些阈值应该更低，不同的标准可能适合不同的种族群体[25]。

最近，国际妇产科联合会（FIGO）[26]也试图制定筛查和诊断标准，仔细研究这些标准如何适应世界各地的医疗保健系统。FIGO 指出，筛选和诊断标准需要根据各种因素进行修改，包括基础生物学（基本上与不同人群患有未确诊糖尿病或发展为 GDM 的倾向有关），但也包括获取实验室葡萄糖测量值的实用问题及葡萄糖或 HbA1c 测量值的潜在质量问题[26]。尽管如此，FIGO 采纳了 WHO 和 IADPSG 的总体建议——特别是通过生化测试而非基于风险因素的筛查进行的普遍筛查，以及这些机构提出的诊断标准[26]。

妊娠期显性糖尿病的重要性

除了修订 GDM 的诊断标准之外，国际机构（IADPSG[19]、WHO[23]及后来的 FIGO[26]）将 GDM 与"妊娠期显性糖尿病"或"妊娠期糖尿病"区分开来。后一类符合妊娠后糖尿病的定义[即禁食血糖≥7.0mmol/L（126mg/dl）或餐后 2h 血糖≥11.1mmol/L（200mg/dl）]，在临床上似乎是一种有用的手段，可以用来识别那些需要更密切管理，而且糖尿病微血管并发症和糖尿病及妊娠严重并发症风险更高的女性，最重要的是有可能发生先天异常，这是妊娠前高血糖更严重的反映[19]。

这种分类的含义是，许多先前存在但未确诊的糖尿病女性可能会被归入显性糖尿病而不是妊娠糖尿病。还应该注意的是，患有显性糖尿病的妇女及被诊断患有 GDM 但葡萄糖水平较高的妇女，由于伦理原因，没有被纳入 HAPO 研究和大规模干预试验。例如，在 HAPO 研究中，OGTT 期间，平均妊娠 28 周，空腹血糖≥5.8mmol/L 或餐后 2h 血糖≥11.1mmol/L 的女性被排除在外。因为基线时空腹或餐后 2h 血糖值升高，这导致 1.7% 的女性被排除在外。另有 1.2% 的女性因随机葡萄糖升高（血糖高于 8.9mmol/L）而被排除在外。

因此，虽然这项观察性研究对于描述孕产妇血糖与各种妊娠结局之间的关系是非常宝贵的，但是约 2.9% 的女性以前没有被诊断患有糖尿病，但是妊娠期间血糖水平最高的人群被排除在观察性研究之外，这可能（并且适当地）减少了一些不良结局。同样，各种排除标准也同样适用于两项大型干预研究，这两项研究被公开设计为对轻度 GDM 的随机研究，排除了妊娠期间血糖水平最高的女性[10, 11]。

诊断妊娠高血糖的理论基础

回顾妊娠高血糖症诊断的历史背景清楚地表明，至少部分争议与 GDM 的诊断结果存在分歧。除妊娠外，诊断的理由更加简单，无论是空腹血糖、负荷后血糖还是 HbA1c，都需要预测人群微血管并发症风险增加的水平[13]。可以确定阈值，如超过该阈值，发生微血管并发症的风险增加，如糖尿病视网膜病变和肾病；超过该阈值，并发症的发生率也显著增加。

这种方法构成了将一部分人群分类为糖尿病的逻辑基础，更重要的是谁将从检测这种微血管并发症的筛查项目中受益。虽然糖尿病患者患大血管疾病的风险也在增加，但是对于微血管疾病来说，还不存在这样的葡萄糖阈值，此外，这个终点并不是糖尿病患者所独有的。

HAPO 分析的一个重要贡献是明确证明了除糖尿病外，妊娠妇女高血糖是不良妊娠结局的预测因素[27]。从数据中还可明显地看出，没有明确的阈值使这些结果显著增加。因此，这种危险因素与临床结果的连续分级关系更类似于胆固醇或血压与缺血性心脏病的关系，而不与糖尿病的非妊娠定义相关联。同样类似于胆固醇和心脏病，妊娠妇女体内的葡萄糖水平可能被认为是几个危险因素之一，而检测和治疗的原理可能会因这些其他危险因素的存在而有所不同。这也是胆固醇管理中很常见的问题，我们可以根据年龄、高血压和糖尿病等其他风险因素接受不同的治疗阈值。值得注意的是，在撰写本报告时，GDM 还没有采用基于其他风险因素的不同诊断或治疗阈值模式——尽管至少南亚妇女[25]已经建议采用这种方法。

这些考虑也提出了命名方面的问题。对于个人来说，糖尿病的诊断标签可能没有帮助，而妊娠高血糖等替代术语可能更有用，可以将妊娠妇女的血糖作为一系列危险因素之一[28]。这种差异可能不仅仅是语义上的，因为长期以来，人们一直认为给患者贴上 GDM 标签会增加手术分娩的可能性，并可能对妊娠妇女产生负面影响，即使这在最近的文献中并没有完全得到证实[10, 11]。

接下来，我们将考虑可能支持诊断的具体结果，关键为是否已经证明干预可以降低这些结果的风险。

以改善治疗结果为基础

妊娠期间的高血糖显然与母亲和孩子身体健康状况的风险增加有关。对母亲来说，结果可以分为妊娠和产后立即出现的症状（如先兆子痫或器械辅助分娩的风险）及长期影响，最显著的是母亲将来有患2型糖尿病的风险。同理，对于孩子来说，妊娠和分娩也可能存在风险，包括巨大儿（有潜在的创伤性分娩）和新生儿低血糖，从长远来看，还包括发展为肥胖和2型糖尿病的可能。

HAPO研究表明，巨大儿、脐带胰岛素大于第90百分位、临床新生儿低血糖和剖宫产的可能性[27]与新生儿肥胖[29]之间存在持续的分级关系，而与新生儿血糖的关系不大[30]。HAPO的次要结果中，肩难产和先兆子痫与母亲空腹和负荷后血糖呈正相关，而早产、高胆红素血症和新生儿重症监护与负荷后血糖无关[27]。

HAPO数据在很大程度上与以前文献中少数的研究一致，最显著的是Sacks的研究[31]。HAPO的研究没有证明也没有显示出与围产期死亡率有任何显著的关系——也许与血糖最高的母亲被排除在外有关，正如"妊娠期显性糖尿病的重要性"部分[27]所讨论的。更广泛地说，文献并没有令人信服的证据证明GDM与死产或围产期死亡率之间的联系，只有少数研究证明了这种联系[32,33]。

然而，至关重要的是，不仅关键结果与诊断相关，而且干预也能改善这些结果。为此，对轻度GDM的两项里程碑式的干预研究显示，胎儿生长[平均出生体重和大于胎龄儿（LGA）后代的比例]明显下降（表5.1）[10,11]。尽管研究的数量和规模都很小[34]，但是即使血糖水平低于GDM的阈值，随着血糖水平的降低，胎儿生长也会下降。

妊娠高血糖的治疗会降低母亲和新生儿的更严重的不良结局吗？如表5.1所示，先兆子痫的风险持续降低，为未治疗组的50%～70%[10,11]。肩难产的发生率似乎也有所降低，尽管这种并发症的发生率很低，而且临床上很难确定这种结果，因此这是一个有争议的结果[10]。然而，澳大利亚孕妇糖类不耐受试验（ACHOIS）和母婴医学协作网（MFMU）的研究与其他可能依赖于医疗行为的结果并不一致。因此，在 MFMU 研究中，剖宫产率降低，新生儿重症监护入院率保持不变，但在 ACHOIS 中，剖宫产率保持不变，其他两项结果增加[10, 11]。鉴于人们长期担心给女性贴上 GDM 标签可能会增加剖宫产率[35]，这在一定程度上是一个令人安心的结果，但治疗是否会最终减少其中的一些不良事件仍不清楚。

表 5.1 ACHOIS 和 MFMU 试验中不良结果的相对风险

项目	ACHOIS	MFMU
主要结局*	↓0.33（0.14~0.75）（$P=0.01$）	↔0.87（0.72~1.07）NS
孕龄大	↓0.62（0.47~0.81）（$P<0.001$）	↓0.49（32~0.76）（$P<0.001$）
巨大儿：出生体重大于 4kg	↓0.47（0.34~0.64）（$P<0.001$）	↓0.41（0.26~0.66）（$P<0.001$）
新生儿脂肪量	—	↓（$P=0.003$）
NICU 入院率	↑1.13（1.03~1.23）（$P=0.04$）	↔0.77（0.51~1.18）（$P=NS$）
肩难产	↔0.46（0.19~1.10）（$P=NS$）	↓0.37（0.14~0.97）（$P=0.02$）
引产	↑1.36（1.15~1.62）（$P<0.001$）	↔1.02（0.81~1.29）（$P=NS$）
先兆子痫	↓0.70（0.51~0.95）（$P=0.02$）	↓0.46（0.22~0.97）（$P=0.02$）
剖宫产	↔0.97（0.81~1.16）（$P=NS$）	↓0.79（0.64~0.99）（$P=0.02$）

*ACHOIS 的主要结局是死亡、肩难产、骨折和神经麻痹。MFMU 的主要结局是死产、新生儿死亡、新生儿低血糖、高胆红素血症、高胰岛素血症和出生创伤。

注：所有数据均以干预组与对照组各自研究的相对风险（95%置信区间）给出。

ACHOIS，澳大利亚孕妇糖类不耐受试验；MFMU，母婴医学协作网；NICU，新生儿重症监护病房；NS，无显著差异。

在最严重的并发症中，患 1 型和 2 型糖尿病的产妇与围产期死亡率增加有关，死产和新生儿早期死亡率都增加了[36]。荟萃分析显示 GDM 围产期死亡率没有显著增加[32]。应该注意的是，一些全国性调查显示有所增加[33]，这可能是由于未确诊的妊娠前糖尿病的影响。在 ACHOIS 研究中，该研究的主要结果，包括死亡（表 5.1），有显著减少，尽管所有这些结果的比例都很低[10]。相比之下，在 MFMU 研究中，主要结果没有显著减少[11]。值得注意的是，MFMU 研究人群中没有死产——这可能反映出血糖水平较高的人群已经被排除在外[11]。综上所述，轻度 GDM 的治疗似乎不会导致围产期死亡率的增加。与此同时，在筛查项目中发现血糖较高的妇女，特别是在未确诊的 2 型糖尿病高发人群中，这些益处可能会显现出来。

母亲患有糖尿病也被认为会增加后代肥胖和 2 型糖尿病的风险[37, 38]。这些后期影响通常被认为是宫内环境反映在子宫的"程序化"中，最有可能的是高血糖症。这是一个重要的领域，因为尽管妊娠前患糖尿病的母亲对这种影响描述得最清楚，但由于涉及的人数较多，妊娠期糖尿病将对公众健康产生更大的影响。正如美洲印第安人早期研究中所描述的，2 型糖尿病母亲的后代明显肥胖增加，糖耐量异常[37, 38]，1 型糖尿病母亲的后代也观察到类似的影响[39, 40]，这支持了正在发生的进展效应观点。患有 GDM 母亲的后代的数据不太清楚——部分原因是血糖进展对后代的影响可能会更小。迄今为止，HAPO 研究[41]和干预研究中对母亲所生的两个孩子的长期随访并没有表明长期依赖治疗的儿童的健康有所改善[42, 43]，但进一步的研究正在进行中。

对于下一步的研究，建议不仅通过检测和治疗妊娠糖尿病来改善临床结果，而且诊断和干预项目也应该显示出成本效益[24]。基于对母亲和婴儿最重要的临床结局（肩难产、剖宫产、新生儿黄疸、先兆子痫、引产和新生儿重症监护病房入院）及基于这些结果的筛查和治疗成本的分析，NICE 建议了一套单独的阈值，空腹血糖≥5.6mmol/L，餐后 2h 血糖≥7.8mmol/L 代表筛查成本的最佳截止值。相比之下，其他团队的建议，如 IADPSG 截止值可以从健康经济学的角度得到支持[44]，尽管所使用的模型仍有争议[45]。

妊娠高血糖早期诊断

另一个重要领域是早期妊娠高血糖状态的诊断潜力。传统上，由于中期和晚期胰岛素抵抗的发展，GDM 的筛查目标是妊娠 24～28 周，只有在妊娠早期进行 GDM 检测的妊娠妇女例外。IADPSG 共识指出，对于妊娠早期行 OGTT 缺乏证据，因此不建议在 24～28 周（18 周）之前例行进行 OGTT。然而，有学者建议空腹血糖≥5.1mmol/L 被归类为 GDM[19]。大约在同一时间（2008 年）对文献进行系统回顾时发现，在 24 周之前，没有筛选和治疗的随机对照试验[46]。从广义上来说，通过各种措施提高血糖似乎可以预测不良后果。在观察性研究中，妊娠早期空腹血糖可预测晚期 GDM、LGA 和剖宫产[在"正常"范围内研究，最高为 5.8mmol/L][47]。妊娠早期诊断为 GDM 的女性（本研究中按照 Carpenter-Coustan 标准）与晚期诊断的女性[48]相比，包括高血压和先兆子痫在内的并发症有所增加，新生儿低血糖和围产期死亡率也有所增加，尽管基数很小[48]。比较连续观察组在 24~28 周接受筛查或额外早期筛查的妇女，结果显示某些结果（羊水过多和早产）可能减少，但早期筛查的妇女的孩子出生体重没有总体差异[49]。类似的，在患有 GDM 的妇女中，虽然诊断时 HbA1c 较高（5.9%~6.6%）是不良后果（先兆子痫和早产）风险增加的标志，但与后来开始治疗的妇女相比，在 24 周之前诊断和治疗的这一亚组妇女的先兆子痫有所减少[50]。总的来说，这些数据给人一种感觉，即早期治疗可能是有利的，但它们远没有确定什么是最好的指标（葡萄糖或 HbA1c）或阈值，而且所有的警告通常都只适用于观察数据。特别的是，大部分数据都没有解决是否从早孕开始治疗轻度 GDM 的争议。显然，进一步的随机对照试验将是关键。

这方面的一个重要例外是那些在妊娠期间被诊断出可能有 GDM 的人群。因此，在妊娠早期 HbA1c 明显升高的情况下（大于 6%~6.5%），预计现有 1 型和 2 型糖尿病患者先天异常和流产的早期风险数据，以及妊娠前糖尿病的管理计划和咨询将是合适的。

结论

GDM 还没有统一的定义。然而，IADPSG/WHO 标准公布以来，已经取得了重大进展，并且朝着达成全球共识的方向又迈进了一大步。不应忽视 2 型糖尿病和肥胖症的长期急剧增加，而且似乎有必要定义一组血糖非常高的女性，她们有特别高的不良母体胎儿结局风险，需要特别监管。目前这一组最接近 GDM 的类型，反映出妊娠前未检测到的糖尿病。在这一类型之下，有一大群妇女的胎儿生长从后期妊娠高血糖症的检测和管理中获益。这一群体的血糖确切下限仍有争议，这一目标到底是纯临床的还是由健康经济学来控制的将被改进，并且在不同的医疗保健环境中可能会变得不同[26]。特别是对那些糖耐量异常最轻微的人来说，人们有理由担心妊娠"医疗化"的可能性[51]，但是也应该认识到对许多妇女来说，非侵入性的医疗干预对胎儿生长和先兆子痫是会产生正向影响的。在这些轻度 GDM 的研究中，绝大多数（80%～90%）女性可以通过饮食干预单独控制[10, 11]。正如其他人所述，如果这些妇女被认为不是妊娠时患有某种疾病，而是一个有多种危险因素之一的群体，那么 GDM 这个术语可能无用。

选择题

1. 可诊断为妊娠期显性糖尿病或妊娠糖尿病空腹血糖水平是（　　）
   A. 5.1mmol/L　　　　　　　　B. 5.3mmol/L
   C. 5.6mmol/L　　　　　　　　D. 7.0mmol/L
   正确答案是 D。
2. 在妊娠中期，HbA1c 达到或超过哪项标准是公认的妊娠糖尿病诊断标准（WHO）（　　）
   A. 5.8%　　　　　　　　　　B. 6.5%
   C. 7.0%　　　　　　　　　　D. 以上都不对
   正确答案是 D。

（孙　焱　译，朱海清　校）

参 考 文 献

1　Hadden DR. A historical perspective on gestational diabetes. Diabetes Care 1998;21(Suppl 2):B3–B4.
2　Evers IM, de Valk HW, Visser GH. Risk of complications of pregnancy in women with type 1 diabetes: nationwide prospective study in the Netherlands. BMJ 2004 Apr 17;328:915.
3　Wilkerson HL, Remein QR. Studies of abnormal carbohydrate metabolism in pregnancy; the significance of impaired glucose tolerance. Diabetes 1957 Jul;6(4):324–329.
4　Hoet JP, Lukens FD. Carbohydrate metabolism during pregnancy. Diabetes 1954 Jan;3(1):1–12.
5　O'Sullivan JB, Mahan CM. Criteria for the oral glucose tolerance test in pregnancy. Diabetes 1964 May;13:278–285.
6　O'Sullivan JB, Charles D, Mahan CM, Dandrow RV. Gestational diabetes and perinatal mortality rate. Am J Obstet Gynecol 1973 Aug 1;116(7):901–904.
7　O'Sullivan JB. Long term follow up of

gestational diabetes. In: Camerini-Davalos RA, Cole HS (eds). Early Diabetes in Early Life. Academic Press: New York, 1975.

8 WHO Expert Committee on Diabetes Mellitus: second report. World Health Organ Tech Rep Ser 1980;(646):1–80.

9 American Diabetes Association Workshop-Conference on gestational diabetes: summary and recommendations. Diabetes Care 1980;3(3):499–501.

10 Crowther CA, Hiller JE, Moss JR, McPhee AJ, Jeffries WS, Robinson JS. Effect of treatment of gestational diabetes mellitus on pregnancy outcomes. N Engl J Med 2005 Jun 16;352(24):2477–2486.

11 Landon MB, Spong CY, Thom E, Carpenter MW, Ramin SM, Casey B, et al. A multicenter, randomized trial of treatment for mild gestational diabetes. N Engl J Med 2009 Oct 1;361(14):1339–1348.

12 Gabbe SG. Definition, detection, and management of gestational diabetes. Obstet Gynecol 1986 Jan;67(1):121–125.

13 World Health Organization. Definition, Diagnosis and Classification of Diabetes Mellitus and its Complications. Report No. WHO/NCD/NCS/99.2. World Health Organization: Geneva, 1999.

14 Martin FI. The diagnosis of gestational diabetes. Ad Hoc Working Party. Med J Aust 1991 Jul 15;155(2):112.

15 Berger H, Crane J, Farine D, Armson A, De La Ronde S, Keenan-Lindsay L, et al. Screening for gestational diabetes mellitus. J Obstet Gynaecol Can 2002 Nov;24(11):894–912.

16 Scott DA, Loveman E, McIntyre L, Waugh N. Screening for gestational diabetes: a systematic review and economic evaluation. Health Technol Assess 2002;6(11):1–161.

17 Waugh N, Royle P, Clar C, Henderson R, Cummins E, Hadden D, et al. Screening for hyperglycaemia in pregnancy: a rapid update for the National Screening Committee. Health Technol Assess 2010 Sep;14(45):1–183.

18 Practice Bulletin No. 137: Gestational diabetes mellitus. Obstet Gynecol 2013 Aug;122(2 Pt 1):406–416.

19 Metzger BE, Gabbe SG, Persson B, Buchanan TA, Catalano PA, Damm P, et al. International association of diabetes and pregnancy study groups recommendations on the diagnosis and classification of hyperglycemia in pregnancy. Diabetes Care 2010 Mar;33(3):676–682.

20 Standards of medical care in diabetes. Diabetes Care 2011 Jan;34(Suppl 1):S11–S61.

21 Ryan EA. Diagnosing gestational diabetes. Diabetologia 2011 Mar;54(3):480–486.

22 Thompson D, Berger H, Feig D, Gagnon R, Kader T, Keely E, et al. Diabetes and pregnancy. Can J Diabetes 2013 Apr;37(Suppl 1):S168–S183.

23 World Health Organization. Diagnostic Criteria and Classification of Hyperglycaemia First Detected in Pregnancy. Report No. WHO/NMH/MND/13.2. Geneva: WHO, 2013.

24 National Institute for Clinical Excellence (NICE). Diabetes in Pregnancy: Management of Diabetes and Its Complications from Preconception to the Postnatal Period. NICE: London, 2015.

25 Farrar D, Fairley L, Santorelli G, Tuffnell D, Sheldon TA, Wright J, et al. Association between hyperglycaemia and adverse perinatal outcomes in south Asian and white British women: analysis of data from the Born in Bradford cohort. Lancet Diabetes Endocrinol 2015 Oct;3(10):795–804.

26 Hod M, Kapur A, Sacks DA, Hadar E, Agarwal M, Di Renzo GC, et al. The International Federation of Gynecology and Obstetrics (FIGO) Initiative on gestational diabetes mellitus: a pragmatic guide for diagnosis, management, and care. Int J Gynaecol Obstet 2015;131(3).

27 Metzger BE, Lowe LP, Dyer AR, Trimble ER, Chaovarindr U, Coustan DR, et al. Hyperglycemia and adverse pregnancy outcomes. N Engl J Med 2008 May 8;358(19):1991–2002.

28 Murphy HR, Hadden DR. Hyperglycaemia in pregnancy: what's in a name? Diabet

29 Hyperglycemia and Adverse Pregnancy Outcome (HAPO) Study: associations with neonatal anthropometrics. Diabetes 2009 Feb;58(2):453–459.
30 Metzger BE, Persson B, Lowe LP, Dyer AR, Cruickshank JK, Deerochanawong C, et al. Hyperglycemia and adverse pregnancy outcome study: neonatal glycemia. Pediatrics 2010 Dec;126(6):e1545–e1552.
31 Sacks DA, Greenspoon JS, Abu-Fadil S, Henry HM, Wolde-Tsadik G, Yao JF. Toward universal criteria for gestational diabetes: the 75-gram glucose tolerance test in pregnancy. Am J Obstet Gynecol 1995 Feb;172(2 Pt 1):607–614.
32 Wendland EM, Torloni MR, Falavigna M, Trujillo J, Dode MA, Campos MA, et al. Gestational diabetes and pregnancy outcomes – a systematic review of the World Health Organization (WHO) and the International Association of Diabetes in Pregnancy Study Groups (IADPSG) diagnostic criteria. BMC Pregnancy Childbirth 2012;12:23. doi:10.1186/1471-23 93-12-23.:23-12
33 Wendland EM, Duncan BB, Mengue SS, Schmidt MI. Lesser than diabetes hyperglycemia in pregnancy is related to perinatal mortality: a cohort study in Brazil. BMC Pregnancy Childbirth 2011 Nov 11;11:92. doi:10.1186/1471-2393-11-92.:92-11
34 Han S, Crowther CA, Middleton P. Interventions for pregnant women with hyperglycaemia not meeting gestational diabetes and type 2 diabetes diagnostic criteria. Cochrane Database Syst Rev 2012 Jan 18;1:CD009037. doi:10.1002/14651858. CD009037.pub2.:CD009037
35 Sermer M, Naylor CD, Gare DJ, Kenshole AB, Ritchie JW, Farine D, et al. Impact of increasing carbohydrate intolerance on maternal-fetal outcomes in 3637 women without gestational diabetes. The Toronto Tri-Hospital Gestational Diabetes Project. Am J Obstet Gynecol 1995 Jul;173(1):146–156.
36 Macintosh MC, Fleming KM, Bailey JA, Doyle P, Modder J, Acolet D, et al. Perinatal mortality and congenital anomalies in babies of women with type 1 or type 2 diabetes in England, Wales, and Northern Ireland: population based study. BMJ 2006 Jul 22;333(7560):177.
37 Pettitt DJ, Baird HR, Aleck KA, Bennett PH, Knowler WC. Excessive obesity in offspring of Pima Indian women with diabetes during pregnancy. N Engl J Med 1983 Feb 3;308(5):242–245.
38 Pettitt DJ, Aleck KA, Baird HR, Carraher MJ, Bennett PH, Knowler WC. Congenital susceptibility to NIDDM. Role of intrauterine environment. Diabetes 1988 May;37(5):622–628.
39 Lindsay RS, Nelson SM, Walker JD, Greene SA, Milne G, Sattar N, et al. Programming of adiposity in offspring of mothers with type 1 diabetes at age 7 years. Diabetes Care 2010 May;33(5):1080–1085.
40 Clausen TD, Mathiesen ER, Hansen T, Pedersen O, Jensen DM, Lauenborg J, et al. High prevalence of type 2 diabetes and pre-diabetes in adult offspring of women with gestational diabetes mellitus or type 1 diabetes: the role of intrauterine hyperglycemia. Diabetes Care 2008 Feb;31(2):340–346.
41 Pettitt DJ, McKenna S, McLaughlin C, Patterson CC, Hadden DR, McCance DR. Maternal glucose at 28 weeks of gestation is not associated with obesity in 2-year-old offspring: the Belfast Hyperglycemia and Adverse Pregnancy Outcome (HAPO) family study. Diabetes Care 2010 Jun;33(6):1219–1223.
42 Landon MB, Rice MM, Varner MW, Casey BM, Reddy UM, Wapner RJ, et al. Mild gestational diabetes mellitus and long-term child health. Diabetes Care 2015 Mar;38(3):445–452.
43 Gillman MW, Oakey H, Baghurst PA, Volkmer RE, Robinson JS, Crowther CA. Effect of treatment of gestational diabetes mellitus on obesity in the next generation. Diabetes Care 2010 May;33(5):964–968.
44 Duran A, Saenz S, Torrejon MJ, Bordiu E, Del VL, Galindo M, et al. Introduction of IADPSG criteria for the screening and diagnosis of gestational diabetes mellitus

results in improved pregnancy outcomes at a lower cost in a large cohort of pregnant women: the St. Carlos Gestational Diabetes Study. Diabetes Care 2014 Sep;37(9):2442-2450.
45 Bilous R. Diagnosis of gestational diabetes, defining the net, refining the catch. Diabetologia 2015 Sep;58(9):1965-1968.
46 Hillier TA, Vesco KK, Pedula KL, Beil TL, Whitlock EP, Pettitt DJ. Screening for gestational diabetes mellitus: a systematic review for the U.S. Preventive Services Task Force. Ann Intern Med 2008 May 20;148(10):766-775.
47 Riskin-Mashiah S, Younes G, Damti A, Auslender R. First-trimester fasting hyperglycemia and adverse pregnancy outcomes. Diabetes Care 2009 Sep;32(9):1639-1643.
48 Bartha JL, Martinez-Del-Fresno P, Comino-Delgado R. Gestational diabetes mellitus diagnosed during early pregnancy. Am J Obstet Gynecol 2000 Feb;182(2):346-350.
49 Bartha JL, Martinez-Del-Fresno P, Comino-Delgado R. Early diagnosis of gestational diabetes mellitus and prevention of diabetes-related complications. Eur J Obstet Gynecol Reprod Biol 2003 Jul 1;109(1):41-44.
50 Rowan JA, Budden A, Ivanova V, Hughes RC, Sadler LC. Women with an HbA1c of 41-49 mmol/mol (5.9-6.6%): a higher risk subgroup that may benefit from early pregnancy intervention. Diabet Med 2016 Jan;33(1):25-31.
51 Moynihan R. Medicalization: a new deal on disease definition. BMJ 2011 May 3;342:d2548. doi:10.1136/bmj.d2548.:d2548

第六章 生活方式的干预

Christina Anne Vinter[2,3] and Dorte Møller Jensen[1,2,3]

1 Department of Endocrinology, Odense University Hospital, Odense, Denmark
2 Department of Gynecology and Obstetrics, Odense University Hospital, Odense, Denmark
3 Department of Clinical Research, Faculty of Health Sciences, University of Southern Denmark, Odense, Denmark

实践要点

- 妊娠期肥胖被认为是妊娠期间健康受损的主要因素之一。
- 在一些发达国家，约 50% 的女性在妊娠期间受到超重和肥胖的影响。
- 肥胖会增加孕妇妊娠糖尿病、先兆子痫、早产、死产和生产巨大儿的风险。
- 妊娠期间的生活方式干预试验已被证明可以减少妊娠期体重的增加并改善饮食质量。
- 生活方式干预试验对临床妊娠和新生儿结局的影响有限。
- 目前正等待来自个体患者数据（IPD）荟萃分析的亚组分析结果，以确定是否有任何人群可能从特定干预措施中受益。
- 对参与妊娠期生活方式干预试验的母亲的后代进行随访，这对于证明长期结果的影响和安全性非常重要。
- 早期母体代谢条件从受孕时起调控胎盘功能和基因表达。
- 未来的干预试验需要在妊娠前的肥胖妇女中进行，以检查随后的妊娠中生活方式干预对孕产妇和新生儿结局的影响。

病 例

Linda 是一名 29 岁的初产妇，妊娠前 BMI 为 31kg/m^2。妊娠时没有任何并发症。在妊娠第 28 周，进行口服葡萄糖耐量试验，其中餐后 2h 血糖为 8.4mmol/L，刚好低于妊娠糖尿病的阈值。妊娠期间她的体重增加了 18kg。在分娩时，有 5min 的肩难产，但婴儿在持续气道正压通气（CPAP）数分钟后恢复，出生体重为 4300g。之后母乳喂养失败。20 个月后，Linda 再次妊娠。她没有减掉第一次妊娠时增加的体重，发现妊娠时的 BMI 为 34kg/m^2。由于尿糖阳性，口服葡萄糖耐量试验在妊娠 24 周时进行，Linda 被诊断患有妊娠糖尿病，并被建议向专业医师和护理人员寻求干预计划。诊断

> 为妊娠糖尿病时,她的体重已经增加了 5kg,需要通过干预将总体重增加限制在 8kg。从妊娠第 35 周开始,添加胰岛素治疗,并且由于婴儿腹围的快速增加而在 4 周后催产,出生体重为 4650g,分娩时肛门括约肌 3°裂伤。

概述

妊娠期肥胖已被确定为当代产科实践中的重要临床问题。发达国家和发展中国家的肥胖患病率都在迅速上升[1],这种全球流行病给公共卫生和临床实践带来了沉重的负担[2, 3]。在美国 20~39 岁的女性中,肥胖（BMI≥30kg/m^2）的患病率已达到 36%[4],而在英国,约有 16%的妊娠妇女肥胖[5]。

上述这种情况会对妊娠期间的葡萄糖代谢产生深远的影响,并与 2 型糖尿病、多囊卵巢综合征和 GDM 相关。

研究表明,潜在可改变的母体因素,如妊娠前 BMI,妊娠期体重增加（GWG）和不同程度的葡萄糖耐受不良与不良妊娠结局相关[6]。最重要的是,不利的宫内环境可预示出生时的巨大儿,未来妊娠时的 GDM,以及后代的肥胖、糖尿病和其他代谢问题,从而形成代际恶性循环。

在改变行为和提高健康意识方面,妊娠一直被视为"机会之窗"。此外,由于在妊娠期间经常与医疗保健专业人员接触,因此很容易找到专业治疗。尽管最近有大量关于妊娠期生活方式干预的临床试验,但其临床影响的证据有限,特别是在 GDM 方面。本章重点介绍了肥胖女性的不同生活方式干预试验,并讨论了将妊娠期作为治疗肥胖的一个时间是具有挑战性的原因。

生活方式干预在肥胖妊娠妇女中的作用

妊娠提供了管理或预防肥胖的机会,因为许多女性都关注婴儿的健康状况,并经常与她们的医疗保健专业人士接触。2009 年,美国医学研究所（IOM）建议肥胖女性在妊娠期间体重增长控制在 5~9kg。

对于超重和体重正常的女性，推荐的体重增长分别为 7～11.5kg 和 11.5～16kg[7]。生活方式干预有可能通过限制 GWG 和改善母体葡萄糖代谢与胰岛素敏感性来改善胎儿-母体结局。过量的 GWG 与孕产妇和胎儿并发症及产后体重潴留的风险增加有关。大部分肥胖女性超过推荐的 GWG。因此，在丹麦国家出生队列中，58%的肥胖女性体重增加超过 10kg，平均总 GWG 为（10.5±8.3）kg[8]。最近的一项荟萃分析发现，即使是体重正常的女性，过度的 GWG 也会影响短期和长期的后代肥胖[9]。

目前，公布了很多关于 GDM 风险增加的超重或肥胖女性生活方式干预的临床试验。其中大部分都集中在改变饮食习惯、身体活动或两者的结合，以及许多人使用 GWG 作为主要结果和（或）女性是否获得低于、等于或高于国际移民组织对 GWG 的建议[7]。一些研究还涉及了母体代谢参数，如高血糖、胰岛素和血脂谱[10, 11]。到目前为止，只有一项研究公布了后代的详细儿童随访数据[12]。一些最新的研究已经足以检验临床孕产妇和新生儿的结局，包括 GDM 和巨大儿[11, 13-15]。

澳大利亚 LIMIT 研究是迄今为止最大的已发表的试验 [随机对照试验（RCT）]，包括 2212 名超重或肥胖的非糖尿病妊娠妇女，她们随机接受生活方式干预或标准产前保健。参与者入组时间在妊娠 10～20 周[16]。生活方式干预包括饮食建议、个人饮食计划和鼓励锻炼。行为策略由专业营养师在入选后和妊娠第 28 周与第 36 周进行面对面访问时提供，并在妊娠第 22 周、24 周和 32 周电话随访三次。与标准治疗相比，该研究没有显著降低生活方式组中出生时大于胎龄儿（LGA）的婴儿风险（19% vs 21%，$P=0.24$），这是主要结果。此外，各组之间 GWG 没有显著降低：干预组增加 9.39kg，而对照组为 9.44kg，$P=0.89$。出生体重超过 4.5kg 的婴儿的风险降低；然而，这项措施没有考虑孕龄。后代的后续随访正在进行中。

在英国妊娠改善饮食和活动试验（UPBEAT）中，1555 名具有不同背景的肥胖妊娠妇女（$BMI \geqslant 30kg/m^2$）在妊娠 15～18 周被随机分为针对饮食和身体活动的行为干预组或标准产前保健组[11]。分配到干预组的妇女与健康教练进行单独面谈，然后进行为期 8 周的每周 1 次会谈（控制理论和社会认知疗法的要素）。主要结果是，GDM 和 LGA

发生率在两组中相似（分别为 25% vs 26% 和 8% vs 9%），以及其他一些产科并发症发生率也相似。干预组的女性在妊娠期间体重增加的程度低于对照组（7.19kg vs 7.76kg；$P=0.04$），并且她们达到了减少饮食血糖负荷和提高身体活动的目标[11]。

在爱尔兰的 ROLO 研究（降低血糖指数饮食的随机对照试验以预防正常血糖妇女的巨大儿症）中，800 名具有先前孕育巨大儿（出生体重＞4000g）的 BMI 正常血糖妊娠妇女随机分为干预组（妊娠 22 周前的小组课程介绍低升糖指数和健康饮食指导）或标准对照组[17]。基于每 3 个月的 3d 食物日记，干预组能量摄入量显著降低，高升糖指数食物摄入量减少。与干预组相比，干预组的 GWG（kg）显著降低对照组（平均为 11.5kg±4.2kg vs 12.6kg±4.4kg，$P=0.003$），干预组中超过了 IOM 对 GWG 建议的妊娠妇女比例较低，出生体重（主要结果）、身长或新生儿腹围没有差异。在丹麦 LiP（妊娠期生活方式）研究中，共有 360 名肥胖孕妇（BMI≥30kg/m^2）在妊娠 14 周前被随机分配到干预组或对照组[18]。干预组的妇女在妊娠期间接受了 4 次单独的饮食健康课程，并参加了一项有氧课程（每周 1h），妊娠期间被给予免费健身俱乐部会员资格及锻炼激励计划。与对照组相比，干预组的 GWG（kg）显著降低[中位数（四分位范围）：7.0（4.7～10.6）vs 8.6（5.7～11.5），$P=0.01$]。先兆子痫、妊娠高血压、妊娠糖尿病、剖宫产、LGA 婴儿或入住新生儿重症监护病房的风险没有显著差异。该研究测量了整个妊娠期间的一些代谢结果，发现生活方式干预导致生理性妊娠诱导的胰岛素抵抗减弱[10]。干预对母乳喂养持续时间或产后体重保持没有影响[19]。该研究是第一个在后代发表详细随访的妊娠干预试验，显示在 2.5～3 岁时没有人体测量指标或代谢影响[12, 20]。

TOP 研究（妊娠期肥胖症治疗）是丹麦 RCT 研究，425 名肥胖孕妇（BMI≥30kg/m^2）被随机分配到两个干预组，包括体力活动组（PA 组）和计步器组，体力活动和饮食咨询(营养师每周提供 1h 饮食指导)(PAD)组或对照组[21]。各个干预组的 GWG 中位值（范围）[PAD 组：8.6（-9.6～34.1）kg，PA 组：9.4（-3.4～28.2）kg]与对照组相比[10.9（-4.4～28.7）kg（PAD 组 vs 对照组；$P=0.01$ 和 PA 组 vs 对照组；$P=0.042$）]较低。研究发现任何组产科或新生儿结局均无差异。

糖尿病及妊娠期维生素 D 和生活方式干预（DALI）研究是一项针对肥胖孕妇的欧洲多中心研究（BMI≥29kg/m²）。DALI 旨在通过生活方式干预（动机访谈）和（或）补充维生素 D 来预防肥胖女性发生 GDM[22]。在 DALI 生活方式研究中，根据肥胖和葡萄糖耐量选择妊娠早期的女性并随机分为 4 个干预组：健康饮食（HE）组（113 名女性）、体力活动（PA）组（110 名）、HE+PA 组（108 名）和接受常规治疗的对照组（105 名）。在 HE+PA 组中，但不是单独的 HE 或 PA，女性在妊娠 35～37 周时实现的 GWG 显著低于对照组（−2.02kg，95%CI：−3.58～−0.46）。尽管有这种减少，但禁食或葡萄糖负荷没有改善胰岛素抵抗的水平、胰岛素浓度或稳态模型评估（HOMA-IR）。出生体重与胎龄大小的比例相似[14]。

芬兰妊娠糖尿病预防研究（RADIEL）选择 293 名妊娠妇女，BMI≥30kg/m² 和（或）以前有 GDM 的妊娠妇女在妊娠 20 周之前入组[23]。这些妇女被随机分配到关于饮食和身体活动的个人咨询组或标准产前保健组。与对照组相比，干预组的 GDM 发生率较低（13.9% vs 21.6%，$P=0.097$ 未调整，基线数据调整后 $P=0.044$）。因此，只有在调整基线数据后，这一发现才有意义。此外，干预措施对饮食质量和身体活动产生了有利影响。

许多其他 RCT 研究都集中在 GWG 上，并发现了不同的结果。Phelan 等的"适合分娩研究"[24]是低强度的行为干预，410 例正常体重和超重至肥胖的美国妇女在妊娠 10～16 周随机进行干预或标准治疗。他们发现，干预措施显著降低了超过 IOM 推荐 GWG 的正常体重妊娠妇女的百分比，但对超重和肥胖女性的 GWG 没有显著影响。Luoto 等在芬兰的 NELLI 研究中发现，至少有一种 GDM 危险因素的患者在饮食和运动方面进行个体咨询后新生儿出生体重明显减少。营养学家在比利时进行的低强度生活方式教育的 RCT 中没有显著影响 GWG；然而，后来的 RCT 表明，接受产前身心健康生活方式干预的干预组 GWG 明显减少。最近 5 年内主要研究的结果见表 6.1[11, 14, 16, 18, 21, 23-32]。

表 6.1 生活干预试验

文献研究	设计	人口总数	介入	结果
Simmons（2017）[14] DALI	RCT 3 组：健康饮食（HE）、体力活动（PA）和 HE+PA	BMI≥29kg/m²，欧洲 9 国（n=436）	5 个面对面和 4 个可选的电话辅导课程，基于动机性访谈的原则	HE 女性的 GWG 显著降低[-2.02kg（95%CI：-3.58～-0.46）]，空腹血糖和胰岛素抵抗无显著差异，HE+PA 与其他组之间未观察到显著差异。所有干预组的 GDM 患病率相似
Koivusalo 2015)[23] RADIEL	RCT 干预对照	BMI≥30kg/m²，芬兰（n=293）	研究护士和一组营养师任饮食、体力活动和体重控制方面进行个性化咨询	在调整基线特征后，干预组的 GDM 发生率为 13.9%，对照组为 21.6%（95%CI：0.40%～0.98%；P=0.044），GWG 显著降低：0.58kg（95%CI：-1.12～-0.04）；调整后 P=0.037
Poston（2015）[11] UPBEAT	RCT 干预对照	BMI≥30kg/m²，美国（n=1555）	行为干预，每周 8 次由健康教练主持，分组或个性化	干预和对照之间的 GDM 没有差异：25% vs 26%，P=0.68。LGA 无差异：9% vs 8%，P=0.40。GWG 显著降低：7.19kg vs 7.76kg，P=0.041
Dodd（2014）[13] LIMIT	RCT 干预对照	BMI≥25kg/m²，澳大利亚（n=2212）	由营养师和助理在 2 次面对面的拜访中提供饮食、运动和行为建议，随后进行 3 次私人电话	干预和对照之间的 LGA 没有减少：19% vs 21%，P=0.24；显著降低巨大儿儿（>4000g）的发病率：15% vs 19%，P=0.04。GWG 无差异：9.39kg vs 9.44kg，P=0.89
Renault（2014）[21] TOP	RCT 3 组：体力活动（PA）+饮食（D）、PA 和对照	BMI≥30kg/m²，丹麦（n=425）	每 2 周由营养师提供膳食建议面对面和电话）。PA 包括使用计步器，敦励每天要求 11 000 步	与对照组相比，两个干预组的 GWG 显著降低：8.6kg vs 9.4kg 与 10.9kg，P=0.01。对出生体重、LGA 或 GDM 无影响

续表

文献研究	设计	人口总数	介入	结果
Bogaerts (2013)[30]	RCT 3 组：生活方式的干预和对照	BMI≥29kg/m², 比利时 (n=205)	手册小组收到了有关健康生活方式的书面信息，生活方式小组进行了 4 次产前干预，并对助产士进行了动机访谈培训	与对照组相比，干预组的 GWG 显著降低：9.5kg vs 10.6kg vs 13.5kg，P=0.007。仅在积极的生活方式组中显著降低焦虑水平。对出生体重或 GDM 没有影响
Walsh (2012)[32] ROLO	RCT 干预/对照	第一次妊娠，先前分娩的婴儿>4000g, 爱尔兰 (n=800)	妊娠早期的低血糖指数饮食（与营养师进行小组讨论），书面材料随访，并进行两次强化训练	出生体重或巨大儿无明显差异。GWG 显著降低：-1.3kg（95%CI：-2.4～-0.2），P=0.01
Vinter (2011)[18] LiP	RCT 干预/对照	BMI≥30kg/m² 丹麦 (n=360)	与营养师进行 4 次面对面访问，每周接受物理治疗师及计步器和免费健身俱乐部的培训	GWG 显著降低：7.0kg vs 8.6kg，P=0.01；对出生体重、LGA 或 GDM 没有影响
Luoto (2011)[28] NELLI	Cluster-RCT 干预/对照	所有 BMI 组，正常血糖但至少有1个 GDM 危险因素，芬兰 (n=399)	与护士进行 5 次面对面的产前检查，并提供个人饮食和运动咨询	对 GWG 没有影响：13.8kg vs 14.2kg，P=0.52；干预组与对照组的出生体重：3532g vs 3659g，P=0.008；出生体重/周和 LGA 显著减少。对 GDM 或巨大儿无影响
Phelan (2011)[24] Fit for Delivery	RCT 干预/对照	BMI 为 19.8~40kg/m²，美国 (n=401)	低强度的行为干预，在研究开始时与干预者进行面对面的接触，并提供 3 个简短的电话支持	超过1990年IOM标准的GWG显著减少：40.2% vs 52.1%，P=0.003（仅正常体重）；超重/肥胖对 GWG 没有显著影响

干预试验的系统评价

近年来已经进行了许多系统评价和荟萃分析[33-36],由此可以得出结论,尽管认识到肥胖是一个严重的临床问题并且已经做出相当大的努力来预防并发症,但尚未确定具体的基于证据的生活干预方式。这种知识差距对于未来的研究很重要。最新的系统评价一致认为,产前干预与GWG受限有关,饮食干预似乎与GWG的最大减少有关。如上所述,这不是后来发布的大型LIMIT试验中的发现。此外,结论是现有的研究,质量低至中等,结果应谨慎解释。一项从2015年开始的循证医学也评估了综合饮食和运动干预措施的影响,特别是预防GDM[37]。该评价包括了13项随机对照试验,涉及4983名妇女及其婴儿。将接受饮食和运动干预的妊娠妇女与对照组相比,发生GDM的风险是否有显著差异。该评价的结论是,鉴于这些试验的质量不同,干预措施和人群特征及结果定义不可能得出任何明确的结论。因此,根据目前可获得的数据,没有确凿的证据表明生活方式干预能够阻止GDM的发展。

干预可能会有危害吗?

重要的是,任何生活方式干预的有益效果与潜在的不良后果相平衡,如小于胎龄儿(SGA)、低出生体重、早产和死产。根据观察性研究的结果,IOM在2009年关于GWG的建议表明孕期体重增加最少5kg。到目前为止,已经发表的RCT研究中还没有发现干预计划的不良反应,甚至在体重增加不到5kg的妊娠妇女中也没有。Hinkle等根据超过122 000名肥胖女性的肥胖等级,研究了GWG与胎儿生长之间的关联[38]。对于肥胖Ⅰ级,与5~9kg的GWG相比,妊娠期体重减轻与SGA婴儿的风险显著增加相关。肥胖Ⅰ级和GWG的妊娠期体重增加0.1~4.9kg,肥胖Ⅱ级和Ⅲ级的GWG为-4.9~4.9kg,与SGA风险增加无关,但降低了巨大儿的风险。在另一项研究中,Blomberg等于2004年评估了46 000名来自瑞典的肥胖妊娠妇女,其中有GWG低于IOM的建议[39],结果显示妊娠期减肥的肥胖Ⅱ级和Ⅲ级女性剖宫产率与LGA的风险降低,并且没有显著增加先兆子痫、低 Apgar 评分和胎儿窘迫风险。SGA 婴儿的风险增加了 2 倍,但肥胖女性的风险较低(3.7%)。如果肥胖Ⅲ级女性体重增加较低(0~4.9kg),SGA 风险增加就会消失。这些研究的结果表明,低于 IOM 标准的 GWG 对于肥胖Ⅱ级和Ⅲ级的女性来说是相当安全的。尽管如此,这些结论仍然是基于观察数据,还没有关于这些婴儿长期后果的报道。在 Catalano 等的一项后来的观察性研究中发现,与体重增长超过 5kg 的肥胖产妇的新生儿相比,体重增长低于 5kg 的肥胖女性的 GWG 与婴儿的出生体重、脂肪量和体长显著降低有关[40]。这些初步调查结果需要在未来的试验中得到确认或否定,因为干预措施需要保证对母亲和后代的短期与长期结果都不会造成伤害。

正在进行的研究和 Meta 分析

目前正在进行有效和全面的干预试验,结果尚未完成。澳大利亚 SPRING 研究(益生菌预防妊娠糖尿病的研究)是对 540 名超重和肥胖妊娠妇女预防 GDM 的随机对照研究[41]。在最近的一项随机对照试验中,正常体重妊娠妇女使用益生菌可降低 GDM 的发生率[42]。国际孕期体重管理协作网络(iWIP)目前监督着正在进行的 IPD 荟萃分析,涉及 36 名作者的汇总数据[43],将包括超过 9000 名参加妊娠期体重管理 RCT 的妇女的结果。该研究的主要结果是关于 GWG,但也将分析一些次要结果。IPD 荟萃分析将允许识别和随后将干预目标定位到那些可能受益于迄今为止最大样本量的妊娠干预的群体。最后,iWIP 还计划将该研究扩展到这些研究中后代的后续数据。

比较研究

肥胖妊娠妇女的生活方式干预可能限制 GWG,这对于减少产后体重和限制随后妊娠期间的妊娠前体重非常重要。此外,有限的 GWG 可能对未来的体重轨迹产生积极影响。本章引用的 RCT 使用了不同的妊娠期间的生活方式干预,他们提供了不同的行为改变、饮食习惯和体力活动的组合，从低强度行为研究到更密集的干预，包括重复的个人咨询和锻炼课程。研究设置、BMI、干预设计和强度的不一致使得比较变得困难。干预研究的另一个限制是研究者无法始终如一地正确监测对饮食和（或）体力活动要求的依从性。缺乏临床效果的其他原因可能与干预试验吸引最健康的女性有关，这些女性不能代表超重和肥胖妊娠妇女的背景人群。对干预对象进行盲法试验是不可能的，并且由于控制措施是积极的，并能意识到正在进行的干预，可能会改善妊娠妇女的妊娠行为，从而可能降低空腹血糖和 GWG[14]。干预研究结果之间的差异可能部分是由于入选研究中代谢状态的入选标准的差异（BMI 分级，纳入 GDM 后的女性被排除等）。这应该在未来的研究中解决。尽管如此，有希望通过芬兰 RADIEL 研究中的生活方式干预来预防 GDM，其中女性有 GDM 的高风险并有约 30%有既往 GDM[23]。然而，大多数研究并未成功地减少临床孕产妇和新生儿不良结局，如 GDM、先兆子痫、巨大儿和早产。这些并发症可能都与妊娠早期不利的代谢环境有关，因此在妊娠中期开始的干预可能为时已晚，并且持续时间不足以克服早期代谢紊乱状况的负面影响。研究已经表明，妊娠前 BMI 是孕产妇和新生儿妊娠结局的一个比 GWG 更强的预测因子[44]。与体重较轻的妇女相比，妊娠期前肥胖的女性胰岛素抵抗更多，从妊娠开始就有更高的三酰甘油水平[45]。有学者提出，早期母体代谢条件会影响胎盘功能和基因表达，这两种因素都可能影响胎儿的后期生长。一些观察性研究表明，妊娠期体重变化对于下一次妊娠并发症的风险很重要[46-48]。即使轻微的体重增加也会增加超重和肥胖女性在随后妊娠期间患 GDM、先兆子痫和巨大儿的风险，但在正常体重的女性中也是如此[46, 49]。

在肥胖女性中，轻度至中度的体重减轻已被证明可显著降低随后 LGA 婴儿在观察性研究中的风险，但增加 SGA 婴儿的风险[48]。总之，这些发现强调了在妊娠前优化母体体重和代谢条件的重要性。在未来的研究中，妊娠间隔可能是肥胖女性体重减轻的关键时期。

未来的方向

妊娠期肥胖给公共健康和临床实践带来巨大压力，伴随着巨大的健康问题及孕产妇和新生儿并发症,但是我们在如何有效处理这些问题方面存在知识空白。为了解决临床面临的问题,我们需要更好地理解肥胖潜在的代谢、生理、行为和心理机制。一代又一代的肥胖恶性循环,究竟在什么时间及如何干预这个问题还有待研究。在妊娠期间对母亲进行生活方式干预后,对后代的随访非常重要,以进一步了解宫内环境的重要性及其对后代的新陈代谢和长期健康的影响。大规模干预研究的后代的详细随访结果,如 LIMIT 和 UPBEAT 试验正在进行中。由于妊娠期间行为干预对孕产妇和新生儿并发症的影响有限,我们现在面临的事实是,在妊娠前优化代谢状态可能需要进行妊娠前干预。这些研究的实施难度更大,因为非妊娠妇女不易获取,大部分妊娠是无计划的。大规模研究尚未发表。基于现有知识,显然要实现母亲和子孙后代健康的实质性改善,这种方法需要扩展到妊娠期以外。

至少,在任何基于证据的饮食健康和身体活动方案之前,医疗保健专业人员应鼓励(超重或肥胖)妊娠妇女避免过多的体重增加;保持健康多样的饮食,并注意运动,应支持女性在产后进行母乳喂养和减肥。

选择题

1. 在肥胖妊娠妇女中进行了许多生活方式干预研究,以下陈述正确的是(   )
   A. 生活方式干预一直表明可降低巨大儿的风险
   B. 生活方式干预可以减少妊娠期体重增加
   C. 生活方式干预一直表明可降低 GDM 风险
   D. 干预不影响妊娠期体重增加

正确答案是 B。

2. 下列在这一领域进一步研究可能是一个很好策略的是(   )
   A. 前瞻性荟萃分析汇总临床数据,以确定受益于不同干预措施的亚组
   B. 对肥胖妊娠妇女进行饮食和运动干预的更大规模随机对照
   C. 仅限运动干预
   D. 以上均不正确

正确答案是 A。

（王凯亮 译，朱海清 校）

参 考 文 献

1. Mitchell S, Shaw D. The worldwide epidemic of female obesity. Best Pract Res Clin Obstet Gynaecol 2015;29(3):289-299.
2. Webber L, Divajeva D, Marsh T, McPherson K, Brown M, Galea G, et al. The future burden of obesity-related diseases in the 53 WHO European-Region countries and the impact of effective interventions: a modelling study. BMJ Open 2014;4(7):e004787.
3. Wang YC, McPherson K, Marsh T, Gortmaker SL, Brown M. Health and economic burden of the projected obesity trends in the USA and the UK. Lancet 2011;378(9793):815-825.
4. Flegal KM, Carroll MD, Kit BK, Ogden CL. Prevalence of obesity and trends in the distribution of body mass index among US adults, 1999-2010. JAMA 2012;307(5):491-497.
5. Heslehurst N, Rankin J, Wilkinson JR, Summerbell CD. A nationally representative study of maternal obesity in England, UK: trends in incidence and demographic inequalities in 619 323 births, 1989-2007. Int J Obes (Lond) 2010;34(3):420-428.
6. Nelson SM, Matthews P, Poston L. Maternal metabolism and obesity: modifiable determinants of pregnancy outcome. Hum Reprod Update 2010;16(3):255-275.
7. Institute of M. Weight gain during pregnancy: reexamining the guidelines. National Academies Press: Washington, DC, 2009.
8. Nohr EA, Vaeth M, Baker JL, Sorensen TI, Olsen J, Rasmussen KM. Combined associations of prepregnancy body mass index and gestational weight gain with the outcome of pregnancy. Am J Clin Nutr 2008;87(6):1750-1759.
9. Mamun AA, Mannan M, Doi SA. Gestational weight gain in relation to offspring obesity over the life course: a systematic review and bias-adjusted meta-analysis. Obes Rev 2014;15(4):338-347.
10. Vinter CA, Jorgensen JS, Ovesen P, Beck-Nielsen H, Skytthe A, Jensen DM. Metabolic effects of lifestyle intervention in obese pregnant women: results from the randomized controlled trial 'Lifestyle in Pregnancy' (LiP). Diabet Med 2014;31(11):1323-1330.
11. Poston L, Bell R, Croker H, Flynn AC, Godfrey KM, Goff L, et al. Effect of a behavioural intervention in obese pregnant women (the UPBEAT study): a multicentre, randomised controlled trial. Lancet Diabetes Endocrinol 2015;3(10):767-777.
12. Tanvig M, Vinter CA, Jorgensen JS, Wehberg S, Ovesen PG, Beck-Nielsen H, et al. Effects of lifestyle intervention in pregnancy and anthropometrics at birth on offspring metabolic profile at 2.8 years - results from the Lifestyle in Pregnancy and Offspring (LiPO) study. J Clin Endocrinol Metab 2014:jc20142675.
13. Dodd JM, McPhee AJ, Turnbull D, Yelland LN, Deussen AR, Grivell RM, et al. The effects of antenatal dietary and lifestyle advice for women who are overweight or obese on neonatal health outcomes: the LIMIT randomised trial. BMC Med 2014;12(1):163.
14. Simmons D, Devlieger R, van Assche A, Jans G, Galjaard S, Corcoy R, Adelantado JM, Dunne F, Desoye G, Harreiter J, Kautzky-Willer A, Damm P, Mathiesen ER, Jensen DM, Andersen L, Lapolla A, Dalfrà MG, Bertolotto A, Wender-Ozegowska E, Zawiejska A, Hill D, Snoek FJ, Jelsma JG, van Poppel MN. Effect of physical activity and/or healthy eating on

GDM risk: the DALI Lifestyle Study. J Clin Endocrinol Metab 2017 Mar 1;102(3):903-913.
15. de Wit L, Jelsma JG, van Poppel MN, Bogaerts A, Simmons D, Desoye G, et al. Physical activity, depressed mood and pregnancy worries in European obese pregnant women: results from the DALI study. BMC Pregnancy Childbirth 2015;15:158.
16. Dodd JM, Cramp C, Sui Z, Yelland LN, Deussen AR, Grivell RM, et al. The effects of antenatal dietary and lifestyle advice for women who are overweight or obese on maternal diet and physical activity: the LIMIT randomised trial. BMC Med 2014;12(1):161.
17. McGowan CA, Walsh JM, Byrne J, Curran S, McAuliffe FM. The influence of a low glycemic index dietary intervention on maternal dietary intake, glycemic index and gestational weight gain during pregnancy: a randomized controlled trial. Nutrition J 2013;12(1):140.
18. Vinter CA, Jensen DM, Ovesen P, Beck-Nielsen H, Jorgensen JS. The LiP (Lifestyle in Pregnancy) Study: A randomized controlled trial of lifestyle intervention in 360 obese pregnant women. Diabetes Care 2011;34(12):2502-2507.
19. Vinter CA, Jensen DM, Ovesen P, Beck-Nielsen H, Tanvig M, Lamont RF, et al. Postpartum weight retention and breastfeeding among obese women from the randomized controlled Lifestyle in Pregnancy (LiP) trial. Acta Obstet Gynecol Scand 2014;93(8):794-801.
20. Tanvig M, Vinter CA, Jorgensen JS, Wehberg S, Ovesen PG, Lamont RF, et al. Anthropometrics and body composition by dual energy X-ray in children of obese women: a follow-up of a randomized controlled trial (the Lifestyle in Pregnancy and Offspring [LiPO] study). PLoS One 2014;9(2):e89590.
21. Renault KM, Norgaard K, Nilas L, Carlsen EM, Cortes D, Pryds O, et al. The Treatment of Obese Pregnant Women (TOP) study: a randomized controlled trial of the effect of physical activity intervention assessed by pedometer with or without dietary intervention in obese pregnant women. Am J Obstet Gynecol 2014;210(2):134.e1-e9.
22. Jelsma JG, van Poppel MN, Galjaard S, Desoye G, Corcoy R, Devlieger R, et al. DALI: vitamin D and lifestyle intervention for gestational diabetes mellitus (GDM) prevention: an European multicentre, randomised trial – study protocol. BMC Pregnancy Childbirth 2013;13:142. doi:10.1 186/1471-2393-13-142.:142-13
23. Koivusalo SB, Rono K, Klemetti MM, Roine RP, Lindstrom J, Erkkola M, et al. Gestational diabetes mellitus can be prevented by lifestyle intervention: the Finnish Gestational Diabetes Prevention Study (RADIEL): a randomized controlled trial. Diabetes Care 2016;39(1):24-30.
24. Phelan S, Phipps MG, Abrams B, Darroch F, Schaffner A, Wing RR. Randomized trial of a behavioral intervention to prevent excessive gestational weight gain: the Fit for Delivery Study. Am J Clin Nutr 2011;93(4):772-779.
25. Olson CM, Strawderman MS, Reed RG. Efficacy of an intervention to prevent excessive gestational weight gain. Am J Obstet Gynecol 2004;191(2):530-536.
26. Quinlivan JA, Lam LT, Fisher J. A randomised trial of a four-step multidisciplinary approach to the antenatal care of obese pregnant women. Aust NZ J Obstet Gynaecol 2011;51(2):141-146.
27. Asbee SM, Jenkins TR, Butler JR, White J, Elliot M, Rutledge A. Preventing excessive weight gain during pregnancy through dietary and lifestyle counseling: a randomized controlled trial. Obstet Gynecol 2009;113(2 Pt 1):305-312.
28. Luoto R, Kinnunen TI, Aittasalo M, Kolu P, Raitanen J, Ojala K, et al. Primary prevention of gestational diabetes mellitus and large-for-gestational-age newborns by lifestyle counseling: a cluster-randomized controlled trial. PLoS Med 2011;8(5):e1001036.
29. Guelinckx I, Devlieger R, Mullie P, Vansant G. Effect of lifestyle intervention on dietary habits, physical activity, and gestational

30. Bogaerts AF, Devlieger R, Nuyts E, Witters I, Gyselaers W, Van den Bergh BR. Effects of lifestyle intervention in obese pregnant women on gestational weight gain and mental health: a randomized controlled trial. Int J Obes (Lond) 2013;37(6): 814-821.
29. weight gain in obese pregnant women: a randomized controlled trial. Am J Clin Nutr 2010;91(2):373-380.
31. Stafne SN, Salvesen KA, Romundstad PR, Eggebo TM, Carlsen SM, Morkved S. Regular exercise during pregnancy to prevent gestational diabetes: a randomized controlled trial. Obstet Gynecol 2012;119(1):29-36.
32. Walsh JM, McGowan CA, Mahony R, Foley ME, McAuliffe FM. Low glycaemic index diet in pregnancy to prevent macrosomia (ROLO study): randomised control trial. BMJ 2012;345:e5605.
33. Tanentsapf I, Heitmann BL, Adegboye AR. Systematic review of clinical trials on dietary interventions to prevent excessive weight gain during pregnancy among normal weight, overweight and obese women. BMC Pregnancy Childbirth 2011;11(1):81.
34. Oteng-Ntim E, Varma R, Croker H, Poston L, Doyle P. Lifestyle interventions for overweight and obese pregnant women to improve pregnancy outcome: systematic review and meta-analysis. BMC Med 2012;10:47. doi:10.1186/1741-7015-10-47.: 47-10
35. Thangaratinam S, Rogozinska E, Jolly K, Glinkowski S, Roseboom T, Tomlinson JW, et al. Effects of interventions in pregnancy on maternal weight and obstetric outcomes: meta-analysis of randomised evidence. BMJ 2012;344:e2088. doi:10.1136/bmj.e2088.:e2088
36. Agha M, Agha RA, Sandell J. Interventions to reduce and prevent obesity in pre-conceptual and pregnant women: a systematic review and meta-analysis. PLoS One 2014;9(5):e95132.
37. Bain E, Crane M, Tieu J, Han S, Crowther CA, Middleton P. Diet and exercise interventions for preventing gestational diabetes mellitus. Cochrane Database System Rev 2015;4:Cd010443.
38. Hinkle SN, Sharma AJ, Dietz PM. Gestational weight gain in obese mothers and associations with fetal growth. Am J Clin Nutr 2010;92(3):644-651.
39. Blomberg M. Maternal and neonatal outcomes among obese women with weight gain below the new Institute of Medicine recommendations. Obstet Gynecol 2011;117(5):1065-1070.
40. Catalano PM, Mele L, Landon MB, Ramin SM, Reddy UM, Casey B, et al. Inadequate weight gain in overweight and obese pregnant women: what is the effect on fetal growth? Am J Obstet Gynecol 2014;211(2):137.e1-e7.
41. Nitert MD, Barrett HL, Foxcroft K, Tremellen A, Wilkinson S, Lingwood B, et al. SPRING: an RCT study of probiotics in the prevention of gestational diabetes mellitus in overweight and obese women. BMC Pregnancy Childbirth 2013;13:50.
42. Luoto R, Laitinen K, Nermes M, Isolauri E. Impact of maternal probiotic-supplemented dietary counselling on pregnancy outcome and prenatal and postnatal growth: a double-blind, placebo-controlled study. Br J Nutr 2010;103(12):1792-1799.
43. Ruifrok AE, Rogozinska E, van Poppel MN, Rayanagoudar G, Kerry S, de Groot CJ, et al. Study protocol: differential effects of diet and physical activity based interventions in pregnancy on maternal and fetal outcomes-individual patient data (IPD) meta-analysis and health economic evaluation. System Rev 2014;3(1):131.
44. Catalano PM, Ehrenberg HM. The short- and long-term implications of maternal obesity on the mother and her offspring. BJOG 2006;113(10):1126-1133.
45. Catalano P, deMouzon SH. Maternal obesity and metabolic risk to the offspring: why lifestyle interventions may have not achieved the desired outcomes. Int J Obes (Lond) 2015;39(4):642-649.
46. Villamor E, Cnattingius S. Interpregnancy weight change and risk of adverse pregnancy outcomes: a

population-based study. Lancet 2006;368(9542):1164−1170.
47 Classification and diagnosis of diabetes mellitus and other categories of glucose intolerance. National Diabetes Data Group. Diabetes 1979;28(12):1039−1057.
48 Jain AP, Gavard JA, Rice JJ, Catanzaro RB, Artal R, Hopkins SA. The impact of interpregnancy weight change on birthweight in obese women. Am J Obstet Gynecol 2013;208(3):205.e1−e7.
49 Bogaerts A, Van den Bergh BR, Ameye L, Witters I, Martens E, Timmerman D, *et al.* Interpregnancy weight change and risk for adverse perinatal outcome. Obstet Gynecol 2013;122(5):999−1009.

第七章　妊娠期肥胖和糖尿病

H. David McIntyre[1], Marloes Dekker Nitert[2], Helen L. Barrett[3] and Leonie K. Callaway[3]

1 Department of Obstetric Medicine, Mater Health Services and Mater Research, Faculty of Medicine, The University of Queensland, Brisbane, Queensland, Australia
2 School of Chemistry and Molecular Biosciences, The University of Queensland, Brisbane, Queensland, Australia
3 UQ Centre for Clinical Research, Faculty of Medicine, The University of Queensland, Brisbane, Queensland, Australia

实践要点

- GDM 和肥胖均为独立的危险因素，与妊娠期并发症发生风险增加相关，应该受到临床的关注。
- 应当谨防 GDM 患者为避免使用胰岛素而采用过度控制饮食的方法。GDM 确诊后的 2~3 周应该频繁观察体重的高值。如果出现持续体重下降，应进行尿检以确定是否有酮症，同时密切观察进食情况。
- 出生前，在应用糖皮质激素促进胎儿肺成熟治疗的 2~3d，要避免行口服葡萄糖耐量试验，因为结果可能异常升高引起误判。

病　例

Suzies 是一位 38 岁的厨师，孕 3 产 1，流产 2 次，进行妊娠前保健咨询。她最近再婚，新任丈夫 25 岁，这对夫妻想生一个孩子。她的产科病史包括 15 年前妊娠后被确诊为 GDM 和先兆子痫，这导致她妊娠 36 周时剖宫产产下一个重 3980g 的女婴。在这之前，曾有 2 次早期流产病史。童年期就处于肥胖和超重的状态，18 岁时被确诊为多囊卵巢。23 岁起，她的体重增长了 25kg，目前为 105kg（身高 168cm，BMI 为 37.2kg/m^2）。5 年前，她被确诊为 2 型糖尿病，采用早晨服用 5mg 利格列汀，睡前服用 2g 二甲双胍治疗。近期测糖化血红蛋白为 7.0%（53mmol/mol）。她还有 3 年的原发性高血压、高胆固醇血症和微量白蛋白尿（800mg/24h）病史，每天服用厄贝沙坦 300mg，瑞舒伐他汀 10mg，近期检测指标大体满意。每天吸烟 30 支。曾经，每次试图戒烟时，体重都会增加 10kg，最近开始应用尼古丁透皮贴剂来试图减少香烟的摄入。没有避孕措施，月经周期正常，而且黄体期孕酮水平提示有排卵。体格检查显示肥胖，血压为 140/90mmHg，腋窝和颈部可见黑棘皮征。

- 列出导致 Suzies 不容易妊娠的因素。
- Suzies 在这个阶段妊娠合适吗？在治疗期间是不是应该选择合适的避孕方法？如果是这样，你推荐什么避孕方法？
- 需要优先解决哪方面的健康问题？
- 如果计划妊娠，Suzies 现有的血糖控制水平令人满意吗？
- 糖尿病治疗方面有什么变更？
- 如果计划妊娠，现有的药物治疗哪种需要停止，替代方案是什么？
- 肥胖和糖尿病有哪些潜在的并发症需要特殊关注，需要进一步做什么检查？
- 在这个临床病例中，肥胖症的手术治疗有哪些优缺点？

概述

在世界范围内，肥胖症和糖尿病变得越来越常见，在高中低收入水平的国家均明显增加[1]。伴随着两种疾病流行的另一现状是，女性计划妊娠的年龄增长，尤其在发达国家更为明显。这些因素导致妊娠期和妊娠前糖尿病的发病率增加[2]。母体糖尿病和母体肥胖妊娠期并发症的发病率相似[3]。本章既单独考虑了这些风险，也从几个方面综合列举出它们的流行病学、发病率和对妊娠期总体不利的危险因素：①临床病例讨论；②潜在的生理和病理生理机制；③流行病学；④目前治疗的依据，尤其参照随机对照试验的结果；⑤妊娠期间的这些因素对后代健康的重要性。

定义

关于 GDM 的定义，自从 Carrington 提出这一概念后就一直争论不休[4]。普遍认为，妊娠期间激素水平的变化会让一些血糖水平正常的女性变成高血糖状态。在 GDM 研究的初期就表明妊娠期间确诊为 GDM 的女性有长期的潜在的转化为 2 型糖尿病的风险[5]。

现在的观点认为，在全世界范围内，育龄期女性中的 2 型糖尿病及 IFG 和 IGT 均普遍流行[6]。然而，在 2 型糖尿病发病率高的国家，许多原来诊断为 GDM（妊娠期发现的任何形式的高血糖[7]）的患者或许原来就存在糖耐量异常,只是在妊娠期被确诊。妊娠前就确诊 2 型糖尿病的女性,妊娠期间发生严重并发症的风险更高[8],应该有单独的分类以获得更多的医学关注。

本章作者采用了最新 ADA、IADPSG[9]、WHO[10]关于 GDM 的定义,通过 OGTT 确诊 GDM。这同非妊娠期诊断糖尿病的方法是一致的。后者被描述为显性糖尿病(IADPSG 标准)或单纯妊娠期间的糖尿病(WHO 标准)。确诊 GMD 的血糖标准见表 7.1。

对于肥胖的定义争论较少,大部分作者均认同 WHO 的分类[11],即承认 BMI 作为不太完美的潜在肥胖的衡量标准,但同时也认为这一标准并不适用于所有人群。

表 7.1 妊娠糖尿病和(显性)妊娠期间糖尿病的定义

定义	IADPSG	WHO
"显性糖尿病"(IADPSG)或"妊娠期间糖尿病"(WHO)	空腹血糖≥7.0mmol/L 随机血糖≥11.1mmol/L(确认) 或糖化血红蛋白≥6.5%	空腹血糖≥7.0mmol/L 餐后 2h 血糖≥11.1mmol/L 75g 葡萄糖负荷试验随机血糖≥11.1mmol/L 伴有明显症状
妊娠糖尿病	空腹血糖 5.1~6.9mmol/L 餐后 1h 血糖≥10.0mmol/L 餐后 2h 血糖≥8.5mmol/L	空腹血糖 5.1~6.9mmol/L 餐后 1h 血糖≥10.0mmol/L 餐后 2h 血糖 8.5~11.0mmol/L

生理及病理生理机制

妊娠早期,母体的合成代谢增加,导致母体的脂肪堆积。正常妊娠期中,受胎盘激素的影响,妊娠中期母体的胰岛素抵抗增加,妊娠后期会达到峰值。正常的女性,从妊娠初期到后期胰岛素敏感度会下降 50%~60%[12]。这种胰岛素敏感度的下降(或者说是胰岛素抵抗的增加)通常是通过胰岛素分泌增加来克服的,以确保血糖正常。

胰岛素抵抗的增加使母体从合成代谢转化为分解代谢阶段。在分解代谢阶段,母体的代谢更依赖于脂质和酮体。这确保发育中的胎儿有充足的营养供给。胰岛素敏感度同母体血浆游离脂肪酸水平密切相关[13]。除了游离脂肪酸水平增加以外,母体脂代谢的其他方面也会在妊娠期产生变化。脂肪氧化明显增加，而且妊娠后期会出现明显的高脂血症。极低密度脂蛋白、低密度脂蛋白及高密度脂蛋白中三酰甘油含量会增加。母体的血浆胆固醇水平也会升高。健康女性妊娠期发生的这些代谢变化在妊娠糖尿病或母体肥胖状态时会更加明显[14]。

妊娠糖尿病和肥胖时糖代谢的变化

妊娠前身体肥胖的女性在妊娠后与妊娠相关的胰岛素抵抗会使之前就存在的胰岛素抵抗状态加重。对很多肥胖女性来说，额外增加的胰岛素抵抗可以增加胰岛素分泌并达到平衡状态。但是，胰岛 B 细胞不能代偿增加胰岛素分泌时就会出现高血糖，进而被诊断为 GDM。妊娠造成的胰岛素抵抗在妊娠中期会明显增加，在妊娠中期末达到稳定的高水平，而这个时点正是推荐进行 GDM 检测的时间。

妊娠前 BMI 增加的女性更容易罹患 GDM。其他胰岛素分泌潜能下降的女性，如有遗传性糖耐量低减倾向者（如明确 2 型糖尿病家族史）发展成为 GDM 的风险增加[15]。消瘦的女性发展成 GDM 通常都具有以下特征：发生 GDM 时同非 GDM 的女性相比，胰岛素抵抗指数（稳态模型 HOMA-IR）增加很少，但是胰岛素分泌指数（HOMA-β）却明显降低[16, 17]。在消瘦女性中，家族史和血浆三酰甘油水平同 GDM 相关[16]。有无发展成为 GDM 倾向还有人种差异，不考虑 BMI，南亚地区的女性在妊娠中期的开始和产后其 HOMA-IR 和 HOMA-β 均高于西欧地区的女性[18]。

即使没有伴随 GDM，身体肥胖的女性进行持续血糖监测也会表现为轻度高血糖症[19]。

妊娠糖尿病和妊娠期肥胖时脂质与脂肪组织的代谢

胰岛素敏感性下降不仅影响葡萄糖，脂质的利用率也会增加。在早期妊娠之前，身体肥胖但血糖正常的女性和 GDM 的女性同正常体重、正常糖耐量的女性相比，三酰甘油及 VLDL 胆固醇水平均会增加，HDL 胆固醇水平会下降[20, 21]。GDM 的女性与无 GDM 的女性相比，皮下脂肪组织胰岛素受体底物 1 蛋白表达较低。同非妊娠女性相比，不管她们的葡萄糖耐量状态如何，空腹的妊娠妇女胰岛素受体底物 2 表达增加[13]。胰岛素信号的传导，尤其是介导其靶组织中的代谢效应，主要依赖于胰岛素受体底物，其中胰岛素受体底物 1 是骨骼肌和脂肪组织的主要底物，胰岛素受体底物 2 是肝脏的主要底物[22]。虽然底物具有重叠功能，但它们也调节特定过程，因此不能完全相互补偿[22]。此外，在患有和不患有 GDM 的肥胖妇女的脂肪组织中，许多与脂肪酸代谢有关的基因表达降低[23]。这包括编码与脂肪酸摄取和细胞内转运、三酰甘油合成、脂肪生成和脂肪分解有关的蛋白质的基因。在妊娠晚期，胰岛素通过抑制激素敏感脂肪酶抑制脂肪分解的效果较差。在患有 GDM 的肥胖妊娠妇女中，调节脂质代谢的转录因子（包括 PPARγ）的基因表达也会降低[13, 23]。患有 GDM 的女性脂肪组织中胰岛素信号传导的这些改变导致在 GDM 中可观察到过度胰岛素抵抗。妊娠期脂肪组织中 PPARγ 的低表达可能反映了在妊娠后期禁食的"加速饥饿"。

肥胖和妊娠糖尿病时的炎症反应

胎盘是一种活跃的内分泌器官，有助于调节母亲和发育中胎儿的新陈代谢。胎盘合成并分泌大量激素、细胞因子和代谢信号分子。对患有 GDM 的超重女性的胎盘的微阵列研究表明，炎症和脂质代谢相关的基因表达增加，但与葡萄糖代谢相关的基因表达却没有增加[24]。身体肥胖的女性在妊娠期间，胎盘和脂肪组织均调节母体代谢，尽管它们的调节不太协调。

白色脂肪组织不仅是脂质的储存库，也是活跃的内分泌器官，分泌多种脂肪因子和细胞因子。在肥胖妊娠中，脂肪组织中炎症标志物如白细胞介素-6（IL-6）和 TNF-α 的释放增加，这可能导致肥胖 GDM 女性中胰岛素抵抗水平升高[25]。妊娠前 BMI 是妊娠期代谢燃料被氧化的决定因素。消瘦的女性不管有没有 GDM，基础糖类氧化增加 55%～80%，但脂肪氧化没有变化，而肥胖妊娠妇女增加脂肪而不是糖类氧化[25]。因此，在肥胖 GDM 女性中，脂质可以为胎儿脂质合成提供额外的底物[26]，可以增强胎儿生长并增加巨大儿的风险。

妊娠也是一种低级"变换"炎症状态，胎盘和子宫上皮表达促炎性细胞因子[27]。这种炎症反应的触发因素尚不清楚，但胎盘碎片以微颗粒形式存在，称为合体滋养细胞膜微粒（STBM）[28]或外泌体[29]及胎盘衍生的信号分子与之有关。随着正常妊娠的进展，促炎和抗炎细胞因子之间的平衡向抗炎细胞因子转移[30]。在患有 GDM 的正常体重的女性中，与匹配的对照相比，TNF-α 水平而非 IL-6 水平（均为促炎细胞因子）增加[31]。此外，妊娠早期白细胞计数增加可预测 GDM 的发展，而与母亲 BMI 状况无关[32]。然而，肥胖本身是低度炎症状态，肥胖妊娠妇女有较高的循环 IL-6 水平，这与 GDM 状态无关[33]。肥胖和 GDM 的结合加剧了一些但不是所有研究中的炎症特征[33]，这可能反映了抽样的时机和异质人口。炎症特征因以下事实而进一步复杂化，如胎盘也可以表达和分泌细胞因子。然而，它可以作为缓冲剂来限制胎儿暴露于母体炎症及应对肥胖症和 GDM[33]。

妊娠糖尿病和肥胖——相互关系与共同和不同的机制

胰岛素抵抗

妊娠期肥胖会使中度肥胖的女性患 GDM 的风险增加 3.0 倍，而病态肥胖的女性的患病风险则可增加 5.6 倍[34]。

BMI 每增加 $1kg/m^2$，GDM 的患病率增加 0.92%[34]。胰岛素抵抗是肥胖和 GDM 的标志。在 GDM 中骨骼肌胰岛素受体磷酸化减少 1/3，但在体重偏瘦的女性中受体数量没有变化；而在肥胖女性中，胰岛素受体数量和磷酸化均降低。所有妊娠妇女骨骼肌胰岛素受体[IRS1]的数量和磷酸化均减少，这是骨骼肌中最重要和最丰富的胰岛素受体底物，表明妊娠期胰岛素信号传导能力较低[35]。

胰岛素分泌

对于预先存在胰岛素抵抗的女性，妊娠期胰岛素抵抗的生理上升不可能总是通过增加胰岛素分泌来补偿，这时一些身体肥胖的女性易患 GDM。这种胰岛素分泌能力的降低是可以测量的，如通过计算 HOMA-β 指数或更多直接测量如静脉葡萄糖耐量试验等。

妊娠糖尿病和肥胖的流行病学

许多报道试图从 GDM 和肥胖对妊娠结局及后来的母婴健康的影响中剖析出 GDM 和肥胖对人群健康影响的重要性。它们之间的联系很难分离，尤其是作为两种情况经常共存，肥胖通常是导致高血糖的原因之一。此外，研究人群的异质性、筛选、治疗和分析会使研究的解释复杂化。

幸运的是，这些问题通过高血糖和不良妊娠结局（HAPO）研究已经大部分解决[3, 36]，研究中，护理人员对于妊娠 28 周时平均 75g OGTT 的结果不知情，除非葡萄糖水平上升高于预定义的阈值，导致参与者被排除在研究之外。此外，没有为肥胖女性提供具体的干预措施。

HAPO 研究表明，孕产妇 BMI 和高血糖与妊娠结局的关系相似。两者都与主要结局（大胎龄儿、原发性剖宫产、临床新生儿低血糖和新生儿高胰岛素血症）和重要的次要结局（包括胎儿肥胖和子痫前期）的发生率增加有关。总的来说，母亲体重指数与这些结果的关系倾向于是最高分类中的"高限"，而葡萄糖没有显示出这种趋势[36]。重要的是要记住，出于伦理和安全的原因，如果妇女的葡萄糖水平超过了预先设定的阈值，那么她们就不会被 HAPO 研究所纳入，而 BMI 相关研究则没有这样的限制。

研究还报道了 BMI 和 GDM 与不良妊娠结局的关联（图 7.1）[3]。在 HAPO 研究的未揭盲的人群中，IADPSG 标准[9]的肥胖率为 13.7%，GDM 为 16.1%。只有 25% 的 GDM 女性肥胖。与既没有 GDM 也没有肥胖的女性相比，单纯肥胖的女性和只有 GDM 的女性的大多数妊娠并发症的校正优势比（OR）都有所增加。先兆子痫似乎在"肥胖症"中更为普遍。"胎儿过大和胎儿高胰岛素血症"在单独 GDM 组中比在单独肥胖组中常见。GDM 和肥胖的结合显然是使妊娠并发症的风险显著增加（图 7.2）。HAPO 研究也通过分类来检验，如 BMI 分为正常和体重不足，超重和肥胖，以及将复合 OGTT Z-分数分为正常、中度和 GDM。选择中度血糖是为了接近 HAPO 参与者超重的频率。

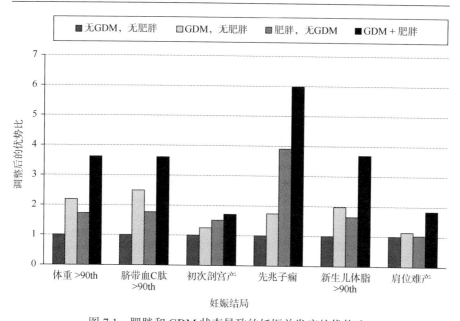

图 7.1 肥胖和 GDM 状态导致的妊娠并发症的优势比

在高血糖和不良妊娠结局（HAPO）研究中，完全调整了所选妊娠并发症的优势比[3]。"无 GDM，无肥胖"类别是所有比较的参照组。其他类别，如图所示，仅指 GDM、肥胖及这两个因素的组合。优势比指的是来源出版物中详细解释的"模型Ⅱ"对潜在的混杂因素进行了充分的调整

其他一些研究也有助于提示肥胖和 GDM 对不良妊娠结局的贡献。来自美国的病例对照研究显示，如果患有 GDM 未经治疗的体重偏瘦的女性（产前很少甚至没有产前护理的女性，在 37 周时被诊断为 GDM），妊娠期合并死产的风险高出 2 倍；大于胎龄儿（LGA）、新生儿低血糖、红细胞增多症和高胆红素血症及代谢并发症增加 7 倍[37]。这些不良后果的增加与没有 GDM 的肥胖女性相似。未经治疗的患有 GDM 的消瘦女性剖宫产的分娩率也高于没有 GDM 的消瘦女性。对于未接受 GDM 治疗的肥胖妇女，综合结果中这些风险增加了 10 倍，LGA 婴儿增加了 3 倍，代谢并发症增加了 5 倍，引产分娩增加了 4 倍，剖宫产分娩率增加了 9 倍。这些结果表明肥胖和 GDM 单独与不良妊娠后果相关，但它们的联合发生显著增加了风险。然而，当接受 GDM 治疗时，一般来说肥胖女性[38]或接受胰岛素治疗的肥胖女性[39]的不良妊娠结局风险不高。

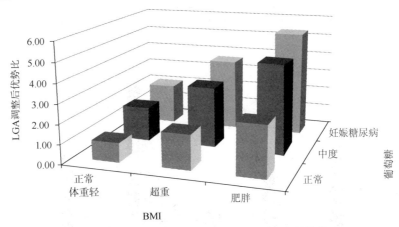

图 7.2　不同血糖和体重指数类型 LGA 婴儿的优势比

在 HAPO 研究参与者中，完全调整了 LGA 婴儿分娩的优势比，其特征是出生体重大于第 90 百分位数[3]。血糖水平正常和体重指数正常或偏低的组作为参照组。根据诊断 OGTT 期间空腹、餐后 1h 和餐后 2h 血糖水平的平均标准差（Z 分数）评分确定中间葡萄糖组。在 HAPO 研究队列[3]中，用于定义这一类别的值被选择来达到相当于超重频率的中间葡萄糖频率。在诊断 OGTT 时测量 BMI，通过回归分析转换为等效的 WHO 类别

总之，有证据表明母体 BMI 和血糖与不良妊娠结局具有独立且基本上相加的关联。鉴于此，这些因素的相对"重要性"受到预防或治疗策略的潜在成本和益处的严重影响。

人口风险与预防

解决肥胖 GDM 女性的另一个考虑因素是它们在整个孕妇人群中的相对重要性。许多研究试图解决这一问题，但妊娠期血糖的确定偏误和积极干预 GDM 导致的治疗混淆仍是主要问题。

一项针对 9835 名超重（32%）和肥胖（28%）高发的南加利福尼亚州女性的研究[40]显示，超重和肥胖在无 GDM 女性中 LGA 的发生率是 21.6%，在 GDM 女性中是 23.3%。在她们的研究对象中，75%的 GDM 患者超重或肥胖。本研究也强调妊娠体重增加的重要性，它是 LGA 的一个决定因素，这也被其他人报道过，是一个潜在的可修改的因素[41, 42]。这些结论在很大程度上取决于背景人群。在全球 HAPO 研究队列中，超

重（22%）和肥胖的患病率（14%）要低得多[43]。

综上所述，很明显的是，在超重和肥胖患病率较高的人群中，这些因素构成了 LGA 人群风险的很大一部分。然而，与"以葡萄糖为中心"的 GDM 治疗的积极结果相比，治疗妊娠期肥胖的策略已被证明是令人失望的（参见第十二章）。

妊娠糖尿病和肥胖治疗的证据基础

两个精心设计的大型前瞻性随机对照研究证实了这一点，GDM 的诊断和治疗对母亲及婴儿双方都有短期益处[44, 45]。澳大利亚（克罗瑟）研究的女性妊娠早期 BMI 为 $22.9 \sim 31.2 kg/m^2$，研究干预组的女性在妊娠期间体重增加较少，与未治疗组相比，巨核细胞减少，LGA 减少，子痫前期发生率降低[44]。在美国（兰登）的研究中，女性的 BMI 招募者治疗组是（30.1 ± 5）kg/m^2，在对照组为（30.2 ± 5.1）kg/m^2。同样，在这项研究中，干预组的女性体重增加更少，婴儿 LGA 和巨细胞症的发病率更低，而且女性患子痫前期的比例低于未治疗组[45]。

目前有两项大型试验足以检验超重和肥胖女性在生活方式干预后的孕产妇与围产儿结局——LIMIT 研究[46]和 UPBEAT 研究[47]。这两项试验的结果都令人失望。本质上，这些研究旨在通过生活方式干预限制超重和肥胖妊娠妇女的体重增加。不过，这两项研究都没有发现 GDM 和出生 LGA 婴儿的比例存在差异。LIMIT 研究确实报道了体重超过 4000g 的婴儿体重下降。此外，EMPRWAR 研究中对妊娠早期肥胖女性使用二甲双胍，旨在检测出生体重百分位数的变化，结果发现，出生体重百分位数或母体葡萄糖或脂质指标没有差异[48]。近期另一项肥胖妊娠妇女服用二甲双胍的随机对照试验显示，治疗组妊娠体重增加减少，子痫前期减少，但出生体重的主要结果没有减少，GDM 患病率也没有降低[49]。

在很多小的随机对照试验（通常是强化的）中发现，超重和肥胖妇女经过生活方式和其他干预措施后其在妊娠期间的体重增加减少，一些试验也已证明新生儿体重也减少。这些研究已在 Meta 分析中得到总结[50, 51]。到目前为止，这些小型研究的益处在转化为人口负担得起的实际干预措施时没有得到复制[46]。

目前，对超重和肥胖妇女诊断及治疗 GDM 在限制体重增加、预防孕产妇不良结局和预防新生儿不良结局方面有最好的证据。然而，需要注意的是，这些干预措施对成年子女健康的长期影响还没有得到证实，需要进一步研究。

在子宫内暴露于肥胖和妊娠糖尿病的后代健康问题

出生体重和身体成分

1952 年首次提出的 Pedersen 假说指出，巨体症（胎儿过度生长和肥胖）是由母体高血糖反应所致的胎儿胰岛肥大引起的胎儿高血糖和高胰岛素血症[52]。即使母体血糖控制似乎令人满意，也可能由母体三酰甘油和其他脂质增加而导致巨细胞症[14, 20]。母亲的肥胖预示着更高的胎儿脂肪量[53]，并与之相关出现胎儿胰岛素抵抗[54]。这些结果表明，母亲的肥胖特别影响胎儿的脂肪，而不是胎儿的整体生长。没有肥胖的 GDM 也与胎儿肥胖有关[55]。出生体重和胎儿脂肪无限制增长均与妊娠晚期母亲胰岛素敏感性相关[12]。

母亲肥胖使儿童肥胖的风险翻倍[56, 57]，并与后代的代谢综合征相关[58]。同样，即使不考虑母体 GDM，出生时 LGA 的儿童发生代谢综合征的风险也会增加[58, 59]。在葡萄糖耐受性强的比马印第安母亲中，她们的基因倾向于在发展为 2 型糖尿病时，妊娠妇女在妊娠晚期的血糖水平与后代患 2 型糖尿病的风险增加密切相关[60]。

这些在后代中增加的风险可能在很大程度上是由易于肥胖的遗传背景及与家庭生活方式有关的出生后环境决定的。然而，据健康和疾病的发展起源（DOHaD）理论所示，一些疾病风险的增加可能由宫内环境改变所致。动物模型已经证明表观遗传调控可以改变后代许多调节和代谢器官，包括大脑、肝脏、胰腺[61]和肾上腺，以应对妊娠期和哺乳期的母亲肥胖与高血糖。在人类中，宫内环境长期的影响已被荷兰冬季饥饿研究中[62]母亲营养不良状态的影响证实。因此，胎儿宫内环境可能会影响胎儿的健康，这种影响甚至远超过胎儿出生后环境的影响。

对于母亲来说，GDM 与未来高血压、糖耐量受损和高脂血症的高风险相关，这些都是代谢综合征的组成部分[59]。这些增加的风险在妊娠前肥胖的女性中尤为明显[59]。

对后代的其他影响

除了宫内过度生长外，糖尿病妇女和肥胖妇女所生婴儿还可能出现其他严重并发症。这些风险有相似之处，也有不同之处，而妊娠妇女的糖尿病和肥胖状况对婴儿的影响是起协同作用的。

糖尿病母亲的后代

先天畸形

孕妇妊娠前糖尿病与先天畸形增加之间的关系早已被认识到。这种风险显然与受孕前后和器官发生期间的血糖控制有关。在 Meta 分析中，妊娠前期糖尿病患者发生重大先天畸形的相对风险增加了 2.7 倍[63]。最近的人口登记研究表明，1 型糖尿病妇女的先天畸形率持续增加，2 型糖尿病妇女的先天畸形率进一步增加[64]。

肥胖母亲的后代

先天畸形

母亲肥胖本身与先天畸形率的增加有关。最近的一项系统回顾显示了母亲肥胖和先天性心脏缺陷两者之间的阳性相关性。中度肥胖与重度肥胖相关性分别增加 1.15 和 1.39，与糖尿病无关。然而，对于超重的女性，只有当有糖尿病的女性被纳入分析[65]时才会有关联（OR：1.08）。佛罗里达州出生缺陷登记处的一项分析显示，这种疾病的发病率使出生缺陷的比例从 3.9% 增加到在 BMI>40kg/m^2 的肥胖妇女中的 5.3%[66]。研究表明，大多数出生缺陷的剂量-效应关系是阳性的，妊娠妇女肥胖除外[66]。此外，在肥胖妇女中，母亲肥胖使产前发现先天异常的概率降低了 23%[67]。

对新生儿并发症的影响

除了过度肥胖，肥胖女性的后代在出生时代谢更加不健康，脐带血中的 HOMA - IR、leptin 和 IL-6 含量更高[54]。使用人体测量方法和全身电导率进行的肥胖评估显示，出生体重略微增加，消瘦体型比例没有变化，但超重或肥胖妇女所生新生儿的体脂百分比显著增加，从9.7%增加到11.6%[53]。LGA的风险随着肥胖母亲体重的增加而增加[68]。经妊娠期体重增加调整后，与正常体重、血糖正常的女性相比，GDM正常体重女性的LGA发病率增加了1.96%，仅肥胖女性增加了2.63%，而GDM肥胖女性的LGA发病率增加了5.47%[69]。出生时肥胖和病态肥胖的婴儿的新生儿低血糖风险增加，病态肥胖妇女的婴儿早产、重症监护和黄疸的风险也增加[70]。

同时患有糖尿病和肥胖母亲的后代

母亲糖尿病和母亲肥胖的影响是相加的和独立的。治疗母亲糖尿病和减少母亲体重增加可能会改善两者对婴儿的影响。

对身体组成和大小的影响

在GDM设置中，OGTT试验中妊娠妇女体重和空腹血糖与出生体重独立相关，只有分娩时妊娠妇女体重显著独立预测LGA[71]。在1型糖尿病妇女中，母亲的BMI与LGA患病率的变化无关，但2型糖尿病妇女、超重妇女和肥胖妇女更可能生产LGA[72]。然而，妊娠妇女妊娠期体重增加会影响1型糖尿病妇女生产LGA的风险，妊娠妇女体重每周增加450g，生产LGA的风险增加4%[72]。在1型糖尿病患者中，婴儿出生体重随着母亲体重的增加而增加，即使在调整母亲体重指数、36周时的糖化血红蛋白、吸烟、体重平衡和种族因素后，体重仍会增加[73]。在2型糖尿病妇女中进行的一项类似研究显示，妊娠期体重过度增加的妇女的婴儿出生体重比常规妊娠期体重增加的妇女的婴儿出生体重高0.5kg[74]。

总结与未来研究

GDM和妊娠妇女肥胖与一系列类似的不良妊娠结局相关，尤其是与胎儿过度生长、肥胖和高血压并发症相关的不良妊娠结局相关。GDM与肥胖共同存在，但并非不可避免，共同的预防和治疗策略的发展似乎是一个诱人的前景。

尽管数据显示 GDM 和肥胖与不良妊娠结局之间存在关联，但我们对这些关联机制的了解仍然有限。Pedersen 假设作为一个有用的框架来考虑妊娠高血糖的发病机制[21]，但即使是我们最积极的达到正常血糖的方法也没有使妊娠结局正常化，尤其是在肥胖作为一种常见病的情况下。针对妊娠期 GDM 和肥胖的血脂异常的特异性治疗看起来很吸引人，但由于安全问题，实际操作起来很困难[14]。对妊娠期代谢性炎症及其后果的探索也可能改善我们对其机制的理解[26, 75, 76]，但目前的治疗方案似乎仍然有限。

在妊娠期间开始的干预措施似乎在预防肥胖并发症方面效果有限。这与肥胖妇女（与正常体重妇女相比）的观察结果一致，妊娠前体重与新生儿肥胖的关系比妊娠期间体重增加更密切[77]。因此，可能需要采取预防和治疗措施来获得积极的效益。相比之下，GDM 的治疗效果得到了很好的证明。有效实施 GDM 诊断和治疗策略[78-80]目前似乎具有最大的整体效益潜力。未来的研究应侧重于通过基础研究和临床研究来阐明肥胖与 GDM 的发病机制，制定针对妊娠前、妊娠期间和妊娠后这两种情况的有效战略，以及有效实施已知有效但目前未得到充分利用的治疗措施。

选择题

1. 以下指标(平均)在妊娠女性肥胖状态比消瘦状态更低的是（　　）
   A. 血清瘦素　　　　　　　　B. 体重指数
   C. 血清脂联素　　　　　　　D. 空腹血清胰岛素
   E. 稳态模型评估-胰岛素抵抗（HOMA-IR）

正确答案是 C。血清脂联素与"健康"代谢谱有关，在妊娠期间和妊娠外的肥胖人群血清中浓度较低。

2. 下列关于妊娠期口服葡萄糖耐量试验（OGTT）的陈述正确的是（　　）
   A. OGTT 前 5 天必须避免糖类摄入过多
   B. OGTT 能明确地鉴别所有孕育 LGA 的女性
   C. 所有 OGTT 值（空腹，餐后 1h、2h 和 3h）一般都是紧密相关的
   D. OGTT 结果具有较高的重复性

E. 使用葡萄糖聚合物比使用葡萄糖单体产生更少的恶心和呕吐

正确答案是 E。虽然葡萄糖单体在 HAPO 研究中使用较多，应用范围更广。

3. 关于肥胖和 GDM，下面表述正确的是（　　　）

　　A. 在缺乏 GDM 的情况下，肥胖与妊娠并发症无关

　　B. 在没有肥胖的情况下，GDM 与妊娠并发症无关

　　C. 肥胖和 GDM 在妊娠并发症的风险方面通常具有叠加效应

　　D. 在人口学基础上，GDM 比肥胖对妊娠时 LGA 的影响更大

　　E. 对妊娠期肥胖可采取有效的治疗方法

正确答案是 C。肥胖和 GDM 都与妊娠并发症的增加有关，其影响通常是累加的（而不是协同或倍增的）。在大多数人群中，肥胖对人群比 GDM 对 LGA 风险的影响更大。

（王　冰　译，朱海清　校）

参 考 文 献

1. Hanson MA, Gluckman PD, Ma RC, Matzen P, Biesma RG. Early life opportunities for prevention of diabetes in low and middle income countries. BMC Public Health 2012;12:1025. PubMed PMID: 23176627.
2. Guariguata L, Linnenkamp U, Beagley J, Whiting DR, Cho NH. Global estimates of the prevalence of hyperglycaemia in pregnancy. Diabetes Res Clin Pract 2014 Feb;103(2):176–185. PubMed PMID: 24300020.
3. Catalano PM, McIntyre HD, Cruickshank JK, McCance DR, Dyer AR, Metzger BE, et al. The Hyperglycemia and Adverse Pregnancy Outcome Study: associations of GDM and obesity with pregnancy outcomes. Diabetes Care 2012 Feb 22;35(4):780–786. PubMed PMID: 22357187.
4. Carrington ER, Shuman CR, Reardon HS. Evaluation of the prediabetic state during pregnancy. Obstetr Gynecol 1957 Jun;9(6):664–669. PubMed PMID: 13431126.
5. O'Sullivan JB, Mahan CM. Criteria for the oral glucose tolerance test in pregnancy. Diabetes 1964 May–Jun;13:278–285. PubMed PMID: 14166677.
6. McIntyre HD. Diagnosing gestational diabetes mellitus: rationed or rationally related to risk? Diabetes Care 2013 Oct;36(10):2879–2880. PubMed PMID: 24065840.
7. Metzger BE, Buchanan TA, Coustan DR, et al. Summary and recommendations of the Fifth International Workshop – Conference on Gestational Diabetes Mellitus. Diabetes Care 2007;30:S251–S260.
8. Omori Y, Jovanovic L. Proposal for the reconsideration of the definition of gestational diabetes. Diabetes Care 2005 Oct;28(10):2592–2593. PubMed PMID: 16186312.
9. Metzger BE, Gabbe SG, Persson B, Buchanan TA, Catalano PA, Damm P, et al. International association of diabetes and pregnancy study groups recommendations on the diagnosis and classification of hyperglycemia in pregnancy. Diabetes Care 2010 Mar;33(3):676–682. PubMed PMID: 20190296.

10 Colagiuri S, Falavigna M, Agarwal MM, Boulvain M, Coetzee E, Hod M, et al. Strategies for implementing the WHO diagnostic criteria and classification of hyperglycaemia first detected in pregnancy. Diabetes Res Clin Pract 2014;103.

11 WHO. Obesity: Preventing and Managing the Global Epidemic: Report of a WHO Consultation. World Health Organization Technical Report series. WHO: Geneva, 2000. PubMed PMID: 11234459.

12 Catalano PM, Ehrenberg HM. The short- and long-term implications of maternal obesity on the mother and her offspring. BJOG 2006 Oct;113(10):1126–1133. PubMed PMID: 16827826.

13 Catalano PM, Nizielski SE, Shao J, Preston L, Qiao L, Friedman JE. Downregulated IRS-1 and PPARg in obese women with gestational diabetes: relationship to FFA during pregnancy. American J Physiol Endocrinol Metabol 2002;282(3):E522–E533.

14 Barrett HL, Dekker Nitert M, McIntyre HD, Callaway LK. Normalizing metabolism in diabetic pregnancy: is it time to target lipids? Diabetes Care 2014 May;37(5):1484–1493. PubMed PMID: 24757231.

15 Lambrinoudaki I, Vlachou SA, Creatsas G. Genetics in gestational diabetes mellitus: association with incidence, severity, pregnancy outcome and response to treatment. Current Diabetes Rev 2010 Nov;6(6):393–399. PubMed PMID: 20879971.

16 Park S, Kim MY, Baik SH, Woo JT, Kwon YJ, Daily JW, et al. Gestational diabetes is associated with high energy and saturated fat intakes and with low plasma visfatin and adiponectin levels independent of prepregnancy BMI. Europ J Clin Nutr 2013 Feb;67(2):196–201. PubMed PMID: 23385969.

17 Moleda P, Homa K, Safranow K, Celewicz Z, Fronczyk A, Majkowska L. Women with normal glucose tolerance and a history of gestational diabetes show significant impairment of beta-cell function at normal insulin sensitivity. Diabetes Metabol 2013 Apr;39(2):155–162. PubMed PMID: 23369626.

18 Morkrid K, Jenum AK, Sletner L, Vardal MH, Waage CW, Nakstad B, et al. Failure to increase insulin secretory capacity during pregnancy-induced insulin resistance is associated with ethnicity and gestational diabetes. Europ J Endocrinol 2012 Oct;167(4):579–588. PubMed PMID: 22889687.

19 Harmon KA, Gerard L, Jensen DR, Kealey EH, Hernandez TL, Reece MS, et al. Continuous glucose profiles in obese and normal-weight pregnant women on a controlled diet: metabolic determinants of fetal growth. Diabetes Care 2011 Oct;34(10):2198–2204. PubMed PMID: 21775754.

20 Barrett HL, Gatford KL, Houda CM, De Blasio MJ, McIntyre HD, Callaway LK, et al. Maternal and neonatal circulating markers of metabolic and cardiovascular risk in the Metformin in Gestational Diabetes (MiG) Trial: responses to maternal metformin versus insulin treatment. Diabetes Care 2013 Mar;36(3):529–536. PubMed PMID: 23048188.

21 Catalano PM, Hauguel-De Mouzon S. Is it time to revisit the Pedersen hypothesis in the face of the obesity epidemic? Am J Obstet Gynecol 2011 Jun;204(6):479–487. PubMed PMID: 21288502.

22 Giovannone B, Scaldaferri ML, Federici M, Porzio O, Lauro D, Fusco A, et al. Insulin receptor substrate (IRS) transduction system: distinct and overlapping signaling potential. Diabetes/Metabol Res Rev 2000 Nov–Dec;16(6):434–441. PubMed PMID: 11114102.

23 Lappas M. Effect of pre-existing maternal obesity, gestational diabetes and adipokines on the expression of genes involved in lipid metabolism in adipose tissue. Metabolism 2014;63(2):250–262.

24 Radaelli T, Varastehpour A, Catalano P, Hauguel-de Mouzon S. Gestational diabetes induces placental genes for

chronic stress and inflammatory pathways. Diabetes 2003;52(12):2951–2958.
25 Catalano PM. Trying to understand gestational diabetes. Diabetic Med 2014 Mar;31(3):273–281. PubMed PMID: 24341419.
26 Radaelli T, Farrell KA, Huston-Presley L, Amini SB, Kirwan JP, McIntyre HD, et al. Estimates of insulin sensitivity using glucose and C-peptide from the hyperglycemia and adverse pregnancy outcome glucose tolerance test. Diabetes Care 2010 Mar;33(3):490–494. PubMed PMID: 20032280.
27 Sacks G, Sargent I, Redman C. An innate view of human pregnancy. Immunology Today 1999;20(3):114–118.
28 Messerli M, May K, Hansson SR, Schneider H, Holzgreve W, Hahn S, et al. Feto-maternal interactions in pregnancies: placental microparticles activate peripheral blood monocytes. Placenta 2010;31(2):106–112.
29 Clifton VL, Stark MJ, Osei-Kumah A, Hodyl NA. Review: The feto-placental unit, pregnancy pathology and impact on long term maternal health. Placenta 2012;33(Suppl, 0):S37–S41.
30 Denney JM, Nelson EL, Wadhwa PD, Waters TP, Mathew L, Chung EK, et al. Longitudinal modulation of immune system cytokine profile during pregnancy. Cytokine 2011;53(2):170–177.
31 Lopez-Tinoco C, Roca M, Fernandez-Deudero A, Garcia-Valero A, Bugatto F, Aguilar-Diosdado M, et al. Cytokine profile, metabolic syndrome and cardiovascular disease risk in women with late-onset gestational diabetes mellitus. Cytokine 2012 Apr;58(1):14–19. PubMed PMID: 22200508.
32 Wolf M, Sauk J, Shah A, Vossen Smirnakis K, Jimenez-Kimble R, Ecker JL, et al. Inflammation and Glucose Intolerance: a prospective study of gestational diabetes mellitus. Diabetes Care 2004;27(1):21–27.
33 Pantham P, Aye IL, Powell TL. Inflammation in maternal obesity and gestational diabetes mellitus. Placenta 2015 Jul;36(7):709–715. PubMed PMID: 25972077.
34 Torloni MR, Betran AP, Horta BL, Nakamura MU, Atallah AN, Moron AF, et al. Prepregnancy BMI and the risk of gestational diabetes: a systematic review of the literature with meta-analysis. Obesity Rev 2009 Mar;10(2):194–203. PubMed PMID: 19055539.
35 Friedman JE, Ishizuka T, Shao J, Huston L, Highman T, Catalano P. Impaired glucose transport and insulin receptor tyrosine phosphorylation in skeletal muscle from obese women with gestational diabetes. Diabetes 1999 Sep;48(9):1807–1814. PubMed PMID: 10480612.
36 HAPO Study Cooperative Research Group. Hyperglycaemia and Adverse Pregnancy Outcome (HAPO) Study: associations with maternal body mass index. BJOG 2010 Apr;117(5):575–584. PubMed PMID: 20089115.
37 Langer O. Obesity or diabetes: which is more hazardous to the health of the offspring? J Matern Fetal Neonat 2015 Jan 8:1–5. PubMed PMID: 25471171.
38 Harper LM, Renth A, Cade WT, Colvin R, Macones GA, Cahill AG. Impact of obesity on maternal and neonatal outcomes in insulin-resistant pregnancy. Amer J Perinatol 2014 May;31(5):383–388. PubMed PMID: 23877768.
39 Langer O, Yogev Y, Most O, Xenakis EM. Gestational diabetes: the consequences of not treating. Amer J Obstetr Gynecol 2005;192(4):989–997.
40 Black MH, Sacks DA, Xiang AH, Lawrence JM. The relative contribution of prepregnancy overweight and obesity, gestational weight gain, and IADPSG-defined gestational diabetes mellitus to fetal overgrowth. Diabetes Care 2013;36(1):56–62. doi:10.2337/dc12-0741
41 Kim SY, Sharma AJ, Sappenfield W, Wilson HG, Salihu HM. Association of maternal body mass index, excessive weight gain, and gestational diabetes mellitus with large-for-gestational-age births. Obstetr Gynecol 2014 Apr;123(4):737–744. PubMed PMID: 24785599.

42 Alberico S, Montico M, Barresi V, Monasta L, Businelli C, Soini V, et al. The role of gestational diabetes, pre-pregnancy body mass index and gestational weight gain on the risk of newborn macrosomia: results from a prospective multicentre study. BMC Pregnancy Childbirth 2014;14:23. PubMed PMID: 24428895.
43 McIntyre HD, Catalano PM. Comment on: Black et al. The relative contribution of prepregnancy overweight and obesity, gestational weight gain, and IADPSG-defined gestational diabetes mellitus to fetal overgrowth. Diabetes Care 2013;36:56–62. Diabetes Care. 2013 Aug;36(8):e127. PubMed PMID: 23881980.
44 Crowther CA, Hiller JE, Moss JR, McPhee AJ, Jeffries WS, Robinson JS. Effect of treatment of gestational diabetes mellitus on pregnancy outcomes. N Engl J Med 2005 Jun 16;352(24):2477–2486. PubMed PMID: 15951574.
45 Landon MB, Spong CY, Thom E, Carpenter MW, Ramin SM, Casey B, et al. A multicenter, randomized trial of treatment for mild gestational diabetes. N Engl J Med 2009 Oct 1;361(14):1339–1348. PubMed PMID: 19797280.
46 Dodd JM, Turnbull D, McPhee AJ, Deussen AR, Grivell RM, Yelland LN, et al. Antenatal lifestyle advice for women who are overweight or obese: LIMIT randomised trial. BMJ (clinical research ed.) 2014;348:g1285. PubMed PMID: 24513442.
47 Poston L, Bell R, Croker H, Flynn AC, Godfrey KM, Goff L, et al. Effect of a behavioural intervention in obese pregnant women (the UPBEAT study): a multicentre, randomised controlled trial. Lancet Diabetes Endocrinol 2015 Oct;3(10):767–777. PubMed PMID: 26165396.
48 Chiswick C, Reynolds RM, Denison F, Drake AJ, Forbes S, Newby DE, et al. Effect of metformin on maternal and fetal outcomes in obese pregnant women (EMPOWaR): a randomised, double-blind, placebo-controlled trial. Lancet Diabetes Endocrinol 2015 Oct;3(10):778–786. PubMed PMID: 26165398.
49 Syngelaki A, Nicolaides KH, Balani J, Hyer S, Akolekar R, Kotecha R, et al. Metformin versus placebo in obese pregnant women without diabetes mellitus. N Engl J Med 2016 Feb 4;374(5):434–443. PubMed PMID: 26840133.
50 Dodd JM, Grivell RM, Crowther CA, Robinson JS. Antenatal interventions for overweight or obese pregnant women: a systematic review of randomised trials. BJOG 2010 Oct;117(11):1316–1326. PubMed PMID: 20353459.
51 Oteng-Ntim E, Varma R, Croker H, Poston L, Doyle P. Lifestyle interventions for overweight and obese pregnant women to improve pregnancy outcome: systematic review and meta-analysis. BMC Med 2012;10:47. PubMed PMID: 22574949.
52 Pedersen J. Diabetes and pregnancy: blood sugar of newborn infants during fasting and glucose administration. Nord Med 1952 Jul 25;47(30):1049. PubMed PMID: 14948109.
53 Sewell MF, Huston-Presley L, Super DM, Catalano P. Increased neonatal fat mass, not lean body mass, is associated with maternal obesity. Am J Obstet Gynecol 2006 Oct;195(4):1100–1103. PubMed PMID: 16875645.
54 Catalano PM, Presley L, Minium J, Hauguel-de Mouzon S. Fetuses of obese mothers develop insulin resistance in utero. Diabetes Care 2009 Jun;32(6):1076–1080. PubMed PMID: 19460915.
55 Catalano PM, Thomas A, Huston-Presley L, Amini SB. Increased fetal adiposity: a very sensitive marker of abnormal in utero development. Am J Obstet Gynecol 2003 Dec;189(6):1698–1704. PubMed PMID: 14710101.
56 Whitaker RC. Predicting preschooler obesity at birth: the role of maternal obesity in early pregnancy. Pediatrics 2004 Jul;114(1):e29–e36. PubMed PMID: 15231970.
57 Reilly JJ, Armstrong J, Dorosty AR, Emmett PM, Ness A, Rogers I, et al. Early life risk factors for obesity in childhood: cohort study. BMJ (clinical research ed) 2005 Jun

11;330(7504):1357. PubMed PMID: 15908441.
58. Boney CM, Verma A, Tucker R, Vohr BR. Metabolic syndrome in childhood: association with birth weight, maternal obesity, and gestational diabetes mellitus. Pediatrics 2005 Mar;115(3):e290–e296. PubMed PMID: 15741354.
59. Vohr BR, Boney CM. Gestational diabetes: the forerunner for the development of maternal and childhood obesity and metabolic syndrome? J Matern Fetal Neonatal Med 2008 Mar;21(3):149–157. PubMed PMID: 18297569.
60. Franks PW, Looker HC, Kobes S, Touger L, Tataranni PA, Hanson RL, et al. Gestational glucose tolerance and risk of type 2 diabetes in young Pima Indian offspring. Diabetes 2006;55(2):460–465.
61. Sandovici I, Smith NH, Nitert MD, Ackers-Johnson M, Uribe-Lewis S, Ito Y, et al. Maternal diet and aging alter the epigenetic control of a promoter-enhancer interaction at the Hnf4a gene in rat pancreatic islets. Proc Natl Acad Sci USA. 2011 Mar 29;108(13):5449–5454. PubMed PMID: 21385945.
62. Roseboom TJ, Painter RC, van Abeelen AFM, Veenendaal MVE, de Rooij SR. Hungry in the womb: what are the consequences? Lessons from the Dutch famine. Maturitas 2011;70(2):141–145.
63. Balsells M, Garcia-Patterson A, Gich I, Corcoy R. Major congenital malformations in women with gestational diabetes mellitus: a systematic review and meta-analysis. Diabetes Metab Res Rev 2012 Mar;28(3):252–257. PubMed PMID: 22052679.
64. Vinceti M, Malagoli C, Rothman KJ, Rodolfi R, Astolfi G, Calzolari E, et al. Risk of birth defects associated with maternal pregestational diabetes. Eur J Epidemiol 2014 Jun;29(6):411–418. PubMed PMID: 24861339.
65. Cai GJ, Sun XX, Zhang L, Hong Q. Association between maternal body mass index and congenital heart defects in offspring: a systematic review. Am J Obstet Gynecol 2014 Aug;211(2):91–117. PubMed PMID: 24631708.
66. Block SR, Watkins SM, Salemi JL, Rutkowski R, Tanner JP, Correia JA, et al. Maternal pre-pregnancy body mass index and risk of selected birth defects: evidence of a dose-response relationship. Paediatr Perinat Epidemiol 2013 Nov;27(6):521–531. PubMed PMID: 24117964.
67. Best KE, Tennant PW, Bell R, Rankin J. Impact of maternal body mass index on the antenatal detection of congenital anomalies. BJOG 2012 Nov;119(12):1503–1511. PubMed PMID: 22900903.
68. Vesco KK, Sharma AJ, Dietz PM, Rizzo JH, Callaghan WM, England L, et al. Newborn size among obese women with weight gain outside the 2009 Institute of Medicine recommendation. Obstet Gynecol 2011 Apr;117(4):812–818. PubMed PMID: 21422851.
69. Black MH, Sacks DA, Xiang AH, Lawrence JM. The relative contribution of prepregnancy overweight and obesity, gestational weight gain, and IADPSG-defined gestational diabetes mellitus to fetal overgrowth. Diabetes Care 2013 Jan;36(1):56–62. PubMed PMID: 22891256.
70. Callaway LK, Prins JB, Chang AM, McIntyre HD. The prevalence and impact of overweight and obesity in an Australian obstetric population. Med J Aust 2006 Jan 16;184(2):56–59. PubMed PMID: 16411868.
71. Ben-Haroush A, Hadar E, Chen R, Hod M, Yogev Y. Maternal obesity is a major risk factor for large-for-gestational-infants in pregnancies complicated by gestational diabetes. Arch Gynecol Obstet 2009 Apr;279(4):539–543. PubMed PMID: 18758799.
72. Feghali MN, Khoury JC, Timofeev J, Shveiky D, Driggers RW, Miodovnik M. Asymmetric large for gestational age newborns in pregnancies complicated by diabetes mellitus: is maternal obesity a culprit? J Matern Fetal Neonatal Med 2012 Jan;25(1):32–35. PubMed PMID: 21957900.

73 Secher AL, Parellada CB, Ringholm L, Asbjornsdottir B, Damm P, Mathiesen ER. Higher gestational weight gain is associated with increasing offspring birth weight independent of maternal glycemic control in women with type 1 diabetes. Diabetes Care 2014 Oct;37(10):2677–2684. PubMed PMID: 25249669.

74 Parellada CB, Asbjornsdottir B, Ringholm L, Damm P, Mathiesen ER. Fetal growth in relation to gestational weight gain in women with type 2 diabetes: an observational study. Diabet Med 2014 Dec;31(12):1681–1689. PubMed PMID: 25081349.

75 Challier JC, Basu S, Bintein T, Minium J, Hotmire K, Catalano PM, et al. Obesity in Pregnancy Stimulates Macrophage Accumulation and Inflammation in the Placenta. Placenta 2008 Feb 8. PubMed PMID: 18262644.

76 Desoye G, Hauguel-de Mouzon S. The human placenta in gestational diabetes mellitus: the insulin and cytokine network. Diabetes Care 2007 Jul;30(Suppl 2):S120–S126. PubMed PMID: 17596459.

77 Waters TP, Huston-Presley L, Catalano PM. Neonatal body composition according to the revised institute of medicine recommendations for maternal weight gain. J Clin Endocrinol Metab 2012;97(10):3648–3654. doi:10.1210/jc.2012-1781

78 Marseille E, Lohse N, Jiwani A, Hod M, Seshiah V, Yajnik CS, et al. The cost-effectiveness of gestational diabetes screening including prevention of type 2 diabetes: application of a new model in India and Israel. J Matern Fetal Neonatal Med 2013;14:14.

79 Jiwani A, Marseille E, Lohse N, Damm P, Hod M, Kahn JG. Gestational diabetes mellitus: results from a survey of country prevalence and practices. J Matern Fetal Neonat 2012 Jun;25(6):600–610. PubMed PMID: 21762003.

80 Lohse N, Marseille E, Kahn JG. Development of a model to assess the cost-effectiveness of gestational diabetes mellitus screening and lifestyle change for the prevention of type 2 diabetes mellitus. Int J Gynaecol Obstet 2011 Nov;115 Suppl 1:S20–25. PubMed PMID: 22099435.

第八章 妊娠糖尿病的代谢异常

Ravi Retnakaran

Leadership Sinai Centre for Diabetes, Mount Sinai Hospital; Division of Endocrinology, University of Toronto; and Lunenfeld-Tanenbaum Research Institute, Mount Sinai Hospital, Toronto, Canada

实践要点

- GDM 女性在未来发展为 2 型糖尿病和心血管疾病的风险较高。
- 与同龄人相比，患有 GDM 的女性在糖尿病或糖尿病之外的多种代谢异常的风险增加。这些异常包括代谢综合征、血脂异常、高血压、亚临床炎症和脂肪因子分泌失调。
- 在有 GDM 病史的妇女中，着重考虑其可改变的心血管代谢危险因素，如血压、血脂和体重。

病 例

一位 41 岁的女性正在向她的新家庭医师进行初步咨询。她目前没有急切的疾病需要治疗，也没有服用过任何药物。既往史是 3 年前第一次妊娠时患有 GDM。她的母亲有 2 型糖尿病（T_2DM）。已婚，有一个孩子，在银行工作。体检时体重 70kg，BMI 为 26.3kg/m^2，血压为 130/80mmHg，心率为 72 次/分。除此之外，体检没有其他异常。

她对自身的医疗保健非常积极，并认识到告知新家庭医师 GDM 病史很重要。她明白，基于既往 GDM 的病史，将来有患 T_2DM 的风险。事实上，她妊娠后还进行过产后葡萄糖耐量试验。她当下的困惑是，GDM 病史是否表明除了 T_2DM 外，还可能有其他代谢紊乱的风险。

妊娠糖尿病：一种慢性代谢紊乱

虽然 GDM 是根据高血糖诊断的一种慢性代谢紊乱，但 GDM 的人群是除了血糖异常外还患有多种代谢异常的女性[1]。重要的是，这些代谢缺陷很多存在于妊娠期间，并可能持续下去。事实上，有 GDM 史的女性和同龄人之间的代谢功能的差异是常有的。此外，越来越多的证据表明，与在妊娠期维持正常糖耐量的妇女相比，GDM 患者在妊娠期间会发展为临床和代谢差异[2]。因此，GDM 很可能是一种慢性病，妊娠时临床上出现的代谢紊乱在妊娠后很长一段时间内持续存在，并可能先于妊娠而出现。这种病理的典型例子是，慢性胰岛 B 细胞功能障碍和胰岛素抵抗会促进 GDM 的发展和增加产后发展为 T_2DM 的风险（参见第九章和第二十七章）[3-5]。在本章中，我们将回顾除了胰岛 B 细胞功能障碍和胰岛素抵抗之外的与 GDM 相关的其他代谢异常。

妊娠糖尿病妇女代谢综合征

代谢综合征是一组描述个体特定心血管代谢危险因素的综合征。尽管不同组织已经提出了代谢综合征的各种定义，但组分危险因素通常包括中心性肥胖、葡萄糖不耐受、高血压、高三酰甘油血症、低高密度脂蛋白（HDL）血症[6]。代谢综合征自从引入以来，其诊断标准、病理生理基础、临床实用性甚至其存在性等就一直存在争议[6]。然而，这些问题仍然清楚地表明，由该综合征所确定的患者人群存在发展成为 T_2DM 和心血管疾病的高风险[6]。因此，GDM 患者是最终发生前两者风险的妇女群体[7-10]。因此，GDM 与代谢综合征之间的关系值得考虑。一些研究表明，有 GDM 病史的妇女代谢综合征的患病率增加[11-14]。例如，在丹麦有 GDM 病史的妇女中，产后 9.8 年代谢综合征的患病率（如 WHO 标准[6]所定义的）为 38.4%，而在没有 GDM 病史的同龄人中，患病率为 11%[11]。有代谢综合征的年龄和 BMI 调整的优势比为 3.4（95% CI：2.5～4.8）[11]。同样，美国的研究人群在产后 11 年，代谢综合征的患病率（由国家胆固醇教育计划-成人治疗小组Ⅲ标准[6]定义）为 27.2%[12]。总体而言，最近的荟萃分析包括 17 项研究，涉及 5832 名妇女，研究证实了妊娠合并糖尿病后具有更高的代谢综合征风险（优势比：3.96；95% CI：2.99～5.26）[13]。重要的是，这种增加的代谢综合征的风险最早在分娩后 3 个月出现，患病率为 20%（国际糖尿病协会标准）或 16.8%（美国心脏协会/国家心肺血液研究所标准）[14]。在调整包括 BMI 的共变量后，有 GDM 病史的妇女代谢综合征的风险仍然增加[14]。因此，在产后早期就存在这种疾病提醒我们需要注意，GDM 妇女是否在妊娠期间也一样存在代谢综合征的风险。由于缺乏在妊娠状态下诊断代谢综合征的标准，因此排除了对这种可能性的直接评价。然而，Clark 等的横断面研究显示，在产前葡萄糖耐量测试时，被诊断 GDM 的女性确实表现出代谢紊乱的特征，包括低 HDL 和高三酰甘油[15]。

总的来说，这些数据导致 GDM 可以代表潜在代谢综合征[2, 15]的假说。因此，GDM 和代谢综合征的各组成部分之间的关系是值得关注的。尽管在第九章和第二十七章中讨论了 GDM 女性的中心性肥胖和血糖异常的风险，但本章接下来将着重介绍血脂异常和高血压及新出现的代谢功能障碍的非传统标志物，即亚临床炎症和脂肪因子分泌失调。

妊娠糖尿病妇女血脂谱的研究

由于胎儿发育中需要胆固醇和必需脂肪酸，脂蛋白会出现生理上调。妊娠期的激素（特别是雌激素）环境导致高脂血症，并向胎盘和胎儿输送脂质[16]。因此，妊娠期血清三酰甘油和低密度脂蛋白（LDL）升高，而妊娠中期 HDL 峰值下降[16]。在此背景下，先前的研究已经报道了 GDM 对妊娠期血脂谱的影响不同，尽管普遍发现 GDM 妇女的三酰甘油较高，HDL 胆固醇较同龄人低[16-18]。然而，这些差异对胎儿的影响仍然不确定。一些研究者报道了较高的母体三酰甘油浓度与胎儿脂肪量或出生体重增加之间的关联，但这在所有研究中都没有被一致地观察到[16, 19, 20]。在此背景下，研究之间的比较受到葡萄糖耐量标准差异的限制。

虽然妊娠期的生理适应可能掩盖了妊娠期 GDM 患者和未妊娠 GDM 患者的血脂差异，但这些差异在妊娠后的数年中是明显的。这些差异包括低密度脂蛋白和高密度脂蛋白、三酰甘油和肝脏脂肪含量[14, 18, 21, 22]。此外，与代谢综合征一样，有和没有 GDM 的妇女之间的血脂差异在产后 3 个月内很容易检测到[18]。事实上，在一项对妊娠期和产后 3 个月的 482 名妇女的各种糖代谢状态的研究中，发现不同糖耐量情况的妊娠妇女（从正常到 GDM）妊娠中期的后期和妊娠晚期的早期血脂谱几乎没有差异，而产后存在明显的梯度[18]。最值得注意的是，在多元线性回归分析中，GDM 作为产后总胆固醇、LDL、三酰甘油、总胆固醇/HDL 比值和载脂蛋白 B（APOB）的独立预测因子，以及 HDL 胆固醇的逆预测因子。而高三酰甘油血症和低 HDL 是 T_2DM 中血脂异常的典型特征，因此在 GDM 妇女中可能是预期的（即鉴于其与 T_2DM 的病理生理和临床关系），LDL 和 APOB 增加尤其值得注意。具体来说，这些观察结果（甚至在产后早期就可以检测到）增加了患有 GDM 妇女患慢性动脉粥样硬化性血脂异常的可能性，这可能是导致其心血管疾病风险增加的因素，这已在产后 11~12 年的研究中得到证实[9, 10]。

GDM 中脂质生理学的其他因素可能支持这一假说。首先，与同龄人相比，GDM 的妇女具有以下特点：①更低的平均 LDL 粒径；②小的、致密的 LDL 颗粒占优势；③LDL 的亚种分布变化的特点是非常小的 LDL ⅣA 和 LDL ⅣB 亚类的比例增加[23, 24]。小而致密的 LDL 已知易被氧化，从而有助于内皮功能障碍和动脉粥样硬化。因此，值得注意的是，GDM 的妇女已经被证明在整个妊娠期内 LDL 对氧化的敏感性增加[25]。虽然绝对 LDL 浓度可能不会明显升高，但从这些数据中得出的结果是，有 GDM 病史的女性多年暴露于高 LDL 水平和增强的氧化易感性的组合中可能有助于增加长期心血管风险[18]。

妊娠高血压综合征患者的血压

妊娠高血压疾病可分为四组：①慢性高血压；②妊娠高血压；③先兆子痫或子痫；④先兆子痫叠加慢性高血压[26, 27]。GDM 和这些疾病之间有几个关联：第一，GDM 和妊娠期高血压疾病共有几种常见的危险因素，包括糖尿病风险的主要临床决定因素，如孕母年龄增加、肥胖、种族和家族史[26]。第二，GDM 本身与妊娠期高血压风险增加有关[27]。第三，妊娠早期血压升高可预测调整后的 GDM 风险，包括年龄、种族、BMI 和产次[28]。虽然 GDM 与高血压关系的病因基础是不确定的，但胰岛素抵抗已经被认为是有助于这两种疾病的病理生理学的因素[29]。

在分娩后的几年中，有几项研究报道了与没有这些病史的女性相比，既往 GDM 女性的血压升高[14, 30, 31]。同代谢综合征及血脂异常一样，这种差异可在产后 3 个月内就被检测到[14]。此外，像 GDM 一样，妊娠期高血压疾病预示着母亲在产后 T_2DM 和心血管疾病的风险增加[32]。因此，综合起来，这些数据支持妊娠期高血压和 GDM 之间的慢性联系，这些代谢异常的存在使心血管代谢疾病的终身风险升高。

妊娠糖尿病患者的炎症反应

慢性低度炎症是中枢性肥胖症（尤其是内脏脂肪块的扩张）的病理效应，其特征是升高的炎性生物标志物如 C 反应蛋白（CRP）的循环浓度。这种亚临床全身炎性反应已被证明可预测 T_2DM 和心血管疾病的未来发展[33]。因此，对女性炎性生物标志物谱与该患者群体未来心脏代谢风险的相关性值得关注。在前瞻性嵌套病例对照研究中，妊娠早期 CRP 浓度升高与 GDM 后续发展的风险增加有关[34, 35]。这种关系在调整 BMI 后不显著，类似于在亚临床炎症与妊娠期 T_2DM[34]的研究中观察到的衰减相似。在妊娠后期，GDM 妇女在一些但不是所有的横断面研究中都显示 CRP 浓度增加[36, 37]。

虽然这些冲突结果的基础是不确定的，但已经表明，它们可能涉及产妇肥胖，这似乎是主导亚临床炎症的决定因素。在这一背景下，应该注意到，在调整协变量（包括 BMI）之后，妊娠期 CRP 浓度与空腹胰岛素（间接肝胰岛素抵抗的检测）独立相关[37]。总而言之，这些数据潜在地表明母体肥胖介导了慢性低度炎性反应，进而导致不良的代谢后遗症，如胰岛素分泌增加、胰岛素抵抗和葡萄糖耐受不良[37]。一些研究已经报道，在妊娠后的数年中，有 GDM 病史的妇女表现出升高的炎性生物标志物的循环水平，包括 CRP、唾液酸和纤溶酶原激活物抑制剂 1[38-41]。这些研究也始终关注 CRP 与中心性肥胖之间的关系。例如，在美国第三次全国健康和营养调查检查中，有和没有 GDM 病史的女性的 CRP 在调整腰围后差异不显著[38]。因此，虽然亚临床炎症似乎是 GDM 妇女的慢性特征，但尚不清楚这一发现是否完全由内脏脂肪和中心性肥胖引起。

妊娠糖尿病妇女脂肪因子的异常调节

另一种已知的肥胖在一般人群中的病理效应是脂肪衍生蛋白或脂肪细胞因子失调。类似于 CRP 在炎症中的主导作用，研究的脂肪因子是脂联素,一种循环中高浓度胶原样蛋白,并具有公认的胰岛素增敏、抗动脉粥样硬化、抗炎作用[42]。体重增加和内脏脂肪增加有助于(或与之相关)循环脂联素水平的降低,其意义通过纵向研究一致显示基线低脂联素血症可预测 T_2DM 的发展[42]。与没有 GDM 的妇女相比,GDM 妇女的循环脂联素水平较低[42-46]。此外,一些证据表明,低脂联素血症可能在 GDM 中起病理作用。第一,妊娠期低脂联素与 B 细胞功能障碍和胰岛素抵抗相关[43, 44]。第二,这些效应与 GDM 妇女脂联素的高分子量(HMW)形式(即脂联素的循环多聚体形式,被认为介导了这种脂肪因子所导致的公认的抗糖尿病作用)[45]特异性地联系在一起。第三,妊娠早期低脂联素血症独立预测妊娠后 GDM 的发展在调整已知的 GDM 危险因素[46]后。

与 GDM 的其他代谢特征一样,脂肪因子失调的存在也可能超出妊娠期。GDM 妇女产后第 1 年脂联素水平低于同龄人[39]。此外,调整协变量(包括肥胖)后的低脂联素血症(即低循环脂联素)与产后升高的血糖、胰岛素抵抗和 B 细胞功能障碍相关[47]。最重要的是,低脂联素被报道为 GDM[48]后 B 细胞功能恶化的独立预测因子。因此,低脂联素血症可能是 T_2DM 在该人群中进展的独立因素。

妊娠前和妊娠早期代谢异常对于妊娠糖尿病的诊断

近年来一个反复出现的主题是,代谢异常在产后一年内的 GDM 妇女中很容易显现,这反映了长期代谢障碍的可能性,这可能是 GDM 临床诊断的先兆。越来越多的证据支持这一主题,证明妊娠早期女性代谢紊乱将继续发展为 GDM。事实上,妊娠 15 周时继续发展为 GDM 的女性已经显示出羊水中检验指标的改变,包括葡萄糖、胰岛素和胰岛素样生长因子结合蛋白 1[49]。此外,在妊娠早期,已经报道了各种生物标志物的血清水平,以预测妊娠晚期 GDM 的后续发展。这些因素包括脂质(高三酰甘油和低 HDL)、CRP、低脂联素及高组织纤溶酶原激活物抗原浓度[17, 28, 34, 35, 46, 50]。因此,最近人们对妊娠前代谢特征产生了相当大的兴趣,这些特征可以识别可能在妊娠期间发展成 GDM 的妇女。

迄今为止,已经报道了下列妊娠前代谢和临床因素在协变量调整后能不同程度地预测 GDM:较高的空腹血糖、空腹胰岛素、BMI、三酰甘油、血压、γ-谷氨酰转移酶水平和较低的脂联素浓度、HMW 水平[28, 51-56]。综上所述，这些数据支持将继续发展为 GDM 的妇女在妊娠前就存在代谢功能障碍的表型[2]。妊娠前、妊娠期间和妊娠后的代谢表型见表 8.1。

表 8.1　代谢性异常在妊娠糖尿病患者中的表现，即妊娠前、妊娠期间和妊娠后的代谢异常

代谢异常	妊娠前	妊娠期间	妊娠后
代谢综合征			+
高密度脂蛋白			+
低密度脂蛋白		+	+
高三酰甘油		+	+
高血压	+	+	+
肥胖	+	+	+
超重	+	+	+
亚临床炎症（CRP）		+	+
低脂联素血症	+	+	+

展望

由于认识到 GDM 妇女代谢功能障碍的慢性性质，这将对未来几年的研究产生影响。首先，预计未来研究兴趣的领域将是该患者群体的代谢组学和蛋白质组学表征。其次，需要仔细的研究设计来识别 GDM 本身的代谢影响，独立于潜在混杂条件，特别是肥胖/超重和糖尿病前期/糖尿病[57]。再次，这项研究可能揭示新陈代谢功能的决定因素，如最近出现的胎儿性别作为一个先前未被认识到的影响妊娠期妇女葡萄糖代谢的因素[58-60]。最后，GDM 女性的详细纵向特征可能会对代谢和血管疾病的病理生理学产生新的见解，从而为该人群代谢风险的改变提供策略。此外，在临床实践中，对存在 GDM 病史妇女的代谢异常的认识强调了筛查心血管危险因素和鼓励高危患者的健康生活方式实践的重要性。

选择题

1. 发展为 GDM 的妇女通常会出现代谢异常的时间点是（　　　）

A. 仅妊娠时

B. 妊娠后

C. 妊娠前后

D. 妊娠前、妊娠期间和妊娠后

正确答案是 D。

2. 与同龄人相比，在妊娠后有 GDM 病史的妇女中已经证实的脂质异常包括（　　）

A. 高三酰甘油和低高密度脂蛋白

B. 高密度脂蛋白

C. 高载脂蛋白 B

D. 以上所有

正确答案是 D。

3. 在产后几年，有 GDM 病史的妇女表现出发病率增加的疾病是（　　）

A. 2 型糖尿病　　　　B. 心血管疾病

C. 代谢综合征　　　　D. 以上所有

正确答案是 D。

（张　焱 译，朱海清　校）

参 考 文 献

1 Retnakaran R. Glucose tolerance status in pregnancy: a window to the future risk of diabetes and cardiovascular disease in young women. Curr Diabetes Rev 2009;5:239–244.

2 Wen SW, Xie RH, Tan H, Walker MC, Smith GN, Retnakaran R. Preeclampsia and gestational diabetes mellitus: pre-conception origins? Medical Hypotheses 2012;79:120–125.

3 Buchanan TA, Xiang AH. Gestational diabetes mellitus. J Clin Invest 2005;115:485–491.

4 Retnakaran R, Qi Y, Sermer M, Connelly PW, Hanley AJ, Zinman B. Beta-cell function declines within the first year postpartum in women with recent glucose intolerance in pregnancy. Diabetes Care 2010;33:1798–1804.

5 Kramer CK, Swaminathan B, Hanley AJ, et al. Each degree of glucose intolerance in pregnancy predicts distinct trajectories of beta-cell function, insulin sensitivity and glycemia in the first 3 years postpartum. Diabetes Care 2014;37:3262–3269.

6 Alberti, KG, Eckel RH., Grundy SM, et al. Harmonizing the metabolic syndrome: a joint interim statement of the international Diabetes Federation Task Force on Epidemiology and Prevention; National Heart, Lung, and Blood Institute; American Heart Association; World Heart Federation; International Atherosclerosis Society; and

International Association for the Study of Obesity. Circulation 2010;120:1640-1645.
7 Retnakaran R, Qi Y, Sermer M, Connelly PW, Hanley AJ, Zinman B. Glucose intolerance in pregnancy and future risk of pre-diabetes or diabetes. Diabetes Care 2008;31:2026-2031.
8 Bellamy L, Casas JP, Hingorani AD, Williams D. Type 2 diabetes after gestational diabetes a systematic review and meta-analysis. Lancet 2009;373:1773-1779.
9 Shah BR, Retnakaran R, Booth GL. Increased risk of cardiovascular disease in young women following gestational diabetes. Diabetes Care 2008;31:1668-1669.
10 Retnakaran R, Shah BR. Mild glucose intolerance in pregnancy and risk of cardiovascular disease in young women: population-based cohort study. CMAJ 2009;181:371-376.
11 Lauenborg J, Mathiesen E, Hansen T, et al. The prevalence of the metabolic syndrome in a Danish population of women with previous gestational diabetes mellitus is three-fold higher than in the general population. J Clin Endocrinol Metab 2005;90:4004-4010.
12 Verma A, Boney CM, Tucker R, Vohr BR. Insulin resistance syndrome in women with prior history of gestational diabetes mellitus. J Clin Endocrinol Metab 2002;87:3227-3235.
13 Xu Y, Shen S, Sun L, Yang H, Jin B, Cao X. Metabolic syndrome risk after gestational diabetes: a systematic review and meta-analysis. PLoS One 2014;9:e87863.
14 Retnakaran R, Qi Y, Sermer M, Connelly PW, Zinman B, Hanley AJ. Glucose intolerance in pregnancy and postpartum risk of metabolic syndrome in young women J Clin Endocrinol Metab 2010;95:670-677.
15 Clark CM Jr, Qiu C, Amerman B, et al. Gestational diabetes: should it be added to the syndrome of insulin resistance? Diabetes Care 1997;20:867-871.
16 Knopp RH, Chan E, Zhu X, Paramsothy P, Bonet B. Lipids in gestational diabetes: abnormalities and significance. In: Kim C & Ferrara A (eds.), Gestational Diabetes During and After Pregnancy. Springer-Verlag: London, 2010, 155-169.
17 Ryckman K, Spracklen C, Smith C, Robinson J, Saftlas A. Maternal lipid levels during pregnancy and gestational diabetes: a systematic review and meta-analysis. BJOG 2015;122:643-651.
18 Retnakaran R, Qi Y, Connelly PW, Sermer M, Hanley AJ, Zinman B. The graded relationship between glucose tolerance status in pregnancy and postpartum levels of LDL cholesterol and apolipoprotein B in young women: implications for future cardiovascular risk. J Clin Endocrinol Metab 2010;95:4345-4353.
19 Herrera E, Ortega-Senovilla H. Lipid metabolism during pregnancy and its implications for fetal growth. Curr Pharm Biotechnol 2014;15:24-31.
20 Retnakaran R, Ye C, Hanley AJ, et al. Effect of maternal weight, adipokines, glucose intolerance and lipids on infant birthweight in women without gestational diabetes mellitus. CMAJ 2012;184:1353-1360.
21 Meyers-Seifer CH, Vohr BR. Lipid levels in former gestational diabetic mothers. Diabetes Care 1996;19:1351-1356.
22 Forbes S, Taylor-Robinson SD, Patel N, Allan P, Walker BR, Johnston DG. Increased prevalence of non-alcoholic fatty liver disease in European women with a history of gestational diabetes. Diabetologia 2011;54:641-647.
23 Qiu C, Rudra C, Austin MA, Williams MA. Association of gestational diabetes mellitus and low-density lipoprotein (LDL) particle size. Physiol Res 2007;56:571-578.
24 Rizzo M, Berneis K, Altinova AE, et al. Atherogenic lipoprotein phenotype and LDL size and subclasses in women with gestational diabetes. Diabet Med 2008;25:1406-1411.
25 Sánchez-Vera I, Bonet B, Viana M, et al. Changes in plasma lipids and increased low-density lipoprotein susceptibility to oxidation in pregnancies complicated by gestational diabetes: consequences of obesity. Metabolism 2007;56:1527-1533.

26 Sibai B, Habli M. Blood pressure in GDM. In: Kim C & Ferrara A (eds.), Gestational Diabetes During and After Pregnancy. Springer-Verlag: London, 2010, 171–180.
27 Sibai BM, Ross MG. Hypertension in gestational diabetes mellitus: pathophysiology and long-term consequences. J Matern Fetal Neonatal Med 2010;23:229–233.
28 Hedderson MM, Ferrara A. High blood pressure before and during early pregnancy is associated with an increased risk of gestational diabetes mellitus. Diabetes Care 2008;31:2362–2367.
29 Mastrogiannis DS, Spiliopoulos M, Mulla W, Homko CJ. Insulin resistance: the possible link between gestational diabetes mellitus and hypertensive disorders of pregnancy. Curr Diab Rep 2009;9:296–302.
30 Tobias DK, Hu FB, Forman JP, Chavarro J, Zhang C. Increased risk of hypertension after gestational diabetes mellitus: findings from a large prospective cohort study. Diabetes Care 2011;34:1582–1584.
31 Bentley-Lewis R, Powe C, Ankers E, Wenger J, Ecker J, Thadhani R. Effect of race/ethnicity on hypertension risk subsequent to gestational diabetes mellitus. Am J Cardiol 2014;113:1364–1370.
32 Lykke JA, Langhoff-Roos J, Sibai BM, Funai EF, Triche EW, Paidas MJ. Hypertensive pregnancy disorders and subsequent cardiovascular morbidity and type 2 diabetes mellitus in the mother. Hypertension 2009;53:944–951.
33 Ziegler D. Type 2 diabetes as an inflammatory cardiovascular disorder. Curr Mol Med 2005;5:309–322.
34 Wolf M, Sandler L, Hsu K, et al. First-trimester C-reactive protein and subsequent gestational diabetes. Diabetes Care 2003;26:819–824.
35 Qiu C, Sorensen TK, Luthy DA, et al. A prospective study of maternal serum C-reactive protein (CRP) concentrations and risk of gestational diabetes mellitus. Paediatr Perinat Epidemiol 2004;18:377–384.
36 Leipold H, Worda C, Gruber CJ, et al. Gestational diabetes mellitus is associated with increased C-reactive protein concentrations in the third but not second trimester. Eur J Clin Invest 2005;35:752–757.
37 Retnakaran R, Hanley AJG, Raif N, Connelly PW, Sermer M, Zinman B. C-reactive protein and gestational diabetes: the central role of maternal obesity. J Clin Endocrinol Metab 2003;88:3507–3512.
38 Kim C, Cheng YJ, Beckles GL. Inflammation among women with a history of gestational diabetes mellitus and diagnosed diabetes in the Third National Health and Nutrition Examination Survey. Diabetes Care 2008;31:1386–1388.
39 Winzer C, Wagner O, Festa A, et al. Plasma adiponectin, insulin sensitivity, and subclinical inflammation in women with prior gestational diabetes mellitus. Diabetes Care 2004;27:1721–1727.
40 Farhan S, Winzer C, Tura A, et al. Fibrinolytic dysfunction in insulin-resistant women with previous gestational diabetes. Eur J Clin Invest 2006;36:345–352.
41 Sriharan M, Reichelt AJ, Opperman ML, et al. Total sialic acid and associated elements of the metabolic syndrome in women with and without previous gestational diabetes. Diabetes Care 2002;25:1331–1335.
42 Retnakaran A, Retnakaran R. Adiponectin in pregnancy: implications for health and disease. Curr Med Chem 2012;19:5444–5450.
43 Retnakaran R, Hanley AJ, Raif N, Connelly PW, Sermer M, Zinman B. Reduced adiponectin concentration in women with gestational diabetes: a potential factor in progression to type 2 diabetes. Diabetes Care 2004;27:799–800.
44 Retnakaran R, Hanley AJ, Raif N, Hirning CR, Connelly PW, Sermer M, Kahn SE, Zinman B. Adiponectin and beta-cell dysfunction in gestational diabetes: pathophysiologic implications. Diabetologia 2005;48:993–1001.
45 Retnakaran R, Connelly PW, Maguire G, Sermer M, Zinman B, Hanley AJ. Decreased high molecular weight

adiponectin in gestational diabetes: implications for the pathophysiology of type 2 diabetes. Diabet Med 2007;24:245-252.
46 Williams MA, Qiu C, Muy-Rivera M, et al. Plasma adiponectin concentrations in early pregnancy and subsequent risk of gestational diabetes mellitus. J Clin Endocrinol Metab 2004;89:2306-2311.
47 Retnakaran R, Qi Y, Connelly PW, Sermer M, Hanley AJ, Zinman B. Low adiponectin concentration during pregnancy predicts postpartum insulin resistance, beta-cell dysfunction and fasting glycaemia Diabetologia 2010;53:268-276.
48 Xiang AH, Kawakubo M, Trigo E, Kjos SL, Buchanan TA. Declining beta-cell compensation for insulin resistance in Hispanic women with recent gestational diabetes mellitus: association with changes in weight, adiponectin, and C-reactive protein. Diabetes Care 2010;33:396-401.
49 Tisi DK, Burns DH, Luskey GW, Koski KG. Fetal exposure to altered amniotic fluid glucose, insulin, and insulin-like growth factor-binding protein 1 occurs before screening for gestational diabetes mellitus. Diabetes Care 2011;34:139-144.
50 Savvidou M, Nelson SM, Makgoba M, Messow CM, Sattar N, Nicolaides K. First-trimester prediction of gestational diabetes mellitus: examining the potential of combining maternal characteristics and laboratory measures. Diabetes 2010;59:3017-3022.
51 Gunderson EP, Quesenberry CP Jr, Jacobs DR Jr, Feng J, Lewis CE, Sidney S. Longitudinal study of prepregnancy cardiometabolic risk factors and subsequent risk of gestational diabetes mellitus: the CARDIA study. Am J Epidemiol 2010;172:1131-1143.
52 Hedderson MM, Darbinian JA, Quesenberry CP, Ferrara A. Pregravid cardiometabolic risk profile and risk for gestational diabetes mellitus. Am J Obstet Gynecol 2011;205:55.e1-e7.
53 Harville EW, Viikari JS, Raitakari OT. Preconception cardiovascular risk factors and pregnancy outcome. Epidemiology 2011;22:724-730.
54 Hedderson MM, Darbinian J, Havel PJ, Quesenberry CP, Sridhar S, Ehrlich S, Ferrara A. Low prepregnancy adiponectin concentrations are associated with a marked increase in risk for development of gestational diabetes mellitus. Diabetes Care 2013;36:3930-3937.
55 Sridhar SB, Xu F, Darbinian J, Quesenberry CP, Ferrara A, Hedderson MM. Pregravid liver enzyme levels and risk of gestational diabetes mellitus during a subsequent pregnancy. Diabetes Care 2014;37:1878-1884.
56 Catalano PM, Tyzbir ED, Wolfe RR, et al. Carbohydrate metabolism during pregnancy in control subjects and women with gestational diabetes. Am J Physiol 1993;264:E60-E67.
57 Kew S, Swaminathan B, Hanley AJ, et al. Postpartum microalbuminuria following gestational diabetes: the impact of current glucose tolerance status. J Clin Endocrinol Metab 2015;100:1130-1136.
58 Retnakaran R, Kramer CK, Ye C, et al. Fetal sex and maternal risk of gestational diabetes: the impact of having a boy. Diabetes Care 2015;38:844-851.
59 Retnakaran R, Shah BR. Fetal sex and the natural history of maternal risk of diabetes during and after pregnancy. J Clin Endocrinol Metab 2015;100:2574-2580.
60 Jaskolka D, Retnakaran R, Zinman B, Kramer CK. Sex of the baby and risk of gestational diabetes mellitus in the mother: a systematic review and meta-analysis. Diabetologia 2015;58:2469-2475.

第九章 妊娠糖尿病母亲的风险

Lisa Chasan-Taber[1] and Catherine Kim[2]

1 Department of Biostatistics & Epidemiology, University of Massachusetts, Amherst, Massachusetts, USA
2 Departments of Medicine and Obstetrics & Gynecology, University of Michigan, Ann Arbor, Michigan, USA

实践要点

- GDM 妇女在以后妊娠期发生 GDM 的风险增加，发生 1 型糖尿病和 2 型糖尿病的风险也会增加。
- 产后血糖检测应在分娩后立即进行。然而传统的检测在产后 6 周随访时进行，如果妇女不能参加此次随访，应更早接受血糖检测。
- 关于最佳产后血糖检测的建议各不相同，包括敏感性、依从性和成本。对根据餐后血糖水平诊断为 GDM 的妇女在产后检测餐后血糖可以获益。
- 通过增加体力活动和改善饮食质量来减轻体重，可以降低产后血糖水平。
- 选择计划生育和母乳喂养可能改变妇女再次发生 GDM 和随后发生 2 型糖尿病的风险。

问题

- 患有 GDM 的女性需要告知她们产后患糖尿病的风险增加。
- 在妊娠早期经常用糖化血红蛋白作为糖尿病检测标准，但糖化血红蛋白在妊娠数周时可能降低发现糖尿病的敏感性。
- 产后立即改变生活方式，并未被证明能降低以后发生糖尿病的风险。然而产后体重与糖尿病发病风险之间有着明显的正相关，所以鼓励通过积极的体育锻炼和健康的饮食来降低体重。
- 由于担心联合避孕药对母乳产生的影响，产后常常开具孕激素避孕药，但这种避孕方式可能会增加哺乳期闭经妇女的糖尿病风险。

病例

一名 34 岁的白种人孕妇，产 2 孕 2，产后 8 周。此次妊娠前，BMI 为 28kg/m^2（依据 IOM 指南[1]为肥胖），无其他病史。GDM 使妊娠变得复杂，在妊娠 25 周时进行常规筛查、口服 75g 葡萄糖耐量试验。空腹血糖为 4.8mmol/L，餐后 1h 血糖为 10.5mmol/L，餐后 2h 血糖为 8.3mmol/L。在剩下的妊娠期间，她自我监测毛细血管血糖水平，积极控制饮食和适当活动，使血糖控制在达标范围内。由于先前的剖宫产，婴儿在 38 周时按计划行剖宫产分娩。

在产后随访时，她的 BMI 为 31kg/m²（依据 IOM 指南[1]为肥胖）。她自述剖宫产后母乳喂养困难，使用吸奶器能成功。术后不能做运动。她和她的爱人还没有进行性生活，但是她更有兴趣尝试除避孕套外的其他避孕方式。她打算在 1 年内再次妊娠。

- 由于她的 GDM 诊断，她有哪些并发症的风险？
- 你推荐哪种产后避孕方法？
- 你建议怎么做餐后血糖检测？
- 你建议什么样的产后生活方式？

概述

分娩后，对于母亲来说不良的健康后果与 GDM 有关。这些后果包括将来再发生 GDM、1 型糖尿病和 2 型糖尿病的可能性，以及异常心血管危险因素和心血管事件。因此，推荐进行葡萄糖耐量试验与改变生活方式以减少不良后果的发生。然而，实施这些做法的最有效方法还不是很清楚。在这一章中，我们总结了在 GDM 患者分娩后发生糖代谢异常的风险，推荐糖耐量试验检测，还有一些关于生活方式改变的好处的科学文献。

妊娠糖尿病分娩后的后遗症

GDM 患者在未来再次妊娠后有发生 GDM 的风险[2]。在一项约 6500 名妇女的研究中[3]，初次妊娠时发生 GDM 的女性第二次妊娠时 GDM 的患病率达 41%，初次妊娠未发生 GDM 的女性第二次妊娠时的患病率仅为 4%。

GDM 的女性产后发生糖尿病的主要类型为 2 型糖尿病。在一项荟萃分析中[4]，与没有 GDM 的女性相比，既往有 GDM 的女性发生糖尿病的风险增加 7 倍。产后第 5 年发生糖尿病的风险差异显著[5]，这反映了一部分女性在妊娠前有未被发现的糖尿病。相当多的空腹血糖水平或餐后血糖水平升高的女性[6, 7]及非白种人妇女（尤其是亚洲女性）[3, 8]和 GDM 时使用胰岛素治疗的女性,是以后发生糖尿病的危险人群[9]。有 GDM 病史的妇女其他心血管危险因素会升高,包括血压[6, 10-13]和血脂[6, 10-14]水平的不良变化。GDM 也与未来发生心血管事件风险增加有关[15-17],虽然风险似乎主要在糖尿病患者中。

分娩后,有 GDM 的女性也增加了发生 1 型糖尿病的风险,患病率反映了其种族 1 型糖尿病的患病率[18]。因此,1 型糖尿病报道最多的是北欧女性[19]。例如,在一个队列研究中,随访芬兰的女性产后 6 年的情况,5%以上者患 1 型糖尿病,5%以上者患 2 型糖尿病[19]。在妊娠期间[20, 21]及分娩后 1～2 年能检测出血清胰岛细胞抗体[22],发生 1 型糖尿病风险显著升高,提示为胰岛素分泌缺陷,而不是以胰岛素抵抗为特点的 2 型糖尿病[22]。

产后血糖筛查建议

由于糖耐量受损的风险增加,有 GDM 的女性应在产后进行血糖检测。推荐的检查包括仅做空腹血糖、75g 口服葡萄糖耐量试验、糖化血红蛋白或这些检查都要做[23-27],因为这些检查更方便、更精准。这些策略在区分产后有不良后果女性的能力方面还没有进行比较：OGTT 将诊断出糖负荷试验后高血糖症的妇女,患糖尿病的妇女比例更高,但不知道这些妇女一旦被识别和治疗是否会降低微血管和大血管并发症及未来妊娠并发症的风险。

因为产后访视通常安排在第 6 周,建议对于葡萄糖的筛选主要关注于此时间,然后定期检查。但要注意的是,关于产后的报道很少见,至少有一项报道表明在此之前进行测试与 6 周前的血糖值相似[28]。FPG 与 OGTT 相比,只需一次抽血即可。目前,美国糖尿病协会没有建议在产后 6 周访视时进行 HbA1c 检测,因为它与并发血糖水平的相关性较弱,并且需要考虑到产前治疗、体液转移和其他因素造成混杂-母体红细胞周转率的变化[29]。此外,在一项报道中,与产后 1 年的单个 75g OGTT 相比,HbA1c 没有改善 FPG 的敏感性和特异性[30]。相比之下，NICE 推荐 HbA1c 或空腹血糖，注意 HbA1c 测定不需要禁食，因此依从性可能会提高[27]。

目前还不清楚 2h 75g OGTT 与 3h 100g OGTT 对产后糖耐量的影响。我们可以预期，降低 GDM 诊断所需的阈值导致产后使用 WHO 常规标准诊断糖尿病的风险降低，从而减少产后加强检测的益处。有报道[31]说明了这一原则，该报道比较了按照 Carpenter 和 Coustan 标准及国家糖尿病数据组标准诊断为 GDM 的妇女产后血糖调节受损的发病率，虽然 GDM 的发病率增加了约 50%，但新增人口的风险往往较低，在年龄小于 25 岁的妇女（70%）和白种人（58%）中观察到发病率增加。自 2013 年 WHO 标准使用以来诊断为患有 GDM 的女性比之前的报道都多[32]，而产后糖尿病发病率甚至更低。

建议改变行为方式

母乳喂养

观察性研究表明，母乳喂养可降低未来产妇患糖尿病的风险[33-35]。有 GDM 病史的母乳喂养妇女患糖尿病的平均时间是 12.3 年，没有母乳喂养的妇女是 2.3 年[20]。母乳喂养时间延长导致糖尿病的患病风险显著降低[20]。目前缺少对非白种人群体的研究。

与上述研究结果相反，纯母乳喂养导致的乳汁性闭经，再加上仅含孕激素的避孕药物，可能会增加某些种族（民族）人群患糖尿病的风险[36]。哺乳期可能会引起一种相对的孕产状态，再加上仅含孕激素的避孕药物，会导致血糖升高。在拉丁裔（西班牙裔）和包括纳瓦霍人在内的美洲土著部落中，口服和注射孕激素都观察到这种风险，而且这种风险还通过体重变化和除了体重变化外的因素产生影响[14,36,37]。值得注意的是，在最近的研究报道中，避孕药的种类（单独使用孕激素与联合使用雌激素-孕激素药物）似乎与母乳产量的差异无关[38]。因此，应该鼓励母乳喂养，但在哺乳期闭经的情况下，仅含孕激素的避孕药物可能不是糖尿病高危妇女的最佳选择。

产后减肥

妊娠期母体高体重会增加产后患糖尿病的风险[9]。然而，很少有研究检测体重减轻干预对产后 GDM 妇女的影响。最近的一项系统综述确定了 11 项有 GDM 病史的女性生活方式干预的随机对照试验（总结见表 9.1）。每一项试验都涉及饮食摄入和身体活动，只有一项试验只关注饮食的改变[39]。试验的体育锻炼目标是适度的，主要目标是每周 150min[40-45]，或者每周 5d，每天 10 000 步[40, 46]。膳食调整的目标也同样适度，目标是减少膳食脂肪的摄入，通常低于总热量摄入的 30%[35, 42, 45]。大多数试验都是预试验，没有足够的能力检测干预措施对意外发生的产后糖尿病结局的影响，只有一项试验发现干预措施对这一结局有保护作用[45]。然而，其中三项试验表明，如果在分娩后尽早实施生活方式干预可以降低血糖和（或）胰岛素水平[42, 44, 47]。

这项成功的试验是对糖尿病预防项目的一项二级分析，这是一项多中心随机试验，针对空腹和餐后血糖浓度升高的成年人进行强化生活方式干预。这项试验并不是专门针对 GDM 的女性，而是针对所有葡萄糖耐受不良的成年人。随机改变生活方式的女性患糖尿病的风险比随机服用安慰剂的女性低 53%（$P=0.002$），随机服用二甲双胍的女性患糖尿病的风险比随机服用安慰剂的女性低 50%（$P=0.006$）。

表 9.1 中的试验还检验了干预措施对产后体重减轻的影响。妇女产后可立即迅速减轻体重。生活方式的改变导致其中 5 项试验[42, 44, 47-49]的受试者体重显著下降，而 4 项试验发现干预对产后体重减轻没有影响。

虽然这些试验取得一定效果，但目前尚不清楚产后数年是否可以通过改变生活方式来避免糖尿病。目前正在进行几项更大规模的研究，这些研究可能有助于确定预防糖尿病发展所需的最佳分娩方式和行为改变的强度[50-54]。

表 9.1 生活方式干预降低 GDM 妇女患 2 型糖尿病风险的随机试验及研究设计

作者(年份)	随访时间	人群	干预	方式	对糖尿病的影响	对血糖的影响	对体重的影响	对身体的影响	对饮食的影响
Cheung 等 (2011)[40]	12 个月	43 例既往有 GDM, 4 年内, 澳大利亚	锻炼干预与常规治疗控制	个性化; 电话; 邮件	NA	NA	BMI (kg/m²): 28 (95% CI: 23.9~34.3) vs 25.5 (95% CI: 22.5~28.7), P=0.14	步骤 (实现目标): 30.8% vs 17.6%, P=0.34; PA (实现目标): 70.0% vs 57.9%, P=0.51	NA
Ferrara 等 (2011)[41,52]	12 个月	179 例腔前证发生 GDM, 加利福尼亚州	生活方式干预(饮食, 运动, 母乳喂养)与常规治控制	个性化; 电话	NA	NA	体重 (实现目标): 37.5% vs 21.4%, P=0.07	PA (平均变差, 分钟/周): 25.3, P=0.91	脂肪 (平均变化率, %): -3.6, P=0.002
Hu 等 (2012)[42]	12 个月	404 例既往 (2005~2009 年) 有 GDM 的女性, 中国	生活方式干预(饮食, 锻炼)与常规治疗控制	个性化	NA	空腹血糖 (mmol/L): (-0.09±0.52) vs (-0.09±0.60), P=0.97	体重变化 (kg): (-1.4±3.44) vs (-0.21±3.52) (0.3%), P=0.001 BMI 变化 (kg/m²): (-0.50±1.41) vs (-0.09±1.37), P=0.004	LTPA 增加: 59.4% vs 26.9%, P<0.001	脂肪 (减少): 71.1% vs 68.9% 中, P=0.064; 纤维增加: 59.5% vs 47.4%, P=0.012

续表

作者（年份）	随访时间	人群	干预	方式	对糖尿病的影响	对血糖的影响	对体重的影响	对身体的影响	对饮食的影响
Kim 等（2012）[46]	13 周	49 例既往有（3 年内）有 GDM 的女性，密歇根	锻炼干预与常规治疗控制	网络	NA	空腹血糖（mmol/L）: −0.046 vs 0.038, P=0.65; OGTT 餐后 2h 血糖（mmol/L）: −0.48 vs −0.42, P=0.91	体重变化（kg）: −0.14 vs −1.5, P=0.13	PA（中等强度）: 58 岁 vs 47 岁, P=0.51	NA
McIntyre 等（2012）[43]	12 周	28 例既往有 GDM 产后 6 周的女性，澳大利亚	锻炼干预与常规治疗控制	个性化；电话	NA	空腹血糖（mmol/L）: (0.25±0.56) vs (0.12±0.42), NS	体重变化（kg）: (0.97±3.7) vs (0.22±4.2), NS	PA（中位数（范围）计划 PA 增长中位数，分钟/周）: 60(0~540) vs 0 (0~580), P=0.234; 行走: NS	NA
Nicklas 等（2014）[49]	12 个月	75 例既往有 GDM 产后 6 周的女性，美国	生活方式干预与常规治疗控制	个性化网络干预	NA	NA	体重变化（kg）: −2.6 (−4.4, −0.8) vs 1.4 (−0.4, 3.1), P=0.003	NA	NA
Peacock 等（2015）[47]	12 周	既往有 GDM，产后 6~24 个月的女性，澳大利亚	生活方式干预（饮食和锻炼）vs 腰围控制	个性化网络干预；营养支持	NA	空腹血糖（mmol/L）: (0.35±0.5) vs (−0.1±0.6), P=0.052	体重变化（kg）: (−2.5±1.4) vs (0+2.3), P=0.002	PA（臀围的区别）: 135 分钟/周干预-控制, NS	总脂肪变化（g/日）: (0.2±0.40) vs (2±0.5), NS

续表

作者（年份）	随访时间	人群	干预	方式	对糖尿病的影响	对血糖的影响	对体重的影响	对身体的影响	对饮食的影响
Ratner 等（2008）[45]	2.8年	350例既往有GDM，目前血糖水平偏高的女性，美国	生活方式干预（饮食和锻炼）vs安慰剂	个性化；团队会议	糖尿病：风险降低53%减少风险与安慰剂组比较，$P=0.002$	NA	6个月，干预组体重变化为（−5.13±0.43）kg，与安慰剂组比较，$P<0.01$；3年，干预组体重变化为（−1.6±0.80）kg，与安慰剂组比较，$P=0.021$	PA（变化，小时/周）：1.5 小时/周，1年之后随机选择，$P<0.01$ 和0.5小时/周，3年后第3周随机选择，NS	NA
Reinhardt 等（2012）[48]	6个月	38例诊断GDM的女性，澳大利亚	生活方式干预（饮食和运动）vs常规治疗控制	电话；邮件	NA	NA	BMI差异改变（kg/m²）：−2.8～−0.1，$P<0.05$；体重改变kg：−7.6～−0.5，差异95%CI：−4.0（95%CI：−0.5），$P<0.05$	LTPA（变化，分钟/天）：11（95% CI：1～22）	总脂肪（变化，g/d）：−19（95% CI：−37，−1），$P<0.05$；GL（变化，U）=−26（95% CI：−48，−4），$P<0.05$

· 132 ·

续表

作者（年份）	随访时间	人群	干预	方式	对糖尿病的影响	对血糖的影响	对体重的影响	对身体的影响	对饮食的影响
Shyam 等（2013）[44]	6个月	77 例既往有 GDM 的女性2个月内，马来西亚	低 GI 饮食 vs 常规治疗控制	个人，短信、邮件	NA	葡萄糖 2h 后 75g OGTT（中位数 mmol/L）：−0.2（2.8）vs 0.8（2.0），$P=0.025$	重量（实现目标）：33% vs 8%，$P=0.01$	PA（代谢当量，中位数，分钟/周，IQR）：933（1403）vs 965（857），$P=0.908$	脂肪（g）：(58±18) vs (53±16)，$P=0.695$；纤维（g）：(17±4) vs (13±4)，$P=0.02$；GI：(57+5) vs (64+6)，$P=0.033$
Wein 等（1999）[39]	51 个月	796 人（中位数 200 例既往有 GDM 的女性，89～91 曾患有 IGT 的女性）	饮食干预与控制	电话、邮件	糖尿病/年度 IR：6.1% vs 7.3%（IRR=0.83，95%CI：0.47～1.48），$P=0.50$	NA	NA	NA	NA

注：LTPA，业余体育活动；PA，体力活动

总结

虽然已经确定 GDM 妇女是妊娠后葡萄糖耐受不良的高危人群，但如何降低这一风险尚不清楚。DPP 证明，有 GDM 病史的女性即使在分娩 10 年后实施干预措施也能改变她们的行为，但对育龄妇女产后阶段的研究效果较差。与此同时，应该将产后的护理标准告知有 GDM 病史的妊娠妇女：第一，产后血糖失调的风险性与她们的 GDM 诊断结果息息相关。第二，通过增加体育锻炼和减少从脂肪中摄入的能量占比来减轻体重十分重要。第三，定期针对妊娠期间特定的代谢紊乱进行葡萄糖筛查是十分必要的。第四，要讨论计划生育方法。女性在妊娠之前接受葡萄糖测试，随后在妊娠期间应进行密切监测，并每隔 1~3 年重复筛查一次。

展望

正在进行的试验和正在测试几种降低风险的策略，可以为妇女降低产后风险的最佳实践提供指导。正在进行的研究也在检验妊娠期间的体重管理干预是否能在不影响妊娠结局的情况下使产后体重下降。未来的研究还应包括产后筛查策略的比较，以确定特定策略是否影响未来妊娠和产妇健康。

选择题

1. 患有 GDM 的妇女除下列哪种情况外，风险都会增加（　　）
   A. 复发 GDM　　　　　　B. 1 型糖尿病
   C. 心血管疾病　　　　　D. 甲状腺功能减退

正确答案是 D。患有 GDM 的妇女复发的风险、1 型及 2 型糖尿病和心血管疾病的风险增加。

2. 以下与减少 GDM 后糖耐量异常风险无关的是（　　）
   A. 母乳喂养　　　　　　B. 孕激素避孕
   C. 减肥　　　　　　　　D. 增加体力活动

正确答案是 B。以孕激素为基础的避孕，结合哺乳期闭经，实际上可能增加妊娠后糖尿病的风险。

3. 常规产后访视时，不建议进行哪项血糖检测（　　）
   A. 仅空腹血糖
   B. 2h 葡萄糖耐量试验
   C. 糖化血红蛋白

正确答案是 C。产后访视时的糖化血红蛋白可能反映产前血糖控制，以及缺铁、贫血和其他可能干扰产后血糖水平的因素。A 和 B 都是由不同的医疗机构推荐的。

（韩　旸　译，朱海清　校）

参 考 文 献

1. Rasmussen K, Yaktine A, Committee to Reexamine Institute of Medicine Weight Guidelines. Weight Gain During Pregnancy: Reexamining the Guidelines. National Academies Press: Washington, DC, 2009.
2. Kim C, Berger D, Chamany S. Recurrence of gestational diabetes mellitus: a systematic review. Diabetes Care 2007;30(5):1314–1319.
3. Getahun D, Nath C, Ananth C, Chavez M, Smulian J. Gestational diabetes in the United States: temporal trends 1989 through 2004. Am J Obstet Gynecol 2008;198:525.
4. Bellamy L, Casas J, Hingorani A, Williams D. Type 2 diabetes mellitus after gestational diabetes: a systematic review and meta-analysis. Lancet 2009;373:1773–1779.
5. Kim C, Newton K, Knopp R. Gestational diabetes and incidence of type 2 diabetes mellitus: a systematic review. Diabetes Care 2002;25(10):1862–1868.
6. Pallardo F, Herranz L, Garcia-Ingelmo T, Grande C, Martin-Vaquero P, Janez M, et al. Early postpartum metabolic assessment in women with prior gestational diabetes. Diabetes Care 1999;22:1053–1058.
7. Golden S, Bennett W, Baptiste-Roberts K, Wilson L, Barone B, Gary T, et al. Antepartum glucose tolerance test results as predictors of type 2 diabetes mellitus in women with a history of gestational diabetes mellitus: a systematic review. Gend Med 2009;6(Suppl 1):109–122.
8. Wang Y, Chen L, Horswell R, Xiao K, Besse J, Johnson J, et al. Racial differences in the association between gestational diabetes mellitus and risk of type 2 diabetes. J Womens Health (Larchmt) 2012;21(6):628–633.
9. Baptiste-Roberts K, Barone B, Gary T, Golden S, Wilson L, Bass E, et al. Risk factors for type 2 diabetes among women with gestational diabetes: a systematic review. Am J Med 2009;122(3):207–214.
10. Cho N, Jan J, Park J, Cho Y. Waist circumference is the key risk factor for diabetes in Korean women with history of gestational diabetes. Diabetes Res Clin Pract 2006;71(2):177–183.
11. Pallardo L, Herranz L, Martin-Vaquero P, Garcia-Ingelmo T, Grande C, Janez M. Impaired fasting glucose and impaired glucose tolerance in women with prior gestational diabetes are associated with a different cardiovascular profile. Diabetes Care 2003;26:2318–2322.
12. Rivero K, Portal V, Vieria M, Behle I.

Prevalence of the impaired glucose metabolism and its association with risk factors for coronary artery disease in women with gestational diabetes. Diabetes Res Clin Pract 2008;79(3):433–437.

13 Kousta E, Efstathiadou Z, Lawrence N, et al. The impact of ethnicity on glucose regulation and the metabolic syndrome following gestational diabetes. Diabetologia 2006;49(1):36–40.

14 Xiang A, Kawakubo M, Kjos S, Buchanan T. Long-acting injectable progestin contraception and risk of type 2 diabetes in Latino women with prior gestational diabetes mellitus. Diabetes Care 2006;29(3):613–617.

15 Kessous R, Shoham-Vardi I, Pariente G, Sherf M, Sheiner E. An association between gestational diabetes mellitus and long-term maternal cardiovascular morbidity. Heart 2013;99(15):1118–1121.

16 Shah B, Retnakaran R, Booth G. Increased risk of cardiovascular disease in young women following gestational diabetes. Diabetes Care 2008;31(8):1668–1669.

17 Carr D, Utzschneider K, Hull R, Tong J, Wallace T, Kodama K, et al. Gestational diabetes mellitus increases the risk of cardiovascular disease in women with a family history of type 2 diabetes. Diabetes Care 2006;29:2078–2083.

18 de Leiva A, Mauricio D, Corcoy R. Diabetes-related autoantibodies and gestational diabetes. Diabetes Care 2007;30:S127–S133.

19 Jarvela I, Juutinen J, Koskela P, Hartikainen A, Kulmala P, Knip M, et al. Gestational diabetes identifies women at risk for permanent type 1 and type 2 diabetes in fertile age: predictive role of autoantibodies. Diabetes Care 2006;29(3):607–612.

20 Ziegler A, Wallner M, Kaiser I, Rossbauer M, Harsunen M, Lachmann L, et al. Long-term protective effect of lactation on the dvelopment of type 2 diabetes in women with recent gestational diabetes mellitus. Diabetes 2012;61(12):3167–3171.

21 Fuchtenbusch M, Ferber K, Standl E, Ziegler A. Prediction of type 1 diabetes postpartum in patients with gestational diabetes mellitus by combined islet cell autoantibody screening: a prospective multicenter study. Diabetes 1997;46:1459–1467.

22 Papadopolou A, Lynch K, Anderberg E, Landin-Olsson M, Hansson I, Agardh C, et al. HLA-DQB1 genotypes and islet cell autoantibodies against GAD65 and IA-2 in relation to development of diabetes postpartum in women with gestational diabetes mellitus. Diabetes Res Clin Pract 2012;95(2):260–264.

23 ACOG Committee on Obstetric Practice. Postpartum screening for abnormal glucose tolerance in women who had gestational diabetes mellitus. Obstet Gynecol 2009;113(6):1419–1421.

24 World Health Organization. Definition and diagnosis of diabetes mellitus and intermediate hyperglycemia: a report of WHO/IDF consultation. World Health Organization: Geneva, 2006.

25 Thompson D, Berger H, Feig D, Gagnon R, Kader T, Keely E, et al. Diabetes and Pregnancy: Canadian Diabetes Association Clinical Practice Guidelines Expert Committee 2013. May 22, 2013. http://guidelines.diabetes.ca/Browse/Chapter36

26 International Diabetes Federation. International Diabetes Federation Diabetes Atlas. International Diabetes Prevention: Brussels, 2012.

27 National Institute for Health and Care Excellence. Diabetes in pregnancy: management of diabetes and its complications from preconception to the postnatal period 2015. https://www.nice.org.uk/guidance/ng3/chapter/key-priorities-for-implementation

28 Lawrence J, Contreras R, Chen W, Sacks D. Trends in the prevalence of pre-existing diabetes and gestational diabetes mellitus among a racially/ethnically diverse population of pregnant women, 1999–2005. Diabetes Care 2010;33(3):569–576.

29 Kim C, Herman W, Cheung N, Gunderson E, Richardson C. Comparison of hemoglobin A1c with fasting plasma

glucose and 2-h post-challenge glucose for risk stratification among women with recent gestational diabetes mellitus. Diabetes Care 2011;34(9):1949–1951.
30. Picon M, Murri M, Munoz A, Fernandez-Garcia J, Gomez-Huelgas R, Tinahones F. Hemoglobin A1c versus oral glucose tolerance test in postpartum diabetes screening. Diabetes Care 2012;35:1648–1653.
31. Ferrara A, Hedderson M, Quesenberry C, Selby J. Prevalence of gestational diabetes mellitus detected by the National Diabetes Data Group or the Carpenter and Coustan plasma glucose thresholds. Diabetes Care 2002;25(9):1625–1630.
32. American Diabetes Association. Standards of medical care in diabetes: position statement. Diabetes Care 2014;37(S):S14–S80.
33. O'Reilly M, Avalos G, Dennedy M, O'Sullivan E, Dunne F. Atlantic DIP: high prevalence of abnormal glucose tolerance post-partum is reduced by breast-feeding in women with prior gestational diabetes mellitus. Eur J Endocrinol 2011;165(6):953–959.
34. Gunderson E, Hedderson M, Chiang V, Crites Y, Walton D, Azevedo R, et al. Lactation intensity and postpartum maternal glucose tolerance and insulin resistance in women with recent GDM: the SWIFT cohort. Diabetes Care 2012;35(1):50–56.
35. Ferrara A, Hedderson M, Albright C, Ehrlich S, Quesenberry Jr. C, Peng T, et al. A pregnancy and postpartum lifestyle intervention in women with gestational diabetes mellitus reduces diabetes risk factors: a feasibility randomized controlled trial. Diabetes Care 2011;34(7):1519–1525.
36. Kjos S, Peters R, Xiang A, Thomas D, Schaefer U, Buchanan T. Contraception and the risk of type 2 diabetes mellitus in Latina women with prior gestational diabetes mellitus. JAMA 1998;280(6):533–538.
37. Kim C, Seidel K, Begier E, Kwok Y. Diabetes and depot medroxyprogesterone contraception in Navajo women. Arch Intern Med 2001;161(14):1766–1771.
38. Espey E, Ogburn T, Leeman L, Singh R, Ostrom K, Schrader R. Effect of progestin compared with combined oral contraceptive pills on laactation: a randomized controlled trial. Obstet Gynecol 2012;119(1):5–13.
39. Wein P, Beischer N, Harris C, Permezel M. A trial of simple versus intensified dietary modification for prevention of progression to diabetes mellitus in women with impaired glucose tolerance. Aus N Z J Obstet Gynaecol 1999;39(2):162–166.
40. Cheung N, Smith B, van der Ploeg H, Cinndaio N, Bauman A. A pilot structured behavioural intervention trial to increase physical activity among women with recent gestational diabetes. Diabetes Res Clin Pract 2011;92(1):e27–e29.
41. Ferrara A, Ehrlich S. Strategies for diabetes prevention before and after pregnancy in women with GDM. Curr Diab Rev 2011;7:75–83.
42. Hu G, Tian H, Zhang F, Liu H, Zhang C, Zhang S, et al. Tianjin gestational diabetes mellitus prevention program: study design, methods, and 1-year interim report on the feasibility of lifestyle intervention program. Diabetes Res Clin Pract 2012;98(3):508–517.
43. McIntyre H, Peacock A, Miller Y, Koh D, Marshall A. Pilot study of an individualised early postpartum intervention to increase physical activity in women with previous gestational diabetes. Int J Endocrinol 2012. doi:10.1155/2012/892019
44. Shyam S, Arshad F, Abdul Ghani R, Wahab N, Safii N, Nisak M, et al. Low glycaemic index diets improve glucose tolerance and body weight in women with previous history of gestational diabetes: a 6 months randomized trial. Nutr J 2013;12:68.
45. Ratner R, Christophi C, Metzger B, Dabelea D, Bennett P, Pi-Sunyer X, et al. Prevention of diabetes in women with a history of gestational diabetes; effects of metformin and lifestyle interventions. J Clin Endocrinol Metab

2008;93(12):4774-4779.
46. Kim C, Draska M, Hess M, Wilson E, Richardson C. A web-based pedometer program in women with recent histories of gestational diabetes. Diabet Med 2012;29(2):278-283.
47. Peacock A, Bogossian F, Wilkinson S, Gibbons K, Kim C, McIntyre H. A randomised controlled trial to delay or prevent type 2 diabetes after gestational diabetes: walking for Exercise and Nutrition to Prevent Diabetes for You (WENDY). Int J Endocrinol 2015; epub ahead of print.
48. Reinhardt J, van der Ploeg H, Grzegrzulka R, Timperley J. Implementing lifestyle change through phone-based motivational interviewing in rural-based women with previous gestational diabetes mellitus. Health Promot J Austr 2012;23(1):5-9.
49. Nicklas J, Zera C, England L, Rosner B, Horton E, Levkoff S, et al. A web-based lifestyle intervention for women with recent gestational diabetes mellitus. Obstet Gynecol 2014;124:563-570.
50. Berry D, Neal M, Hall E, Schwartz T, Verbiest S, Bonuck K, et al. Rationale, design, and methodology for optimizing outcomes in women with gestational diabetes mellitus and their infants study. BMC Pregnancy Childbirth 2013. doi:10.1186/1471-2393-13-184
51. Chasan-Taber L, Marcus B, Rosal M, Tucker K, Hartman S, Pekow P, et al. Estudio Parto: postpartum diabetes prevention program for Hispanic women with abnormal glucose tolerance in pregnancy: a randomised controlled trial-study protocol. BMC Pregnancy Childbirth 2014. doi:10.1186/1471-2393-14-100
52. Ferrara A, Hedderson M, Albright C, Brown S, Ehrlich S, Caan B, et al. A pragmatic cluster randomized clinical trial of diabetes prevention strategies for women with gestational diabetes: design and rationale of the Gestational Diabetes Effects on Moms (GEM) study. BMC Pregnancy Childbirth 2014. doi:10.1186/1471/2393-14-21
53. Infanti J, Dunne F, O'DEA A, Gillespie P, Gibson I, Glynn L, et al. An evaluation of Croi MyAction community lifestyle modification programme compared to standard care to reduce progression to diabetes/pre-diabetes in women with prior gestational diabetes mellitus (GDM): study protocol for randomised controlled trial. Trials 2013. doi:10.1186/1745-6215-14-121
54. Shih S, Davis-Lameloise N, Janus E, Wildey C, Versace V, Hagger V, et al. Mothers After Gestational Diabetes in Australia Diabetes Prevention Program (MAGDA-DPP) postnatal intervention: an update to the study protocol for a randomized controlled trial. Trials 2014. doi:10.1186/1745-6215-15-259

第三篇 妊娠糖尿病相关问题

第十章 1型和2型糖尿病患者的妊娠前护理

Rosemary C. Temple [1] and Katharine P. Stanley [2]

1 Elsie Bertram Diabetes Centre, Norfolk and Norwich University Hospital NHS Trust, Norwich, UK
2 Department of Obstetrics, Norfolk and Norwich University Hospital NHS Trust, Norwich, UK

实践要点

- 妊娠前护理（PPC）是为患糖尿病的女性妊娠时提供的额外支持，其主要目的是为糖尿病女性提供相关医学建议及支持，使其在妊娠前达到最佳的血糖控制目标。
- 给予1型糖尿病女性PPC可以使其在妊娠初期改善血糖控制，并降低其后代发生先天畸形的风险。
- PPC包括以下方面：开始服用叶酸（5mg/d），终止使用可能的致畸药物（如他汀类药物、血管紧张素转换酶抑制剂和某些降糖药物），戒烟。此外需重视饮食控制，其目的为鼓励妊娠前保持健康的体重，并将血糖控制到最佳水平。
- 2型糖尿病女性的妊娠结局与1型糖尿病女性类似甚至更糟，但2型糖尿病女性获得正规PPC的可能性小得多。
- 除PPC外，糖尿病女性应定期进行常规妊娠前咨询，并贯穿整个生育年龄。咨询包括讨论未来的妊娠计划，避孕建议，关于意外妊娠导致风险增加的相关教育，如何尽量减少意外妊娠，如何获得PPC。

病 例

25岁的Mary很高兴地发现自己再次妊娠。她第一次妊娠时出现妊娠糖尿病，当时接受了饮食治疗。尽管被告知需减重，但由于她在妊娠后出现抑郁，体重反而增加了9kg。两年后她被诊断为2型糖尿病。她发现很难坚持节食，因此服用二甲双胍和磺脲类药物控制血糖。近来，她还开始服用血管紧张素转换酶抑制剂来控制血压。妊娠约8周时，她的家庭医师紧急将她转诊到糖尿病产前诊所，在那里她惊讶地发现，自己在妊娠期间可能需要接受胰岛素治疗，因为她的 HbA1c 在就诊时是 8.4%。她后来说，以前从来没有接受过相关咨询，包括关于未来妊娠可能面临的风险，以及可能将需要停止口服降糖药而开始行胰岛素治疗等。她开始每天注射两次胰岛素，并停止了口服降糖药物，同时停止服用血管紧张素转换酶抑制剂，并开始服用拉贝洛尔和叶酸片。她在妊娠 20 周扫描时发现胎儿有异常的室间隔缺损。此后，她的血糖变得更加难以控制，需要一天注射 4 次胰岛素。在 28 周时又增加了另一种降压药。在 35 周时，由于出现了子痫前期，于是实施了紧急剖宫产。婴儿由于低血糖被送入新生儿监护病房，故不能进行母乳喂养，而且这个婴儿后续还需要进一步行心脏手术治疗。

- 对于妊娠前 1 型和 2 型糖尿病的女性患者，PPC 如何有效减少妊娠并发症？
- 对于 1 型和 2 型糖尿病的女性患者，PPC 的基本内容是什么？
- 严格血糖控制的目的是什么？
- 为什么有些女性没接受 PPC？
- 妊娠前咨询是什么，它应该包括什么？

背景

为糖尿病女性患者进行 PPC 出现于 40 年前，其目的是改善妊娠结局。然而，仅有 1/3 的女性能够获得 PPC，因此糖尿病女性的妊娠结局仍然欠佳。在世界范围内，2 型糖尿病是妊娠时最常见糖尿病类型，而且 2 型糖尿病的女性在妊娠时可能更多合并肥胖，更多可能服用致畸药物。但与 1 型糖尿病的女性患者相比，2 型糖尿病女性患者却更少可能获得 PPC。所有提供糖尿病护理的卫生保健专业人士都应该了解 PPC 的重要性，并能够提供专业的妊娠前咨询，包括避孕措施的建议。

妊娠前护理的历史

早在 1964 年，Molsted-Pedersen 就描述了一种现象，糖尿病女性患者生产的婴儿先天畸形发生率高达 6.4%，而没有糖尿病的女性生产的婴儿先天畸形发生率仅为 2.1%[1]。动物研究和人类研究均发现，高血糖可能是导致畸形的原因之一[2, 3]。Pedersen 观察到血糖控制和畸形的关系，胎儿畸形的母亲在妊娠前 3 个月低血糖反应和胰岛素昏迷的发生率较低,提示妊娠早期高血糖与胎儿畸形的相关性。此后,针对糖尿病女性患者提出了 PPC 的概念[4]。

妊娠前护理有效吗

先天畸形

神经管在妊娠 6 周时关闭,胎儿心脏在妊娠 8 周时形成。因此,要影响这些事件,必须在妊娠前改善血糖控制。

Fuhrmann 在 1983 年对 420 名 1 型糖尿病女性患者进行研究发现,妊娠前控制血糖可显著减少先天畸形的发生(0.8% vs 7.5%)[5]。20 世纪 80 年代早期,在一些医疗中心妊娠前诊所已成为日常保健的一部分,如 Edinburgh 的 Steel[6]。此外,多个研究也证实了 PPC 的有效性,妊娠早期血糖改善能使畸形风险降低(表 10.1)[5-15]。然而,这些研究都是前瞻性或回顾性队列研究,而且只有 5 项研究包括糖化血红蛋白的数据。

目前已知的两个 PPC 相关的 Meta 分析,一个纳入 2500 多名妊娠妇女[16],另一个纳入 12 个队列研究[17],其结果表明以下两种相关性:缺乏 PPC 与先天畸形风险增加 3～4 倍相关,PPC 与妊娠前 3 个月 HbA1c 水平平均下降 1.9% 相关。

表 10.1　1 型糖尿病患者妊娠前护理和先天畸形的相关性

作者	年份	PPC 例数	畸形发生率(%)	无 PPC 例数	畸形发生率(%)	P 值
Fuhrmann[5]	1983	128	0.8	292	7.5	0.01
Steel[6]	1994	196	1.5	117	12.0	<0.005
Goldman[7]	1986	44	0	31	9.7	NS
Mills[8]	1988	347	4.9	279	9.0	0.03
Kitzmiller[9]	1991	84	1.2	110	10.9	0.01
Rosenn[10]	1991	28	0	71	1.4	NS
Cousins[11]	1991	27	0	347	6.6	NS
Drury[12]	1992	100	1.0	244	4.1	NS
Willhoitte[13]	1993	62	1.6	123	6.5	NS
Temple[14]	2006	110	1.8	180	6.1	0.07
Murphy[15]	2010	107	0.9	230	5.7	0.02

围产期死亡率

一个纳入 5 项队列研究的 Meta 分析发现，PPC 与围产期死亡率降低相关（RR：0.35；95% CI：0.15～0.82）[17]。而众所周知，围产期死亡可能与畸形有关，在排畸扫描出现之前的研究中尤其如此。

自然流产

在没有 PPC 和早期诊断的妊娠女性中，自然流产的记录比较少，很难评估 PPC 对自然流产的影响，因此 PPC 对女性自然流产的影响目前也知之不多。有关研究表明，在妊娠早期血糖控制不佳的女性中，自然流产的风险增加了 3～4 倍[18,19]。另一项早期研究表明，PPC 与自然流产风险降低相关（8.4% vs 28%）[19]。但另一项纳入 7 项 PPC 和自然流产研究的 Meta 分析发现，PPC 对自然流产没有影响[20]。

围产期发病率

PPC 对围产儿发病率或产科并发症的影响研究较少。一项纳入 290 名 1 型糖尿病女性患者的研究表明，PPC 与 34 周前分娩显著减少有关（5.0% vs 14.2%）[14]。最近一项有关 PPC 研究的 Meta 分析也表明，PPC 在降低早产风险（定义为 37 周前分娩）方面是有效的，其风险比为 0.70（95% CI：0.55～0.90）[21]。相比之下，研究表明 PPC 与巨大儿、子痫前期、早产或剖宫产的风险没有关系，表明这些并发症可能更多地与妊娠后期的血糖控制有关，而非妊娠早期（表 10.2）[14,22-25]。

表 10.2　1 型糖尿病的妊娠前护理和妊娠结局[14]

	妊娠前护理	无妊娠前护理	P 值
人数	110	180	
妊娠并发症			
早产＜34 周（%）	5.0	14.2	0.02

续表

	妊娠前护理	无妊娠前护理	P 值
巨大儿（%）	44.0	43.4	NS
先兆子痫（%）	13.1	12.7	NS
妊娠结局			
自然流产（%）	5.7	14.0	0.056
畸形（n）	2	11	0.065
不良结局*（%）	2.9	10.2	0.026

* 不良结局包括先天畸形、死产和新生儿死亡

妊娠前护理对 2 型糖尿病的疗效

大多妊娠前保健的研究很少将患 2 型糖尿病女性纳入其中，大多数只纳入 1 型糖尿病的女性患者。到目前为止，还没有针对 2 型糖尿病女性患者的 PPC 研究。

英格兰东部的一个区域性妊娠项目报道了 680 例妊娠病例，其中 2 型糖尿病患者 274 例（40.2%）[15]。只有 27% 的女性接受 PPC（1 型糖尿病占 31%，2 型糖尿病占 20%）。在整个队列中，PPC 与畸形风险（0.7% vs 5.6%，$P=0.02$）和不良结局风险（畸形或围产期死亡的综合因素）（1.3% vs 7.8%，$P=0.0009$）的显著降低相关。此外，在 2 型糖尿病患者中，接受 PPC 的患者无不良反应，而未接受 PPC 的患者不良反应发生率为 6.8%，但这些结果的差异无显著性。

为什么有些女性没有参加妊娠前护理

对于女性不选择 PPC 的原因现在也越来越明确。没有接受 PPC 的女性可能更多为 2 型糖尿病患者，她们可能更年轻，体重更重，大多来自于收入较低的社会阶层或少数民族[25, 26]，也很少有机会获得妊娠前咨询（表 10.3）[15]。

表 10.3　1 型和 2 型糖尿病女性的特征及 PPC 的应用比例[15]

项目	PPC	无 PPC	P 值
人数	181	499	
年龄（岁）	33	31	0.002
种族（白种人比例）（%）	91.7	77.6	0.000 5
贫困：五分位中的第四、五分位数（%）*	41.2	55.1	0.01
BMI（kg/m²）	26.1	27.9	0.005
妊娠前咨询（%）	82.1	31.7	<0.000 1
非吸烟者（%）	83.9	71.4	0.000 2

*来源于 IMD（英格兰东部多重贫困指数）评分中的居住地邮政编码。

最近的一个研究通过采访女性探讨了女性为什么没有接受 PPC 这一问题，该研究纳入了 29 名未参加 PPC 的妊娠女性，她们在妊娠风险宣教（90%）或以往的妊娠前咨询（38%）时并没有被提醒或鼓励参加 PPC，而之前妊娠结局不佳的妇女在发生流产、畸形或死胎经历（41%）时也没有被提醒或鼓励参加 PPC。未接受 PPC 的其他原因还包括妊娠速度快于预期（45%）、生育问题（31%）、与卫生专业人员沟通的负面经历（21%）、对"正常"妊娠的渴望（17%）和对需定期随诊的反感（10%）[27]。另一项研究纳入 15 名女性 40 次妊娠的研究结果表明，计划妊娠和计划外妊娠之间的二分法是有问题的[28]。对于女性来说，在控制葡萄糖水平或被葡萄糖水平所影响之间似乎存在挑战。一名女性在接受妊娠前检查后感到恐惧，她说："这是一次非常非常消极的经历。"一项纳入 14 名女性（大多数为 1 型糖尿病患者）的进一步研究发现，她们不接受 PPC 的理由为害怕和担心被说教[29]。

妊娠前服务的组成部分

生殖健康教育分为两个单独的组成部分。首先是妊娠前咨询，这应该是女性生殖健康教育的一部分，在整个生育期应该定期参加。咨询内容应包括关于避孕药物及工具使用指导、宣教计划妊娠的重要性等。其次是妊娠前护理即 PPC，该护理专门针对希望在不久的将来妊娠的糖尿病女性，其目的是将其妊娠风险降到最低。

妊娠前咨询

妊娠前咨询是针对育龄妇女进行有关妊娠和避孕的教育与讨论。它是初级和（或）专科护理咨询的一个基本组成部分。

在整个生育期应定期进行妊娠前咨询。它包括以下方面。
- 讨论未来的妊娠计划。
- 对避孕措施和相关建议进行记录，相关风险评估，包括糖尿病并发症、吸烟状态和体重。
- 宣教①：血糖控制不佳与不良妊娠结局风险增加密切相关。
- 宣教②：PPC 是什么，以及 PPC 如何改善妊娠结局。
- 建议如何访问 PPC，包括自我推荐时的联络细节。
- 宣教③：应停止服用具有潜在致畸作用的口服降糖药物，如磺酰脲类或 DPP4 抑制剂。
- 宣教④：妊娠前及妊娠早期需补充叶酸。
- 宣教⑤：妊娠期间应避免使用他汀类药物和血管紧张素转换酶抑制剂。
- 宣教⑥：妊娠期间吸烟的风险。
- 宣教⑦：不良妊娠结局与肥胖症和糖尿病妊娠的相关性。
- 如果意外妊娠，告知如何向 PPC 自我推荐。
- 文档记录的任何相关讨论和教育。

妊娠前护理

PPC 是为患有糖尿病的女性做好妊娠准备所需要的额外护理，需要女性患者与医疗专业人员密切合作。其内容包括优化血糖控制、补充叶酸、避免可能致畸的药物、体重管理、戒烟、评估任何糖尿病相关并发症（如眼睛或肾脏并发症），以及讨论妊娠风险。

PPC 最好在糖尿病女性患者妊娠前至少 6 个月开始。表 10.4 显示了 PPC 的内容摘要。

PPC 最好由多学科的团队提供，在患者妊娠期间予以照护，因此团队需要在患者妊娠前即与患者建立联系。

表 10.4　1 型或 2 型糖尿病妇女的妊娠前护理目标

避孕
（1）有效地避孕
（2）避孕直到达到最佳糖化血红蛋白水平

优化血糖控制
（1）使糖化血红蛋白尽可能接近正常范围，而无明显低血糖
（2）建议餐前和餐后 1h 监测血糖，偶尔在夜间监测
- 餐前血糖＜5.8mmol/L
- 餐后（1h）血糖＜7.8mmol/L

（3）如果血糖控制不佳，停止口服降糖药并开始胰岛素治疗
（4）如果血糖改善超过潜在风险，考虑使用二甲双胍
（5）对低血糖的管理予以建议

饮食、锻炼和有组织的教育
（6）推荐营养师针对常规但少量到中度低血糖指数糖类的摄入进行指导
（7）体重指数大于 $27kg/m^2$ 时进行减肥教育
（8）鼓励经常锻炼
（9）提供戒烟、戒酒建议

开具叶酸补充剂
补充剂量：每天 5mg（一些国家的低剂量）

审核其他药物
（10）停止 ACE 抑制剂（ACEI）、血管紧张素受体阻滞剂、他汀类药物或利尿剂
（11）用甲基多巴或拉比他洛尔治疗高血压

筛查糖尿病并发症
（12）在初次访视时评估视网膜病变（除非在过去 6 个月内进行过评估），然后每年评估一次。如果有视网膜病变，考虑转诊给眼科医师
（13）如果出现蛋白尿或肾小球滤过率降低，咨询肾病专家
（14）评估心脏状况并考虑转诊心脏病专家

筛查风疹免疫

对妊娠合并糖尿病和肥胖的风险予以建议
（15）胎儿可能出现：流产、畸形、死产、新生儿死亡、巨大儿
（16）妊娠可能出现：子痫、早产、剖宫产
（17）糖尿病并发症的进展

考虑转诊产科医师或糖尿病专科助产士
（18）评估产科风险
（19）进一步教育和支持

血糖的控制目标

优化血糖控制可降低先天畸形的风险。应鼓励和支持女性在妊娠前降低糖化血红蛋白水平，但始终应注意平衡妊娠妇女发生严重低血糖的风险。在确定目标糖化血红蛋白水平时，应告知女性患者，糖化血红蛋白水平任何程度的减少均可降低胎儿的畸形风险。最近的一项研究表明，当糖化血红蛋白水平高于 10.4% 时，畸形风险约为 10%；当糖化血红蛋白水平低于 6.3% 时，畸形风险线性下降至 3% 左右。糖化血红蛋白降低 1%，风险降低 30%[30]。一个研究糖化血红蛋白与先天畸形相关性的 Meta 分析显示，随着糖化血红蛋白水平的下降，畸形风险逐步下降，糖化血红蛋白为 12% 时，畸形风险为 12%，糖化血红蛋白为 9.0% 时，畸形风险为 9%，糖化血红蛋白为 6.0% 时，畸形风险为 3%[31]。在没有糖尿病的普通人群中，先天畸形的风险约为 3%。

- 在英国，2015 年出版的国家临床优化研究所制定的指南推荐，如果可以实现且没有低血糖风险，妊娠前糖化血红蛋白目标值为 6.5%[32]。
- 相比之下，美国糖尿病协会推荐，建议妊娠前糖化血红蛋白控制在 7.0%[33]。

对于长期患有 1 型糖尿病的女性而言，将糖化血红蛋白控制在 6.5% 以下且不发生低血糖这一目标可能很难实现。对这些女性来说，在向她们表达风险时的措辞很重要，这样才能使患者明白那些罕见但是很严重的后果。女性可能会认为"个体风险比率"的概念更有帮助，尤其是对患有或没有糖尿病的女性进行比较时。例如，33 个没有糖尿病的女性中有 1 个在妊娠时可能发生畸形，但在患有糖尿病的女性中，如果糖化血红蛋白控制在 6.5% 以内，这个比例也是 1：33。但如果糖化血红蛋白大于 7.0%，这个比例为 1：26。糖化血红蛋白大于 7.5%，这个比例为 1：20。如果糖化血红蛋白大于 10%，这个比例为 1：9。

尽管与患者讨论畸形的风险很重要，但医疗保健专业人员必须认识到，给予"不可能达到的"糖化血红蛋白目标可能会妨碍女性参加 PPC[27-29]。为了达到这些目标，应鼓励女性密切地监测血糖，包括每日快速的餐前和餐后血糖测量，并将结果记录在家庭血糖监测日记或记录仪中。门诊血糖仪或远程血糖监测系统有助于进行血糖监测。如果血糖过高或女性身体不适，应检查血液中的酮体。持续的血糖监测系统对某些患者非常有帮助，尤其是那些想明确是否存在夜间血糖不稳定或餐后血糖高的患者，或是那些糖化血红蛋白控制不理想而想明确是否存在餐后血糖高的患者。

低血糖

必须告知所有女性，尤其是 1 型糖尿病女性患者，她们可能不会出现常见的低血糖警告信号，或者这些信号可能很弱。女性在驾车前应常规检测血糖。如果患者无法感受到低血糖，应建议其停止驾驶。应指导家庭成员学会使用胰高血糖素。虽然没有人类研究的证据表明低血糖对胎儿有害，但低血糖对母亲有潜在的危害，会限制母亲实现最佳血糖控制。

研究表明，严重低血糖的风险在妊娠早期最为常见。Evers 和其同事发现，糖化血红蛋白水平较低和糖尿病病史较长的女性发生严重低血糖的风险增加[34]。最近的一项研究显示，尽管接受 PPC 的患者糖化血红蛋白含量较低，但他们发生严重低血糖的风险并未增加[14]。

糖尿病的并发症

一般来说，妊娠与微血管并发症风险的增加无关，因此女性患者不必担心这一点[35]。妊娠和血糖控制的加强都会增加视网膜病变进展的风险。因此，在妊娠前进行视网膜成像很重要。如果有必要，在开始严格的血糖控制和受孕前，对所有视网膜病变进行评估和治疗（参见第二十一章）。糖尿病病史较长和妊娠早期即有视网膜病变的女性在妊娠期间发生视网膜病变恶化的风险最大[36]。

轻度肾脏病的女性其妊娠结局应通过对血糖和血压的最佳控制来优化。但需要提醒这些女性，她们出现子痫前期或肾病恶化的风险增加，进而导致早产的风险增加。早期积极的抗高血压治疗可以降低这些风险[37]。所有女性在妊娠前都应该对白蛋白和肌酐清除率进行评估。患有缺血性心脏病的女性应转诊给心脏病专家进行评估。

血糖控制以外的因素

患有糖尿病的女性生出先天畸形婴儿的概率更高，尤其是先天性心脏缺陷和神经管缺陷。妊娠前补充叶酸可以降低这种风险，在英国，建议所有1型或2型糖尿病女性在妊娠前服用5mg叶酸[32]。所有正在服用的药物都应被重新检视，潜在的致畸药物（包括他汀类药物和血管紧张素转换酶抑制剂）应停止使用。必要时，应将血压治疗更改为适合妊娠期使用的药物。应该为糖尿病女性制订戒烟计划。如果女性的体重指数超过27kg/m^2，应该提供体重管理建议。

2型糖尿病女性PPC的其他因素

导致2型糖尿病患者不良结局的情况是复杂的，包括其他医学合并症、肥胖、血糖控制欠佳、潜在致畸药物、高龄、社会经济地位低和种族因素，其中有许多问题可以用PPC解决（表10.4）。2型糖尿病患者通常比1型糖尿病患者更容易实现严格的血糖控制。肥胖问题必须通过强化饮食管理来解决，鼓励在妊娠前达到最佳BMI（＜27kg/m^2）。必须告知女性，肥胖会增加各种妊娠风险，包括先天畸形、围产期死亡率、子痫、早产、剖宫产和血栓栓塞性疾病。

研究前景

已证实PPC能改善糖尿病患者的妊娠结局，特别是能够有效减少胎儿畸形。但许多问题仍然存在。我们需要进一步理解为什么只有很少的女性能参加PPC。这需要在不同的人群中进行研究，可能需要深入的访谈来加深我们对这个问题的理解。随着2型糖尿病患者的迅速增加，再加上肥胖，目前迫切需要研究如何使更多这样的女性（其中许多妇女仅接受初级保健）参加PPC，并确定PPC对2型糖尿病一样有效。

选择题

1. 应为所有计划妊娠的糖尿病妇女提供妊娠前护理。应告知女性，妊娠前护理将降低以下哪些妊娠并发症的风险（　　）

    A. 视网膜病变　　　　　　B. 先兆子痫
    C. 先天畸形　　　　　　　D. 巨大儿
    E. 宫内生长迟缓

    正确答案是 C。到目前为止，研究表明，妊娠前护理和其他并发症之间没有任何关系。

2. 没有妊娠前护理的糖尿病妇女更有可能具有以下哪些特征（　　）

    A. 来自较高的社会经济阶层　　B. 有视网膜病变病史
    C. 年龄较大　　　　　　　　　D. 来自少数民族
    E. 曾有吸烟史

    正确答案是 D。一些研究表明，接受妊娠前护理的妇女通常来自社会经济地位较高的群体、年龄较大的人群和不吸烟的人群。

（汪　琦　译，朱海清　校）

参 考 文 献

1. Pedersen LM, Tygstrup I, Pedersen J. Congenital malformations in newborn infants of diabetic women. Lancet 1964;1:1124–1126.
2. Karlsson K, Kjellemer I. The outcome of diabetic pregnancies in relation to the mother's blood sugar level. Am J Obstet Gynecol 1972;112:213–220.
3. Morii K, Watanabe G, Ingalls TH. Experimental diabetes in pregnant mice: prevention of congenital malformations in the offspring by insulin. Diabetes 1966;15:194–204.
4. Pedersen J. Congenital malformations. In: The Pregnant Diabetic and Her Newborn, 2nd ed. Munksgaard: Copenhagen, 1977, 196.
5. Fuhrmann K, Reiher H, Semmler K. Prevention of malformations in infants of insulin-dependent diabetic mothers. Diabetes Care 1983;6:219–223.
6. Steel JM. Personal experience of pre-pregnancy care in women with insulin-dependent diabetes. Aust NZ J Obstet Gynaecol 1994;34(2):135–139.
7. Goldman JA, Dicker D, Feldberg D, et al. Pregnancy outcome in patients with insulin-dependent diabetes mellitus with preconceptional diabetic control: a comparative study. Am J Obstet Gynaecol 1986;155:293–297.
8. Mills JL, Knopp RH, Simpson JL, Jovanovic-Peterson L, Meyzger BE, Holmes

LB, Aarons JH, Brown Z, Reed GF, Bieber FR, et al. Lack of relation of increased malformation rates in infants of diabetic mothers to glycaemic control during organogenesis. N Engl J Med 1988;318:671-676.
9 Kitzmiller JL, Gavin LA, Gin GD, Jovanovic-Peterson L, Main EK, Zigrang WD. Pre-conception care of diabetes: glycaemic control prevents congenital anomalies. JAMA 1991;265:731-736.
10 Rosenn B, Miodovnik M, Combs CA, Khoury J, Siddiqi TA. Pre-conception management of insulin dependent diabetes: improvements in pregnancy outcome. Obstet Gynecol 1991;77:846-849.
11 Cousins L. The California Diabetes and Pregnancy Programme: a statewide collaborative program for the pre-conception and prenatal care of diabetic women. Ballieres Clin Obstet Gynecol 1991;5:443-459.
12 Drury PL, Doddridge M. Pre-pregnancy clinics for diabetic women. Lancet 1992;340:919.
13 Willhoite MB, Bennert HW Jr, Palomaki GE, Zaremba MM, Herman WH, Williams JR, Spear NH. The impact of pre-conception counselling on pregnancy outcomes. Diabetes Care 1993;16:450-455.
14 Temple RC, Aldridge VJ, Murphy HR. Prepregnancy care and pregnancy outcomes in women with type 1 diabetes. Diabetes Care 2006;29:1744-1749.
15 Murphy HR, Roland JM, Skinner TC, Simmons D, Gurnell E, Morrish NJ, Soo SC, Kelly S, Lim B, Randall J, Thompsett S, Temple RC. Effectiveness of a regional prepregnancy care program in women with type 1 and type 2 diabetes: benefits beyond glycemic control. Diabetes Care 2010;12:2514-2520.
16 Ray JG, O'Brien TE, Chan WS. Preconception care and the risk of congenital anomalies in the offspring of women with diabetes mellitus: a meta-analysis. Q J Med 2001;94:435-444.
17 Wahabi, HA, Alzeidan RA, Esmaeil SA. Pre-pregnancy care for women with pre-gestational diabetes: a systemic review and meta-analysis. BMC Public Health 2012;12:792.
18 Combs CA, Kitzmiller JL. Spontaneous abortion and congenital malformations in diabetes. Ballieres Clin Obstet Gynaecol 1991;5:315-331.
19 Temple R, Aldridge V, Greenwood R, Heyburn P, Sampson M, Stanley K. Association between outcome of pregnancy and glycaemic control in early pregnancy in type 1 diabetes: population based study. BMJ 2002;325:1275-1276.
20 Dicker D, Feldberg D, Samuel N, Yeshaya A, Karp M, Goldman GA. Spontaneous abortions in patients with insulin-dependent diabetes mellitus: the effect of preconceptional diabetic control. Am J Obstet Gynecol 1988;158:1161-1164.
21 Wahabi HA, Alzeidan RA, Bawazeer GA, Alansari LA, Esmaeil SA Preconception care for diabetic women for improving maternal and fetal outcomes: a systematic review and meta-analysis. BMC Pregnancy Childbirth 2010;10:63.
22 Gold AE, Reilly R, Little J, Walker JD. The effect of glycaemic control in the pre-conception period and early pregnancy on birth weight in women with IDDM. Diabetes Care 1998;21:535-538.
23 Hanson U, Persson B. Epidemiology of pregnancy-induced hypertension and preeclampsia in type 1 (insulin-dependent) diabetic pregnancies in Sweden. Acta Obstet Gynecol Scand 1998;77:620-624.
24 Evers IM, de Valk HW, Visser GH. Risk of complications of pregnancy in women with type 1 diabetes: nationwide prospective study in the Netherlands. BMJ 2004;328:915.
25 Janz NK, Herman WH, Becker MP, Charron-Prochownik D, Shayna VL, Lesnick TG, Jacober SJ, Fachnie JD, Kruger DF, Sanfield JA, Rosenblatt SI, Lorenz RP. Diabetes and pregnancy: factors associated with seeking pre-conception care. Diabetes

Care 1995;18:157-165.
26 Holing EV, Beyer CS, Brown ZA, Connell FA. Why don't women with diabetes plan their pregnancies? Diabetes Care 1998;21:889-895.
27 Murphy HR, Temple RC, Ball VE, Roland JM, Steel S, Zill-E-Huma R, Simmons D, Royce LR, Skinner TC. Personal experiences of women with diabetes who do not attend pre-pregnancy care. East Anglia Study group for Improving Pregnancy Outcomes in Women with Diabetes (EASIPOD). Diabet Med 2010;27(1):92-100.
28 Griffiths F, Lowe P, Boardman F, Ayre C, Gadsby R. Becoming pregnant: exploring the perspectives of women living with diabetes. Br J Gen Pract 2008;58(548):184-190.
29 O'Higgins S, McGuire BE, Mustafa E, Dunne F. Barriers and facilitators to attending pre-pregnancy care services: the ATLANTIC-DIP experience. Diabet Med 2014;31(3):366-374.
30 Bell R, Glinianaia SV, Tennant PW, Bilous RW, Rankin J. Peri-conception hyperglycaemia and nephropathy are associated with risk of congenital anomaly in women with pre-existing diabetes: a population-based cohort study. Diabetologia 2012;55:936-947.
31 Guerin A, Nisenbaum R, Ray JG. Use of maternal GHb concentration to estimate the risk of congenital anomalies in the offspring of women with prepregnancy diabetes. Diabetes Care 2007;30:1920-1923.
32 National Institute for Clinical Excellence. Diabetes in pregnancy: management of diabetes and its complications from preconception to the postnatal period. Guideline NG3. National Institute for Clinical Excellence: London, 2015.
33 American Diabetes Association. Standards of medical care in diabetes. Diabetes Care 2015;37(Suppl 1):S77.
34 Evers IM, ter Braak EW, de Valk HW, van Der Schoot B, Janssen N, Visser GH. Risk indicators predictive for severe hypoglycaemia during the first trimester of type 1 diabetic pregnancy. Diabetes Care 2002;25:554-559.
35 Verier-Mine O, Chaturvedi N, Webb D, Fuller JH. Is pregnancy a risk factor for microvascular complications? The EURODIAB Prospective Complications Study. Diabet Med 2005;22:1503-1509.
36 Temple RC, Aldridge VJ, Sampson MJ, Greenwood RH, Heyburn PJ, Glenn A. Impact of pregnancy on progression of retinopathy in Type 1 diabetes. Diabet Med 2001;18:573-577.
37 Nielsen LR, Muller C, Damm P, Mathiesen ER. Reduced prevalence of early preterm delivery in women with Type 1 diabetes and microalbuminuria-possible effect of early antihypertensive treatment during pregnancy. Diabet Med 2006;23:426-431.

第十一章 先天畸形

Montserrat Balsells[1], Apolonia García-Patterson[2], Juan María Adelantado[3] and Rosa Corcoy[2, 4, 5]

1 Department of Endocrinology and Nutrition, Hospital Universitari Mútua de Terrassa, Terrassa, Spain
2 Department of Endocrinology and Nutrition, Hospital de la Santa Creu i Sant Pau, Barcelona, Spain
3 Department of Obstetrics and Gynaecology, Hospital de la Santa Creu i Sant Pau, Barcelona, Spain
4 CIBER Bioengineering, Biomaterials and Nanotechnology (CIBER-BBN), Instituto de Salud Carlos III, Zaragoza, Spain
5 Department of Medicine, Universitat Autònoma de Barcelona, Bellaterra (Cerdanyola del Vallès), Spain

实践要点

- 定期询问患糖尿病的育龄妇女的妊娠意图,并提供咨询:关于妊娠期间产妇血糖与先天畸形(CM)的发病率之间的关系,持续避孕直到血糖得到合理控制的重要性及相关内容。
- 建议在妊娠前开始补充叶酸。
- 2型和1型糖尿病女性发生先天畸形的风险是相似的。
- 在不能保证良好控制血糖的情况下,在妊娠的前3个月不要停用磺脲类药物或二甲双胍。
- 确保糖尿病妇女得到适当的先天畸形的筛查检测和相应的建议。

病 例

一名32岁的患有1型糖尿病的妇女对一次意外妊娠进行咨询。她在12岁时被诊断出患有1型糖尿病,应用胰岛素类似物作为基础及餐前大剂量模式治疗,她的HbA1c控制在7%~8%(53~63.9mmol/mol)。并发糖尿病视网膜病变和糖尿病肾病;接受过眼科激光手术治疗,现口服依那普利20mg/d。第一次咨询时,她的孕龄为12^{+2}周,HbA1c为7.5%(58.5mmol/mol)。第一次B超扫描也证实了这一日期,眼底检查提示稳定的糖尿病视网膜病变。妊娠18周时行高分辨率超声检查提示心脏畸形(单心室)。1周后,患者被安排进行胎儿超声心动图检查,检查时没有检测到胎儿心跳。行人工流产,对胎儿的尸检证实了超声发现的心脏缺陷。与患者讨论了避孕方式的选择,并询问了患者的妊娠意向。当她表达了想再次妊娠的愿望时,被给予提前的妊娠期保健。

尽管临床实践指南和糖尿病管理及产科监测均得到改进,但先天畸形仍然是糖尿病妊娠的一个严重问题。

流行病学

患病率

自 20 世纪 60 年代起，已经明确患糖尿病的母亲分娩先天畸形婴儿的风险明显增加[1]，与对照组相比，报道的优势比（OR）高达 7.9。

在 21 世纪发表的基于人口学的研究中，综合统计数据显示，糖尿病妇女妊娠后，婴儿发生先天畸形的风险增加[2, 3]。大多数基于时间趋势的文章没有发现显著的差异，除了 Feig 的研究[4]，该报道指出从 1996～2010 年相对风险比（RR）减少了 23%。

虽然关于糖尿病导致先天畸形的信息最初均来自于 1 型糖尿病患者，但是在过去的 10 年中，一些作者也报道了 2 型糖尿病患者妊娠后先天畸形的风险升高。一项发表于 2009 年[5]的 Meta 分析得出结论，虽然患有 2 型糖尿病的女性在妊娠早期 HbA1c 相对较低，但妊娠后期发生先天畸形的风险与 1 型糖尿病的女性相似（RR 为 1.19）。

类型

无论是相对于糖尿病本身还是相对于糖尿病类型，患糖尿病女性后代的先天畸形的发生情况均没有特异性。有些先天畸形发生率较高，而有些则更为独特[6]。

糖尿病女性后代中最常见的先天畸形是心脏缺陷（CD），占所有异常的 40%。神经管畸形（NTD）、骨骼肌肉系统先天畸形和泌尿生殖系统先天畸形的发生率紧随其后，尽管具体的顺序可能因系列而异。有高达 20% 的畸形婴儿存在多重先天畸形。

表 11.1 为妊娠糖尿病妇女和非糖尿病母亲婴儿先天畸形发生风险比较的大型研究。尽管尾部的退化非常少见，但与非糖尿病妊娠相比，糖尿病妊娠导致该畸形的风险大大增加（RR 为 26），这也是糖尿病妊娠中最具特征性的先天畸形。多重先天畸形也是糖尿病导致先天畸形的特征，与非糖尿病女性相比，其 RR 可达 12。尽管有一些例外，但

心脏和中枢神经系统缺陷的 RR 值大约升高两倍。对于其他先天畸形，RR 更加多样。

表 11.1　妊娠前患糖尿病妇女的后代的主要先天畸形

分类	类型	澳大利亚[7] RR（95%CI）	美国[8] RR（95%CI）	欧洲[9] OR（95%CI）	英国[10] PR*（95%CI）	加拿大[11] RR（95%CI）
中枢神经系统		3.16（1.02~9.85）	8.38（3.99~17.64）	1.23（0.96~1.57）	2.7（1.5~4.4）	2.65（0.64~10.9）
心脏		2.84（1.89~4.26）	8.43（3.49~20.4）	2.20（1.88~2.58）	3.4（2.5~4.6）	1.32（0.59~2.98）
肌肉、骨骼和结缔组织	肢体	1.34（0.85~2.12）	0.77（0.11~5.53）	0.61（0.49~0.77）	1.4**（0.8~2.1）	1.33（0.50~3.59）
	脐膨出			2.28（1.13~3.97）		
	其他的骨骼肌			1.5（1.11~2.02）		
尾部退化				26.4（8.98~77.64）		
泌尿生殖系统	肾发育不全/阻塞性缺陷	2.34（1.64~3.33）	9.47（3.02~29.7）	0.88（0.70~1.11）	1.2（0.6~2.2）	0.56（0.08~4.01）
	尿道下裂			0.73（0.50~1.07）	1.5（0.5~3.4）	
胃肠道		0.98（0.37~2.61）	6.15（2.30~16.45）	0.8（0.59~1.08）	0.8（0.2~2.5）	3.27（0.79~13.56）
多系统			12.4（6.86~22.5）	13.6 vs 6.1%***	21 vs 6.1%***	

特定类型的患病率基于在 21 世纪发表的研究人群中确定。*基于 EUROCAT 2002；**适用于所有类型的肌肉、骨骼和结缔组织畸形；***参考的是来自 EUROCAT 的非糖尿病患者的随机样本；PR，比值比；OR，优势比；RR，风险比

使用发展的方法，Mills 推测糖尿病母亲的婴儿发育异常在妊娠的第 8 周之前出现[12]。由于囊胚发育发生在妊娠后的第 5~9 天[6]，这些婴儿有更多的胚原性和中线异常这一事实支持了这一结论。

发病机制

高血糖

现今,妊娠妇女高血糖在先天畸形发病中的作用是无可争议的。早期的数据提示了这一规律后,HbA1c 的出现提供了更明确的证据。2007 年,一项 Meta 分析研究了关于 HbA1c 和先天畸形关系的 7 个队列研究结果,显示两值之间呈指数相关:HbA1c 每增加 1%,CM 的 OP 值增加 1.71[13]。

体内和体外的动物实验研究清楚地证明了妊娠早期高血糖的致畸潜力。其潜在的致病机制将在"介质"(mediators)部分中描述。

低血糖

胰岛素休克疗法(以诱导胰岛素昏迷作为精神疾病的治疗方法)在非糖尿病妊娠早期妇女应用的报道表明低血糖可能是先天畸形的致病因素[14]。患有糖尿病的母亲的信息并不支持这种可能性。例如,Rowland 报道称,患有先天畸形婴儿的糖尿病母亲在妊娠期低血糖发生率低于无先天畸形婴儿的糖尿病母亲[15]。此外,在优化降血糖时经常发生的轻度低血糖与先天畸形没有关系[16]。

上述信息似乎与动物实验数据不符,动物实验表明妊娠早期的低血糖是致畸的危险因素[17]。

人类和动物的实验数据的不同是可以理解的,因为在动物模型中持续低血糖的时间 1~48h,相当于人类持续低血糖的时间 14h~28d,但在临床实践中并没有被观察过。

酮体

在患有 T_1DM 的女性中,妊娠早期 β-羟基丁酸高于无糖尿病的女性,但与先天畸形没有关系[18]。这与动物实验研究结果一致,该实验为证明酮体与先天畸形之间存在因果关系的动物研究,该实验中 β-羟基丁酸的浓度要高 20 倍。动物模型中与先天畸形有关的 β-羟基丁酸的浓度

(>8mmol/L)在糖尿病酮症酸中毒中可以出现,而饥饿酮症则无法达到。

胰岛素

在动物实验中,胰岛素过量或缺乏都会导致先天畸形[19, 20]。胰岛素和胰岛素原水平在发育过程中得到了精细的调节,因为过量会干扰胚胎形态发生,减少引发细胞自然地凋亡。因此,胰岛素在人类妊娠中的致畸作用是可能的[21]。因此,胰岛素在人类妊娠中可能有致畸的作用[21]。

在缺乏特异性抗体的情况下,胰岛素通常是不能穿透人的胎盘的,但在妊娠早期胰岛素是否穿过胎盘仍不清楚。有趣的是,一项病例对照研究发现肥胖和高胰岛素血症是神经管畸形的危险因素;当纠正肥胖后,与高胰岛素血症相关的畸形风险只有轻微降低[22]。

肥胖

在一般人群中,体重指数和先天畸形之间存在正相关性。在一项研究神经管畸形风险的荟萃分析中,有证据表明,神经管畸形与体重指数存在量效关系(OR 值在超重人群中为 1.20,在肥胖人群中为 1.87,均是有意义的)[23]。在针对 CD 的荟萃分析中,风险也与 BMI 呈剂量-反应关系:OR 值在超重人群中为 1.08,在肥胖人群中为 1.23,在重度肥胖人群中为 1.39 人,差异均有显著性意义[24]。肥胖诱发先天畸形的可能机制包括营养过剩、高胰岛素血症和叶酸缺乏。

在患有 T_1DM 的女性中,DM 和 BMI 类别之间存在相互作用[25]。在没有糖尿病的女性中,正常体重组(参照组)观测到的先天畸形的 RR 值为 1.00,超重组为 1.10,肥胖组为 1.15。在 T_1DM 患者中的相应数据分别为正常体重组 2.28、超重组 2.34 和肥胖组 4.11。

介质

在体外模型中,糖尿病动物的血清可导致畸形。在血清成分中,过量的葡萄糖是第一个被检测并被证明是致畸剂因素,随后是酮体和氨基酸。已经证明了存在剂量依赖性效应,不同致畸因素产生协同效应[26]。

导致糖尿病胚胎病变的最后阶段中的一项是细胞过度凋亡，这是胚胎发生的一个重要事件[27]。过量的燃料通过氧化应激导致细胞过度凋亡，该作用通过修改以下数个信号传导通路得以实现：①激活蛋白激酶C，该作用直接或通过脂质过氧化和花生四烯酸的改变导致细胞凋亡。②有丝分裂原激活蛋白激酶信号，该作用抑制细胞增殖，诱发线粒体功能障碍。③Jun N-端激酶的激活，该作用诱导内质网应激。④激活凋亡信号调节激酶-1。肌醇的消耗也可以通过蛋白激酶C信号传导促进致畸。高血糖诱导的缺氧可以通过增加氧化应激来促进先天畸形。

药物

为了治疗高血压和糖尿病肾病，妊娠前糖尿病患者经常使用血管紧张素转换酶抑制剂（ACEI）和血管紧张素受体阻滞剂（ARB）。在妊娠的中期和晚期它们是禁用的，因为在这一时期子宫中的暴露与严重的肾发育和肾功能的损害、羊水过少、肢体挛缩、肺发育不全、胎儿宫内生长发育迟缓和死亡相关，称为ACEI/ARB胎儿病[28, 29]。

在一项队列研究中，在妊娠早期接受ACEI治疗的非糖尿病女性中，先天畸形的发生增多（与未服用抗高血压药物的女性相比，RR为2.71），而在服用其他药物的女性中则没有观察到这一点[30]。然而，一项荟萃分析显示，与健康对照相比，服用ACEI观察到的先天畸形风险增加（RR为1.78）与其他降压药（RR为1.45）风险增加[31]相似。事实上，即使没有治疗，妊娠妇女高血压本身也会显著增加先天畸形的风险（OR为1.20）[32]。因此，与高血压本身或其他降压药物相比，仅限妊娠的前3个月使用ACEI似乎并不增加先天畸形风险。

他汀类药物

他汀类药物被认为是潜在的致畸因子，在妊娠期间禁止使用他汀类药物。胆固醇是Sonic Hedgehog（Shh）蛋白的激活剂，该蛋白对脊椎动物胚胎的形态发生至关重要。在动物模型中，对脂质组织具有高亲和力的他汀类药物到达胚胎，通过降低Sonic Hedgehog（Shh）蛋白来下调内源性胆固醇生物合成，导致畸形发生[33]。在一个包括所有FDA报道的妊娠期间暴露于他汀类药物的不受控制的病例系列中，妊娠初期暴露于他汀类药物导致的重要畸形的发生比例为 31.4%，所有的这些妊娠妇女均为妊娠早期服用了亲脂性他汀类药物。一种特殊的模式被描述，包括不常见的畸形，如全颅畸形、肢体缺陷和 VACTERL[其含义为：V，脊柱畸形（vertebral anomaly）；A，肛门畸形（anal atresia）；C，心脏畸形（cardiac anomaly）；T，气管（tracheo），E，食管瘘（esophageal fistula）；R，肾脏或桡骨畸形（renal or radial anomaly）；L，limb，代表肢体畸形]相关联畸形，这种畸形已经被一些研究报道，但并不是所有的。然而，最近的荟萃分析得出结论，在妊娠期间暴露于他汀类药物时，先天畸形的患病率没有增加（RR：1.15），尽管研究结果受到质量差、样本量小、混淆因素不加调整的限制[34]，但是这些研究并不仅限于患有糖尿病的女性。

根据现有资料，建议妇女在妊娠前停止服用他汀类药物似乎是审慎的。然而，在妊娠初期无意中使用它们不应成为终止妊娠的理由。

口服制剂（降糖药物）

一项针对 T_2DM 妇女妊娠前 3 个月口服药物（主要是第一代磺胺类药物）控制血糖的研究报道显示，先天畸形的患病率为 50%（包括主要和次要畸形）。而相对的，在使用胰岛素治疗的血糖控制相似的 T_2DM 妇女中，畸形的发生率为 15%[35]。然而在包含更大数量女性的更多研究中，并没有报道在胚胎形成过程中暴露于磺脲类药物会导致后代中先天畸形的发生率增加[36]。

尽管有报道称，在小鼠胚胎的培养过程中，苯甲双胍诱导了先天畸形，但二甲双胍并不是致畸的。在人类中，大多数的信息来自于对多囊卵巢综合征的女性在妊娠的前 3 个月给予二甲双胍的研究，研究结果也是让人放心的。在最近的荟萃分析中，暴露于二甲双胍后的女性仅有无意义的低的先天畸形发生率[37]。在患有 T_2DM 的女性中，信息非常有限，但二甲双胍似乎与先天畸形没有关联[35, 38]。

2015 年 ADA 糖尿病指南中没有提及在已有糖尿病的女性中使用格列苯脲或二甲双胍[39]。相反，指南建议口服降糖药物的妇女在妊娠时应尽快开始注射胰岛素行降糖治疗，但可以继续服用二甲双胍和格列苯脲，直到开始胰岛素治疗，以避免发生严重的高血糖症，而严重的高血糖症是一种已知的致畸因素。NICE 2015 建议当改善血糖控制可能带来的好处超过了潜在的危害时，可以考虑在备孕和妊娠期间使用二甲双胍（但需要知情同意,因为药品说明书指出妊娠或计划妊娠的妇女不应该使用二甲双胍治疗)[40]。

胰岛素和胰岛素类似物

胰岛素本身作为致畸因素在病理生理学中有过讨论。目前,没有明确的证据表明胰岛素剂量或类型与先天畸形有关。

尽管缺乏使用胰岛素类似物改善妊娠结局的证据,最近的指南建议优先使用 FDA 和欧洲药品管理局(EMEA)批准的短期作用胰岛素类似物(优泌乐和甘精胰岛素),而不是普通胰岛素[41, 42],因为它们更有可能减少餐后血糖波动。在甘精胰岛素的试验中,与常规胰岛素相比,甘精胰岛素组在妊娠第一和第三个月结束时,餐后血糖增量显著降低。优泌乐的信息主要来自售后监控。

在长效胰岛素类似物的情况下,地特胰岛素(detemir)试验表明,与 NPH 胰岛素相比,地特胰岛素(FDA 和 EMEA 批准)在妊娠 24 周和 36 周时空腹血糖较低,但妊娠结局没有差异。对于甘精胰岛素,目前还没有应用于妊娠的对照临床试验的临床数据,但作为上市后监测报告的应用于妊娠的数据表明没有不良影响。目前建议已经成功地应用这些长期作用胰岛素类似物进行血糖控制的患有糖尿病的妇女继续应用治疗[41]。

预防

妊娠前保健

由于与 DM 相关的先天畸形发生在妊娠早期,此时妇女甚至不知道自己妊娠,所以在妊娠前就采取预防措施是至关重要的。PPC 与先天畸形率降低有关,参加者与非参加者相比仅有 1/3 的风险[43]。随机临床试验尚未进行,而且可能永远也不会进行,因为支持 PPC 有益作用的数据使这项试验不道德。基本的预防措施有:①妊娠前期及早期血糖控制的优化;②避免使用致畸药物;③补充叶酸。体重指数的优化也应该包括在内。这些预防措施意味着患有妊娠前糖尿病的妇女应该计划妊娠并使用有效的避孕方法,直到她们处于最佳受孕状态。

补充叶酸

自 20 世纪 90 年代起,在围妊娠期补充叶酸被用来预防先天畸形。它可以防止神经管畸形的发生(总体 RR 为 0.28),并对其他先天畸形有预防作用,但没有得到证实[44]。由于大量妊娠妇女未能遵循补充叶酸的建议,世界上许多国家已开始使用强制性叶酸强化食品配方。这些项目在没有不良影响的证据的情况下,大幅减少了神经管畸形。

尽管糖尿病妇女妊娠时并非叶酸缺乏状态[45],但在过去的 20 年中,大多数糖尿病妇女妊娠护理指南都包含了补充叶酸的具体建议(表 11.2)。除了少数例外[39],指南建议在围受孕年龄补充高剂量的叶酸(4~5mg/d)。它的依据是包括神经管畸形在内的先天畸形的高风险,动物研究支持该依据[51],一项数学模型研究表明补充叶酸对母体叶酸浓度的影响和叶酸浓度与神经管畸形的关系也支持该依据[52]。然而,建议的措辞是谨慎的,而且建议的力度参差不齐。

表 11.2 妊娠糖尿病妇女补充叶酸的建议

学会	推荐剂量或证据水平和(或)强度的建议	时期
Australian Diabetes in Pregnancy Society 2005[46]	· 5mg/d · 没有提及建议的强度	在妊娠开始前
Endocrine Society 2013[41]	· 5mg/d · 证据 2 ++;强烈建议少	在停止避孕措施或试图妊娠前 3 个月开始……在妊娠 12 周时,叶酸剂量降低到 0.4~1.0mg/d
Canadian Diabetes Association 2013[42]	· 5mg/d · D 级,最有力的证据是共识,临床试验或队列研究除外	妊娠前至少 3 个月,持续到妊娠后至少 12 周
American College of Obstetricians and Gynecologists 2005 on Pregestational Diabetes[47]	· 至少 400μg,大剂量的叶酸可能是在某些情况下有益的,特别是在神经管缺陷的其他风险因素存在时 · 建议的强度没有给出	应该给予所有考虑妊娠的妇女
American College of Obstetricians and Gynecologists 2003/2013 on Neural Tube Defects[48]	· 神经管畸形的高危妇女,推荐每天 4mg 叶酸 · A 级,基于良好的和一致的科学证据	围妊娠期

续表

学会	推荐剂量或证据水平和（或）强度的建议	时期
Royal College of Obstetricians and Gynaecologists 2014[49]	·可能被建议 5mg/d ·建议的强度没有给出	在……之前开始服用额外的叶酸，直到妊娠第 13 周
Society of Obstetricians and Gynaecologists of Canada 2015[50]	·需要叶酸量丰富的食物的饮食，每日口服补充维生素含有 1.0mg 叶酸，测量红细胞叶酸水平可作为妊娠前评估的一部分，以确定复合维生素和叶酸的补充剂量策略（红细胞叶酸＜906nmol/L，1.0mg；红细胞叶酸＞906nmol/L；0.4～0.6mg） ·A 级；有很好的证据推荐临床预防措施	妊娠前至少 3 个月开始直到妊娠 12 周
American Diabetes Association 2008/2016[39]	·至少 400μg/d ·建议强度没有给出	围妊娠期
National Institute for Health and Care Excellence 2015[40]	·建议 5mg/d ·证据级别 3～4 级（非分析研究/专家意见）	从计划妊娠开始到妊娠 12 周

  补充叶酸对已有糖尿病的妇女发生先天畸形风险的影响数据仅限于观察性数据，包括少于 700 例妊娠，而且还不是结论性的。

  由于叶酸在营养指南中推荐的最高摄入量水平是 1mg/d[53]，上述建议应该被认为是在药理学范围的，并且可能有潜在的副作用。掩盖维生素 B_{12} 缺乏是首要问题之一，但 2009 年美国预防措施服务工作组没有发现任何证据来支持或反驳这一点[54]。在最近的 Meta 分析中，虽然大多数研究使用的剂量＜1mg/d，暴露时间＜5 年[55]，但未证实癌症（总体或特定类型）的发生增加。在调整了体外受精的数据后，补充叶酸与双生子没有相关性[54]。关于补充叶酸与哮喘和过敏性疾病之间可能存在联系，一项系统性综述得出结论，大多数研究没有报道与补充叶酸有关，而那些支持正相关的研究发现在妊娠晚期补充叶酸的哮喘和过敏性疾病风险略有增加，且一般局限于幼儿时期[56]。最后，在维生素 B_{12} 缺乏症高发且补充大量叶酸的人群中，母体叶酸浓度高预示了后代的胰岛素抵抗和肥胖[57]。

  可能的机制是推测性的，包括表观遗传修饰和随着脂肪生成增加而减少瘦体重。蛋白质合成的减少是由于缺乏维生素 B_{12}，阻止了同型半胱氨酸合成蛋氨酸的过程，而 5-甲基四氢叶酸的增加会促进这种效果。与此同时，维生素 B_{12} 的缺乏会阻断甲基丙二酰-辅酶 A 变位酶，而甲基丙二酰-辅酶 a 水平的升高会阻断脂肪酸的氧化，促进脂肪生成。

检测和管理

先天畸形的筛查使母亲和家庭有机会为意外事件做好准备，允许产前咨询、治疗，并根据母亲的决定进行适当的产科管理。一旦证实妊娠，妇女应该联系产科医师以确认胎儿情况和预产期。在糖尿病患者中染色体异常的风险并不会增加，并且应该像没有糖尿病的女性一样对异倍体进行筛查。然而，对于妊娠早期的生化筛选，必须考虑到患糖尿病母体可能会影响 AFP（降低）、未结合雌激素（降低）、β-HCG（在一些研究中降低）和妊娠相关血浆蛋白-A 的浓度（降低）。其他参数如颈部透明带似乎不受糖尿病的影响[40]。因此，AFP+雌三醇+β-HCG 或妊娠相关血浆蛋白-A+β-HCG+颈部透明带的筛查结果需要结合母亲患糖尿病的情况进行调整，以便对风险类别提出建议。胎盘活检或羊膜穿刺术的适应证与一般人群没有区别。

进行异倍体筛查的超声扫描可以检测出大部分（30%~70%）的重大异常。然而，在 18~22 周，仍应该为所有妊娠妇女提供高分辨率的超声波扫描，尤其是那些患有糖尿病的妊娠妇女。其目的是检测出妊娠早期无法识别的结构异常，但应该警告妇女注意筛查的局限性，尤其是在存在肥胖的情况下。胎儿身体的器官和结构，特别是中枢神经系统应该被描述，神经管畸形应该被排除（图 11.1）。超声扫描是检测心脏先天畸形的最佳方法，胎儿超声心动图应采用四维超声，流出道需要可视化描述。这种方法的成本效益在敏感度分析中被描述为鲁棒性。如有疑问或发现异常，超声检查应在数周内重复进行，并应与儿科心脏病专家一起告知该妇女异常的重要性。

如果诊断出严重的先天畸形，应该就终止或继续妊娠做出决定。为母亲和家庭提供咨询与支持是必要的，应该确保母亲不会感到内疚。如果决定终止妊娠，可以通过前列腺素诱导和硬膜外麻醉来完成；应提供避孕建议，并在妊娠前提供适当的建议来评估未来的妊娠意向。如果决

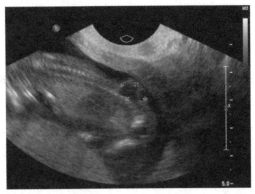

图 11.1　一位妊娠 13 周的糖尿病妇女的超声波扫描显示胎儿腰椎脊髓脊膜膨出

定继续妊娠，应就婴儿的预后和出生后的手术提出建议，婴儿出生后需要进行手术；手术计划需要多学科参与规划，并应该在一个设施完善的三级中心进行。

选择题

1. 以下关于人类先天畸形的陈述之一不正确的是（　　）
    A. 1 型糖尿病和 2 型糖尿病妇女的患病率相似
    B. 心脏异常是最常见的类型
    C. 低血糖是一种强力致畸因素
    D. 高体重指数是致畸的

正确答案是 C。虽然在动物模型中，低血糖是一种强有力的致畸因素，但它在人类糖尿病患者妊娠中的作用仍不清楚；最可能的原因是，人类妊娠期间的暴露时间并不等同于动物模型。的确，在 T_1DM 和 T_2DM 的女性中，先天畸形的患病率是相似的，心脏异常是最常见的类型，高体重指数是致畸性的。

2. 以下关于妊娠期补充叶酸的说法不正确的是（　　）
    A. 1mg/d 叶酸是成年人推荐的最高摄入量
    B. 在动物模型中，叶酸可以防止高血糖诱导的畸形
    C. 糖尿病妊娠是叶酸缺乏状态
    D. 在糖尿病妊娠的人群中补充叶酸的证据很少

正确答案是 C。糖尿病妊娠不是叶酸缺乏状态。的确，1mg/d 是成年人的叶酸摄入量上限。在动物模型中，叶酸可以预防高血糖引起的畸形。在糖尿病妊娠的人群中补充叶酸的证据也很少。

（刘长春 译，王 冰 校）

参 考 文 献

1. Pedersen LM, Tygstrup I, Pedersen J. Congenital malformations in newborn infants of diabetic women: correlation with maternal diabetic vascular complications. Lancet 1964;23:1124-1126.
2. Banhidy F, Acs N, Puho, et al. Congenital abnormalities in the offspring of pregnant women with type 1, type 2 and gestational diabetes mellitus: a population-based case-control study. Congenit Anom 2010;50:115-121.
3. Correa A, Gilboa SM, Besser LM, et al. Diabetes mellitus and birth defects. Am J Obstet Gynecol 2008;199:237-245.
4. Feig DS, Hwee J, Shah BR, et al. Trends in incidence of diabetes in pregnancy and serious perinatal outcomes: a large, population-based study in Ontario, Canada, 1996-2010. Diabetes Care 2014;37:1590-1596.
5. Balsells M, Garcia-Patterson A, Gich I, et al. Maternal and fetal outcome in women with type 2 versus type 1 diabetes mellitus: a systematic review and meta-analysis. J Clin Endocrinol Metab 2009;94:4284-4291.
6. Martínez-Frías ML. Epidemiological analysis of outcomes of pregnancy in diabetic mothers: identification of the most characteristic and most frequent congenital anomalies. Am J Med Genet 1994;51:108-113.
7. Sharpe PB, Chan A, Haan EA, et al. Maternal diabetes and congenital anomalies in South Australia 1986-2000: a population-based cohort study. Birth Defects Res A ClinMol Teratol 2005;73:605-611.
8. Sheffield JS, Butler-Koster EL, Brian Casey BM, et al. Maternal diabetes mellitus and infant malformations. Obstet Gynecol 2002;100:925-930.
9. Garne E, Loane M, Dolk H, et al. Spectrum of congenital anomalies in pregnancies with pregestational diabetes. Birth Defects Res A Clin Mol Teratol 2012;94:134-140.
10. Macintosh MC, Fleming KM, Bailey JA, et al. Perinatal mortality and congenital anomalies in babies of women with type 1 or type 2 diabetes in England, Wales, and Northern Ireland: population based study. BMJ 2006;333:177.
11. Peticca P, Keely EJ, Walker MC, et al. Pregnancy outcomes in diabetes subtypes: how do they compare? A province-based study of Ontario,2005-2006. J Obstet Gynaecol Can 2009;31:487-496.
12. Mills JL, Baker L, Goldman AS. Malformations in infants of diabetic mothers occur before the seventh gestational week: implications for treatment. Diabetes 1979;28:292-293.
13. Guerin A, Nisenbaum R, Ray JG. Use of maternal GHb concentration to estimate the risk of congenital anomalies in the offspring of women with prepregnancy diabetes. Diabetes Care 2007;30:1920-1925.
14. Wickes IG. Foetal defects following insulin coma therapy in early pregnancy. Br Med J 1954;2:1029-1030.
15. Rowland TW, Hubbell JP Jr, Nadas AS. Congenital heart disease in infants of diabetic mothers. J Pediatr 1973;83:815-820.
16. Kitzmiller JL, Gavin LA, Gin GD, et al. Preconception care of diabetes: glycemic

control prevents congenital abnormalities. JAMA 1991;265:731-736.
17 Buchanan TA, Schemmer JK, Freinkel N. Embryotoxic effects of brief maternal insulin-hypoglycemia during organogenesis in the rat. J Clin Invest 1986;78:643-649.
18 Jovanovic L, Metzger BE, Knopp RH, et al. The Diabetes in Early Pregnancy Study: beta-hydroxybutyrate levels in type 1 diabetic pregnancy compared with normal pregnancy. Diabetes Care 1998;21:1978-1984.
19 Landauer W. Rumplessness of chicken embryos produced by the injection of insulin and other chemicals. J Exp Zool 1945;98:65-77.
20 Travers JP, Exell L, Huang B, et al. Insulin and insulin like growth factors in embryonic development: effects of a biologically inert insulin (guinea pig) on rat embryonic growth and development in vitro. Diabetes 1992;41:318-324.
21 Hernández-Sánchez C, Mansilla A, de la Rosa EJ, et al. Proinsulin in development: new roles for an ancient prohormone. Diabetologia 2006;49:1142-1150.
22 Hendricks KA, Nuno OM, Suarez L, et al. Effects of hyperinsulinemia and obesity on risk of neural tube defects among Mexican Americans. Epidemiology 2001;12:630-635.
23 Stothard KJ, Tennant PWG, Bell R, et al. Maternal overweight and obesity and the risk of congenital anomalies: a systematic review and meta-analysis. JAMA 2009;301:636-650.
24 Cai GJ, Sun XX, Zhang L, et al. Association between maternal body mass index and congenital heart defects in offspring: a systematic review. Am J Obstet Gynecol 2014;211:91-117.
25 Persson M, Pasupathy D, Hanson U, et al. Prepregnancy body mass index and the risk of adverse outcome in type 1 diabetic pregnancies: a population-based cohort study. BMJ Open 2012;Feb 14;2(1):e000601.
26 Eriksson UJ, Borg LA. Diabetes and embryonic malformations. Role of substrate-induced free-oxygen radical production for dysmorphogenesis in cultured rat embryos. Diabetes 1993;42:411-419.
27 Yang P, Reece EA, Wang F, et al. Decoding the oxidative stress hypothesis in diabetic embryopathy through proapoptotic kinase signaling. Am J Obstet Gynecol 2014. (Epub ahead of print)
28 Tabacova SA, Kimmel CA. Enalapril: pharmacokinetic/dynamic inferences for comparative developmental toxicity: a review. Reprod Toxicol 2001;15:467-478.
29 Schaefer C. Angiotensin II-receptor-antagonists: further evidence of fetotoxicity but not teratogenicity. Birth Defects Res A Clin Mol Teratol 2003;67:591-594.
30 Cooper WO, Hernandez-Diaz S, Arbogast PG, et al. Major congenital malformations after first-trimester exposure to ACE inhibitors. N Engl J Med 2006;354:2443-2451.
31 Walfisch A, Al-maawali A, Moretti ME, et al. Teratogenicity of angiotensin converting enzyme inhibitors or receptor blockers. J Obstet Gynaecol 2011;31:465-472.
32 Bateman BT, Huybrechts KF, Fischer MA, et al. Chronic hypertension in pregnancy and the risk of congenital malformations: a cohort study. Am J Obstet Gynecol 2014. (Epub ahead of print)
33 Edison RJ, Muenke M. Mechanistic and epidemiologic considerations in the evaluation of adverse birth outcomes following gestational exposure to statins. Am J Med Genet A 2004;131:287-298.
34 Zarek J, Koren G. The fetal safety of statins: a systematic review and meta-analysis. J Obstet Gynaecol Can 2014;36:506-509.
35 Piacquadio K, Hollingsworth D, Murphy M. Effects of in-utero exposure to oral hypoglycaemic drugs. Lancet 1991;338:866-869.
36 Towner D, Kjos SL, Leung B, et al. Congenital malformations in pregnancies complicated by NIDDM. Diabetes Care 1995;18:1446-1451.
37 Cassina M, Donà M, Di Gianantonio E, et al. M. First-trimester exposure to metformin and risk of birth defects: a

systematic review and meta-analysis. Hum Reprod Update 2014;20:656–669.
38 Coetzee EJ, Jackson WP. Oral hypoglycaemics in the first trimester and fetal outcome. S Afr Med J 1984;65:635–637.
39 American Diabetes Association. 12. Management of diabetes in pregnancy. Diabetes Care 2016;39(Suppl):S94–S98.
40 NICE guideline ng3. Diabetes in pregnancy: management of diabetes and its complications from preconception to the postnatal period 2015. http://nice.org.uk/guidance/ng3
41 Blumer I, Hadar E, Hadden DR, et al. Diabetes and pregnancy: an Endocrine Society Clinical Practice Guideline. J Clin Endocrinol Metab 2013;98:4227–4249.
42 Canadian Diabetes Association Clinical Practice Guidelines Expert Committee. Diabetes and pregnancy. Can J Diabetes 2013;37(Suppl 1):S168–S183.
43 Ray JG, O'Brien TE, Chan WS. Preconception care and the risk of congenital anomalies in the offspring of women with diabetes mellitus: a meta-analysis. QJM 2001;94:435–444.
44 De-Regil LM, Fernández-Gaxiola AC, Dowswell T, et al. Effects and safety of periconceptional folate supplementation for preventing birth defects. Cochrane Database Syst Rev 2010;Oct 6(10):CD007950.
45 Kaplan JS, Iqbal S, England BG, et al. Is pregnancy in diabetic women associated with folate deficiency? Diabetes Care 1999;22:1017–1021.
46 McElduff A, Cheung NW, McIntyre HD, et al. The Australasian Diabetes in Pregnancy Society consensus guidelines for the management of type 1 and type 2 diabetes in relation to pregnancy. Med J Aust 2005;183:373–377.
47 American College of Obstetricians and Gynecologists. Pregestational diabetes mellitus. ACOG Practice Bulletin No. 60. Obstet Gynecol 2005;105:675–685.
48 American College of Obstetricians and Gynecologists. Neural tube defects. ACOG Practice Bulletin No. 44. Int J Gynecol Obstet 2003;83:123–133. Reaffirmed in 2013.
49 Fraser RB, Rees G on behalf of RCOG. Nutrition in pregnancy. Paper No. 18. 2010. https://www.rcog.org.uk/en/guidelines-research-services/guidelines/sip18/
50 Pre-conception folic acid and multivitamin supplementation for the primary and secondary prevention of neural tube defects and other folic acid-sensitive congenital anomalies. SOGC Clinical Practice Guideline No. 324. May 2015.
51 Wentzel P, Gäreskog M, Eriksson UJ. Folic acid supplementation diminishes diabetes- and glucose-induced dysmorphogenesis in rat embryos in vivo and in vitro. Diabetes 2005;54:546–553.
52 Wald NJ, Law MR, Morris JK, et al. Quantifying the effect of folic acid. Lancet 2001;358:2069–2073. Review. Erratum in: Lancet 2002;359:630.
53 IOM Committee on Improving Birth Outcomes, Bale JR, Stoll BJ, Lucas, AO, eds. Reducing birth defects: meeting the challenge in the developing world. National Academies Press: Washington, DC, 2003.
54 Wolf T. Folic acid supplementation for the prevention of neural tube defects: an update of the evidence for the U.S. Preventive Services Task Force. Ann Intern Med 2009;150:632–639.
55 Vollset SE, Clarke R, Lewington S, et al. B-Vitamin Treatment Trialists' Collaboration. Effects of folic acid supplementation on overall and site-specific cancer incidence during the randomised trials: meta-analyses of data on 50,000 individuals. Lancet 2013;381:1029–1036.
56 Brown SB, Reeves KW, Bertone-Johnson ER. Maternal folate exposure in pregnancy and childhood asthma and allergy: a systematic review. Nutr Rev 2014;72:55–64.
57 Yajnik CS, Deshpande SS, Jackson AA, et al. Vitamin B12 and folate concentrations during pregnancy and insulin resistance in the offspring: the Pune Maternal Nutrition Study. Diabetologia 2008;51:29–38.

第十二章 妊娠期护理

Jenny Myers[1,2], Susan Quinn[1], Gretta Kearney[1], Susan Curtis[3], Prasanna Rao-Balakrishna[3] and Michael Maresh

1 St Mary's Hospital, Central Manchester University Hospitals NHS Foundation Trust, Manchester Academic Health Sciences Centre, Manchester, UK

2 Maternal & Fetal Health Research Centre, University of Manchester, Manchester, UK

3 Manchester Diabetes Centre, Central Manchester University Hospitals NHS Foundation Trust, Manchester Academic Health Sciences Centre, Manchester, UK

实践要点

- 在妊娠糖尿病管理方面缺乏国际共识,尤其是妊娠糖尿病的治疗。
- 英国2002~2003年的一项调查显示,患有糖尿病的女性患者妊娠结局并不理想,最近在英格兰和威尔士的调查显示仍没有显著改善。
- 在英国,糖尿病妇女的护理质量参差不齐,妊娠前护理严重缺乏。而在美国,还缺乏统一的医疗保健服务。
- 研究制定一项国际指导方针,以及改进妊娠前护理,应用多学科团队的治疗方法可改变对糖尿病妇女的护理质量。

病 例

Emma是一位32岁的初产妇,5岁时患1型糖尿病,20岁时出现视网膜病变、蛋白尿。有长期吸烟史,每日20支左右。未咨询糖尿病护理团队时已打算结婚。在她参加糖尿病中心的年度检查时,报告显示BMI为28kg/m^2,HbA1c为9.3%,医师经常提醒她计划妊娠时优化血糖控制的重要性,并告知血糖指标对胎儿潜在并发症的影响,妊娠前必须停止服用赖诺普利和辛伐他汀,及时开始服用叶酸(5mg)及服用禁忌证。随后她还咨询了营养师,并留取了该中心产科团队的联系电话,以方便妊娠时联系。

接下来的6个月里,Emma经常跟她的糖尿病专科护士和营养师沟通。当她的HbA1c低于7%且无显著低血糖时,医师建议她可以停止避孕。2个月后,孕检测试呈阳性,她立即联系了糖尿病产前小组,医师建议她开始每日服用阿司匹林75mg以降低先兆子痫的风险。

妊娠期间，Emma 每 3 周来诊所进行一次检查，诊所也会对她进行电话随访，及时了解妊娠期间糖尿病的控制情况。她的血糖控制良好，HbA1c 降至 6%，无明显低血糖。常规超声检查显示胎儿生长正常，视网膜评估也显示无恶化，血压平稳，无蛋白尿。到 35 周后，Emma 出现了高血压和蛋白尿。接下来的数周里，情况越来越严重，需要在 37 周时生产。按照标准方案进行葡萄糖胰岛素输注治疗后，分娩出了一个体重 3.3kg 的健康婴儿，不需要进入新生儿病房住院治疗。在分娩后将皮下注射的胰岛素剂量减少至低于妊娠前的胰岛素剂量，考虑她是母乳喂养，所以继续低剂量治疗。产后 6 周复查时，医师建议她采取避孕措施，并为她置入了宫内节育器。告知她母乳喂养结束后继续服用血管紧张素转换酶抑制剂（ACEI）和他汀类药物，并继续回糖尿病中心接受治疗。

- 糖尿病妇女产前护理的具体目标是什么？
- 产前护理的关键要素是什么？
- 一个成功的多学科团队由哪些成员组成？
- 影响有效妊娠护理的因素有哪些？
- 产后护理的主要内容是什么？

背景

在二级或三级保健系统中，普遍采用多学科团队运作的模式，为糖尿病妇女提供妊娠期保健服务[1]。我们的诊所始于 20 世纪 60 年代，多年来不断从实践中更新变革，以适应患者人群的变化、临床发展及当地资源的变化。这也是英国其他地方的做法。在这里，我们会提供符合英国国家卫生和临床技术优化研究所（NICE）指南推荐的妊娠糖尿病服务标准的实用建议[2]。

提供护理指导方针

在 2006 年发表的 12 项国际妊娠糖尿病妇女护理指南[3]中，糖尿病妇女妊娠前服用的叶酸剂量相似，每日剂量在 0.4～5mg。虽然在妊娠时血糖指标、产前预约频率、超声检查及剖宫产胎龄等方面的差异显著，但产前护理指南很少区分 1 型和 2 型糖尿病。对分娩和产后管理的建议也是相似的。

对于妊娠糖尿病，不同国家之间甚至同一国家内部，在筛选过程、筛查方法、诊断标准、口服葡萄糖耐量试验及试验所采集的样本数等方面都存在较大的差异。例如，筛选的纳入标准从无到仅限于特定群体到所有妇女不等。筛选包括在 24 周和 28 周期间进行 50g 非空腹葡萄糖耐量试验，在 28 周时进行 75g 口服葡萄糖耐量试验。诊断阈值包括空腹血糖为 5.1~6.0mmol/L 和（或）75g 口服葡萄糖负荷下 2h 血糖为 7.8~11.1mmol/L[4-6]。

在妊娠糖尿病的治疗管理中，空腹血糖目标为 5.3~6.0mmol/L，餐后 1h 血糖值：<7.0mmol/L，餐后 2h 血糖值：<8.0mmol/L，分娩时间为 38~41 周，分娩后检查的时间为 4~26 周。检查项目为空腹血糖、OGTT、HbA1c 测定。但通常是在 6 周时进行葡萄糖测试，12 周后检测 HbA1c[4]。

对于妊娠糖尿病妇女的管理，尤其是妊娠糖尿病的诊断和治疗，国际上没有共识。然而，WHO 和国际妇产科联合会（FIGO）已经试图去解决与妊娠糖尿病有关的一些问题（参见第四章和第五章）。

糖尿病多学科联合产前诊断及护理的目的

总体目标是让母亲有一个良好的妊娠体验，将血糖控制良好，并正常分娩一个健康的婴儿。

妊娠前护理

读者可参阅第十章。

妊娠期护理

妊娠糖尿病妇女的护理目标：当通过自我检测或体检报告发现妊娠时，快速转诊到联合（糖尿病和产科）诊所。妊娠期间，在保证安全的情况下将血糖维持在接近正常的水平，餐前血糖：4.0~5.3mmol/L；餐后 1h 血糖：小于 7.8mmol/L[2]；餐后 2h 血糖：小于 6.4mmol/L[2]。停止在妊娠前使用任何可能致畸的药物（通常是处方类的他汀类药物和影响肾素-血管紧张素的药物）。

- 妊娠早期根据处方每日服用叶酸 5mg。
- 测定 HbA1c，评估胎儿畸形的风险。
- 监测和适当管理任何与糖尿病相关的并发症，包括快速转诊和进行视网膜评估（参见第二十一章）。
- 通过超声检查准确确定妊娠天数。
- 提供例行产前筛查/检测（如血型、抗体）。
- 约 20 周或更早行超声检查以发现胎儿畸形。
- 通过常规超声检查妊娠中期和晚期胎儿的健康状况。
- 通过 HbA1c 测定，对妊娠早期或妊娠中晚期风险进行评估。
- 确定最合适的分娩时间和方式。
- 妊娠 34 周以下高危产妇在医院内使用类固醇时应进行血糖监测和胰岛素强化治疗（参见第二十三章）。
- 最迟在妊娠 36 周前制订出个性化的血糖管理方案。
- 根据患者的教育、文化、宗教和社会背景，提供以患者为中心的护理和支持。
- 限制护理目标实现的主要因素：①因初级保健服务差或妊娠诊断延迟而延误转诊；②因产妇健康意识欠缺或其他社会经济因素影响导致不能定期及时就诊；③低血糖意识不足是 1 型糖尿病妇女的主要危险因素，尤其是在妊娠初期因恶心、呕吐和自主神经病变加重时导致严重的低血糖。

产后护理

产后护理的目的：
- 根据临床情况，及时调整治疗方案并定期监测血糖。
- 在出生后 1h 内鼓励母婴接触和母乳喂养。
- 除非有新生儿并发症，否则应一律让婴儿留在母亲身边。
- 鼓励产后早期母乳喂养，并监测新生儿血糖（参见第二十四章）。
- 控制产妇血糖水平并维持在可接受范围内：空腹血糖 4～7mmol/L

为非妊娠目标，但是要特别注意的是运动时血糖水平应略高，以防止发生低血糖，尤其是哺乳期妇女，在产后 4～6 周避免低于 5mmol/L。如果母乳喂养，密切监测血糖。

- 在产后 5～6 周时，提供避孕建议（如口服或注射，或放置宫内节育器）（参见第二十五章）。
- 安排产后 6 周的随访。
- 提供妊娠糖尿病保健服务。
    - 妊娠 6 周内监测空腹血糖或 75g 口服葡萄糖耐量试验，12 周后则进行 HbA1c 检查。
    - 提供关于体重管理、饮食和锻炼的建议。
    - 结合社区血糖监测对糖尿病患者进行年度筛查访问，并进行 HbA1c 检查。
    - 讨论未来是否有妊娠计划，在停止避孕措施之前进行血糖评估。

多学科团队成员的组成

临床多学科团队的组成因当地情况而异。该团队的主要成员包括一名产科医师、一名糖尿病医师、一名接受过糖尿病训练的助产士、一名糖尿病专科护士和一名专职的营养师。在美国，可能还包括围产期医师和社会工作者。根据临床经验，一个多学科团队应该具备以下特征：成员具有良好的人际交往能力，对团队工作有高度的亲和力及进取心，成员最好经过动机性访谈和行为改变方面的培训。团队成员应该定期开会讨论服务的组织、国家标准、不良事件、有关研究和教育等。

团队的成员有一些特定的角色，也有一些共享和（或）可交换的角色。团队成员之间沟通良好、团队目标明确能够相互分担任务。表 12.1 总结了根据我们自己的临床经验发展起来的核心成员分工。

糖尿病专科助产士和糖尿病专科护士为优化血糖提供电话支持，必要时每天都有随访。产科医师和其他医师都有一个随时待命系统，为紧急情况提供持续保障。

诊所的架构将因地制宜。我们诊所有 7 间独立的诊疗室，可以让团队成员根据孕周和前一次访问评估的情况对妇女进行（一对一）筛查。

表 12.1 多学科团队成员的角色

成员	角色
团队领导	主持每月小组会议
	与初级保健师联络
	协调区域政策和程序
	负责临床管理包括不良事件
产科医师	针对与糖尿病有关的母婴风险问题提供咨询
	进行有关唐氏综合征筛查和其他检查的健康教育
	评估胎儿的健康状况，包括异常情况和生长发育监测
	确定分娩的时间、方式及产后管理
	针对不良事件向员工和家属提供咨询
	与糖尿病医师一起在制订诊疗计划中发挥主导作用
糖尿病医师	确定育龄妇女进行产前护理
	给出妊娠前的建议，包括药物、检查
	优化妊娠前期、中期、后期血糖控制
	治疗并发症，如视网膜病变或肾病等
	管理胰岛素：处方、教育和剂量调整
	为患者及其伴侣/朋友/支持者提供有关低血糖的诊断、治疗及使用胰高血糖素的教育支持
	提供紧急支持（如确诊低血糖和酮症酸中毒）
糖尿病专科助产士（相当于美国的糖尿病教育工作者，为注册护士）	在妊娠前、产前和产后阶段提供教育支持
	向母亲和婴儿解释潜在风险
	提供有关血糖监测、胰岛素使用、低血糖、高血糖、酮症酸中毒和疾病的建议
	优化血糖控制
	与患者或家人保持联系，提供电话支持
	为产房医护人员提供有关糖尿病患者分娩管理方面的建议
	针对新生儿的喂养给出建议
糖尿病专科护士	在妊娠前、产前和产后阶段提供教育支持
	提供有关血糖监测、胰岛素使用、低血糖、高血糖、酮症酸中毒等疾病的宣教
	优化血糖控制
	提供胰岛素泵和监测仪器方面的专家建议
	与患者或家人保持联系，提供电话支持

续表

成员	角色
营养师	在妊娠前、产前和产后阶段提供饮食建议
	提供关于健康均衡饮食、糖类计数、体重管理、叶酸及应对疾病的策略和建议
	优化血糖控制
	促进和鼓励母乳喂养
初级护理团队	确定育龄糖尿病妇女进行产前护理
	告知有关避孕和妊娠前疾病管理的情况
	及时推荐多学科专家团队
病房普通工作人员	为住院患者提供高质量的糖尿病和产科护理
	产程中优化血糖控制（如葡萄糖-胰岛素输注）

一对一小组成员根据妊娠周数和以前的访问评估对妇女进行临床会诊（图12.1）。在每次临床检查结束时，确定下次就诊时所需的检查项目，以一个支持个体差异的标准模板为基础，从而减少静脉穿刺和超声检查的等待时间。

日期	糖尿病类型
姓名	诊断日期
医院代码	记录日期
	结果：禁食2h
出生日期	年龄
产科病史	
妊娠期体重指数（BMI）	初次妊娠
既往病史	药物（叶酸5mg）
社会/家族史/吸烟史	过敏
糖尿病前期治疗	糖尿病并发症
低血糖（频率/严重程度/意识）	
预防护理	叶酸5mg
专家：日期和研究结果	1.　　　2.　　　3.
胰高血糖素处方	尿酮体处方
高风险：是/否——原因	日期　　　措施
糖尿病管理：用于自然分娩、引产或剖宫产和产后，参照当地指南的具体说明	
新生儿管理：参照当地指南的具体说明	

血糖指标：餐前 4.0~5.3mmol/L；餐后 1h <7.8mmol/L；餐后 2h<6.5mmol/L

周	特殊项目	体重（kg）	HbA1c	血糖:餐前/餐后				胰岛素名称及剂量			
				早餐	午餐	晚餐	睡前				
1											
2											
3	采血检查										
4	记录7~8周										
5	叶酸，尿素氮及电解质										
6	肝功能检查，甲状腺功能检查										
7	视网膜筛查（如果在之前的3个月未做筛查）										
8	HbA1c										
9	胰高血糖素										
10	尿酮体、唐氏筛查										
11											
12											
13											
14											
15											
16											
17	首次视网膜筛查异常										
18											
19											
20	异常扫描										
21											
22											
23											
24	扫描										
25											
26											
27											
28	抗-D 扫描视网膜屏幕										
29											
30											
31											
32											
33											

34									
35									
36	扫描								
37									
38									
39									
40									

图 12.1　妊娠糖尿病临床会诊

妊娠期糖尿病实用手册

当护理质量参差不齐且标准往往不理想时，国家指导标准尤其有用[7]。在这里，介绍一个符合 NICE 2015 指南的本地做法[2]。

妊娠前护理工具

这将取决于所服务人口的具体需要和当地资源。像我们这样的诊所，女性来自多种族的城内人口，可以通过以下方法改善她们获得护理的机会。

- 招聘相关种族的专家成为团队成员。
- 制作教育海报，在初级和二级糖尿病诊所发放。
- 制作教育 DVD，由医师或专科护士向育龄期糖尿病妇女发出[8, 9]。
- 每年向所有育龄期的糖尿病妇女发放教育宣传单。
- 每年由医师或糖尿病专科护士向所有育龄期的糖尿病妇女提供教育短信和电子邮件提醒。
- 开发支持糖尿病的智能手机应用程序，以帮助优化预防治疗。

为妊娠糖尿病妇女提供护理

医疗安排

一旦确定受孕（如约妊娠 5 周），我们将采取鼓励妇女打电话给女性朋友、向任何医疗专业人员求助等方式，促进早期临床就诊。在中心，由糖尿病专科助产士与妇女进行直接电话联系。在其他中心，也可能是糖尿病专科护士进行电话联系。

提供的建议包括每天在家至少进行 7 次血糖监测（三餐前、三餐后和睡前）；告知血糖指标和良好血糖控制的基本原则、叶酸的使用、停止使用潜在的致畸药物，并留下联系电话。对于既往妊娠期间有糖尿病病史的妇女（妊娠小于 12 周），我们将直接转介她向糖尿病专科助产士进行预约咨询，并给予相应的建议。

妊娠期第一次访谈

根据 2016 年 NICE 质量标准[10]，要在转诊后 1 周内进行（通常是与糖尿病专科助产士一起）首次评估。这是第一次病例资料收集，目的是获得该妇女详细的糖尿病病史，评估她对自己病情的理解和管理，并探讨有利于改善其妊娠期间血糖水平的管理新方案，并为她提供一套个性化的教育套餐。

这将会包括以下内容。

1. 糖尿病治疗，包括胰岛素治疗、注射技术和注射部位。

2. 指导和（或）检查血糖、酮体和神经系统，鼓励定期监测，以改善糖尿病的整体控制。

3. 教育妇女和家庭成员有关低血糖发生的时间、机制、发生低血糖时的临床表现及治疗低血糖时如何使用胰高血糖素。

4. 介绍有关中心假期的规定及妊娠期间何时入院。

5. 妊娠期间视网膜检查的重要性。

这种访谈很费时，但有助于妇女为其妊娠做好准备。访谈后就可以安排一次门诊预约，组织所有团队成员为其进行检查，并进行一次超声检查来确诊是否妊娠。

营养师意见

初次访问时，我们了解患者的饮食习惯和生活方式，并提供合理的饮食建议，以改善营养状况。2 型糖尿病妇女在妊娠期间，不妨减轻体重或尽量减少体重增加。糖类的比例对 2 型糖尿病女性很重要。无论是胰岛素治疗或联合二甲双胍治疗都是为了优化血糖控制。对 1 型糖尿病妇女的自我管理知识及糖类计数的技能进行评估，指导患者主要选择血糖指数低的食物，并在需要时及时提供指导。

妊娠护理计划

从妊娠开始到产后6周，所有妇女都有一个护理计划（图12.1）。这份计划包括血糖指标、视网膜及肾脏筛查和随访、胎儿监测（包括胎儿异常和发育状况）、分娩计划和产后糖尿病管理。护理计划是妊娠女性医疗记录的一部分，所有团队成员都可以使用。

初次就诊时，妇女需要检查是否存在与糖尿病有关的所有并发症。在英国，有一个全国性的视网膜检查项目取代了糖尿病医师在诊所进行检眼镜检查的需要。这项检查应尽早安排（在妊娠前3个月内完成），如果发现有任何异常，应在妊娠16~20周进行复查。所有妇女在妊娠约28周时都应进行进一步评估。患有增生型视网膜病变的妇女可以去看眼科医师。另外，还要通过蛋白尿基线筛查评估肾功能，并使用阈值为30mg/mmol的蛋白质-肌酐比值（PCR）进行定量。如果有尿蛋白-肌酐比值大于30mg/mmol，或总蛋白排泄量超过0.5g/d，或血清肌酐异常（≥120mmol/L）、蛋白尿（≥300mg/mmol）等严重肾损害表现及高血压的妇女，应该考虑转诊给肾病科医师作进一步评估和治疗。她们还将被建议进行血栓预防。

随访

对于患有1型或2型糖尿病的妇女，早期在血糖控制达标之前应每周门诊检查一次。妊娠期内，通常至少每1~3周就诊一次，到36周时每周就诊一次，直到分娩。目前的指南建议，应该每隔1~2周[2]通过电话随访，必要时可以随时通过电话联系。也可以通过家庭数据表格远程下载，及时检查血糖情况，从而减少频繁的医院随访。

对于那些经饮食干预及治疗但仍未能达到良好血糖控制的妇女，以及早孕期HbA1c＞85mmol/mol的妇女，我们建议入院接受治疗。补充静脉胰岛素输注并每小时监测血糖，以确定合适的胰岛素治疗方案[11]。我们有时进行两周血糖监测，以便于更好地控制血糖。在英国，建议所有女性在妊娠20周前进行胎儿异常超声筛查，包括心脏四维超声检查、超声心动图检查[7]，定期进行胎儿健康监测和脐动脉多普勒超声检查，直到分娩。血糖控制良好、胎儿没出现生长过快，可遵循每4周检测一次的标准[2]。如果胎儿生长出现偏差或母亲的血糖状态发生变化，那么就需要增加检查次数。如果胎儿生长速度迟缓，那么可以通过胎儿检测（大脑中动脉和静脉导管多普勒）来加强监护，增加胎儿的存活率，这对于没有糖尿病的女性也是一样的。

如果预计在35周之前早产，则建议住院接受皮质类固醇治疗，以提高胎儿肺的成熟度，第二次类固醇治疗后，建议静脉注射胰岛素治疗，持续24h（参见第二十三章）。

预计胎儿是巨大儿，则要制订明确的管理计划，包括胎儿监测、分娩时机和分娩方式。

在妊娠期的最后几周，需要讨论分娩的时机、方式及糖尿病的治疗方案，如果有必要会安排一次麻醉评估。在一切正常的情况下，我们的目标是在妊娠不超过40周时自然分娩，几乎所有的产妇都在39周前完成分娩，这也符合指南要求[2]。产后管理主要包括根据糖尿病的类型减少或停止使用胰岛素、防治新生儿低血糖、确定母乳喂养的起始时间、评价喂养效果等影响血糖的因素。

分娩

对确定分娩的妇女一律提供持续的胎儿电子监护（参见第二十二章）。每小时进行血糖监测。出现血糖波动的情况时，通过静脉注射葡萄糖-胰岛素来维持正常血糖（参见第二十三章）。越来越多的女性在妊娠期间持续使用皮下胰岛素注射泵（CSII），并定期进行剂量调节，同时也想在分娩中继续使用。建议妊娠妇女（或她们的生育伴侣）能够对泵进行必要的调整，以维持血糖正常，那么就可以在分娩中继续使用，并做好记录（参见第十七章）。同样，对于计划剖宫产的女性，在手术前后对基础率进行仔细的计划，保持分娩前、中、后的血糖控制良好。

产后护理

在出院前讨论血糖指标、血糖管理和避孕措施。如果患有糖尿病的女性对血糖控制有焦虑情绪，则在分娩后6周左右或更早时接受检查。她们将得到关于避孕和未来再次妊娠前护理的进一步建议。如果在出院时没有提供避孕建议，那么这次就诊时会建议妇女在血糖未控制达标前不要停止避孕，以降低与糖尿病相关的出生缺陷。然后，将她们转回妊娠前接受保健服务的机构。

为妊娠糖尿病妇女提供护理

在诊断为妊娠糖尿病时，妇女通常会被转介到多学科联合诊所。在妊娠26周时进行葡萄糖耐量试验，如果检验结果为阳性，需要在试验后1周内进行预约[10]，团队成员将教会女性如何进行血糖监测，并在诊断后1周内进行复查。营养师会评估她们的饮食情况，对于依从性差、血糖值持续高于目标的妇女，在第一次检查时就建议口服二甲双胍治疗。然而，如果血糖值显著升高[如餐前血糖＞6.5mmol/L或餐后血糖＞11.0mmol/L]，则需要启动胰岛素与二甲双胍联合治疗。随后的管理与先前患有糖尿病的妇女一样（如本章所讨论）。在妊娠36周时会告知降糖治疗将在分娩时停止。考虑到增加了2型糖尿病的患病风险，会告知她们注意调整生活方式。

在分娩前，建议重视体重管理、饮食和锻炼。妊娠糖尿病妇女在产后接受对葡萄糖耐受性的评估。在此之前，我们在产后6周左右提供了75g OGTT，与2015年的NICE指南[2]相一致。我们在初级保健中只提供空腹血糖检测，但这样会使在葡萄糖负荷试验后应诊断为糖尿病的一小部分妇女漏诊。如果在6周以后才检查，那么可以检测糖化血红蛋白。根据国家指导方针，妇女还应该每年接受初级保健中的糖化血红蛋白检查。如果妊娠妇女有符合OGTT糖尿病诊断标准的，在妊娠后应该建议其进行OGTT检查。

特殊需求

一些因素限制了女性在妊娠期间得到高质量的糖尿病护理。这些因素包括社会经济地位、卫生保健系统及医疗机构专业人员的态度等外部因素。例如，社会因素，包括群体压力、偏见、家庭、工作需求、沟通困难和缺乏支持；心理因素，包括文化、宗教信仰、健康状况、动机不佳、自我效能低下及焦虑和抑郁等问题。

社会阶层影响

导致糖尿病的原因包括饮食不合理、心理压力较大、低水平的体育运动、文化程度低、就业率低。不同阶层人群所处的生存状态不同，那些在贫困地区患糖尿病的患者往往得到低质量的糖尿病护理。

研究显示，社会底层人群对糖尿病干预的依从性较差，对糖尿病知识的知晓率也较低[12]，2型糖尿病患病率也较高，66%的妇女处于贫困的第4或第5等级[13]，这一点将在第十四章中进一步讨论。

种族

与白色人种相比，2型糖尿病和妊娠糖尿病在少数种族群体中更为常见。在英国和欧洲，有大量来自南亚和中东的高危女性。在美国，许多南亚人、拉丁美洲人尤其是墨西哥和中美洲地区的人群，是妊娠糖尿病的高风险群体。

不同种族的人可能不会说或不懂当地语言，以及有不同的文化和健康理念。例如，孟加拉移民与当地白色人种相比，在糖尿病尤其是饮食和运动方面的保健理念就非常不同。

英国的南亚籍移民户外活动水平低于一般的水平，尤其是女性和老年人活动更少[14]。社会规则和文化差异可以在一定程度上解释这一点，如他们限制女性外出参加社交活动和其他户外活动等。少数种族成员与本地人相比，糖尿病知识普及率更低。不讲英语的患者可能自己的母语读写能力也较差，所以用其可以理解的语言及符合本种族文化的方式来进行糖尿病教育对患者是很有帮助的。对于读写能力较弱的患者，提供DVD和互联网资源可能更合适。

提供产科护理和临床管理

2002~2003年英国母婴健康调查机构（CEMACH）调查结果显示，与没有糖尿病的妇女相比，患有1型或2型糖尿病的女性产后预后较差[7]。只有不到 1/5 的 NHS 医院没有任何先入为主的概念。2014 年一项对英格兰和威尔士生育情况的调查显示[13]，婴儿出生情况改善甚微，只有 55%的患有 1 型糖尿病女性和 33%的 2 型糖尿病女性在妊娠前服用叶酸。妊娠前的血糖控制也很差，妊娠早期 HbA1c 评估时只有 8%的 1 型糖尿病患者和 22%的 2 型糖尿病患者 HbA1c＜43mmol/mol（6.1%）。所有这些因素都取决于是否获得高质量的妊娠前护理。

尽管对患有 1 型糖尿病的妇女进行了多学科的二级护理，但早产率（43%）和剖宫产率（67%）仍然很高，死胎率也较高。然而，接受特殊照顾的婴儿数量较前下降，目前只有 33%的婴儿在出生时与母亲分离。

未来的方向

最紧迫的问题是有效提高妊娠前护理质量，尽管英国和其他国家已经提出了建议，但为数不多。对于患有 2 型糖尿病的妇女来说，在初级保健中，医疗保健专业人员必须定期提供有关妊娠风险的建议，并向所有的育龄期妇女提供适当的预防措施建议。在贫困严重和少数种族妇女人数较多的地区，可能需要采取创新的办法。然而，即使是对患有 1 型糖尿病的妇女，她们的大部分护理等级为二级护理，数据表明类似的方法仍然需要。为了维持和提高妊娠糖尿病护理标准，需要定期审定地方、区域和国家的各级标准。有些医疗机构和保健人员能够以区域/国家的标准为基准，这对于推动和改进护理发展非常有用，还可以作为获得额外资源的一种方法。现在有足够的理论来指导实践，只要普遍应用就可以改变妊娠糖尿病妇女的结局。我们的挑战是向所有糖尿病妇女提供这种高质量的护理。

编者注：美国视角

首先，在向糖尿病的妇女提供医疗保健方面，大西洋两岸存在相似之处。妊娠前血糖控制、妊娠前和妊娠期叶酸的使用、视网膜状况评估和肾功能检测、妊娠期血糖控制、胎儿健康评估等，这些都是糖尿病妇女护理的目标。还必须指出的是，美国的医疗政策是由一些非政府机构制定的，这些权威机构并不总是在患者护理的某些方面达成一致，其中包括妊娠糖尿病的定义和为治疗糖尿病妇女推荐的目标血糖值[15, 16]。

自从该书第一版出版以来，美国的医疗保健服务已经发生了重大变化。2010 年《患者保护与平价医疗法案》(ACA)条款生效后，拥有医疗保险的美国成年人数量增加了 1600 万[17]，没有医疗保险的成年人比例从 2013 年第三季度的 18%下降至 2016 年第一季度的 11%。产科和新生儿护理列为本法规的基本健康福利之一。妊娠前护理也是产妇保健的一项福利，提供避孕建议、药物、设备和措施都是法律规定的。然而，对于认为这些护理保健服务有违于他们宗教信仰的群体，则不受这种要求和约束。评估这些变化对糖尿病妇女护理的影响需要持续的努力。必须指出的是，在农村地区，某些制药商对药物（包括紧急避孕的产后避孕）的持续药效拒绝提供法律担保，还有一些州对医疗和外科手术的实施设置了限制条件，使得 ACA 的某些条款的启动遇到障碍。但在英国，这些障碍大多微不足道或根本不存在，提供医疗保健时出现的问题大多与患者的依从性有关。美国和英国有一个共同点，都需要学习如何有效地提高糖尿病妇女妊娠前和产前护理的依从性。

选择题

1. 下列哪一项是正确的（　　　）
   A. 患有 1 型糖尿病的妇女在妊娠时应将餐前血糖值目标定为 3.5～5.0mmol/L
   B. 社会贫困并不是影响产前护理的一个因素
   C. 视网膜检查应在妊娠早期进行，在妊娠前 2 个月也要进行检查
   D. 患有 1 型糖尿病的妇女的家庭成员（如伴侣或母亲）应被告知何时及如何向她注射胰高血糖素
   E. 饮食建议应包括如何避免低血糖指数食物

   正确答案是 D。

2. 以下正确的是（　　　）（多选题）
   A. 一般不建议将胎儿胎心监测作为糖尿病妇女胎儿畸形筛查的一个组成部分

B. 控制蛋白尿通常被认为是预防血栓形成的一项关键因素
C. 有了适当的产前准备，许多妇女能够使用胰岛素泵来控制分娩前和分娩中的血糖
D. 应建议妇女产后保持妊娠前的血糖指标，尤其是母乳喂养的女性
E. 患有妊娠糖尿病的妇女产后检查无特殊异常时，应该每 1～3 年进行一次葡萄糖耐量测试，以减少未来的健康风险

正确答案是 B、C 和 E。

（侯淑敏　译，朱海清　校）

参 考 文 献

1. Dornhorst A & Hadden D. Diabetes and Pregnancy: An International Approach to Diagnosis and Management. John Wiley & Sons Ltd: Chichester, 1996.
2. National Institute for Health and Care Excellence (NICE). Diabetes in pregnancy: management from preconception to the postnatal period. 2015. http://www.nice.org.uk/guidance/ng3/resources/diabetes-in-pregnancy-management-from-preconception-to-the-postnatal-period-51038446021
3. Cutchie WA, Cheung NW, & Simmons D. Comparison of international and New Zealand guidelines for the care of pregnant women with diabetes. Diabetic Med 2006;23(5):460–468.
4. Agarwal MM, et al. Gestational diabetes: dilemma caused by multiple international diagnostic criteria. Diabetic Med 2005;22(12):1731–1736.
5. National Institutes of Health Consensus Development Conference Statement. Diagnosing Gestational Diabetes Mellitus Conference 2013. http://prevention.nih.gov/cdp/conferences/2013/gdm/resources.aspx
6. Metzger BE, et al. The diagnosis of gestational diabetes mellitus: new paradigms or status quo? J Matern-Fetal Neonat Med 2012;25(12):2564–2569.
7. Confidential Enquiry into Maternal and Child Health (CEMACH). Diabetes in Pregnancy: Are We Providing the Best Possible Care? Findings of a National Enquiry. CEMACH: London, 2007. http://www.cemach.org.uk
8. Gough A, et al. Preconception counselling resource for women with diabetes. BMJ Qual Improv Rep 2015;4(1).
9. Holmes VA, et al. Evaluation of a DVD for women with diabetes: impact on knowledge and attitudes to preconception care. Diabetic Med 2012;29(7):950–956.
10. National Institute for Health and Care Excellence (NICE). Diabetes in Pregnancy. Quality standard. 2016. http://www.nice.org.uk/guidance/qs109
11. Kaushal K, et al. A protocol for improved glycaemic control following corticosteroid therapy in diabetic pregnancies. Diabetic Med 2003;20(1):73–75.
12. Department of Health. National Service Framework for Diabetes: Standards. 2001. http://www.dh.gov.uk/en/Publicationsandstatistics/Publications/PublicationsPolicyAndGuidance/DH_4002951
13. Healthcare Quality Improvement Partnership. National Pregnancy in Diabetes Audit Report, 2014. 2015. http://www.hscic.gov.uk/catalogue/PUB19042/nati-preg-in-diab-audi-rep-2014.pdf
14. Bachmann MO, et al. Socio-economic inequalities in diabetes complications,

control, attitudes and health service use: a cross-sectional study. Diabetic Med 2003;20(11):921–929.
15 American Diabetes Association. Management of diabetes in pregnancy. Diabetes Care 2016;39(Suppl 1): S94–S98.
16 American College of Obstetricians and Gynecologists (ACOG). Pregestational diabetes mellitus. Clinical Management Guidelines for Obstetrician-Gynecologists. ACOG Practice Bulletin No. 60, March 2005. Obstetr Gynecol 2005;105(3):675–685.
17 Wallace J & Sommers BD. Health insurance effects on preventive care and health: a methodologic review. Am J Prev Med 2016;50(5 Suppl 1):S27–S33.

第十三章 1型糖尿病女性更常遇到的问题

Una M. Graham [1], *Michael Maresh* [2] *and David R. McCance* [1]

1 Regional Centre for Endocrinology and Diabetes, Royal Victoria Hospital, Belfast, Northern Ireland, UK

2 St Mary's Hospital, Central Manchester University Hospitals NHS Foundation Trust, Manchester Academic Health Sciences Centre, Manchester, UK

实践要点

- 母体低血糖对于患者和临床医师实现妊娠期间接近正常血糖水平仍然是一项重大挑战。
- 低血糖无意识可与妊娠相关或作为自主神经病变的表现,是临床医师特别关心的问题。管理可能需要更新的技术,包括持续皮下注射胰岛素(CSII)和使用报警装置进行血糖检测。
- 糖尿病胃轻瘫作为自主神经病变的一种表现形式,在其他糖尿病微血管并发症和血糖控制不佳或波动的情况下,尤其是当常规推荐的治疗无效时,应予以怀疑。这些患者面临相当大的管理困难。
- 妊娠糖尿病酮症酸中毒与胎儿死亡率显著相关。关于病假规则和24h热线的母亲教育是预防的关键。
- 1型糖尿病妊娠妇女发生死产的概率是一般妊娠妇女的3倍,而且很可能是多因素导致的。
- 现在越来越多的妇女使用糖类计数来指导妊娠期胰岛素的剂量;需要进一步的研究来评估有组织的患者教育对产妇胎儿结局的影响。

概述

本章的重点是1型糖尿病(T_1DM)患者比2型糖尿病(T_2DM)患者更容易遇到的问题。虽然低血糖包括在这一章中,但很明显,这种并发症也会发生在使用胰岛素的T_2DM妇女身上。此外,糖尿病酮症酸中毒(DKA)通常与T_1DM有关,但也有与T_2DM甚至妊娠糖尿病有关的报道。

低血糖

低血糖（血糖<4.0mmol/L）是 T$_1$DM 患者在妊娠期血糖控制方面面临的主要挑战。它可分为轻度（由患者自主治疗）或重度（需要另一方协助），这两种情况在妊娠期间发生的频率更高。在一项对 108 名患有 T$_1$DM 母亲的研究中，45%的妇女在妊娠的某个阶段有严重的低血糖事件，妊娠前一年的 1.1 个事件/（患者·年）在第 1 年、2 年、3 年的发生率分别为 5.3%、2.4%和 0.5%[1]。轻度低血糖在早期妊娠中也很常见，通常归因于妊娠前 3 个月后期引起的恶心和呕吐及胰岛素需求的下降。严重低血糖的预测指标包括低血糖意识受损、既往有严重低血糖史、糖尿病持续时间长、早孕 HbA1c 低、血糖波动、餐间过量补充胰岛素[2]。

迄今为止，没有任何已知的低血糖的孕产妇的后代随访至 5 岁的长期后果[3]。相反，严重低血糖的孕产妇后果很重要，包括意识丧失、癫痫发作和住院[2]。在许多国家，发生过严重低血糖者要禁忌驾驶长达 12 个月。T$_1$DM 的女性在妊娠期间死亡率显著增加，正如芬兰的一项研究报道，T$_1$DM 的妊娠妇女比没有 T$_1$DM 的妊娠妇女死亡率增加了 100 多倍（0.51% vs 0.004 7%）[4]。在孕产妇死亡队列研究中，2/5 的报道是由于低血糖（其余 3/5 的死亡是由于 DKA、脑干梗死和出血）[4]。最近的一个回顾显示，英国从 2009 年到 2012 年确定为 T$_1$DM 的 5 名孕产妇在妊娠期间死亡，其中 1 名不知道自己妊娠了，死于胰腺炎[5]。剩下的 4 名女性死亡原因分别为低血糖死于溺水（1 名）、DKA（2 名）和糖尿病并发症（1 名）。这 4 名妇女一直在接受糖尿病产前服务，并在试图优化控制过程中经历过低血糖发作[5]。这突出了在妊娠期间对患者和临床医师优化血糖控制的持续挑战，以及避免低血糖的重要性。这是通过密切的末梢血糖自我监测，并通过糖尿病专家小组对妊娠妇女低血糖风险及其管理进行专门的教育来实现的。如果低血糖持续，应考虑使用现有的技术，如胰岛素泵治疗或具有低血糖报警特征的血糖监测传感器。

有指南建议症状性低血糖治疗首选 15～20g 的速效糖类（如 150ml 纯果汁），其次是长效糖类（如一片面包）与重复剂量的速效糖类，直到末梢血糖恢复正常[6]。治疗还包括胰岛素剂量调整，以避免未来低血糖反复发作。

未察觉的低血糖

未察觉的低血糖是临床医师试图优化妊娠期血糖控制的主要问题。对失去预警症状的一种可能解释是自主神经病变，它可能减弱了儿茶酚胺对低血糖的反应。在妊娠期的研究是有限的，但有证据表明，妊娠本身与损坏低血糖负反馈反应相关联，这种影响在糖尿病妊娠妇女中更为明显[7]。然而，在 Airaksinen 研究中，尽管血糖控制水平相当，但患有心血管自主神经病变的妊娠妇女与未患心血管自主神经病变的妊娠妇女相比，发生低血糖的比例没有显著增加[8]。无论低血糖是否为自主神经病变的结果，急性期低血糖的处理是相同的。对于具有低血糖报警功能的血糖监测传感器的适用性可能对这些具有挑战性的患者有用（参见第十六章）。

自主神经病变

自主神经病变是糖尿病患者的长期并发症之一，尤其是在血糖控制不够理想的情况下。虽然本病可发生在 T_2DM 妊娠妇女中，但更常见的是发生在 T_1DM 妊娠妇女中。它可能影响许多器官系统，包括心血管、胃肠、泌尿和视觉系统。此外，低血糖意识可能受损。在妊娠之外，关于患病率的不确定性，部分与诊断标准的变化有关。然而，据估计约有50%的长期糖尿病患者，特别是在其他微血管并发症的情况下，有胃排空延迟（胃轻瘫）。自主神经病变的症状可以在没有神经病变的妊娠妇女中出现，使诊断变得困难。因此，这种疾病在妊娠期的流行程度不确定，但几乎可以肯定的是，它被低估了。关于这一主题的文献（出于实际需要）主要限于小型研究或偶尔的案例报道。

对胃肠道的影响

最常出现的自主神经病变表现是胃延迟排空，因迷走神经受损而引起。症状包括早期饱腹、恶心、呕吐、上腹部不适、腹胀。恶心和呕吐在妊娠早期很常见，通常在妊娠中早期消失。这些症状的持续，或在妊娠后期出现或重新出现，应增加潜在自主神经病变意识的可能性。标准的止吐治疗是第一道防线，但很少有效。也可以考虑使用促胃肠动力药物如胃复安和多哌立酮或红霉素等药物。红霉素静脉注射比口服更有效。关于这个主题的文献主要局限于病例报道，结果往往很差[9, 10]。类固醇治疗（如 30mg/d 的泼尼松龙）也被报道是有益的[11]，尽管这通常会干扰血糖控制，但由于胃肠运输的改变而变化的营养吸收，再加上恶心和呕吐，已经严重干扰血糖控制。严重的胃轻瘫可能导致营养耗尽和脱水，患者需要住院补充水分和维持血糖稳定。在严重病例中，可能需要肠外营养，这与症状改善有关，尽管这可能在一定程度上是心理作用[10]。母体代谢的波动主要增加了胎儿在子宫内死亡的风险，因此需要对可能发生胃轻瘫的病例有较高的怀疑指数和补救措施。

其他不太严重的胃肠道症状仍然困扰妇女，这可能是由自主神经病变引起的便秘和腹泻。如果标准治疗不能缓解便秘，那么应该尝试一种促胃肠动力剂（如已讨论的）。有时候，便秘和腹泻是交替发生的，甲硝唑等抗生素可能会有帮助，因为肠停滞可能导致细菌过度生长。

对心血管的影响

对心脏和血管的自主神经损伤可能影响心率控制，导致心动过速和血压变化，引起直立性低血压或高血压。同样，这些问题在正常妊娠中很常见，导致诊断混乱。这些心血管变化可能限制运动耐受性，增加运动期间不良心血管事件的风险。温度调节也可能受到影响，因此需要特别注意避免在任何极端温度下进行剧烈运动。研究认为妊娠期正常的血流动力学改变是由亚临床自主神经功能障碍所致。在一项妊娠纵向研究中，Airaksinen 等发现 T_1DM 妊娠妇女与未患糖尿病的妊娠妇女相比，其母亲心率的正常生理增长较少，导致心输出量减少[12]。然而，在另一项研究中，没有发现心血管功能的改变[13]。另一项研究表明[8]，有自主神经病变影响心血管系统的客观证据的女性，与没有此类证据的女性相比，不良妊娠事件有所增加。一份病例报道指出，一名因自主神经病变继发直立性低血压的妇女在妊娠期间有改善，可能继发于血容量增加，分娩后立即消退[14]。由心血管自主神经病变引起的孕产妇死亡病例已被报道[9]。如果心血管症状和体征提示自主神经病变，评估包括心电图、体位血压和随呼吸频率变化的心率（尽管这项测试还没有在妊娠中使用）。治疗应以对症治疗为基础。

糖尿病酮症酸中毒

糖尿病酮症酸中毒（DKA）定义为酮血症、高血糖和酸中毒的三联生化反应。回顾性研究显示，在患有糖尿病的母亲中，有1%～2%发生妊娠期DKA[15, 16]。随着血糖控制和随访的加强，目前DKA的发病率可能降低。虽然DKA通常与T_1DM有关，但它也发生在T_2DM的妇女中，并已在妊娠糖尿病中报道。同样值得注意的是，当妊娠妇女在妊娠期间出现DKA时，由于胎儿和胎盘对母体葡萄糖的利用，血糖通常低于预期[17, 18]。因此，对于妊娠期间出现不适的糖尿病患者，即使血糖正常或较低，也应考虑DKA[18-21]。

DKA发生在胰岛素绝对或相对缺乏的情况下。胰岛素缺乏会导致高血糖和血浆胰高血糖素升高，进而刺激肝糖异生和脂解作用，继而引发酮反应（图13.1）。妊娠期间发生的生理变化会增加酮症和随后的酸中毒

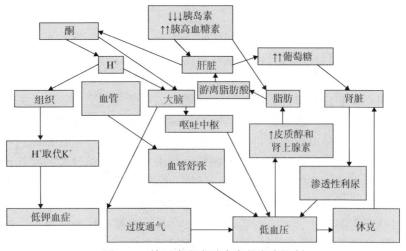

图13.1 糖尿病酮症酸中毒的发病机制

的风险。人胎盘催乳素（hPL）是由滋养细胞合成并释放到母体中血液，降低母体对胰岛素敏感性，增加餐后血糖水平。妊娠妇女也更容易受到禁食的影响，尤其是在妊娠中期和晚期。在妊娠晚期，胎盘和胎儿消耗大量作为主要能量来源的葡萄糖，导致母亲空腹血糖降低。这致使脂肪酸释放用作母体代用能量，随后合成酮。最后，在妊娠晚期发生呼吸性碱中毒，由于呼吸速率增加，导致碳酸氢盐经肾脏排泄增加，从而降低了酮酸的缓冲能力。因此，T_1DM 患者如果病情控制不理想，并且暴露在诱发因素下，可能会发展为 DKA。妊娠期 DKA 与妊娠期外 DKA 类似，包括感染、全身性疾病、呕吐、脱水和胰岛素缺失。妊娠并发症期间服用的药物，即糖皮质激素和抗抑郁药，也与诱发 DKA 有关[18, 20]。

DKA 是一种急症。在过去的 20 年中，孕产妇死亡率从 7.96%下降到 0.67%，这反映了治疗方案的改进和对预防 DKA 并发症的重视[22]。治疗方案在不同的中心有所不同，但都涉及对患者的意识水平、血流动力学状态和可能诱发疾病的初步评估。图 13.2 给出了一个方案示例。管理集中在五个关键领域。

1）液体：在高血糖的情况下，初始选择的液体是 0.9%氯化钠溶液（如果患者也有高钠血症，则用 0.45%氯化钠溶液），考虑到患者的低容量状态，分娩率在开始时通常很高，在入院的前数小时内降低到维持率。

2）胰岛素：目前的指南推荐一种固定的、根据重量调整的静脉注射（IV）胰岛素，输注速率为 0.1U/（kg·h）[23]。这是从静脉输液开始，直到末梢血酮正常为止。为了达到这个目的，通常需要额外输注 10%葡萄糖以避免低血糖。患者继续用长效胰岛素皮下注射。这对于帮助患者在酮症酸中毒消退后迅速转变为常规皮下胰岛素是很重要的。一旦没有酮，就开始进行可变速率胰岛素输注，或胰岛素和葡萄糖输注，以维持正常血糖，直到患者能够进食时用皮下胰岛素替代。

3）钾：严重低钾血症是 DKA 治疗过程中最常见的危及生命的电解质紊乱[24]。DKA 管理的一个重要部分是前瞻性钾替代，即使血清浓度正常[23]。为了确保足够的钾替代，血清钾测量为每小时 2~4 次。

4）沉淀剂：需要识别和处理潜在的原因（请参阅本节前文讨论的沉淀剂）。

5）并发症的预防：DKA 的并发症包括高/低钾血症（也在本节中讨论）、脑水肿和肺水肿及血栓栓塞性疾病。脑水肿的病因是脑灌注不足后再灌注[25]，虽然在成人中很少见，但在患有 DKA 的儿童中，占了死亡人数的 70%～80%[26]。肺水肿也是 DKA 与短时间快速输液相关的罕见并发症[27]。严格遵守液体治疗方案，定期评估液体平衡和患者意识水平，以及对 18 岁以下患者使用可适应的液体治疗方案是避免这些并发症的关键[28]。妊娠和 DKA 均增加血栓栓塞风险，因此对于所有出现 DKA 的患者，都需要使用肝素或低分子量肝素进行预防[29]。

调查	
基线	末梢血糖和酮体
	实验室葡萄糖、尿素氮和电解质
	静脉血气分析
	如果怀疑是高渗性高血糖，则需要检测血清渗透压
	格拉斯哥昏迷量表（GCS）
检测方案	常规观测资料
	每小时末梢血糖和血酮
	在 0h、1h、2h 测静脉的碳酸氢盐和钾，直到 2h 后酮清除
	每小时测 GCS
其他调查	全血计数、血培养、尿培养、心电图和脑部 X 线检查

静脉输注 0.9%氯化钠溶液：

1000ml	在第 1h
2000ml	接下来的 4h
2000ml	接下来的 8h
1000ml	每 6h 1 次

如果初始收缩压小于 90mmHg，则给予 0.9%氯化钠溶液 500ml，持续 10～15min，必要时重复，并考虑其他原因，如心力衰竭或败血症。如果血钠>155mmol/L，考虑初始使用 0.45%的氯化钠溶液

胰岛素：
开始固定静脉注射 50U 可溶性胰岛素+50ml 0.9%氯化钠溶液，以 0.1U/（kg·h）的量（根据患者的体重）估计。如果启动胰岛素有延迟，则给予 20U 可溶性胰岛素肌内注射，如果患者常规服用长效胰岛素，则继续按常规时间和剂量操作。

钾：
在开始胰岛素时开始使用钾，如下：

钾浓度	补钾
>5.5mmol/L	无
3.5～5.5mmol/L	40mmol/L 的 0.9%氯化钠溶液
<3.5mmol/L	暂时停止胰岛素，因为需要补钾，应立即询问上级大夫

其余方法：
- 如果患者昏迷或持续呕吐，必须下鼻胃管。
- 如果尿失禁或 1h 无尿，考虑导尿。
- 酌情用低分子量肝素进行血栓预防。
- 考虑 DKA 的诱发原因。
- 末梢血酮下降 0.5mmol/（L·h），末梢血糖下降至少 3mmol/（L·h）。如果没有，考虑增加 1U/h 的胰岛素输注量。

结果：
- 当末梢血糖＜14mmol/L：在 125ml/h 加入 10%的葡萄糖溶液，并根据需要进行调整，以葡萄糖 5~10mmol/L 为目标。静脉输注胰岛素和 0.9%氯化钠溶液与钾溶液应继续。
- 当末梢血酮＜0.3mmol：停止静脉注射胰岛素和 10%葡萄糖溶液。在准备进食前，开始使用 5%葡萄糖溶液 500ml 和 8U 可溶性胰岛素静脉滴注大于 6h，必要时调整以保持血糖在 5~10mmol/L。必要时继续输注 0.9%氯化钠溶液。
- 转化为皮下注射胰岛素，在临床条件允许的情况下开始进食。第一次皮下注射胰岛素后，持续静脉注射葡萄糖/胰岛素至少 30min。

图 13.2　贝尔法斯特糖尿病酮症酸中毒成人治疗方案

糖尿病酮症酸中毒的胎儿后果

20 多年前的研究报道显示，DKA 患者的胎儿死亡率为 9%~35%，如果诊断和治疗延迟，死亡率会更高[15, 16, 30]。近几年，这些数字可能会随着产前护理的改善而有所改善。在 DKA 治疗的过程中，母亲开始在临床和生化方面进行改进，需要通过超声和胎心监护（CTG）对胎儿进行评估。无论胎儿的状况如何，对胎儿健康的评估都要推迟到母亲处于恢复阶段，因为在母亲的状况稳定下来之前不能采取任何措施。除了胎儿死亡外，还有一些证据表明，宫内接触酮增多与后代的行为和智力发育有不利关系[3]。这进一步加深了避免妊娠期 DKA 的重要性。

预防糖尿病酮症酸中毒

DKA 可以通过频繁的血糖监测、积极的胰岛素调节和在产前类固醇给药等情况下使用胰岛素滴定算法进行预防。必须指导 T_1DM 母亲如何监测尿液或毛细血管的酮类物质，并经常提醒她们注意"生病期间的法则"，包括在强化血糖监测指导下补充胰岛素的需要（图 13.3）。与此相辅相成的是可以 24h 接触的糖尿病小组。

疾病和糖尿病

当你生病时，即使你不吃东西，你的血糖也会升高。控制血糖比较困难，你应该联系糖尿病中心寻求帮助和建议。

你该怎么做呢？

- 永远不要停止服用胰岛素。
- 经常检测血糖。
- 经常检查血液中的酮类——如果有，立即联系你的糖尿病中心。
- 如果反复呕吐或酮类增多，应尽快就医。
- 增加你喝的液体量。
- 如果你不想吃，那就把固体食物换成甜的饮料，如果汁。牛奶饮料、普通的水果酸奶和冰淇淋也提供糖类。

如有疑问，请与您的糖尿病中心联系（应向每位患者提供24h联系电话）

图 13.3　生病期间的法则

死胎

对于 T_1DM 患者和照顾她们的临床医师来说，产前胎死腹中仍然是所有结果中最严重的。大多数 T_1DM 患者意识到死胎风险的增加，监督的临床医师有责任确保母亲得到充分的信息。这种风险通常是普通人群的 3 倍左右，在 2009~2011 年，英国每 100 名妊娠妇女中就有 1 人会受到影响[31]。因此，一个普通的大型妇产医院可能每 1~2 年就会有一次死产。小医院可能有更少的死产，因此可能不知道他们有一个相对高的比例。如此高的比例在今天是不可接受的，尽管不幸的是，英国的比例在过去 10 年里几乎没有变化[32, 33]。长期以来，为了降低宫内死亡的风险，妊娠妇女倾向于提前分娩，目前的建议是在妊娠 37 周或更早时分娩，如果妊娠妇女或胎儿有特殊的风险[34]。然而研究表明，糖尿病妊娠妇女在分娩前死产的风险增加，发生在妊娠 32 周时[35]。

虽然在一般人群中已探讨了死产的危险因素[36]，但很难确定与 T_1DM 具体相关的原因，因为从数字上讲，这些妊娠相对不常见，幸运的是，死亡是罕见的。T_1DM 的胎儿死亡很可能是多因素的，但是有很多因素使一些女性的风险增加，包括胎盘的血管供应问题与子痫前期、肾脏和大血管疾病的风险增加有关。这也可能导致妊娠早期胎盘不良，在妊娠的不同阶段可能出现胎儿生长受限。此外，令人沮丧的是，在一项研究中，仍然有高达 19% 的糖尿病女性吸烟[37]，这可能也会减少胎盘的氧气供应。妊娠晚期 HbA1c 的评估与死产和不良妊娠结局的风险增加有关[38, 39]，而且似乎需要 HbA1c 低于 6.0% 才能将风险降至最低。母亲高血糖与胎儿酸中毒的增加有关[40]，与对照组相比，糖尿病妇女的羊水促红细胞生成素升高，提示存在缺氧，羊水促红细胞生成素与母体 HbA1c 呈正相关，与脐动脉 pH 呈负相关[41]；这部分可能由 2，3-DPG 活性受损所致。如果胎儿是大体型的，可能会有心肌肥大和增加氧气需求。胎儿也可能易患心律失常。在妊娠晚期发现的子宫收缩力增加会导致短暂的缺氧发作，这是正常胎儿能够承受的，没有困难。然而，对于胎儿的氧需求量增加，已有轻度酸血症，并有边缘胎盘血管供应不足，可能不太容易。一项对患有糖尿病的妇女进行的对照死胎研究报道称，胎盘重量较轻，子代胸腺变化的发生率增加，这可能归因于严重的亚急性代谢紊乱[42]。

总之，戒烟、超声监测胎儿的生长、妊娠中期子宫动脉多普勒测量，以及多学科小组的努力使血糖水平接近正常，并意识到具体的危险因素，减少妇女及其家庭发生这些悲剧的风险，因为她们几乎总是在妊娠期间投入大量时间和精力。但集中治疗是否能改善这些结果仍不确定。

糖类计数和 1 型糖尿病

建议对所有 T_1DM 患者进行糖类计算的结构化教育[43]。英国正常饮食剂量调整（DAFNE）课程是一项经过验证的有益处的结构化教育计划，T_1DM 患者可以根据膳食或零食中的糖类含量来调整胰岛素（图 13.4）[44]。

午餐
一片面包：15g 糖类
1 个煮鸡蛋：0g 糖类
一杯牛奶：15g 糖类
总计：30g 糖类
10g 糖类=1 糖类点
因此，这顿饭是 3 糖类点。如果患者的胰岛素和糖类的比例是 1：1，他们需要 3U 的胰岛素

图 13.4 根据膳食中糖类含量调整胰岛素

因此，胰岛素剂量是用个性化的胰岛素-糖类比例来计算的。越来越多的 T_1DM 孕妇将接受糖类计数的培训。照顾这些妇女的糖尿病学家要

熟悉在妊娠期间需要定期调整胰岛素和糖类的比例。已经发表的关于妊娠期 1 型糖尿病妇女糖类计数经验的研究很少。在贝尔法斯特，一项针对 28 名 T_1DM（14 名在达夫尼接受训练）女性的小型研究发现，达夫尼训练过的女性能更好地控制妊娠前血糖，也更有可能参加妊娠前咨询并服用适当剂量的叶酸（未发表的数据）。这反映出围绕妊娠期的强化教育计划可能会被纳入结构化教育里。我们的研究没有能力去评估妊娠结果，这需要进行更大规模的研究以评估结构化教育对母婴结局的影响。

选择题

1. 关于 1 型糖尿病患者妊娠期的低血糖（可选择适用项）（　　　）
   A. 它仍然是孕产妇死亡的一个重要原因
   B. 目前英国的 NICE 指南建议血糖≥3.5mmol/L
   C. 低血糖意识可能因自主意识而降低
   D. 当妇女妊娠时，严重的低血糖事件会减少
   E. 治疗低血糖事件应包括短期和长期作用的糖类

正确答案是 A、C、E。

2. 关于 DKA（　　　）
   A. DKA 与超过 40% 的胎死腹中风险相关
   B. 在 DKA 时，如果 CTG 呈病理性，应迅速行剖宫产术
   C. 如果血糖正常，则不应诊断 DKA
   D. DKA 可发生于 2 型糖尿病和妊娠糖尿病
   E. 妊娠晚期正常呼吸性碱中毒部分缓解 DKA 的发展

正确答案是 D。

致谢

本章的部分内容从第一版的各个章节中摘录和修改，包括 Bob Young 教授撰写的关于 DKA 的部分。

（任　歆　译，朱海清　校）

参 考 文 献

1. Nielsen RL, Pendersen-Bjergaard U, Thorsteinsson B, et al. Hypoglycaemia in pregnant women with type 1 diabetes: predictors and role of metabolic control. Diabetes Care 2008;31:9–14.
2. Ringholm L, Pedersen-Bjergaard U, Thorsteinsson B, Damm P, & Mathiesen ER. Hypoglycaemia during pregnancy in women with type 1 diabetes. Diabetic Med 2012;29:558–566.
3. Rizzo T, Metzger BE, Burns WJ, & Burns K. Correlations between antepartum maternal metabolism and child intelligence. N Engl J Med 1991;325:911–916.
4. Leinonen PJ, Hiilesmaa VK, Kaaja RJ, & Teramo KA. Maternal mortality in type 1 diabetes. Diabetes Care 2001;24:1501–1502.
5. Knight M, Kenyon S, Brocklehurst P, et al. on behalf of MBRRACE. Saving lives, improving mothers' care. Lessons learned to inform future maternity care from the UK and Ireland confidential enquiries into maternal deaths and morbidity 2009–2012. National Perinatal Epidemiology Unit, University of Oxford: Oxford, 2014.
6. Joint British Diabetes Societies. The Hospital Management of Hypoglycaemia in Adults with Diabetes Mellitus. 2013. https://www.diabetes.org.uk/Documents/About%20Us/Our%20views/Care%20recs/JBDS%20hypoglycaemia%20position%20(2013).pdf
7. Rosenn BM, Miodovnik M, Khoury JC, & Siddiqi TA. Counterregulatory hormonal responses to hypoglycemia during pregnancy. Obstet Gynecol 1996;87:568–574.
8. Airaksinen KE, Anttila LM, Linnaluoto MK, Jouppila PI, Takkunen IT, & Salmela PI. Autonomic influence on pregnancy outcome in IDDM. Diabetes Care 1990;13:756–761.
9. Steel JM. Autonomic neuropathy in pregnancy. Diabetes Care 1989;12:170–171.
10. Macleod AF, Smith SA, Sonksen PH, & Lowy C. The problem of autonomic neuropathy in diabetic pregnancy. Diabetic Med 1990;7:80–82.
11. Myers JM. Autonomic neuropathy in diabetes in pregnancy. In: A Practical Manual of Diabetes in Pregnancy, Eds: McCance DR, Maresh M, & Sacks DA. Wiley-Blackwell: Chichester, 2010, 176–183.
12. Airaksinen KE, Ikaheimo MJ, Salmela PI, Kirkinen P, Linnaluoto MK, & Takkunen IT. Impaired cardiac adjustment in pregnancy in type 1 diabetes. Diabetes Care 1986;9:376–383.
13. Lapolla A, Cardone C, Negrin P, Midena E, Marini S, Gardellin C, Bruttomesso D, & Fedele D. Pregnancy does not induce or worsen retinal and peripheral nerve dysfunction in insulin-dependent diabetic women. J Diabetic Complic 1998;12:74–78.
14. Scott AR, Tattersall RB, & McPherson M. Improvement of postural hypotension and severe diabetic neuropathy during pregnancy. Diabetes Care 1988;11:369–730.
15. Cullen MT, Reece EA, Homko CJ, et al. The changing presentations of diabetic ketoacidosis during pregnancy. Am J Perinatol 1996;13:449–451.
16. Kilvert JA, Nicholson HO, & Wright AD. Ketoacidosis in diabetic pregnancy. Diabetic Med 1993;10:278–281.
17. Chico M, Levine SM, & Lewis DF. Normoglycaemia diabetic ketoacidosis in pregnancy. J Perinatol 2008;28:310–312.
18. Graham UM, Cooke IE, & McCance DR. A case of euglycaemic diabetic ketoacidosis in a patient with gestational diabetes mellitus. Obstetric Medicine 2014;7:174–176.
19. Alexandre L, Shipman KE, Brahma A, et al. Diabetic ketoacidosis following steroid treatment in a patient with gestational diabetes mellitus. Practical Diab Int 2011;28:21–23.
20. Betalov A & Balasubramanyam A.

Glucocorticoid induced ketoacidosis in gestational diabetes: sequela of the acute treatment of preterm labor. Diabetes Care 1997;20:922–924.

21 Madaan M, Aggarwal K, Sharma R, & Trivedi SS. Diabetic ketoacidosis with lower blood glucose levels in pregnancy: a report of two cases. J Reprod Med 2012;57:452–455.

22 Lin SF, Lin JD, & Huang YY. Diabetic ketoacidosis: comparison of patient characteristics, clinical presentations and outcomes today and 20 years ago. Chang Gung Med 2005;28:24–30.

23 Joint British Diabetes Societies. The Management of Diabetic Ketoacidosis in Adults. 2013. http://www.diabetologists-abcd.org.uk/jbds/JBDS_IP_DKA_Adults_Revised.pdf

24 Hardern RD & Quinn ND. Emergency management of diabetic ketoacidosis in adults. Emerg Med J 2003;20:210–213.

25 Glaser N, Barnett P, McCaslin I, Nelson D, Trainor J, Louie J, et al. Risk factors for cerebral edema in children with diabetic ketoacidosis. N Eng J Med 2001;344(4):264–269.

26 Edge JA, Ford-Adams ME, & Dunger DB. Causes of death in children with insulin dependent diabetes 1990–1996. Arch Dis Child 1999;81(4):318–323.

27 Dixon AN, Jude EB, Banerjee AK, & Bain SC. Simultaneous pulmonary and cerebral oedema, and multiple CNS infarctions as complications of diabetic ketoacidosis: a case report. Diabetic Med 2006;23(5):571–573.

28 British Society for Paediatric Endocrinology. Guideline for the Management of Children and Young People under the Age of 18 Years with Diabetic Ketoacidosis. 2015. http://www.bsped.org.uk/clinical/docs/DKAguideline.pdf

29 College of Obstetricians and Gynaecologists. Reducing the Risk of Venous Thromboembolism during Pregnancy and Puerperium. 2015. https://www.rcog.org.uk/globalassets/documents/guidelines/gtg-37a.pdf

30 Montoro MN, Myers VP, Mestman JH, et al. Outcome of pregnancy in diabetic ketoacidosis. Am J Perinatol 1993;10:17–20.

31 Gardosi J, Madurasinghe V, Williams M, et al. Maternal and fetal risk factors of stillbirth: population based study. BMJ 2013;346:f108.

32 Confidential Enquiry into Maternal and Child Health. Pregnancy in women with type 1 and type 2 diabetes in 2002–03, England, Wales and Northern Ireland. CEMACH: London, 2005.

33 Healthcare Quality Improvement Partnership. N.D.A., National Pregnancy in Diabetes Audit Report, 2014. 2015. http://www.hscic.gov.uk/catalogue/PUB19042/nati-preg-in-diab-audi-rep-2014.pdf

34 National Institute for Clinical Excellence (NICE). Diabetes in pregnancy: management from preconception to the postnatal period. 2015. http://www.nice.org.uk/guidance/ng3/resources/diabetes-in-pregnancy-management-from-preconception-to-the-postnatal-period-51038446021

35 Holman N, Bell R, Murphy H, & Maresh M. Women with pre-gestational diabetes have a higher risk of stillbirth at all gestations after 32 weeks. Diabetic Med 2014;31:1129–1132.

36 Flenady V, Koopmans L, Middleton P, Froen JF, Smith GC, Gibbons K, Coory M, Gordon A, Ellwood D, McIntyre HD, Fretts R, & Ezzati M. Major risk factors for stillbirth in high-income countries: a systematic review and meta-analysis. Lancet 2011;377:1331–1340.

37 McCance DR, Holmes VA, Maresh MJ, Patterson CG, Walker JD, Pearson DW, & Young IS. Vitamin C and vitamin E for the prevention of pre-eclampsia in women with type 1 diabetes (DAPIT): a multicentre randomized placebo-controlled trial. Lancet 2010;376:259–266.

38 Tennant PW, Glinianaia SV, Bilous RW, Rankin J, & Bell R. Pre-existing diabetes, maternal glycated haemoglobin, and the risks of fetal and infant death: a population-

based study. Diabetologia 2014;57:285–294.
39 Maresh MJ, Holmes VA, Patterson CC, Young IS, Pearson DWM, Walker JD, & McCance DR. Glycemic targets in the second and third trimester of pregnancy for women with type 1 diabetes. Diabetes Care 2015;38:34–42.
40 Salvesen DR, Brudenell JM, Proudler A, et al. Fetal pancreatic beta-cell function in pregnancies complicated by maternal diabetes mellitus. Am J Obstet Gynecol 1993;168:1363–1369.
41 Teramo K, Kari MA, Eronen M, Markkanen H, & Hiilesmaa V. High amniotic fluid erythropoietin levels are associated with an increased frequency of fetal and neonatal morbidity in type 1 diabetic pregnancies. Diabetologia 2004;47:1695–1703.
42 Edwards A, Springett A, Padfield J, Dorling J, Bugg G, & Mansell P. Differences in post-mortem findings after stillbirth in women with and without diabetes. Diabetic Med 2013;30:1219–1224.
43 National Institute for Clinical Excellence (NICE). Type 1 diabetes in adults: diagnosis and management. 2015. https://www.nice.org.uk/guidance/ng17/resources/type-1-diabetes-in-adults-diagnosis-and-management-183727 6469701
44 DAFNE Study Group. Training in flexible, intensive insulin management to enable dietary freedom in people with type 1 diabetes: dose adjustment for normal eating (DAFNE) randomised controlled trial. BMJ 2002;325:746.

第十四章 2型糖尿病女性更常遇到的问题

Lorie M. Harper

Department of Obstetrics and Gynecology, University of Alabama at Birmingham, Birmingham, Alabama, USA

实践要点

- 2型糖尿病的妊娠结局与1型糖尿病相似。
- 2型糖尿病患者可能并发高血压、肾病和（或）视网膜病变。
- 2型糖尿病妇女应针对上述并发症进行评估，而无须考虑确诊时间的长短。
- 2型糖尿病妇女可在妊娠期使用口服药物治疗。大多数药物几乎没有任何关于安全性和有效性的数据。胰岛素是在妊娠期间实现血糖控制的首选药物。

病例

一位33岁的2型糖尿病妇女来进行妊娠前咨询。她在31岁时被诊断为2型糖尿病和高血压，截至目前已经超过一年的时间没有见过她的主治医师。目前服用二甲双胍和血管紧张素转换酶抑制剂。糖化血红蛋白为53mmol/mol（7%），尿蛋白/肌酐值为0.3，血压为145/93mmHg。眼科医师证实有良性增生性视网膜病变。

- 妊娠前推荐的糖化血红蛋白是多少？如何达到目标？
- 肾病是如何影响妊娠结局的？
- 血压目标值是多少，推荐什么药物来实现这些目标？
- 妊娠期视网膜病变筛查的建议是什么？视网膜病变是如何影响妊娠结局的？

2型糖尿病的患病率

2013年，国际糖尿病联合会统计，全球约有8.3%的成年人或3.82亿人患有糖尿病[1]，其中90%是2型糖尿病患者，患病率从20～24岁的2%上升到40～44岁的7%不等。令人震惊的是，这些患者中有45%还未被确诊，年轻患者更容易被漏诊[2]。

一般说来，年轻的妊娠糖尿病患者以1型糖尿病的发病率更高。然而，由于肥胖多发，特别是儿童期肥胖，导致年轻患者2型糖尿病的诊断率也在增加。根据 Dabalea 等的报道，10～19 岁的 2 型糖尿病患病率比 10 岁以下增长了 30%[3]。同时，很多女性选择推迟妊娠时间，导致妊娠妇女年龄增加，妊娠期间 2 型糖尿病的风险也随之增加[4]。因此，女性在妊娠期间 1 型糖尿病与 2 型糖尿病的发病率正在发生变化。在英国，2002～2003 年 2 型糖尿病占妊娠糖尿病的 27%[5]；2014 年这一数字增加到了 47%[6]。

与 1 型糖尿病妇女相比，妊娠合并 2 型糖尿病妇女年龄偏大：在英国，79%的患者在 30 岁或以上，只有 50%的妇女患有 1 型糖尿病。2 型糖尿病在白种人女性中较少见，而更多见于亚洲女性或黑种人女性。2 型糖尿病也更多见于社会经济地位较低的人群[6]。由于 2 型糖尿病与妊娠期 2 型糖尿病的发病率越来越高，产科医师必须了解 2 型糖尿病及 1 型糖尿病的特点。区别在于 2 型糖尿病的常规治疗、并发症和患者对于妊娠期血糖管理的态度。

2 型糖尿病患者的妊娠前咨询

妊娠前咨询的重点应在于血糖控制，评估并发症，并将药物改为避免致畸暴露的药物。妊娠前咨询是有益的，可以有效控制糖尿病患者的妊娠成本[7-14]。虽然大多数研究更多关注 1 型糖尿病，妊娠前咨询对 2 型糖尿病女性同样重要。然而，现实是 2 型糖尿病妇女很少进行妊娠期保健。尽管糖化血红蛋白对于评估 2 型糖尿病妇女的价值较低[5, 6, 15]，而最近一项研究证实，母体患有糖尿病，孩子出生缺陷的发生率会增加[16]。尽管原因不明（未确诊糖尿病导致血糖管理缺乏、叶酸摄入不足、肥胖或致畸暴露），因此 2 型糖尿病患者仍然是高风险人群，应努力确诊并优化妊娠前控制。

2 型糖尿病并发症

比起没有微血管并发症的妊娠糖尿病患者，合并微血管并发症患者预后更差。因此，首次产前检查要筛查微血管并发症。尽管微血管并发症（肾病或视网膜病变）在很大程度上是缘于糖尿病患者长期血糖控制不佳，因此更多见于 1 型糖尿病，而对于 2 型糖尿病妇女也必须进行筛查。有 6%～7% 的 2 型糖尿病妇女有微量蛋白尿，可见于糖尿病发病时及临床诊断时[17, 18]。对于 2 型糖尿病患者，从无肾病到微量白蛋白尿，从微量蛋白尿到大量蛋白尿，从大量蛋白尿到尿肌酐升高，每年以 2%～3% 的速度进展。鉴于这些事实，所有的 2 型糖尿病妇女应在初次产检时筛查肾病。

高达 20% 的 2 型糖尿病妇女在确诊糖尿病时即有视网膜病变[19]。有 26% 的无视网膜病变的患者在 4 年后逐渐出现视网膜病变，大部分为背景性视网膜病、黄斑变性、增生性视网膜病变[20]。值得注意的是，绝大多数患者（91%）没有进行视网膜病变的年度筛查；因此，妊娠前要进行视网膜病变的筛查。所有 2 型糖尿病妇女都应该在妊娠早期进行视网膜病变的筛查，作为初筛监控[21]。

2 型糖尿病常见合并症

高血压

糖尿病患者在确诊时，有 1/3 患者同时患有高血压，在很大程度上与 2 型糖尿病相关的代谢综合征有关[18, 22]。高血压与肾病及视网膜病变进展密切相关，因此严格控制血压对 2 型糖尿病妇女至关重要。美国糖尿病协会推荐控制血压 < 140/90mmHg，年轻患者应更低，血压 < 130/80mmHg[23]。ACEI 与 ARB 常被作为首选药物，因其对肾脏的保护作用。然而，ACEI 和 ARB 与胎儿死亡、心脏缺陷、肾小管发育不全及肺发育不良相关，因此在妊娠期要禁用这两种药物[24-28]。因此，对于育龄女性，ACEI 与 ARB 应慎用。对于准备妊娠的 2 型糖尿病妇女，应使用非致畸性抗高血压药进行合理的血压控制。妊娠期常用钙通道阻滞剂、β 受体阻滞剂和肼屈嗪。要阻止妊娠期妇女选择 ACEI 或 ARB，对其耐心劝告，并推荐药物替代选择，建议根据胎龄进行详细的超声检查。无论哪种糖尿病类型，高血压都会明显增加先兆子痫、胎儿生长受限、早产和不良新生儿事件的风险[29]。让前来咨询的患者认识高血压可以帮助他们区别慢性高血压与先兆子痫。目前还不清楚是否控制高血压可以改变不良妊娠结局的风险。

血脂异常

高达 70%的 2 型糖尿病患者存在血脂异常[30]，具有特征性的三酰甘油升高和高密度脂蛋白（HDL）降低的模式[31]。对于非妊娠状态下的女性患者，如三酰甘油升高（>1.7mmol/L）或 HDL 降低（<1.3mmol/L）推荐使用他汀类药物治疗。而他汀类药物禁用于妊娠期妇女。他汀类药物的作用机制是通过抑制胆固醇的生成实现的，而胆固醇对于胚胎发育是非常重要的。虽然目前针对人体的研究尚未显示致畸作用[32,33]，但是他汀类药物仍应停止用于准备妊娠的妇女和妊娠期妇女。应建议患者改善生活方式以降低心血管疾病危险因素，并降低低密度脂蛋白（LDL）的水平。妊娠可以引起血脂谱的变化，因此在妊娠期无须进行常规血脂监测。

心血管疾病

虽然对于无症状的患者并不推荐进行 2 型糖尿病的筛查，其仍然是心血管事件的一个重要的危险因素[23]。然而，幸运的是，患有 2 型糖尿病的育龄妇女很少发生心脏病。小剂量的阿司匹林常推荐用于糖尿病妇女，妊娠期也可持续使用。

抑郁症

抑郁症与 2 型糖尿病常常共患[34-36]。2 型糖尿病妇女应该进行抑郁症的筛查。抑郁症与围产期不良事件有关（早产、先兆子痫和宫内发育迟缓），应该在妊娠期给予治疗，包括心理治疗及合理的药物治疗[37-42]。

肥胖

高达 80%的 2 型糖尿病患者存在肥胖[43]。肥胖与妊娠期合并症显著相关，包括死产、剖宫产、先兆子痫、巨大儿、肩难产和早产[44-48]。如果妊娠前肥胖，应该建议在妊娠前达到正常体重指数。如果妊娠期间肥胖，应该建议遵循健康饮食和每天 30min 的适量运动。虽然在妊娠期间不建议减肥，根据 IOM 指南应该建议肥胖女性在妊娠期间体重增加 10～20 磅（1 磅=0.4536kg）。糖尿病妇女如果在妊娠期体重增加超过指南推荐，会出现围产期不良事件[49-51]。虽然妊娠期体重增加低于指南并不增加低体重婴儿的风险,但目前针对糖尿病妇女妊娠期间体重低于指南推荐范围方面的研究极少。

阻塞性睡眠呼吸暂停/睡眠呼吸紊乱

睡眠障碍,以睡眠呼吸紊乱或阻塞性睡眠呼吸暂停为特征,在 2 型糖尿病患者中更为普遍[52, 53]。这很可能与 2 型糖尿病患者的肥胖相关。睡眠呼吸紊乱是妊娠高血压综合征及严重母婴并发症的危险因素[54-56]。应该对妊娠前或产前检查的 2 型糖尿病肥胖妇女进行睡眠呼吸紊乱的筛查。然而,对睡眠呼吸障碍进行治疗是否可以改善妊娠结局仍有待确定。

癌症

2 型糖尿病有可能增加肝脏、胰腺、结肠、乳腺、膀胱和子宫内膜肿瘤的风险[57]。应该推荐 2 型糖尿病妇女在妊娠前或产后进行年龄相关的肿瘤筛查[58]。

脂肪肝

2 型糖尿病可能与不明原因的肝氨基转移酶升高相关。这很可能是 2 型糖尿病常出现的代谢综合征的一部分,包括肥胖、腰围增加、三酰甘油和空腹胰岛素升高,HDL-C 降低。治疗高血糖、血脂异常与体重下降,有利于非酒精性脂肪肝的治疗[59, 60]。要注意鉴别非酒精性脂肪肝与急性脂肪肝。

妊娠并发症

不管是那种糖尿病的类型,都会增加多种妊娠合并症的风险,包括死产、围产儿死亡、小于胎龄、大于胎龄、巨大儿、肩难产、早产、先兆子痫和剖宫产。与糖尿病类型相比,糖尿病性血管并发症(肾病、视网膜病变和心脏病)与不良预后的风险有更大相关性[29]。在 468 名糖尿病患者的队列研究中,不伴有血管病变的 1 型糖尿病和 2 型糖尿病组患者的不良结局的风险是相似的,而合并有血管病变的两种类型糖尿病患者组不良结局(除了胎儿过度生长及肩难产)的风险急剧升高(表 14.1)。

然而，伴有血管病变的糖尿病患者发生胎儿过度生长和肩难产的风险是降低的。尽管有血管病变的糖尿病患者发生胎儿过度生长的风险降低，但是剖宫产的风险仍然很高，显示头盆不称是有血管病变糖尿病组剖宫产的唯一原因。

表14.1 妊娠并发症的风险与糖尿病类型及伴或不伴血管病变的关系

项目	无血管病变		伴血管病变（肾、视网膜）	
	1型糖尿病 $n=107$	2型糖尿病 $n=297$	1型糖尿病 $n=40$	2型糖尿病 $n=24$
新生儿/胎儿并发症				
总体新生儿结局	11%	13%	21%	25%
死产	2.8%	7.1%	10%	8.3%
小于胎龄（<10%）	4.7%	5.4%	10%	29%
大于胎龄（>90%）	35%	25%	7.5%	4.2%
巨大儿	28%	19%	2.5%	4.2%
肩难产	7.5%	5.1%	2.5%	0
早产	51%	38%	65%	71%
母体并发症				
先兆子痫	36%	25%	63%	79%
剖宫产术	55%	58%	65%	75%

注：总体新生儿结局包括新生儿死亡、肩难产、产伤、新生儿癫痫、血压支持、产房心肺复苏或插管[29]。

产后管理

产后，大多数女性都可以恢复到自己妊娠前的状态，可以重新开始口服妊娠前的药物，特别是妊娠前服药可以良好控制血糖的患者。在妊娠早期被诊断糖尿病的妇女可试用二甲双胍，它是治疗糖尿病的一线药物。对于剖宫产术后高血糖可能影响伤口愈合和有感染风险的患者，控制血糖尤其重要。要注意本章所列出的合并症，处方选用合理药物，必要时转入适合的管理机构。产后最好避孕，建议女性采取避孕措施。

除非存在禁忌证，应鼓励2型糖尿病妇女母乳喂养婴儿。对于那些有妊娠糖尿病史的妇女，全母乳喂养比配方奶喂养更有利于改善婴儿的血糖曲线[61,62]。对于患有2型糖尿病的母亲也有相似的血糖优化。大多数口服降糖药和胰岛素不是母乳喂养的禁忌药物（参见第十五章和第二十六章）。

选择题

1. 糖尿病妇女妊娠期的推荐药物（　　）
   A. 二甲双胍　　　　　　B. 格列美脲
   C. 胰岛素　　　　　　　D. 以上都是

   正确答案是 C。尽管二甲双胍和格列美脲为非妊娠期的一线药物，一旦患者妊娠，通常都会更换为更安全和有效的胰岛素。目前仍有很多患者在妊娠期使用二甲双胍和格列美脲作为一线用药，有关妊娠期使用这两种药物的研究正在进行中。

2. 糖尿病妇女妊娠前咨询应注意的问题是（　　）
   A. 血糖控制
   B. 优化药物治疗方案，避免致畸因素
   C. 评估糖尿病肾病及视网膜病变
   D. 以上都是

   正确答案是 D。

3. 糖尿病的类型比血管病变更容易影响妊娠的结局是（　　）
   A. 正确的　　　　　　　B. 错误的

   正确答案是 B。1 型和 2 型糖尿病患者有非常相似的预后；然而，如果存在血管病变（肾病或视网膜病变），可以显著增加不良预后的风险。

（任　歆　译，朱海清　校）

参 考 文 献

1 Guariguata L, Whiting DR, Hambleton I, Beagley J, Linnenkamp U, Shaw JE. Global estimates of diabetes prevalence for 2013 and projections for 2035. Diabetes Res Clin Pract 2014;103(2):137–149.

2 Beagley J, Guariguata L, Weil C, Motala AA. Global estimates of undiagnosed diabetes in adults. Diabetes Res Clin Pract 2014;103(2):150–160.

3 Dabelea D, Mayer-Davis EJ, Saydah S, Imperatore G, Linder B, Divers J, et al. Prevalence of type 1 and type 2 diabetes among children and adolescents from 2001 to 2009. JAMA 2014;311(17):1778–1786.

4 Martin J, Hamilton B, MJK O, et al. Births: final data for 2012. Natl Vital Stat Rep 2013;62(9).

5 Confidential Enquiry into Maternal and Child Health (CEMACH) (ed.). Diabetes in Pregnancy: Are We Providing the Best Care? Findings of a National Enquiry: England, Wales and Northern Ireland. CEMACH:

London, 2007.
6 Healthcare Quality Improvement Partnership. The National Pregnancy in Diabetes Audit Report, 2014: England, Wales, and the Isle of Man. Healthcare Quality Improvement Partnership: London, 2015.
7 Fuhrmann K, Reiher H, Semmler K, Fischer F, Fischer M, Glockner E. Prevention of congenital malformations in infants of insulin-dependent diabetic mothers. Diabetes Care 1983;6(3):219–223.
8 Goldman JA, Dicker D, Feldberg D, Yeshaya A, Samuel N, Karp M. Pregnancy outcome in patients with insulin-dependent diabetes mellitus with preconceptional diabetic control: a comparative study. Amer J Obstetr Gynecol 1986;155(2):293–297.
9 Kitzmiller JL, Gavin LA, Gin GD, Jovanovic-Peterson L, Main EK, Zigrang WD. Preconception care of diabetes. Glycemic control prevents congenital anomalies. JAMA 1991;265(6):731–736.
10 Murphy HR, Roland JM, Skinner TC, Simmons D, Gurnell E, Morrish NJ, et al. Effectiveness of a regional prepregnancy care program in women with type 1 and type 2 diabetes: benefits beyond glycemic control. Diabetes Care 2010;33(12):2514–2520.
11 Rosenn B, Miodovnik M, Combs CA, Khoury J, Siddiqi TA. Pre-conception management of insulin-dependent diabetes: improvement of pregnancy outcome. Obstetr Gynecol 1991;77(6):846–849.
12 Steel JM, Johnstone FD, Hepburn DA, Smith AF. Can prepregnancy care of diabetic women reduce the risk of abnormal babies? BMJ 1990;301(6760):1070–1074.
13 Temple RC, Aldridge VJ, Murphy HR. Prepregnancy care and pregnancy outcomes in women with type 1 diabetes. Diabetes Care 2006;29(8):1744–1749.
14 Willhoite MB, Bennert HW, Jr., Palomaki GE, Zaremba MM, Herman WH, Williams JR, et al. The impact of preconception counseling on pregnancy outcomes: the experience of the Maine Diabetes in Pregnancy Program. Diabetes Care 1993;16(2):450–455.
15 Gizzo S, Patrelli TS, Rossanese M, Noventa M, Berretta R, Di Gangi S, et al. An update on diabetic women obstetrical outcomes linked to preconception and pregnancy glycemic profile: a systematic literature review. Sci World J 2013;2013:254901.
16 Vinceti M, Malagoli C, Rothman KJ, Rodolfi R, Astolfi G, Calzolari E, et al. Risk of birth defects associated with maternal pregestational diabetes. Euro J Epidemiol 2014;29(6):411–418.
17 Adler AI, Stevens RJ, Manley SE, Bilous RW, Cull CA, Holman RR, et al. Development and progression of nephropathy in type 2 diabetes: the United Kingdom Prospective Diabetes Study (UKPDS 64). Kidney Intl 2003;63(1):225–232.
18 Molitch ME, DeFronzo RA, Franz MJ, Keane WF, Mogensen CE, Parving HH, et al. Nephropathy in diabetes. Diabetes Care 2004;27(Suppl 1):S79–S83.
19 Fong DS, Aiello L, Gardner TW, King GL, Blankenship G, Cavallerano JD, et al. Retinopathy in diabetes. Diabetes Care 2004;27(Suppl 1):S84–S87.
20 Thomas RL, Dunstan F, Luzio SD, Roy Chowdury S, Hale SL, North RV, et al. Incidence of diabetic retinopathy in people with type 2 diabetes mellitus attending the Diabetic Retinopathy Screening Service for Wales: retrospective analysis. BMJ 2012;344:e874.
21 American Diabetes Association. (12) Management of diabetes in pregnancy. Diabetes Care 2015;38(Suppl):S77–S79.
22 Arauz-Pacheco C, Parrott MA, Raskin P, American Diabetes Association. Hypertension management in adults with diabetes. Diabetes Care 2004;27(Suppl 1):S65–S67.
23 American Diabetes Association. (8) Cardiovascular disease and risk management. Diabetes Care 2015;38(Suppl):S49–S57.

24. Bullo M, Tschumi S, Bucher BS, Bianchetti MG, Simonetti GD. Pregnancy outcome following exposure to angiotensin-converting enzyme inhibitors or angiotensin receptor antagonists: a systematic review. Hypertension 2012;60(2):444-450.
25. Cooper WO, Hernandez-Diaz S, Arbogast PG, Dudley JA, Dyer S, Gideon PS, et al. Major congenital malformations after first-trimester exposure to ACE inhibitors. New Engl J Med 2006;354(23):2443-2451.
26. Spaggiari E, Heidet L, Grange G, Guimiot F, Dreux S, Delezoide AL, et al. Prognosis and outcome of pregnancies exposed to renin-angiotensin system blockers. Prenatal Diag 2012;32(11):1071-1076.
27. Tabacova S, Little R, Tsong Y, Vega A, Kimmel CA. Adverse pregnancy outcomes associated with maternal enalapril antihypertensive treatment. Pharmacoepidemiol Drug Safety 2003;12(8):633-646.
28. Briggs G, Freeman RK, Yaffe SJ. Drugs in Pregnancy and Lactation A Reference Guide to Fetal and Neonatal Risk. Lippincott Williams & Wilkins: Philadelphia, 2011. http://www.columbia.edu/cgi-bin/cul/resolve?clio10982497
29. Bennett S, Tita A, Owen J, Biggio J, Harper LM. Assessing White's classification of pregestational diabetes in a contemporary diabetic population. Obstetr Gynecol 2015;125(5):1217-1223.
30. Dixit AK, Dey R, Suresh A, Chaudhuri S, Panda AK, Mitra A, et al. The prevalence of dyslipidemia in patients with diabetes mellitus of ayurveda Hospital. J Diabetes Metab Disord 2014;13:58.
31. Haffner SM, American Diabetes Association. Dyslipidemia management in adults with diabetes. Diabetes Care 2004;27(Suppl 1):S68-S71.
32. Ofori B, Rey E, Berard A. Risk of congenital anomalies in pregnant users of statin drugs. Brit J Clin Pharmacol 2007;64(4):496-509.
33. Zarek J, Koren G. The fetal safety of statins: a systematic review and meta-analysis. J Obstetr Gynecol Canada 2014;36(6):506-509.
34. Kan C, Silva N, Golden SH, Rajala U, Timonen M, Stahl D, et al. A systematic review and meta-analysis of the association between depression and insulin resistance. Diabetes Care 2013;36(2):480-489.
35. Nanri A. Nutritional epidemiology of type 2 diabetes and depressive symptoms. J Epidemiol 2013;23(4):243-250.
36. American Diabetes Association. (4) Foundations of care: education, nutrition, physical activity, smoking cessation, psychosocial care, and immunization. Diabetes Care 2015;38(Suppl):S20-S30.
37. Kurki T, Hiilesmaa V, Raitasalo R, Mattila H, Ylikorkala O. Depression and anxiety in early pregnancy and risk for preeclampsia. Obstetr Gynecol 2000;95(4):487-490.
38. Orr ST, James SA, Blackmore Prince C. Maternal prenatal depressive symptoms and spontaneous preterm births among African-American women in Baltimore, Maryland. Amer J Epidemiol 2002;156(9):797-802.
39. Larsson C, Sydsjo G, Josefsson A. Health, sociodemographic data, and pregnancy outcome in women with antepartum depressive symptoms. Obstetr Gynecol 2004;104(3):459-466.
40. Diego MA, Field T, Hernandez-Reif M, Schanberg S, Kuhn C, Gonzalez-Quintero VH. Prenatal depression restricts fetal growth. Early Human Devel 2009;85(1):65-70.
41. Steer RA, Scholl TO, Hediger ML, Fischer RL. Self-reported depression and negative pregnancy outcomes. J Clin Epidemiol 1992;45(10):1093-1099.
42. Grigoriadis S, VonderPorten EH, Mamisashvili L, Tomlinson G, Dennis CL, Koren G, et al. The impact of maternal depression during pregnancy on perinatal outcomes: a systematic review and meta-analysis. J Clin Psychiat 2013;74(4):e321-e341.
43. Longo DL, Harrison TR. Harrison's Principles of Internal Medicine, 18th ed. New York: McGraw-Hill, 2012.
44. Cedergren M. Effects of gestational weight

gain and body mass index on obstetric outcome in Sweden. Intl J Gynaecol Obstetr 2006;93(3):269–274.
45 Cedergren MI. Maternal morbid obesity and the risk of adverse pregnancy outcome. Obstetr Gynecol 2004;103(2):219–224.
46 Cnattingius S, Bergstrom R, Lipworth L, Kramer MS. Prepregnancy weight and the risk of adverse pregnancy outcomes [see comment]. New Engl J Med 1998;338(3):147–152.
47 Edwards LE, Hellerstedt WL, Alton IR, Story M, Himes JH. Pregnancy complications and birth outcomes in obese and normal-weight women: effects of gestational weight change. Obstetr Gynecol 1996;87(3):389–394.
48 Sebire NJ, Jolly M, Harris JP, Wadsworth J, Joffe M, Beard RW, et al. Maternal obesity and pregnancy outcome: a study of 287,213 pregnancies in London. Intl J Obes Related Metab Disord 2001;25(8):1175–1182.
49 Egan AM, Dennedy MC, Al-Ramli W, Heerey A, Avalos G, Dunne F. ATLANTIC-DIP: excessive gestational weight gain and pregnancy outcomes in women with gestational or pregestational diabetes mellitus. J Clin Endocrinol Metabol 2014;99(1):212–219.
50 Harper LM, Shanks AL, Odibo AO, Colvin R, Macones GA, Cahill AG. Gestational weight gain in insulin-resistant pregnancies. J Perinatol 2013;33(12):929–933.
51 Siegel A, Tita A, Biggio J, Harper L. 408: Evaluating gestational weight gain recommendations in pregestational diabetes. Amer J Obstetr Gynecol 212(1):S213–S214.
52 Resnick HE, Redline S, Shahar E, Gilpin A, Newman A, Walter R, et al. Diabetes and sleep disturbances: findings from the Sleep Heart Health Study. Diabetes Care 2003;26(3):702–709.
53 Lecomte P, Criniere L, Fagot-Campagna A, Druet C, Fuhrman C. Underdiagnosis of obstructive sleep apnoea syndrome in patients with type 2 diabetes in France: ENTRED 2007. Diabetes Metab 2013;39(2):139–147.

54 Louis J, Auckley D, Miladinovic B, Shepherd A, Mencin P, Kumar D, et al. Perinatal outcomes associated with obstructive sleep apnea in obese pregnant women. Obstetr Gynecol 2012;120(5):1085–1092.
55 Louis JM, Mogos MF, Salemi JL, Redline S, Salihu HM. Obstructive sleep apnea and severe maternal-infant morbidity/mortality in the United States, 1998–2009. Sleep 2014;37(5):843–849.
56 Facco FL. LB2: Prospective study of the association between sleep disordered breathing and hypertensive disorders of pregnancy and gestational diabetes. Amer J Obstetr Gynecol 212(1):S424–S425.
57 Suh S, Kim KW. Diabetes and cancer: is diabetes causally related to cancer? Diabetes Metab J 2011;35(3):193–198.
58 American Diabetes Association. (3) Initial evaluation and diabetes management planning. Diabetes Care 2015;38(Suppl):S17–S19.
59 El-Serag HB, Tran T, Everhart JE. Diabetes increases the risk of chronic liver disease and hepatocellular carcinoma. Gastroenterology 2004;126(2):460–468.
60 American Gastroenterological Association. American Gastroenterological Association medical position statement: nonalcoholic fatty liver disease. Gastroenterology 2002;123(5):1702–1704.
61 Gunderson EP, Hedderson MM, Chiang V, Crites Y, Walton D, Azevedo RA, et al. Lactation intensity and postpartum maternal glucose tolerance and insulin resistance in women with recent GDM: the SWIFT cohort. Diabetes Care 2012;35(1):50–56.
62 O'Reilly MW, Avalos G, Dennedy MC, O'Sullivan EP, Dunne F. Atlantic DIP: high prevalence of abnormal glucose tolerance post partum is reduced by breast-feeding in women with prior gestational diabetes mellitus. Euro J Endocrinol 2011;165(6):953–959.

第十五章　妊娠期口服降糖药的研究进展

Geetha Mukerji[1] and Denice S. Feig[2]

1 University of Toronto, Women's College Hospital; and Mount Sinai Hospital [cross-appointed], Toronto, Canada

2 University of Toronto, Diabetes & Endocrinology in Pregnancy Program; and Mount Sinai Hospital, Toronto, Canada

实践要点

- 二甲双胍和格列苯脲虽然可以透过胎盘，但一般不会导致胎儿畸形。
- 二甲双胍用于妊娠糖尿病的治疗是有效的，并且短期应用安全性良好。一些国际指南推荐二甲双胍作为经生活方式干预血糖不达标的妊娠糖尿病女性的一线用药，还有其他的指南推荐二甲双胍作为胰岛素之后的二线用药。
- 有证据表明，在妊娠期间对于妊娠糖尿病的治疗，格列苯脲不如胰岛素和二甲双胍，但是，对于不能耐受二甲双胍和（或）拒绝应用胰岛素且血糖控制不理想的女性，可将格列苯脲作为三线用药的选择。2型糖尿病女性患者在妊娠期可将格列苯脲换成胰岛素或二甲双胍。
- 对于经生活方式干预（一些指南是二甲双胍）后，血糖控制仍不达标的妊娠糖尿病患者和（或）不能耐受或不能接受二甲双胍治疗的女性，胰岛素仍是主要的治疗手段。
- 在一些非小样本的研究中，阿卡波糖用于妊娠糖尿病的治疗，安全性数据是有限的，耐受性可能是一个主要的问题。
- PPARγ激动剂（噻唑烷二酮类）能透过胎盘，在妊娠期间应避免应用，除非有更多的安全性数据。
- 二甲双胍和格列苯脲能进入乳汁中，但短期的安全性资料表明哺乳期的产妇可以应用二甲双胍和格列苯脲。
- 因为没有人类研究的证据，所以在妊娠和哺乳期间不推荐使用DPP4抑制剂、GLP1激动剂和SGLT-2抑制剂。
- 对于在子宫内和哺乳期间暴露于口服降糖药的婴儿的长期随访研究是缺乏的。

> **病例 1**
>
> 一名 32 岁的女性（孕 2 产 0，自发流产），2 型糖尿病病史 3 年，目前妊娠 9 周。糖化血红蛋白 9%，口服二甲双胍 1.0g/次、每天 2 次，格列苯脲 10mg、每天 2 次。您对她有什么建议吗？

> **病例 2**
>
> 一名 30 岁的女性孕 1 产 0，在妊娠 28 周时诊断为妊娠糖尿病。已经进行了生活方式的干预，采取糖尿病饮食，但血糖仍不达标。害怕打针，询问是否可以口服药物治疗。您对她有什么建议吗？

背景

妊娠期间如血糖控制不达标，妊娠糖尿病与不良妊娠结局是相关的[1]。传统观念认为，妊娠糖尿病及 2 型糖尿病合并妊娠可以给予生活方式干预，包括饮食控制和体育锻炼，如果血糖不达标，可加用胰岛素治疗。但是，随着育龄期女性糖尿病患病率的增加，越来越多的女性正在接受口服降糖药的治疗。然而，有些女性对于每日多次注射胰岛素依从性不好[2]，或者不能正确地储存胰岛素，因此在妊娠期间应用口服降糖药控制血糖也许是必要的。虽然对于口服降糖药存在很多潜在的安全性问题，但是有越来越多的文献支持妊娠期间可以口服降糖药。对于妊娠糖尿病患者，如果生活方式干预不能使其血糖达标，现在许多国家推荐有一些口服降糖药可作为一线治疗。在本章，作者分析了在妊娠糖尿病、多囊卵巢综合征及 2 型糖尿病合并妊娠女性中口服降糖药的安全性和有效性的证据。

磺脲类和格列奈类

磺脲类和格列奈类降糖药是胰岛素促泌剂，与胰岛 B 细胞受体结合（两者结合位点不同），刺激胰岛素分泌。第一代磺脲类药物包括甲苯磺丁脲、氯磺丙脲和妥拉磺脲；第二代磺脲类药物包括格列苯脲、格列吡嗪和格列美脲。第一代磺脲类药物由于不良反应较多，目前较少应用。第二代磺脲类药物安全性更好，与第一代磺脲类药物相比降糖效果更佳[3]。格列奈类降糖药包括瑞格列奈和那格列奈。与磺脲类药物相比，格列奈类药物降血糖快而维持时间短，因此主要用于控制餐后高血糖，其下一餐前低血糖风险更低[4, 5]。

胎盘转移

人类胎盘灌流模型已经用于探索磺脲类药物作用机制的研究，假定新生儿低血糖与应用磺脲类药物有关，那么就说明磺脲类药物是可以透过胎盘的。从分娩的健康母亲处获得胎盘，应用灌流和转移研究测定相关的药物。研究发现，第一代磺脲类药物中等量透过胎盘（甲苯磺丁脲21.5%、氯磺丙脲11%），而第二代磺脲类药物透过胎盘的比例更低（格列吡嗪6.6%、格列苯脲3.9%）[6]。然而，在两项最近的研究中发现，在应用格列苯脲的母亲中，脐带血中的药物浓度是母体的50%~70%；药物的转运具有异质性，一些婴儿的药物浓度甚至比母亲的还要高[7, 8]。格列苯脲转运需要通过各种胎盘转运蛋白[9]，因此推测药物浓度的不同是由于胎盘转运蛋白功能的不同[8]。只有一项研究检测了格列奈类药物的胎盘转移，研究指出瑞格列奈的母婴转移是1.5%，但是婴母转移是6.7%[10]。总之，瑞格列奈的胎盘转移似乎是低的，但这仅是一项研究的推测，然而其他一些研究发现格列苯脲易于透过胎盘。

磺脲类药物应用的临床经验

先天异常

2型糖尿病女性

在合并糖尿病的妊娠期女性间分析药物的潜在致畸性有可能受到干扰，因为在妊娠早期母体高血糖本身也是一个潜在的致畸因素。在妊娠早期应用磺脲类药物的大多数研究中并没有显示先天畸形发病率的增加[11-14]。只有两个小样本研究观察到先天畸形的发生率增加（样本量分别为20例和43例）；然而，在这两项研究中血糖控制不理想[15]或没有提到[16]。在一项大的回顾性队列研究中（n=342），先天畸形的发生与血糖控制差有关，而与应用某种特定的 OAD（格列苯脲或二甲双胍）无关[11]。一项 Meta 分析包括了在妊娠早期应用 OAD[磺脲类和（或）双胍类]的 471 名女性和没有应用 OAD 的 1344 名女性，发现主要畸形的发生率在两组之间没有显著差异[17]。总之，磺脲类药物不太可能致畸。

应用格列奈类导致先天畸形的资料有限，但是在 3 名妊娠早期的女性应用瑞格列奈的两个病例报道中并没有发现任何先天畸形[18, 19]。

围产期结局

合并 2 型糖尿病的女性

在南非的一项包括 379 名妊娠妇女的回顾性队列研究中，在整个妊娠期间应用 OAD（单用格列苯脲或与二甲双胍联用）的女性与在妊娠初期转换为胰岛素或单用胰岛素治疗的女性相比，围产期死亡率增加[11]。然而，单纯服用二甲双胍的女性的围产期死亡风险并没有增加。在两组之间，血糖控制、产妇年龄、BMI、胎次、孕周或伴发病的不同还不能解释这种现象。这种围产期死亡率增加的原因还不清楚。然而，一项 Meta 分析（10 个研究共包括 471 名在妊娠早期应用磺脲类或双胍类的女性），发现妊娠早期应用 OAD 的女性与没有应用 OAD 的女性相比，在主要畸形的发生率或新生儿死亡方面没有显著的差异[17]。

妊娠糖尿病的女性

在 2000 年，Langer 进行了一项里程碑式的研究，包括了 404 名单纯生活方式干预血糖不能达标的 GDM 女性，在妊娠 11～33 周时，被随机分配至胰岛素治疗组或格列苯脲治疗组（以 2.5mg 每天 1 次起始，必要时滴定至每天 20mg）[20]。两组在血糖控制及新生儿结局[大于胎龄儿（LGA）、巨大儿、出生体重、新生儿低血糖、肺部并发症、入住新生儿重症监护病房（NICU）、先天畸形或围产期死亡]方面没有显著的差异。格列美脲组的 8 名（4%）患者需要胰岛素治疗。这项研究支持 GDM 女性应用格列苯脲，但其中主要的问题是这项研究用来评估新生儿结局的力度是不够的。

在一项包括了 9000 多名 GDM 女性的大型回顾性队列研究中，应用格列苯脲女性的新生儿与应用胰岛素女性的新生儿相比，入住 NICU、呼吸窘迫、低血糖、产伤和 LGA 的风险更高[21]。在一项近期的随机对照试验的 Meta 分析中，观察了 GDM 女性在应用 OAD 或胰岛素的不同治疗方案中围产期结局的情况，应用格列苯脲治疗的母亲与胰岛素治疗的母亲生出的婴儿相比出生体重更大、巨大儿更多和新生儿低血糖更多[22]。有两项研究报道了母亲低血糖，一个研究报道了服用格列苯脲组母亲低血糖的发生率低于胰岛素治疗组[20]，而另一项研究报道了类似的发病率[23]。在格列苯脲组平均治疗失败率是 6.4%。

在上面提到的 Meta 分析中，两项研究直接对比了格列苯脲和二甲双胍。在二甲双胍组，母亲体重增加更少、新生儿出生体重更低、巨大儿更少和 LGA 新生儿更少。在这些研究中二甲双胍的平均治疗失败率是 26.8%，格列苯脲的平均治疗失败率是 23.5%[22]。

目前还没有关于 GDM 女性应用格列奈类药物的相关资料。

妊娠期间磺脲类药物的应用总结

格列苯脲能透过胎盘，但并不致畸。在 GDM 女性中，应用格列苯脲的大多数患者血糖控制良好，平均治疗失败率是 6%～24%。然而，有证据表明，应用格列苯脲与胰岛素相比，巨大儿和新生儿低血糖的风险更高。在 GDM 女性患者中，使用格列苯脲与二甲双胍相比，出生体重增加、LGA、巨大儿和母亲体重增加的风险更高。因此，在 GDM 女性中，二甲双胍和胰岛素都是优于格列苯脲的选择。对于合并 2 型糖尿病的妊娠女性，有关磺脲类药物应用的资料还比较少。只有一项回顾性研究中提到在整个妊娠期间继续应用格列苯脲增加了围产期死亡，但是在其他研究中并未得到证实。基于 GDM 女性的资料及最新的资料来看，合并 2 型糖尿病的女性在妊娠期间应该考虑转换为胰岛素或二甲双胍治疗。

二甲双胍

二甲双胍是广泛应用的双胍类药物，它的主要作用是减少肝糖输出，增加骨骼肌和脂肪组织葡萄糖的摄取，减少肠道葡萄糖的吸收，从而改善胰岛素敏感性。二甲双胍不促进胰岛素分泌，因此不引起低血糖或体重增加[24]，但是会引起胃肠道不耐受[25]。

胎盘转移

关于 GDM 女性胎盘转移的研究显示，二甲双胍可以自由透过胎盘[26]。两项研究发现，在整个妊娠期间，脐带血中二甲双胍的浓度是母体血液浓度的 50%～100%，在一些婴儿体内药物水平甚至更高[27, 28]。

二甲双胍的临床经验

排卵诱导、妊娠和活产率

合并多囊卵巢综合征的女性

二甲双胍已广泛应用于合并有多囊卵巢综合征（PCOS）的女性，在受孕前生育能力低下的状态下可以改善排卵，以及在妊娠期间减少并发症[29, 30]。

观察性研究发现二甲双胍也许降低了妊娠早期自发流产的发生率[31, 32]，但是一项包括了 17 个随机对照试验的 Meta 分析并没有证实这一结论，这些患者在妊娠前口服二甲双胍，而在妊娠早期停用了二甲双胍[33]。二甲双胍与克罗米芬对比在改善妊娠和活产率方面的获益证据存在不一致性[29, 34]。一个包括了 38 项随机对照试验的共 3495 名女性的综述发现，二甲双胍单用或与克罗米芬联用在 PCOS 女性中对于改善排卵和妊娠率都是有效的，但并没有改善活产率[35]。在 PCOS 女性中，二甲双胍改善活产率的作用是有限的，但需要更进一步的探索。

先天畸形

合并 2 型糖尿病的女性

在妊娠期间单用二甲双胍或联用磺脲类药物的大多数研究并没有发现先天畸形发生率的增加[11-13, 17, 36, 37]。

合并有多囊卵巢综合征的女性

虽然在调查妊娠早期应用 OAD 的 2 型糖尿病女性生育先天畸形胎

儿的发生率的研究中，高血糖是一个主要的混杂因素，但是在 PCOS 女性中并不涉及这个问题，因为在 PCOS 女性中血糖通常在正常范围内，除非 PCOS 女性先前已存在糖耐量异常。在一项包括了 8 个随机对照研究的系统综述和 Meta 分析中，参与研究的患者为合并有 PCOS 的女性，妊娠早期应用二甲双胍的女性与对照组相比，出生的婴儿中主要生产缺陷的发生率并没有显著增加[38]。

其他发病率和死亡率

合并有 2 型糖尿病的女性

南非的一项回顾性分析发现，单用格列美脲或联用二甲双胍的女性与胰岛素治疗组相比，围产期死亡率更高，而单用二甲双胍组围产期死亡率并没有显著增加[11]。近来的一项随机开放标签的研究中，包括了 206 名合并 2 型糖尿病但先前没有应用胰岛素的女性，在妊娠时对比了二甲双胍和胰岛素，如有必要，二甲双胍组可加用胰岛素；二甲双胍治疗组的女性，母亲体重增加更少、低血糖发作更少、妊娠诱导的高血压更少[39]。然而，在二甲双胍治疗组中 84.9% 的女性在平均妊娠 26 周时需要加用胰岛素治疗，二甲双胍组小于胎龄儿更常见[39]。这个研究存在一些局限性，如开放标签设计，缺乏意向性分析，以及样本量较小。在另一项开放标签的随机试验中，包括了 90 名 GDM 或 2 型糖尿病女性，研究发现当在胰岛素的基础上加用二甲双胍时，新生儿低血糖和 NICU 入住率均下降，该研究样本量较小，后随机化（直至妊娠 34 周时），以及缺乏意向性分析，使得结果不可信[40]。一项大的多中心随机、安慰剂对照试验正在进行中，目的是调查是否加用了二甲双胍对合并有 2 型糖尿病的母亲和她们的后代有益（MiTy Trial 和 MiTy Kids）。

GDM 女性

MiG 试验是一个大型的随机对照研究，其中包括了 751 名 GDM 女性，这些患者经饮食治疗后血糖控制仍不理想，被随机分配至二甲双胍组（500mg 每天 1 次或每天 2 次起始，如有必要滴定至最大剂量 2500mg）或胰岛素治疗组[41]。主要联合结局（包括新生儿低血糖、呼吸窘迫、需要光线疗法、产伤、5min Apgar 评分小于 7 分和早产）的发生率在两组中没有显著差异。严重的新生儿低血糖（血糖＜1.6mmol/L）在二甲双胍组是降低的，但是在二甲双胍组中早产更常见（12.1% vs 7.6%；P=0.04）。在两组之间，血糖控制方面没有差异，虽然二甲双胍组 46.3% 的女性需要加用胰岛素以维持良好的血糖控制。值得注意的是，1.9% 的女性由于胃肠道不良反应而停用二甲双胍，8.8% 的女性由于胃肠道不良反应需要将二甲双胍减量。生物电阻抗法和双能 X 线吸收法（DEXA）评估的总脂肪量及体脂百分比在两组之间没有差别。作者推测二甲双胍也许增加了外周脂肪沉积，减少了内脏脂肪分布，后者引起胰岛素抵抗和炎症细胞因子的产生，但这需要更进一步的研究阐明[42]。

一项包括 6 个开放标签研究的系统综述和 Meta 分析中，在 GDM 患者中对比了二甲双胍和胰岛素，二甲双胍组母亲体重增加更少，分娩时孕龄更小，早产更多[22]。值得注意的是，应用二甲双胍治疗的失败率是 33.8%。

如上所述，在两个研究的荟萃分析中，对比了格列苯脲和二甲双胍，二甲双胍组出生体重更低、LGA 婴儿更少、巨大儿更少和母亲体重增加更少[22]。

合并多囊卵巢综合征的女性

在合并 PCOS 女性中进行的观察性和队列性研究中发现应用二甲双胍对于母亲和婴儿没有不良结局，可能还有一些潜在的获益。例如，如果在整个妊娠期间应用二甲双胍，GDM 的发生率降低[30, 43]。然而，在一项纳入合并 PCOS 的妊娠女性的大的随机安慰剂对照试验中，从妊娠早期开始，二甲双胍治疗没有使得先兆子痫、妊娠糖尿病、早产或上述三项联合结局的发生率下降[44]。总之，对于糖耐量正常的 PCOS 女性，妊娠时应用二甲双胍的获益似乎是有限的。

妊娠时二甲双胍的应用总结

二甲双胍能自由透过胎盘，但并不致畸。二甲双胍改善了排卵率，虽然它在合并 PCOS 的女性中并没有改善活产率或降低先兆子痫、GDM 或早产率。二甲双胍应用于 GDM 女性似乎是有效的和安全的，但是由于治疗失败常常需要加用胰岛素，胃肠道不良反应导致患者不能耐受。

合并 2 型糖尿病的女性妊娠时应用二甲双胍似乎是安全的，早期的资料似乎也证实了这一点，然而，我们也期待强有力的双盲随机试验的结果，同时也期待有更长时间的研究以便评估对儿童的可能影响。

α 糖苷酶抑制剂

α 糖苷酶抑制剂如阿卡波糖和伏格列波糖，通过抑制位于小肠刷状缘的 α 糖苷酶延缓糖类的吸收，降低餐后血糖。这些药物基本不被吸收入血液。妊娠时只有阿卡波糖有相关的研究。在一个案例系列中，6 名合并 GDM 的女性单纯饮食控制时血糖控制不佳,给予阿卡波糖 3 次/天。6 名患者空腹和餐后血糖均降至正常，婴儿是健康的[45]。然而，阿卡波糖导致患者在整个妊娠期间肠道不适。在一个小样本的研究中，经饮食治疗血糖控制不佳的 GDM 女性被随机分配至胰岛素（$n=27$）、格列苯脲（$n=24$）或阿卡波糖（$n=19$）组，研究发现三组在血糖控制、LGA 率或新生儿出生体重等方面没有差异。研究中并没有提到阿卡波糖的耐受性情况[46]，需要更大型的随机对照试验来阐明妊娠时阿卡波糖的获益，以及进一步探索妊娠时阿卡波糖的耐受性。

Pparγ 激动剂

推荐的过氧化物酶体增殖剂激活受体 γ（Pparγ）激动剂是噻唑烷二酮类降糖药，包括罗格列酮、吡格列酮和曲格列酮（由于肝毒性已被撤市）。这些药物与细胞核转录因子 Pparγ 结合，Pparγ 调节脂肪组织、骨骼肌和肝脏的基因表达，导致与葡萄糖转运、脂蛋白酯酶及胰岛素信号传导等相关的代谢通路的改变。它们被称为胰岛素增敏剂，因为它们增强了这些部位胰岛素的作用。这些药物被用于 2 型糖尿病患者，很少引起低血糖，虽然这些药物会导致患者体重增加、液体潴留和心力衰竭。人类胎盘转移研究[47,48]发现罗格列酮可以透过胎盘。然而，少数的临床资料并没有发现其与先天畸形或产科并发症相关[49-52]。考虑到罗格列酮的心血管安全性，对于合并 PCOS 的女性不再推荐其用于诱导排卵。

总之，Pparγ 激动剂可以透过胎盘，妊娠时应用这些药物的安全性的研究较少，因此非妊娠时应用 Pparγ 激动剂。

二肽基肽酶-4（DPP4）抑制剂

DPP4 能够降解胰高血糖素样肽-1（GLP1）和葡萄糖依赖的促胰岛素多肽（GIP）。GLP1 和 GIP 促进了胰岛 B 细胞胰岛素的生物合成及分泌。在动物生殖研究中并没有观察到不良事件[53]；然而，至目前为止还没有在妊娠女性中进行相关的研究，因此不推荐用于妊娠女性。

GLP1 受体激动剂

GLP1 受体激动剂是肠促胰液素类似物，是 GLP1 受体的激动剂。在离体研究中，应用人类胎盘子叶模型发现极少量艾塞那肽透过胎盘[54]。在动物生殖研究中观察到有一些不良事件发生[53]，考虑到目前还没有在妊娠女性中进行相关的研究，不推荐妊娠期间应用 GLP1 受体激动剂。

钠-葡萄糖共转运体-2（SGLT2）抑制剂

SGLT2 是位于肾脏近端小管的葡萄糖转运蛋白，其能促进肾小管葡萄糖的重吸收。SGLT2 被抑制后由于肾脏葡萄糖排泄增加，血糖水平下降。SGLT2 抑制剂由糖尿导致的泌尿道感染（UTI）的风险略有增加[55]。在合并糖尿病的女性中，妊娠期间发生 UTI 与肾盂肾炎、脓毒症及对新生儿潜在的长期影响相关[56]。在动物生殖研究中有一些不良事件发生，包括当 SGLT2 抑制剂用于妊娠中期和妊娠晚期时对胎儿肾脏发育有不良影响，虽然还没有在人类中进行相关研究[53]。因此，不推荐妊娠期间应用 SGLT2 抑制剂。

哺乳

合并 2 型糖尿病的女性通常在妊娠前和分娩后应用 OAD 治疗，那么就会提出下面的问题,什么时间可以安全地重新开始服用 OAD?主要的问题在于 OAD 在乳汁中分泌是否可能对婴儿构成一定的风险。

磺脲类药物

第一代磺脲类药物大部分会进入乳汁中[57]。在一项观察第二代磺脲类药物(格列苯脲或格列吡嗪)能否进入合并 2 型糖尿病的女性乳汁的研究中,发现从产后第一天开始 8 名女性接受单一口服剂量格列苯脲 5mg/d 或 10mg/d,5 名女性给予格列苯脲或格列吡嗪 5mg/d[58],在乳汁中均未检测到上述两种药物。母乳喂养的三个婴儿血糖正常(一位母亲口服格列苯脲,两位母亲口服格列吡嗪)。上述两种药物乳汁中含量极低,考虑与格列苯脲或格列吡嗪与血浆蛋白结合有关。在母乳喂养的婴儿中,母亲应用第二代磺脲类药物似乎不发挥任何有临床意义的药理作用。

二甲双胍

在调查二甲双胍是否进入乳汁的三项研究中,观察到二甲双胍可以进入乳汁,但是量很少[59-61]。估计婴儿体内平均剂量是母亲经体重校正后剂量的 0.65%。此外,三名口服二甲双胍的母亲所生婴儿的血糖水平是正常的[60]。母亲每天口服 1.5~2.5g 二甲双胍,然后进行母乳喂养,婴儿 6 月龄时在身高、体重及运动-社交发育等方面与配方奶粉喂养的婴儿没有差异[62]。总之,二甲双胍能够被分泌进入乳汁,但是在有限的研究中发现其与不良结局无关。

其他 OAD 和母乳喂养

Pparγ 激动剂、糖苷酶抑制剂、DPP4 抑制剂、GLP1 激动剂和 SGLT2 抑制剂与母乳喂养之间的关系还没有相关研究资料,这些降糖药不推荐在围产期使用。

OAD 和母乳喂养总结

格列苯脲、格列吡嗪和二甲双胍虽然可以在哺乳期使用,但是需要进一步的长期安全性研究。

选择题

1. 胎盘转移研究中没有提到的一种口服降糖药是(　　)
   A. 瑞格列奈　　　　　　B. 二甲双胍
   C. 格列苯脲　　　　　　D. 西格列汀

   正确答案是 D。二甲双胍和格列苯脲都能够透过胎盘。只有一个观察格列奈类胎盘转移的研究发现瑞格列奈母亲-胎儿的转移率是1.5%[10]。西格列汀在这方面还没有相关的研究。

2. 下面口服降糖药中,进行了与哺乳关系的研究并且没有发现不良事件的是(　　)
   A. 二甲双胍　　　　　　B. DPP4 抑制剂
   C. 糖苷酶抑制剂　　　　D. Pparγ 激动剂

   正确答案是 A。二甲双胍能够被排泄进入乳汁,但是量极少。短期研究关于生长发育结局未见到不良影响,但目前还没有相关的长期研究。

病例 1 和病例 2 的解答

病例 1

对于合并 2 型糖尿病和 PCOS 的女性,二甲双胍和格列苯脲不可能是致畸因素,然而升高的 HbA1c 使得先天畸形的风险增加。在妊娠 18～20 周时应进行解剖超声的评估。为了更好地控制血糖,应停用格列苯脲,开始胰岛素治疗。一些国际团体建议合并 2 型糖尿病并行胰岛素治疗的女性应继续口服二甲双胍[63],而对于其他个体单用胰岛素仍是主要的治疗方式[64, 65]。有关合并 2 型糖尿病女性妊娠时应用二甲双胍是否获益的研究正在进行中。一些证据表明在妊娠早期或整个妊娠期间继续应用二甲双胍也许降低了 PCOS 女性自发流产的风险,但是近来随机试验和

Meta 分析的数据显示事实并非如此。

病例 2

格列苯脲和二甲双胍均能透过胎盘。随机试验结果表明二甲双胍具有很好的短期的安全性,由于降低了母亲体重的增加,二甲双胍优于胰岛素。然而,对于后代的长期影响需要更进一步的研究。此外,为了获得良好的血糖控制,将近 34%的时间需要加用胰岛素。近来一项 Meta 分析的数据显示,在 GDM 女性患者中应用格列苯脲的效果不如二甲双胍和胰岛素,与胰岛素相比,格列苯脲组巨大儿和新生儿低血糖发生率更高;与二甲双胍相比,格列苯脲组新生儿出生体重更大、母亲体重增加更多,大于胎龄儿和巨大儿比例更高。二甲双胍为一线用药,格列苯脲为二线用药,要考虑二者的风险和获益,并同时参考当地的指南(表 15.1)。

表 15.1 糖尿病管理中 OAD 的国际指南推荐

OAD 的指南推荐	UK NICE 指南[63]	ADA 指南[64]	CDA 指南[65]
2 型糖尿病合并妊娠	用二甲双胍 停用其他 OAD	未说明	首选胰岛素 格列苯脲或二甲双胍可以继续应用,除非妊娠时开始胰岛素治疗
GDM	二甲双胍作为继生活方式干预后的一线治疗 可选择胰岛素,如果二甲双胍存在禁忌、不被接受或血糖控制不佳,如果空腹血糖≥7.0mmol/L 或 6.0~6.9mmol/L,同时合并有妊娠并发症,如巨大儿或羊水过多症 应用二甲双胍血糖控制不达标或拒绝应用胰岛素,或二甲双胍不耐受,可将格列苯脲作为三线药物选择	胰岛素和二甲双胍作为首选,由于应用格列苯脲,新生儿低血糖和巨大儿发生率更高 应告知患者二甲双胍和格列苯脲均可透过胎盘,并且缺乏长期研究的资料	在依从性差或拒绝应用胰岛素的患者中可用格列苯脲或二甲双胍替代,但他们是非适用的
哺乳	产后,二甲双胍和格列苯脲可以继续或重新启用	未说明	哺乳期间可应用二甲双胍和格列苯脲

(张雪冰 译,朱海清 校)

参 考 文 献

1. Blumer I, Hadar E, Hadden DR, Jovanovic L, Mestman JH, Murad MH, et al. Diabetes and pregnancy: an endocrine society clinical practice guideline. J Clin Endocrinol Metab 2013;98(11):4227-4249.
2. Centers for Disease Control and Prevention. Diabetes Public Health Resource: Age-adjusted rates of diagnosed diabetes per 100 civilian, non-institutionalized population, by race and sex, United States, 1980-2014. http://www.cdc.gov/diabetes/statistics/prev/national/figraceethsex.htm
3. Rumboldt Z, Bota B. Favorable effects of glibenclamide in a patient exhibiting idiosyncratic hepatotoxic reactions to both chlorpropamide and tolbutamide. Acta Diabetolog Latina 1984;21(4):387-391.
4. Guardado-Mendoza R, Prioletta A, Jimenez-Ceja LM, Sosale A, Folli F. The role of nateglinide and repaglinide, derivatives of meglitinide, in the treatment of type 2 diabetes mellitus. Arch Med Sci 2013;9(5): 936-943.
5. Fuhlendorff J, Rorsman P, Kofod H, Brand CL, Rolin B, MacKay P, et al. Stimulation of insulin release by repaglinide and glibenclamide involves both common and distinct processes. Diabetes 1998;47(3): 345-351.
6. Elliott BD, Schenker S, Langer O, Johnson R, Prihoda T. Comparative placental transport of oral hypoglycemic agents in humans: a model of human placental drug transfer. Amer J Obstetr Gynecol 1994;171(3): 653-660.
7. Hebert MF, Ma X, Naraharisetti SB, Krudys KM, Umans JG, Hankins GD, et al. Are we optimizing gestational diabetes treatment with glyburide? The pharmacologic basis for better clinical practice. Clin Pharmacol Therap 2009;85(6):607-614.
8. Schwartz RA, Rosenn B, Aleksa K, Koren G. Glyburide transport across the human placenta. Obstetr Gynecol 2015;125(3): 583-588.
9. Gedeon C, Anger G, Piquette-Miller M, Koren G. Breast cancer resistance protein: mediating the trans-placental transfer of glyburide across the human placenta. Placenta 2008;29(1):39-43.
10. Tertti K, Petsalo A, Niemi M, Ekblad U, Tolonen A, Ronnemaa T, et al. Transfer of repaglinide in the dually perfused human placenta and the role of organic anion transporting polypeptides (OATPs). Euro J Pharma Sci 2011;44(3):181-186.
11. Ekpebegh CO, Coetzee EJ, van der Merwe L, Levitt NS. A 10-year retrospective analysis of pregnancy outcome in pregestational type 2 diabetes: comparison of insulin and oral glucose-lowering agents. Diabetic Med 2007;24(3):253-258.
12. Coetzee EJ, Jackson WP. Pregnancy in established non-insulin-dependent diabetics. A five-and-a-half year study at Groote Schuur Hospital. South African Med J 1980;58(20):795-802.
13. Coetzee EJ, Jackson WP. Oral hypoglycaemics in the first trimester and fetal outcome. South African Med J 1984;65(16):635-637.
14. Towner D, Kjos SL, Leung B, Montoro MM, Xiang A, Mestman JH, et al. Congenital malformations in pregnancies complicated by NIDDM. Diabetes Care 1995;18(11):1446-1451.
15. Piacquadio K, Hollingsworth DR, Murphy H. Effects of in-utero exposure to oral hypoglycaemic drugs. Lancet 1991;338 (8771):866-869.
16. Botta RM. Congenital malformations in infants of 517 pregestational diabetic mothers. Annali dell'Istituto superiore di sanita 1997;33(3):307-311.
17. Gutzin SJ, Kozer E, Magee LA, Feig DS, Koren G. The safety of oral hypoglycemic agents in the first trimester of pregnancy: a meta-analysis. Canadian J Clin Pharmacol 2003;10(4):179-183.
18. Napoli A, Ciampa F, Colatrella A, Fallucca F. Use of repaglinide during the first weeks of pregnancy in two type 2 diabetic women. Diabetes Care 2006;29(10): 2326-2327.

19 Mollar-Puchades MA, Martin-Cortes A, Perez-Calvo A, Diaz-Garcia C. Use of repaglinide on a pregnant woman during embryogenesis. Diabetes Obes Metab 2007;9(1):146–147.
20 Langer O, Conway DL, Berkus MD, Xenakis EM, Gonzales O. A comparison of glyburide and insulin in women with gestational diabetes mellitus. New Engl J Med 2000;343(16):1134–1138.
21 Camelo Castillo W, Boggess K, Sturmer T, Brookhart MA, Benjamin DK, Jr., Jonsson Funk M. Association of adverse pregnancy outcomes with glyburide vs insulin in women with gestational diabetes. JAMA Pediatr 2015;169(5):452–458.
22 Balsells M, Garcia-Patterson A, Sola I, Roque M, Gich I, Corcoy R. Glibenclamide, metformin, and insulin for the treatment of gestational diabetes: a systematic review and meta-analysis. BMJ 2015;350:h102.
23 Ogunyemi D, Jesse M, Davidson M. Comparison of glyburide versus insulin in management of gestational diabetes mellitus. Endocrine Pract 2007;13(4):427–428.
24 Setter SM, Iltz JL, Thams J, Campbell RK. Metformin hydrochloride in the treatment of type 2 diabetes mellitus: a clinical review with a focus on dual therapy. Clin Ther 2003;25(12):2991–3026.
25 McCreight LJ, Bailey CJ, Pearson ER. Metformin and the gastrointestinal tract. Diabetologia 2016;59(3):426–435.
26 Nanovskaya TN, Nekhayeva IA, Patrikeeva SL, Hankins GD, Ahmed MS. Transfer of metformin across the dually perfused human placental lobule. Amer J Obstetr Gynecol 2006;195(4):1081–1085.
27 Vanky E, Zahlsen K, Spigset O, Carlsen SM. Placental passage of metformin in women with polycystic ovary syndrome. Fertil Steril 2005;83(5):1575–1578.
28 Charles B, Norris R, Xiao X, Hague W. Population pharmacokinetics of metformin in late pregnancy. Therap Drug Monitor 2006;28(1):67–72.
29 Lord JM, Flight IH, Norman RJ. Metformin in polycystic ovary syndrome: systematic review and meta-analysis. BMJ 2003;327(7421):951–953.
30 Glueck CJ, Wang P, Kobayashi S, Phillips H, Sieve-Smith L. Metformin therapy throughout pregnancy reduces the development of gestational diabetes in women with polycystic ovary syndrome. Fertil Steril 2002;77(3):520–525.
31 Glueck CJ, Phillips H, Cameron D, Sieve-Smith L, Wang P. Continuing metformin throughout pregnancy in women with polycystic ovary syndrome appears to safely reduce first-trimester spontaneous abortion: a pilot study. Fertil Steril 2001;75(1):46–52.
32 Jakubowicz DJ, Iuorno MJ, Jakubowicz S, Roberts KA, Nestler JE. Effects of metformin on early pregnancy loss in the polycystic ovary syndrome. J Clin Endocrinol Metab 2002;87(2):524–529.
33 Palomba S, Falbo A, Orio F, Jr., Zullo F. Effect of preconceptional metformin on abortion risk in polycystic ovary syndrome: a systematic review and meta-analysis of randomized controlled trials. Fertil Steril 2009;92(5):1646–1658.
34 Legro RS, Barnhart HX, Schlaff WD, Carr BR, Diamond MP, Carson SA, et al. Clomiphene, metformin, or both for infertility in the polycystic ovary syndrome. New Engl J Med 2007;356(6):551–566.
35 Tang T, Lord JM, Norman RJ, Yasmin E, Balen AH. Insulin-sensitising drugs (metformin, rosiglitazone, pioglitazone, D-chiro-inositol) for women with polycystic ovary syndrome, oligo amenorrhoea and subfertility. Cochrane Database System Rev 2012;5:CD003053.
36 Coetzee EJ, Jackson WP. Metformin in management of pregnant insulin-independent diabetics. Diabetologia 1979;16(4):241–245.
37 Rai L, Meenakshi D, Kamath A. Metformin – a convenient alternative to insulin for Indian women with diabetes in pregnancy. Indian J Med Sci 2009;63(11):491–497.
38 Gilbert C, Valois M, Koren G. Pregnancy outcome after first-trimester exposure to

metformin: a meta-analysis. Fertil Steril 2006;86(3):658–663.
39　Ainuddin JA, Karim N, Zaheer S, Ali SS, Hasan AA. Metformin treatment in type 2 diabetes in pregnancy: an active controlled, parallel-group, randomized, open label study in patients with type 2 diabetes in pregnancy. J Diabetes Res 2015;2015:325851.
40　Ibrahim MI, Hamdy A, Shafik A, Taha S, Anwar M, Faris M. The role of adding metformin in insulin-resistant diabetic pregnant women: a randomized controlled trial. Arch Gynecol Obstetr 2014;289(5):959–965.
41　Rowan JA, Hague WM, Gao W, Battin MR, Moore MP. Metformin versus insulin for the treatment of gestational diabetes. New Engl J Med 2008;358(19):2003–2015.
42　Rowan JA, Rush EC, Obolonkin V, Battin M, Wouldes T, Hague WM. Metformin in gestational diabetes: the offspring follow-up (MiG TOFU): body composition at 2 years of age. Diabetes Care 2011;34(10):2279–2284.
43　Begum MR, Khanam NN, Quadir E, Ferdous J, Begum MS, Khan F, et al. Prevention of gestational diabetes mellitus by continuing metformin therapy throughout pregnancy in women with polycystic ovary syndrome. J Obstetr Gynaecol Res 2009;35(2):282–286.
44　Vanky E, Stridsklev S, Heimstad R, Romundstad P, Skogoy K, Kleggetveit O, et al. Metformin versus placebo from first trimester to delivery in polycystic ovary syndrome: a randomized, controlled multicenter study. J Clin Endocrinol Metab 2010;95(12):E448–E455.
45　Zarate A, Ochoa R, Hernandez M, Basurto L. [Effectiveness of acarbose in the control of glucose tolerance worsening in pregnancy]. Ginecologia y obstetricia de Mexico 2000;68:42–45.
46　Bertini AM, Silva JC, Taborda W, Becker F, Lemos Bebber FR, Zucco Viesi JM, et al. Perinatal outcomes and the use of oral hypoglycemic agents. J Perinatal Med 2005;33(6):519–523.

47　Chan LY, Yeung JH, Lau TK. Placental transfer of rosiglitazone in the first trimester of human pregnancy. Fertil Steril 2005;83(4):955–958.
48　Holmes HJ, Casey BM, Bawdon RE. Placental transfer of rosiglitazone in the ex vivo human perfusion model. Amer J Obstretr Gynecol 2006;195(6):1715–1719.
49　Haddad GF, Jodicke C, Thomas MA, Williams DB, Aubuchon M. Case series of rosiglitazone used during the first trimester of pregnancy. Reprod Toxicol 2008;26(2):183–184.
50　Kalyoncu NI, Yaris F, Ulku C, Kadioglu M, Kesim M, Unsal M, et al. A case of rosiglitazone exposure in the second trimester of pregnancy. Reprod Toxicol 2005;19(4):563–564.
51　Rouzi AA, Ardawi MS. A randomized controlled trial of the efficacy of rosiglitazone and clomiphene citrate versus metformin and clomiphene citrate in women with clomiphene citrate-resistant polycystic ovary syndrome. Reprod Toxicol 2006;85(2):428–435.
52　Ghazeeri G, Kutteh WH, Bryer-Ash M, Haas D, Ke RW. Effect of rosiglitazone on spontaneous and clomiphene citrate-induced ovulation in women with polycystic ovary syndrome. Fertil Steril 2003;79(3):562–566.
53　UpToDate. Copyright 1978–2015 Lexicomp Online®. Accessed online August 31, 2015.
54　Hiles RA, Bawdon RE, Petrella EM. Ex vivo human placental transfer of the peptides pramlintide and exenatide (synthetic exendin-4). Human Exper Toxicol 2003;22(12):623–628.
55　Johnsson KM, Ptaszynska A, Schmitz B, Sugg J, Parikh SJ, List JF. Urinary tract infections in patients with diabetes treated with dapagliflozin. J Diabetes Complicat 2013;27(5):473–478.
56　Schneeberger C, Kazemier BM, Geerlings SE. Asymptomatic bacteriuria and urinary tract infections in special patient groups: women with diabetes mellitus and pregnant women. Curr Opin Infect Dis 2014;27(1):108–114.

57 Moiel RH, Ryan JR. Tolbutamide orinase in human breast milk. Clinical Pediatr 1967;6(8):480.
58 Feig DS, Briggs GG, Kraemer JM, Ambrose PJ, Moskovitz DN, Nageotte M, et al. Transfer of glyburide and glipizide into breast milk. Diabetes Care 2005;28(8):1851–1855.
59 Hale TW, Kristensen JH, Hackett LP, Kohan R, Ilett KF. Transfer of metformin into human milk. Diabetologia 2002;45(11):1509–1514.
60 Briggs GG, Ambrose PJ, Nageotte MP, Padilla G, Wan S. Excretion of metformin into breast milk and the effect on nursing infants. Obstetr Gynecol 2005;105(6):1437–1441.
61 Gardiner SJ, Kirkpatrick CM, Begg EJ, Zhang M, Moore MP, Saville DJ. Transfer of metformin into human milk. Clin Pharmacol Therap 2003;73(1):71–77.
62 Glueck CJ, Salehi M, Sieve L, Wang P. Growth, motor, and social development in breast- and formula-fed infants of metformin-treated women with polycystic ovary syndrome. J Pediatr 2006;148(5):628–632.
63 NICE guideline 3: Diabetes in pregnancy. Management of diabetes and its compliations from preconception to the postnatal period. http://www.nice.org.uk/guidance/ng3/evidence/full-guideline-3784285
64 American Diabetes Association. Management of diabetes in pregnancy. Diabetes Care 2015;38(Suppl):S77–S79.
65 Cheng AY. Canadian Diabetes Association 2013 clinical practice guidelines for the prevention and management of diabetes in Canada. Introduction. Canadian J Diabetes 2013;37(Suppl 1):S1–S3.

第十六章 胰岛素治疗的进展

Gioia N. Canciani [1], *Zoe A. Stewart* [2] *and Helen R. Murphy* [2]

1 Elsie Bertram Diabetes Centre, Norfolk and Norwich University Hospitals, Norwich, UK
2 University of Cambridge Metabolic Research Laboratories and NIHR Cambridge Biomedical Research Centre, Institute of Metabolic Science, Addenbrooke's Hospital, Cambridge, UK

> **实践要点**
> - 很难预测哪些患者对治疗糖尿病的新技术反应良好。当这些新技术应用于血糖控制不佳的女性时,应该采取更加精确的评估。
> - 治疗糖尿病的技术费用是可观的(应用CSII治疗的费用是3500英镑,MDI治疗的费用是150英镑)。新生儿如果住在监护病房的花费大约需要3500英镑,因此任何母亲和婴儿患病率的下降都将减少治疗带来的额外花费。
> - 糖尿病新技术正在迅速发展,每2~3年就有一批新技术问世。临床试验需要3~5年的时间。因此,有关糖尿病妊娠的研究经常落后于临床实践。对于这些新的技术,我们不应该以替代技术试验或基于非妊娠女性的试验做出假设。DIP的患病率为0.2%~0.4%,主要是产后2型糖尿病。
> - 鲜为人知的是,妊娠女性和(或)她们的卫生保健医师是如何确定在妊娠时应用新技术的。

概述

妊娠妇女的高血糖在糖尿病相关的妊娠并发症的发展中扮演着重要角色[1]。因此,胰岛素治疗的主要目的就是在妊娠前、妊娠中和分娩过程中获得安全、良好的血糖控制[2]。然而,由于妊娠期胰岛素敏感性的变化,皮下注射胰岛素的局限性,以及非常严格的血糖控制目标,大多数1型糖尿病的妊娠女性为了让血糖达标需要付出艰辛努力[3]。来自持续血糖监测研究的纵向数据证实了普遍存在的高血糖和低血糖漂移现象。

强化治疗的主要风险是母亲的低血糖。这种低血糖可能是非常严重的。妊娠妇女严重的低血糖可导致昏迷、癫痫发作甚至死亡[4-6]。

不幸的是，由于这些挑战的存在，与糖尿病相关的妊娠并发症患病率仍然居高不下。为了获得良好的血糖控制，而同时又能避免低血糖的发生，在治疗和监测手段上有了很大的进展。新的技术包括CSII、CGM和闭环式人工胰腺系统。

持续皮下胰岛素输注

胰岛素泵通过放置在皮下的管道系统持续输注短效胰岛素，进餐时给予餐前大剂量[7]。这种给药方式模拟了胰岛素的生理分泌模式，与传统的MDI治疗相比更加方便。

自从胰岛素泵在20世纪70年代面世以来，至今已有了很大的改进。现在的胰岛素泵体积更小、重量更轻，以电池为动力，可以储存数天的胰岛素用量。胰岛素泵的主要优点在于基础率的调整更为灵活、方便。对于非妊娠期的女性，胰岛素的应用有助于血糖的控制，降低了HbA1c水平和血糖的变异率，同时没有增加低血糖的风险[7]。妊娠时，胰岛素的需要量不断变化，低血糖的风险增加，胰岛素泵在这类患者中的应用显示了其独特的优势。

根据NICE的推荐，合并有糖尿病的妊娠女性，如果血糖控制不达标，同时没有显著的低血糖，应该从MDI治疗转换为CSII治疗[8]。2015年，ADA指南推荐采取更严格的血糖控制目标（空腹、餐前、睡前和夜间：3.3~5.4mmol/L；峰值5.4~7.1mmol/L；HbA1c<6.0%），但是没有明确指出MDI或CSII哪种治疗方案更好、更安全[9]。

然而，关于妊娠期女性采用CSII或MDI治疗对比的文献是有限的和过时的。10~20年前曾有随机研究，但那时速效胰岛素类似物还没有应用于临床，且胰岛素泵不方便操作。另外，现在的大多数研究是回顾性的和观察性的，样本量较小，探索母亲和胎儿结局之间的不同缺乏统计学力度。

就母亲和胎儿的结局而言，观察性研究显示CSII和MDI并没有太大的差异[10, 11]，同样可以应用于妊娠妇女[10-18]。对比CSII和MDI治疗的一些研究显示，CSII组血糖控制更佳[12, 14, 18, 19]，妊娠结局更好[12]，胰岛素需要量类似[13]或更低[10, 12, 19]，低血糖发生率更低[10]。

然而，应用CSII也存在许多问题，包括母亲体重的增加、酮症酸中毒和新生儿不良结局[16, 20, 21]。考虑到这些研究是观察性研究，患者人群具有高度的选择性，以及许多混杂因素也许导致了这样的结果。应用CSII的患者，年龄更大，糖尿病病程更长，并且已经合并有糖尿病微血管并发症[11, 12, 18, 19, 20]。在这些患者中观察到的不良结局也许只是反映了更严重的血糖紊乱，而与胰岛素的给药方式无关。

2011年，Cochrane Review[22]发表了一项包括了5项前瞻性的随机试验研究，在T_1DM妊娠女性人群中对比了CSII和MDI，包括共153个妊娠女性，154次妊娠。这项Meta分析显示，就母亲高血糖、低血糖、剖宫产、围产期死亡、巨大儿和小于胎龄儿而言，MDI和CSII治疗没有差异。在应用CSII组的新生儿体重略有增加（$P=0.05$）。在新生儿低血糖发生率方面，二者之间没有显著差异（19% vs 15%）。然而，有作者发现这个Meta分析得出了阴性的结果，也许与纳入的试验数量过少及每个试验的样本量过小有关。

由于存在治疗方式改变后可能出现高血糖的风险，在妊娠早期[2]从MDI治疗改为CSII治疗仍存在一些顾虑。虽然推荐在妊娠前就开始CSII治疗，但是如果有适当的经费投入和技术支持，在妊娠期间，妊娠女性仍是可以安全地过渡至CSII治疗。由于在确认成功妊娠后（妊娠6周），器官形成已基本完成，因此没有理由推迟CSII治疗。此外，倘若CSII治疗失败后[2]，为了避免糖尿病酮症酸中毒的发生，虽然先前一些临床医师建议睡前应用NPH，但是目前除了在反复发作糖尿病酮症酸中毒和（或）依从性差的患者中应用外，这种方案已很少应用。现代的胰岛素泵有很敏感的堵塞报警系统，随时提醒患者是否存在胰岛素输注的中断。对于特定的2型糖尿病患者，胰岛素泵有时是可行的。

总之，有证据显示在妊娠期间应用CSII治疗是安全的，并且与MDI疗效相当。技术的进步使得CSII更精确，使用更方便，不过胰岛素泵比较昂贵，并且需要患者及产前卫生保健团队具备更多的糖尿病管理技巧。目前需要有关CSII治疗和胰岛素类似物MDI方案对比的新的更大规模的随机试验以帮助我们更好地了解CSII对母亲和婴儿结局的影响。

持续血糖监测

血糖监测对于确保足够的胰岛素剂量、避免高血糖和低血糖及相关的并发症是非常重要的。目前，血糖监测的金标准是自我血糖监测（SMBG）。

科技的进步促进了 CGM 的发展。CGM 是由皮下葡萄糖感受装置组成，每 10s 测量一次间质血糖，每 5min 提供一个平均值，每天约提供 288 个血糖读数。CGM 的主要优势在于提供了血糖波动的详细信息，而间断指尖血糖检测可能漏掉这些信息。CGM 于 1999 年首次用于临床实践[23]。起初，CGM 只能回顾性地储存数据，回顾性地提供血糖值（盲 CGM）。盲 CGM 可以佩戴 7d；然后下载被储存的数据，回顾性地分析血糖波动模式，然后相应地调整胰岛素治疗。

近年来，实时持续血糖监测（RT-CGM）已问世。除了皮下感受器（既储存数据，还会发送信号），患者同时携带一个接收器，提供了血糖水平变化趋势的持续信息，包括血糖波动的幅度、频率和持续时间。此外，设置警报预测低血糖和高血糖的发生，允许患者主动进行干预以减少血糖波动[24, 25]。

CGM 相对来说没有不良反应。主要的问题包括皮肤刺激、传感器不准确和使用者不适。由于间质葡萄糖略低于血糖，因此 CGM 需要用 SMBG 进行校准，并且在血糖波动周期不是非常精确。首次使用时，RT-CGM 应选择积极性高的患者佩戴，认为这些患者不可能受到大量 RT-CGM 数据的困扰[24-26]。目前，RT-CGM 被用于更广的患者人群，英国 NICE 指南推荐 CGM 可以用于任何血糖控制不佳的妊娠女性[27]。考虑到合并 1 型糖尿病的妊娠女性在 1 天当中平均 12h 血糖处于不正常范围，因此 RT-CGM 适用于几乎所有的妊娠女性。

在非妊娠人群，包括 1 型或 2 型糖尿病的儿童和成人，RT-CGM 已显示可以改善血糖控制，降低高血糖的时间，同时没有增加低血糖发生率，减少了血糖波动及改善了 HbA1c 水平[24, 25, 28, 29]。一项包括 6 个随机试验共 449 名患者的 Meta 分析显示对总体 HbA1c 水平仅有轻微的影响（下降 0.3%），而在增加传感器使用[29]和基线 HbA1c 水平较高[29]的患者获益更大（最大下降 0.9%）。在应用 CGM 过程中，低血糖暴露中位数下降 23%[25]。

实时动态胰岛素泵（SAP）治疗

技术的进步导致 SAP 治疗的发展。RT-CGM 和胰岛素泵同时佩戴，CGM 提供的葡萄糖读数进入泵中——人工或自动。胰岛素泵依赖特定的内置计算器提供足够的胰岛素剂量。在非妊娠期，SAP 治疗已被证实有益于 1 型糖尿病的治疗。与单纯泵治疗或 MDI 治疗相比，SAP 治疗能够改善血糖控制和降低 HbA1c 水平与低血糖发生频率[30-34]。低血糖暂停（LGS）泵在发生低血糖时能够暂停胰岛素输注。对于睡眠中低血糖风险高的患者来说，低血糖暂停泵提供了额外的安全保护，包括高风险个体的研究显示夜间低血糖（血糖＜2.2mmol/L）的时程从超过 45min 降至不足 2min[35]。期待来自实时动态胰岛素泵研究的数据，当预测发生低血糖时，实时动态胰岛素泵可以暂停胰岛素输注，这也许更进一步降低了发生低血糖的风险。

理论上来讲，当获得良好的血糖控制而又避免发生低血糖比较困难时，CGM 和 SAP 治疗对于妊娠糖尿病的治疗也许是有帮助的。然而，评估妊娠时 CGM 和 SAP 治疗的文献是有限的，并且落后于目前的临床实践。

妊娠时，CGM 已被证实是精确的[36]，在 1 型或 2 型糖尿病女性中可以帮助提高更有针对性的胰岛素剂量[37, 38]。一项包括 46 名 1 型糖尿病女性和 25 名 2 型糖尿病女性的前瞻性、开放标签、随机研究结果显示盲 CGM 改善了妊娠晚期的血糖控制（下降 0.6%），降低了出生体重标准差（s）评分，并且使得出生巨大儿的风险下降 60%[39]。

合并 1 型糖尿病或 2 型糖尿病的女性妊娠时应用 RT-CGM 也是有帮助的，并且耐受性良好[40]。当在妊娠早期应用 RT-CGM 也许有助于降低重度低血糖事件的发生率，尤其是高危女性[41]。与非妊娠人群类似，在血糖波动较大时 RT-CGM 不太精确，如运动时[42]。

到目前为止，只有一个随机临床试验调查了妊娠时间歇应用 RT-CGM 的作用。在对 123 名 1 型糖尿病女性和 31 名 2 型糖尿病女性的检测结果显示,血糖控制或妊娠结局没有改善[43]。这可能是因为 RT-CGM 仅仅是间歇佩戴,以及基线 HbA1c 低于 7%,使得研究很难得到阳性结果。目前的文献显示 RT-CGM 对于 HbA1c 水平更高的患者获益最显著,需要每日佩戴而不是间歇佩戴[24]。一项最新的报道得出了如下的结论,我们需要更进一步的样本量大、设计良好的试验来评估 CGM 对母亲和婴儿健康结局影响的证据[44]。

CONCEPTT（the Continuous Glucose Monitoring in Women with Type 1 Diabetes during Pregnancy Trial；临床试验注册账号 NCT01788527）是一个国际随机试验,目前正在进行中。这个研究将评估在 110 名未妊娠和 224 名已妊娠的 1 型糖尿病女性（总共 334 名女性）中应用持续 RT-CGM 的有效性,这些患者来自加拿大、英国、美国、西班牙、爱尔兰和意大利。主要目标是母亲的血糖控制（在已妊娠女性中是指从基线至妊娠 34 周,在未妊娠女性中是指从基线至 24 周时 HbA1c 的变化）。母亲次要目标包括 CGM 达标时间、低血糖、妊娠高血压/先兆子痫、孕期体重增加和剖宫产的发生率。婴儿次要终点包括流产、死胎、新生儿死亡、新生儿出生体重、产伤、新生儿低血糖、新生儿高胆红素血症、新生儿呼吸窘迫和新生儿入住 ICU。一项应用回顾性 CGM（每 6 周应用 CGM5～7 天）的荷兰多中心随机试验包括 300 名糖尿病妊娠女性（1 型、2 型或应用胰岛素治疗的妊娠糖尿病）,GlucoMOMS（试验注册号 NTR2996）即将完成。这个研究的主要目标是巨大儿（定义为出生体重 > 第 90 百分位数）,次要目标包括血糖控制、母亲和婴儿患病率、成本效益的计算,这对于公共资助的健康保健系统是很重要的。

闭环式胰岛素输注系统

尽管有泵治疗和 RT-CGM 方面的进展及临床医师的不懈努力,合并 1 型糖尿病的妊娠女性仍一天当中有一半时间血糖不正常。为了改善血糖控制、生活质量和长期健康结局,闭环式胰岛素输注或人工胰腺正在开发中。闭环式人工胰腺不同于 LGS 和（或）阈值暂停系统,其对高血糖和低血糖均有反应。更早期的实时动态胰岛素泵在发生低血糖时能够停止胰岛素输注,但是对于短期高血糖并不能增加胰岛素输注。

闭环系统由三部分组成——RT-CGM、控制算法装置和胰岛素泵。在闭环中，通过CGM持续测量血糖，血糖被传送至计算机中，计算机包含一个算法。这个算法就是用个体的血糖信息每隔12~15min计算胰岛素剂量。这种闭环结构与传统的或实时动态胰岛素泵治疗相比，在胰岛素输注方面提供了更高的准确性，消除了患者调整基础胰岛素的需要。这种算法是基于妊娠中餐后高血糖的可能变化和皮下速效胰岛素类似物的药代动力学。支持这个算法的生理学研究显示优化餐后血糖控制具有挑战性。餐后低血糖的持续时间随着妊娠进展而增加，主要是由于葡萄糖吸收入骨骼肌延迟和皮下胰岛素吸收延迟[45]。在妊娠晚期，门冬胰岛素的达峰时间为90min，具有非常显著的随时间变异性，证实了患者每天的经历是不同的[46]。

低血糖暂停

胰岛素自动输注的最简单形式就是LGS。当发生低血糖时，LGS泵通过自动暂停胰岛素输注而减少低血糖风险。

在2009年，第一台LGS问世。在发生低血糖时，虽不能预测低血糖，但这个系统会自动停止胰岛素输注2h。在高危人群，LGS降低了低血糖风险而没有显著增加高血糖时间[47-49]。

在2015年，美敦力公司开发了更先进的阈值暂停系统。当预计发生低血糖时，该系统就暂停胰岛素输注，一旦血糖水平恢复，系统自动重新恢复胰岛素输注。LGS和阈值暂停系统都未在妊娠时进行评估。虽然CONCEPTT试验的受试者都将应用LGS和Medtronic 640G，但是由于样本量较小不能进行亚组分析。

夜间闭环系统

将近一半的重度低血糖发生在晚上。妊娠时，重度低血糖的风险增加2~3倍[5]，这将导致严重的后果包括意识丧失、惊厥发作和死亡。最初闭环技术的合理应用是在夜间，因为夜间是重度低血糖的高发期。

初步可行性研究已显示，不论是在住院期间[50-54]，还是在家中[55, 56]佩戴，闭环系统都是安全的，能有效控制夜间血糖。使用闭环的受试者不仅血糖控制得到改善,并且很少发生低血糖。此外,闭环系统能够很好地应对饮酒和高糖类饮食。

两个小样本量住院患者的研究已经显示,过夜闭环能够获得接近正常的血糖控制,并且在妊娠早期和晚期没有增加低血糖风险[57, 58]。第一个门诊患者妊娠中应用闭环的研究(the Closed-Loop in Pregnancy Overnight Home Feasibility Study;CLIP_03,ISRCTN71510001)即将完成。这将是第一个针对人类妊娠的家庭闭环研究。如果可行,将为更长的妊娠期昼夜闭环系统开发铺平道路。

昼夜(24h)闭环系统

闭环胰岛素输注的最终目的就是开发一个控制血糖的系统,没有人类干预,包括吃饭和锻炼时间。小的概念验证性研究显示,闭环系统能够有效控制血糖,并且低血糖发生率低[59-61]。然而,在完全自动化的闭环系统中,该算法依赖于检测膳食或锻炼中葡萄糖水平的变化,进行计算和改变胰岛素剂量。与传统治疗方法相比,产生了一种固有的延迟,因传统治疗方法是主动给药。不足为奇的是,完全自动系统的研究显示,24h闭环导致长期餐后高血糖和频繁餐后低血糖[62]。

在24h闭环系统中,使用者输入了用餐时间和(或)糖类的数量,是迈向全自动化系统的重要一步。一些研究应用闭环控制基础胰岛素,使用者输入餐时大剂量,效果很好[63, 64]。

对于妊娠女性,24h闭环人工推注大剂量和标准化饮食与锻炼可以使血糖水平接近正常,并且降低了低血糖的发生率[58]。

闭环系统的局限和挑战

闭环系统应用皮下传感器测定间质葡萄糖。当传感器精确度改善时,血液和间质葡萄糖测量之间存在一个固有的滞后[65]。闭环算法中考虑到这个误差,但是不精确的CGM仍旧限制了现有闭环系统的有效性。

此外,皮下注射胰岛素的吸收需要时间,对于速效胰岛素类似物达峰值需要90min[66]。胰岛素的吸收和药代动力学在不同患者之间及同一患者不同时间内也存在不同。妊娠时，随着妊娠时间的推移，胰岛素的吸收变得更慢[46]。

进一步的挑战包括用餐时间和锻炼，这两个时间血糖波动较大[67]。完全自动化闭环系统依靠 CGM 检测血糖的变化，因此在这些时间内，是固有反应而不是主动反应。最可行的办法就是应用混合系统，通过闭环系统自动输入基础胰岛素，手动给予餐前大剂量。妊娠时尤其有必要应用这种混合系统，因为妊娠时血糖控制目标更严格，由于胰岛素吸收更慢，可于餐前 30～60min 给予大剂量。

结论和未来的方向

与糖尿病相关的技术进展有潜力改善合并糖尿病女性妊娠时和她们后代的临床结局和生活质量。持续血糖监测提供了更多有关血糖偏移的信息。正在进行中的试验将揭示这些补充信息是否有助于改善血糖控制和临床结局。胰岛素泵越来越多地被应用于临床实践中，胰岛素剂量更加个体化；然而，缺乏可靠的数据来支持其在妊娠前和妊娠中使用。需要对支持强化治疗所需设备和专业人员花费进行详细经济评估的现代泵给予随机试验。闭环胰岛素输注有可能彻底改变 1 型糖尿病的治疗，并且也许对妊娠是有益的，妊娠时血糖控制目标更严格，但是胰岛素剂量不断变化，难以预测。如果能达到临床疗效，闭环系统的花费不超过标准的实时动态胰岛素泵治疗，并且可在无专业人员和昂贵的人员配备的情况下实行。目前，闭环系统仅适用于 1 型糖尿病妊娠，但是 2 型糖尿病住院患者应用闭环的试验正在进行中，有可能得到更广泛的使用。

选择题

1. 下面的陈述正确的是（　　）
   A. 有明确的证据支持妊娠中使用持续血糖监测
   B. 妊娠中起始胰岛素泵治疗是很安全的
   C. 闭环系统降低了高血糖，但是增加了低血糖

D. 低血糖暂停系统的研究正在进行中，在此之后这些系统在市场上可以买到

正确答案是 B。目前。还没有明确的证据支持妊娠时持续血糖监测的常规使用，虽然两个大型试验即将完成。闭环胰岛素输注系统已被证实降低了高血糖，没有增加低血糖风险。低血糖暂停系统已可买到。妊娠时，从多次胰岛素皮下注射转变为胰岛素泵治疗是很安全的。

2. 下面陈述中正确的是（　　）

   A. 持续血糖监测近年来已快速发展，目前比指尖血糖检测更准确

   B. 持续血糖监测应仅限于受过教育、积极性高的患者，该类患者不大可能被设备提供的大量数据困扰

   C. 持续血糖监测对于 HbA1c 更低的患者益处更大，因为可以对血糖进行微调

   D. 在血糖快速波动时，持续血糖监测不太精确

正确答案是 D。持续血糖监测（CGM）提供了更多关于血糖的信息，但是它没有指尖血糖检测精确，胰岛素剂量应依赖指尖血糖检测。很难预测哪些患者从 CGM 获益最多，英国 NICE 指南推荐 CGM 适用于血糖控制不达标的妊娠女性。与大多数干预措施一样，CGM 可能对于血糖控制更差的患者益处更大。在低血糖和快速血糖波动时，持续血糖监测不太精确。

致谢

ZAS 得到了盖茨剑桥信托基金会和 Jean Hailes 澳大利亚妇女健康基金会的支持。HRM 得到了英国国家卫生研究所（NIHR）研究奖学金（CDF-2013-06-035）的支持。

（张雪冰　译，朱海清　校）

参 考 文 献

1. Ringholm L, Mathiesen E, Kelstrup L, et al. Managing type 1 diabetes mellitus in pregnancy – from planning to breastfeeding. Nat Rev Endocrinol 2012;8:659-667.
2. Castorino K, Paband R, Zisser H, et al. Insulin pumps in pregnancy: using technology to achieve normoglycaemia in women with diabetes. Curr Diab Rep 2012;12:53-59.
3. Murphy HR, Rayman G, Duffield K, et al. Changes in the glycemic profiles of women with type 1 and type 2 diabetes during pregnancy. Diabetes Care 2007;30(11):2785-2791.
4. Ringholm L, Pedersen-Bjergaard U, Thorsteinsson B, et al. Hypoglycaemia during pregnancy in women with Type 1 diabetes. Diabet Med 2012 May;29(5):558-566.
5. Evers IM, ter Braak EWMT, de Valk HW, et al. Risk indicators predictive for severe hypoglycemia during the first trimester of type 1 diabetic pregnancy. Diabetes Care 2002;25(March):554-559.
6. Rosenn BM, Miodovnik M, Holcberg G, et al. Hypoglycemia: the price of intensive insulin therapy for pregnant women with insulin-dependent diabetes mellitus. Obstet Gynecol 1995;85(3):417-422.
7. Pickup JC. Insulin-pump therapy for type 1 diabetes mellitus. N Engl J Med 2012;366:1616-1624.
8. The Guideline Development Group. Management of diabetes from preconception to the postnatal period: summary of NICE guidance. BMJ 2008 Mar 29;336(7646):714-717.
9. American Diabetes Association. Management of diabetes in pregnancy. Diabetes Care 2015;38(Suppl 1):S77-S79.
10. Wender-Ozegowska E, Zawiejska A, Ozegowska K, et al. Multiple daily injections of insulin versus continuous subcutaneous insulin infusion for pregnant women with type 1 diabetes. Aust N Z J Obstet Gynaecol 2013 Apr;53(2):130-135.
11. Lapolla a, Dalfrà MG, Masin M, et al. Analysis of outcome of pregnancy in type 1 diabetics treated with insulin pump or conventional insulin therapy. Acta Diabetol 2003 Oct;40(3):143-149.
12. Talaviya P, Saboo B, Joshi S, et al. Pregnancy outcome and glycemic control in women with type 1 diabetes: a retrospective comparison between CSII and MDI treatment. Diabetes Metab Syndr 2013;7(2):68-71.
13. Giménez M, Conget I, Nicolau J, et al. Outcome of pregnancy in women with type 1 diabetes intensively treated with continuous subcutaneous insulin infusion or conventional therapy: a case-control study. Acta Diabetol 2007 Mar;44(1): 34-37.
14. Gonzalez-Romero S, Gonzalez-Molero I, Fernandez-Abellan M, et al. Continuous subcutaneous insulin infusion versus multiple daily injections in pregnant women with type 1 diabetes. Diabetes Technol Ther 2010;12(4):263-269.
15. Hiéronimus S, Cupelli C, Bongain A, et al. Pregnancy in type 1 diabetes: insulin pump versus intensified conventional therapy. Gynécolog Obs Fertil 2005 Jun;33(6): 389-394.
16. Cyganek K, Hebda-Szydlo A, Katra B, et al. Glycemic control and selected pregnancy outcomes in type 1 diabetes women on continuous subcutaneous insulin infusion and multiple daily injections: the significance of pregnancy planning. Diabetes Technol Ther 2010;12(1):41-47.
17. Gabbe SG, Holing E, Temple P, et al. Benefits, risks, costs, and patient satisfaction associated with insulin pump therapy for the pregnancy complicated by type 1 diabetes mellitus. Am J Obstet Gynecol 2000;182(6):1283-1291.
18. Kallas-Koeman MM, Kong JM, Klinke J, et al. Insulin pump use in pregnancy is associated with lower HbA1c without increasing the rate of severe hypoglycaemia or diabetic ketoacidosis in women with

type 1 diabetes. Diabetologia 2014;57(4):681–689.
19 Bruttomesso D, Bonomo M, Costa S, et al. Type 1 diabetes control and pregnancy outcomes in women treated with continuous subcutaneous insulin infusion (CSII) or with insulin glargine and multiple daily injections of rapid-acting insulin analogues (glargine-MDI). Diabetes Metab 2011;37(5):426–431.
20 Chico A, Saigi I, García-Patterson A, et al. Glycemic control and perinatal outcomes of pregnancies complicated by type 1 diabetes: influence of continuous subcutaneous insulin infusion and lispro insulin. Diabetes Technol Ther 2010;12(12):937–945.
21 Chen R, Ben-Haroush A, Weismann-Brenner A, et al. Level of glycemic control and pregnancy outcome in type 1 diabetes: a comparison between multiple daily insulin injections and continuous subcutaneous insulin infusions. Am J Obstet Gynecol 2007 Oct;197(4):404. e1–e5.
22 Farrar D, Tuffnell DJ, & West J. Continuous subcutaneous insulin infusion versus multiple daily injections of insulin for pregnant women with diabetes. Cochrane Database Sys Rev 2011;(10). doi:10.1002/14651858.CD005542.pub2
23 Mastrototaro J. The MiniMed continuous glucose monitoring system. Diabetes Technol Ther 2000;2:13–18.
24 Klonoff DC. Continuous glucose monitoring: roadmap for 21st century diabetes therapy. Diabetes Care 2005;28(5):1231–1239.
25 Pickup JC, Freeman SC, & Sutton AJ. Glycaemic control in type 1 diabetes during real time continuous glucose monitoring compared with self monitoring of blood glucose: meta-analysis of randomised controlled trials using individual patient data. BMJ 2011 Jan;343:d3805.
26 Hewapathirana N, O'Sullivan E, & Murphy HR. Role of continuous glucose monitoring in the management of diabetic pregnancy. Curr Diab Rep 2013;13:34–42.
27 National Institute for Health and Care Excellence (NICE). Diabetes in pregnancy: management from preconception to the postnatal period. NICE guidelines [NG3]. NICE: London, 2015.
28 Garg S, Zisser H, Schwartz S, et al. Improvement in glycemic excursions with a transcutaneous, real-time continuous glucose sensor: a randomized controlled trial. Diabetes Care 2006;29(1):44–50.
29 Langendam M, Luijf YM, Hooft L, et al. Continuous glucose monitoring systems for type 1 diabetes mellitus. Cochrane Database Syst Rev. 2012;(1).
30 Nørgaard K, Scaramuzza A, Bratina N, et al. Routine sensor-augmented pump therapy in type 1 diabetes: the INTERPRET study. Diabetes Technol Ther 2013 May;15(4):273–280.
31 Bergenstal RM, Tamborlane W V, Ahmann A, et al. Effectiveness of sensor-augmented insulin-pump therapy in type 1 diabetes. N Engl J Med 2010;363:311–320.
32 Hermanides J, Nørgaard K, Bruttomesso D, et al. Sensor-augmented pump therapy lowers HbA1c in suboptimally controlled Type 1 diabetes; a randomized controlled trial. Diabet Med 2011;28(10):1158–1167.
33 Schmidt S & Nørgaard K. Sensor-augmented pump therapy at 36 months. Diabetes Technol Ther 2012;14(12):1174–1177.
34 Battelino T, Conget I, Olsen B, et al. The use and efficacy of continuous glucose monitoring in type 1 diabetes treated with insulin pump therapy: a randomised controlled trial. Diabetologia 2012;55(12):3155–3162.
35 Choudhary P, Shin J, Wang Y, et al. Insulin pump therapy with automated insulin suspension in response to hypoglycemia: reduction in nocturnal hypoglycemia in those at greatest risk. Diabetes Care 2011;34(9):2023–2025.
36 Kerssen A, de Valk HW, & Visser GH. The continuous glucose monitoring system during pregnancy of women with type 1

during pregnancy of women with type 1 diabetes mellitus: accuracy assessment. Diabetes Technol Ther 2004 Oct;6(5): 645–651.
37 Yogev Y, Chen R, Ben-Haroush A, et al. Continuous glucose monitoring for the evaluation of gravid women with type 1 diabetes mellitus. Obstet Gynecol 2003 Apr;101(4):633–638.
38 Yogev Y, Ben-Haroush A, Chen R, et al. Continuous glucose monitoring for treatment adjustment in diabetic pregnancies – a pilot study. Diabet Med 2003;20(7):558–562.
39 Murphy H, Rayman G, & Lewis K. Effectiveness of continuous glucose monitoring in pregnant women with diabetes: randomised clinical trial. BMJ 2008;337:1–8.
40 Secher AL, Madsen A, Ringholm L, et al. Patient satisfaction and barriers to initiating real-time continuous glucose monitoring in early pregnancy in women with diabetes. Diabet Med 2012;29(2):272–277.
41 Secher AL, Stage E, Ringholm L, et al. Real-time continuous glucose monitoring as a tool to prevent severe hypoglycaemia in selected pregnant women with Type 1 diabetes – an observational study. Diabet Med 2013;31:352–356.
42 Kumareswaran K, Elleri D, Allen JM, et al. Physical activity energy expenditure and glucose control in pregnant women with type 1 diabetes. Diabetes Care 2013;36:1095–1101.
43 Secher AL, Ringholm L, Andersen H, et al. The effect of real-time continuous glucose monitoring in pregnant women with diabetes: a randomized controlled trial. Diabetes Care 2013;36(7):1877–1883.
44 Moy F, Ray A, & Buckley BS. Methods for monitoring blood glucose in pregnant women with diabetes to improve outcomes. Cochrane Database Sys Rev 2014;(4).
45 Murphy HR, Elleri D, Allen JM, et al. Pathophysiology of postprandial hyperglycaemia in women with type 1 diabetes during pregnancy. Diabetologia 2012;55(2):282–293.
46 Goudie RJB, Lunn D, Hovorka R, et al. Pharmacokinetics of insulin aspart in pregnant women with type 1 diabetes: every day is different. Diabetes Care 2014 Jun;37(6):e121–e122.
47 Ly T, Nicholas J, Retterath A, et al. Effect of sensor-augmented insulin pump therapy and automated insulin suspension vs standard insulin pump therapy on hypoglycemia in patients with type 1 diabetes: a randomized clinical trial. JAMA 2013;310(12):1240–1247.
48 Agrawal P, Welsh JB, Kannard B, et al. Usage and effectiveness of the low glucose suspend feature of the Medtronic Paradigm Veo Insulin Pump. J Diabetes Sci Technol 2011;5(5):1137–1141.
49 Agrawal P, Zhong A, Welsh JB, et al. Retrospective analysis of the real-world use of the threshold suspend feature of sensor-augmented insulin pumps. Diabetes Technol Ther 2015;17(5).
50 Kumareswaran K, Elleri D, Allen JM, et al. Meta-analysis of overnight closed-loop randomized studies in children and adults with type 1 diabetes: the Cambridge Cohort. J Diabetes Sci Technol 2011 Nov 1;5(6):1352–1362.
51 Hovorka R, Kumareswaran K, Harris J, et al. Overnight closed loop insulin delivery (artificial pancreas) in adults with type 1 diabetes: crossover randomised controlled studies. BMJ 2011;342:1855.
52 Steil GM, Rebrin K, Darwin C, et al. Feasibility of automating insulin delivery for the treatment of type 1 diabetes. Diabetes 2006;55(12):3344–3350.
53 O'Grady MJ, Retterath AJ, Keenan DB, et al. The use of an automated, portable glucose control system for overnight glucose control in adolescents and young adults with type 1 diabetes. Diabetes Care 2012 Nov;35(11):2182–2187.
54 Nimri R, Atlas E, Ajzensztejn M, et al. Feasibility study of automated overnight closed-loop glucose control under MD-logic artificial pancreas in patients with type 1 diabetes: the DREAM Project.

Diabetes Technol Ther 2012 Aug;
14(8):728-735.
55 Hovorka R, Elleri D, Thabit H, et al.
Overnight closed-loop insulin delivery in
young people with type 1 diabetes: a free-
living, randomized clinical trial. Diabetes
Care 2014;37(5):1204-1211.
56 Thabit H, Lubina-Solomon A, Stadler M,
et al. Home use of closed-loop insulin
delivery for overnight glucose control in
adults with type 1 diabetes: a 4-week,
multicentre, randomised crossover study.
Lancet Diabetes Endocrinol
2014;2(9):701-709.
57 Murphy HR, Elleri D, Allen JM, et al.
Closed-loop insulin delivery during
pregnancy complicated by type 1 diabetes.
Diabetes Care 2011;34:406-411.
58 Murphy HR, Kumareswaran K, Elleri D,
et al. Safety and efficacy of 24-h closed-
loop insulin delivery in well-controlled
pregnant women with type 1 diabetes: a
randomised crossover case series. Diabetes
Care 2011;34:2527-2529.
59 Atlas E, Nimri R, Miller S, et al. MD-Logic
artificial pancreas system: a pilot study in
adults with type 1 diabetes. Diabetes Care
2010;33(5):1072-1076.
60 Steil GM, Rebrin K, Darwin C, et al.
Feasibility of automating insulin delivery
for the treatment of type 1 diabetes.
Diabetes 2006;55(12):3344-3350.
61 Dassau E, Zisser H, Harvey R, et al. Clinical
evaluation of a personalized artificial
pancreas. Diabetes Care 2013;36:801-809.
62 Steil GM, Rebrin K, Darwin C, Hariri F, &
Saad MF. Feasibility of automating insulin
delivery for the treatment of type 1
diabetes. Diabetes 2006;55(12):3344-3350.
63 Kovatchev B, Cobelli C, Renard E, et al.
Multinational study of subcutaneous
model-predictive closed-loop control in
type 1 diabetes mellitus: summary of the
results. J Diabetes Sci Technol
2010;4(6):1374-1381.
64 Elleri D, Allen JM, Kumareswaran K, et al.
Closed-loop basal insulin delivery over 36
hours in adolescents with type 1 diabetes.
Diabetes Care 2013;36:838-844.
65 Castle JR & Ward WK. Amperometric
glucose sensors: sources of error and
potential benefit of redundancy. J Diabetes
Sci Technol 2010 Jan 1;4(1):221-225.
66 Hovorka R. Continuous glucose
monitoring and closed-loop systems.
Diabet Med 2006 Jan;23(1):1-12.
67 Hovorka R. Closed-loop insulin delivery:
from bench to clinical practice. Nat Rev
Endocrinol 2011 Jul;7(7):385-395.

第十七章 糖尿病合并妊娠的胰岛素泵治疗

Peter Hammond

Harrogate District Hospital, Harrogate, UK

实践要点

- 当存在妊娠期使用胰岛素泵治疗的适应证时,如果条件允许应尽量选择在受孕前就开始接受胰岛素泵治疗。
- 妊娠期开始胰岛素泵治疗,胰岛素初始每日总剂量(TDD)通常应为每日多次注射胰岛素(MDI)时的85%。
- 妊娠期间开始胰岛素泵治疗时,如果 $HbA1c>8.5\%$,初始泵治疗胰岛素 TDD 与 MDI 时 TDD 相同;如果妊娠期胰岛素泵治疗的指征为低血糖,初始泵治疗胰岛素 TDD 为 MDI 时 TDD 的75%。
- 到妊娠晚期,预计基础胰岛素输注率增加了约50%,而大剂量胰岛素的剂量增加了约4倍。
- 妊娠后期,如果餐后高血糖症控制不佳,考虑在餐前45~60min给予大剂量,在大量糖类饮食时采取超大餐前剂量。
- 妊娠期间至少每48h更换一次胰岛素输注装置,以降低因胰岛素输注装置阻塞而导致的高血糖和酮症风险。
- 如果输注部位有问题,考虑使用腹部替代部位和(或)更换为不同的输注装置。
- 使用类固醇促进胎肺成熟时及分娩期间可以继续进行胰岛素泵治疗,不一定要常规地转为静脉注射胰岛素治疗。
- 确保在围产期有针对胰岛素泵治疗管理的指南。
- 如果对产后胰岛素剂量不确定,那么使用 0.3U/kg 的基础量;如果母乳喂养,则降至 0.2U/kg。

注意事项:

- 有一种错误观点是担心从 MDI 换为胰岛素泵治疗的过程中会出现血糖控制恶化,不要因为这种错误观点而延迟启动胰岛素泵治疗的时间。
- 随着孕周增加,妊娠妇女调整胰岛素基础率和餐前大剂量时不要过于保守。
- 如果从妊娠前或妊娠早期就开始胰岛素泵治疗,要考虑到妊娠后期胰岛素需要量大幅增加,并选择适当容量的胰岛素储药器。
- 母乳喂养时,胰岛素剂量应减少约1/3,以防止低血糖的风险增加。

> **病 例**
>
> Kate 从 11 岁起就患有 1 型糖尿病，且还患有甲状腺功能减退症。28 岁第一次妊娠，也是一次计划妊娠，每天两次注射精蛋白锌胰岛素并在餐前注射赖脯胰岛素，HbA1c 为 6.3%。在妊娠的前 3 个月，她经常发生严重低血糖症，并伴有癫痫发作和一次车祸。她在整个妊娠期间血糖控制良好，但出现了严重的羊水过多，因此被转院到地区中心，在妊娠 34 周时产下一名巨大儿。
>
> 2 年后，第二次妊娠时也采取了之前的胰岛素治疗方案，与上次妊娠时类似，在妊娠的前 3 个月她再次出现低血糖发作，尽管血糖控制接近目标值，但她再次出现了羊水过多，并在妊娠 36 周时产下了一名巨大儿。
>
> 她第三次妊娠是计划外的，当时 HbA1c 为 7.7%，胰岛素治疗方案与之前相同，但妊娠 8 周时低血糖发作越来越严重。因此，她立即被改成胰岛素泵治疗，起始每日总剂量为以前每日总剂量的 75%。在剩余的孕程当中她没有进一步的严重低血糖，只有很少的轻微低血糖发作。从胰岛素泵治疗开始，她的血糖水平得到更好地控制，妊娠 30 周时 HbA1c 为 4.8%，羊水量略有增加，但羊水过多不明显。她在妊娠 38 周时剖宫产一个正常的婴儿。
>
> 这一案例说明了胰岛素泵疗法在实现严格的血糖控制同时降低了低血糖风险。对于 MDI 治疗的过程中曾出现过问题的妊娠妇女来说应该采取胰岛素泵治疗。妊娠期间尝试过这两种疗法的妇女通常反映对胰岛素泵治疗效果更满意，理由是血糖控制更佳，灵活性更强，胰岛素注射更容易，饮食可控性更好。

概述

胰岛素泵治疗作为一种强化胰岛素治疗的方法，与 MDI 疗法相比具有潜在优势。胰岛素通过泵输注更灵活，可以提供可变的基础率、不同类型的大剂量输注模式，需要频繁使用校正剂量时更加方便。

胰岛素泵的主要组成部分包括含有胰岛素溶液的储药器（通常使用可以快速起效的胰岛素类似物，如门冬胰岛素或赖脯胰岛素），以规定的速率输注胰岛素的机械泵，以及将胰岛素从泵输送到皮下组织的管路和输注装置。传统胰岛素泵（图 17.1A）被称为拴系式泵，输液装置包括连接到位于皮下组织的塑料或金属套管上的较长的管路。传统的胰岛素泵可以由远程设备控制，也可以直接通过按钮和菜单控制。目前，一体式泵（图 17.1B）已经出现，它是直接安装于皮肤的较小装置，没有管路而输送装置直接位于泵下方，或管路很短，这样输注部位就位于胰岛素泵附近。一体式泵储液罐容量有限，没有任何内置软件来控制胰岛素输送，依赖于手持遥控器发出的信号。输注部位通常位于腹壁，其他可替代的位置包括侧腰、大腿和臀部；一体式泵还可以置于上臂。

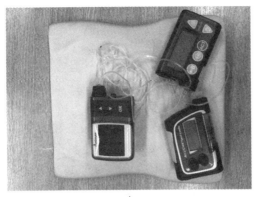

A

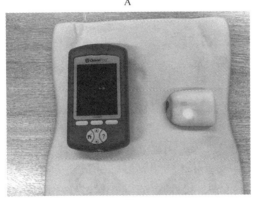

B

图 17.1 胰岛素泵
A. 传统泵；B. 一体式泵

胰岛素泵能够以每 30～60min 调节一次的速率输送基础胰岛素，具体取决于装置型号。虽然被称为连续输注，但实际上是每几分钟弹丸式推注一次规定的累积剂量。胰岛素泵可以多种方式输注大剂量胰岛素。使用胰岛素泵治疗的患者不需要额外的皮下注射，使得加餐时补充大剂量和纠正高血糖时给予校正大剂量更容易。除了提供与传统胰岛素注射所提供的大剂量注射相似的标准大剂量外，还可以通过在预先规定的时间内注入大剂量胰岛素分为方波注射或双波团注；或标准和方波的混合，由使用者确定每种形式中给出的大剂量比例。胰岛素泵的软件包括一个大剂量计算器，有时被称为向导。不同厂家基于的数学算法不同，但大剂量计算器（向导）向使用者提供的信息类似。该功能会根据给定的血糖水平、糖类摄入量及之前大剂量残留的活性胰岛素量计算出此次大剂量的建议值。

在非妊娠的糖尿病患者中，胰岛素泵治疗在降低 HbA1c、改善血糖控制情况、降低低血糖风险方面已被证明优于 MDI[1]。尽管缺乏妊娠期胰岛素泵疗法优于 MDI 的证据（特别是在母体/胎儿结局方面而非血糖方面的证据）（参见第十六章），胰岛素泵对于那些想妊娠前或妊娠期优化血糖控制的 1 型或 2 型糖尿病患者来说是一个有价值的选择，尤其是妊娠期间 MDI 受到低血糖症的限制时（如 NICE 指南中指出的）[2]。在本章中会具体讨论妊娠期胰岛素泵使用的一些实际问题。

起始胰岛素泵治疗

理想状态下，胰岛素泵治疗应该在备孕时就开始。准备妊娠的糖尿病妇女在接受了每日多次胰岛素注射治疗后仍然不能够达到受孕前血糖控制目标或为了达到严格的血糖控制目标而出现频繁低血糖时，胰岛素泵治疗可能是更好的选择。因为受孕前的血糖控制情况会影响妊娠期的血糖控制，任何问题都可能持续到妊娠的早期关键阶段。对于达到受孕前血糖控制目标的女性，如果之前的妊娠过程中出现过血糖控制不佳或与之相关的不良妊娠结局，也可以考虑提前开始胰岛素泵治疗（参见本章病例部分）。

大部分糖尿病患者都是在发现妊娠后才来就诊，而不是在备孕的阶段，所以经常会因为各种不同的原因必须采取胰岛素泵治疗。最常见的原因是 MDI 不能够达到理想的血糖控制目标或是出现低血糖，特别是在妊娠早期。其他起始胰岛素泵治疗的原因包括妊娠剧吐，胰岛素泵可以小剂量频繁输注，有助于达到更加稳定的血糖水平，在我们的临床经验中可以减少呕吐的剧烈程度。在妊娠晚期，胰岛素抵抗进一步加重导致更加明显的黎明现象，胰岛素泵可以按需在清晨就增加胰岛素基础量，这样可以控制由黎明现象导致的高血糖。有一些妊娠糖尿病患者使用胰岛素泵的报道[3]，但是由于妊娠糖尿病通常是在妊娠后期才诊断的，而制订强化胰岛素治疗方案需要花费时间，所以在妊娠糖尿病中使用胰岛素泵的机会不多。

受孕前开始胰岛素泵治疗的女性应当遵循非妊娠妇女的标准治疗方案。一种确定胰岛素泵治疗每日胰岛素总量的方法是在之前每日多次注射胰岛素总剂量的基础上减少 25%，其中的 50% 作为基础胰岛素剂量。起始治疗时可以选择单一的基础率，其计算方法是将每日总的基础胰岛素剂量除以 24（表 17.1）；也可以将基础率在 24h 内分为几个不同的速率，根据患者一天的血糖谱来确定，一般来说不超过 4 段，动态血糖监测的结果可以帮助明确血糖轮廓；也可以使用泵预设的针对典型成年人的基础输注率，如 Accu-Chek 泵。每日多次注射胰岛素的患者中有不少人需要很大剂量的基础胰岛素，所以在根据上述基础量确定胰岛素泵治疗的基础率时需要用估算基础量来核对，对于 1 型糖尿病女性一般为 0.3U/（kg·d），也可以作为一种确定起始基础胰岛素量的方法。

表 17.1　妊娠前从 MDI 转换为胰岛素泵治疗

一名 25 岁的女性，体重 70kg，每天 2 次注射地特胰岛素 16U，IC 比值为 1∶3（1U 胰岛素可以平衡 10g 糖类），每天餐前胰岛素共 32U。她的 HbA1c 为 7.4%。她一直在努力加强血糖控制，但苦于不断增加的低血糖发作和无症状低血糖
全天总胰岛素剂量（TDD）=64U
75%TDD=48U
起始基础胰岛素剂量=24U/d=1U/h[基础率核对：基础量预计值 0.3U/（kg·d）×70kg=21U/d]
糖类系数（ICR）=500/48=10.4（1U 胰岛素可以平衡 10.4g 糖类）
胰岛素敏感系数（ISF）=100/48=2.08（1U 胰岛素可以降低血糖 2.08mmol/L）

餐前大剂量最好根据进食糖类的量来确定。胰岛素泵的大剂量向导可以事先规定糖类系数（IC：每 1U 胰岛素所能平衡的糖类克数，每天的不同时间段该值可能不同）。一个主要的计算糖类系数的方法是 500 法则，即 IC 约等于 500/每日胰岛素总量。与之类似的胰岛素敏感系数[每 1U 胰岛素能降低的血糖（mmol/L）值]的计算方法是 100 法则（100/每日胰岛素总量）（表 17.2）。

表 17.2 基础向大剂量转换

一名 32 岁妇女妊娠 28 周,早餐后 1h 血糖水平通常在 9～12mmol/L。她使用的 IC 比值为 1∶3(1U 胰岛素可以平衡 3g 糖类),并一直尽量限制她的糖类摄入量。如果她尝试在 8∶00 早餐前大剂量多给予 2～3U 的胰岛素,那么她会在 11∶00～12∶00 出现低血糖

建议她尝试基础向大剂量转换。她通常在 8∶00 注射餐前大剂量,她的基础率从 8∶00～13∶00 为 1.6U/h。如果她早餐含 30g 糖类,那么她通常会给 10U 餐前大剂量。在基础向大剂量转换后,她应该在餐前注射 12U 胰岛素,从接下来的 5h 内从基础胰岛素中减去 2U,因此从 8∶00～13∶00 她的基础率为 1.2U/h。这可以通过在这 5h 内将临时基础率设置为原本基础率的 75%来实现

妊娠期的胰岛素泵治疗可以在任何孕龄开始。没有证据表明起始胰岛素泵治疗时血糖控制会恶化。因此,没有理由将开始胰岛素泵治疗的时间推迟至妊娠 12 周以后。这一点对于在妊娠早期有严重低血糖和妊娠剧吐的妇女尤为重要,因为积极地在这些妊娠妇女中使用胰岛素泵治疗可使得患者有较大的获益。起始胰岛素泵的治疗应当遵循在本章中提到的主要原则。起始胰岛素泵治疗时每日总剂量为 MDI 时总剂量的 85%。在有严重低血糖的患者中,起始剂量为之前 MDI 总剂量的75%。相应地,如果血糖控制特别差,糖化血红蛋白大于 8.5%,起始剂量为之前 MDI 的100%,之后需要用0.3U/(kg·d)的估算值来核对基础胰岛量。

尽管 24h 单一的基础率可能就足以满足要求,一些权威专家仍建议将基础率分为 3～4 段[4,5],举例如下:

• 时间段 0∶00～4∶00 的 4h 内胰岛素量为 0.1×胰岛素泵每日基础胰岛素量(TDBD)。

• 时间段 4∶00～8∶00 的 4h 内胰岛素量为 0.2×TDBD。

• 时间段 8∶00～16∶00 的 8h 内胰岛素量为 0.3×TDBD。

• 时间段 16∶00～0∶00 的 8h 内胰岛素量为 0.4×TDBD[5]。

妊娠期胰岛素需要量的变化

妊娠妇女随着孕龄增加,胰岛素抵抗也逐渐加重,导致对胰岛素的需要量也发生改变。因此,妊娠期胰岛素泵的基础率和大剂量都需要有相应改变。随着孕龄增加,餐前大剂量明显增加。最近的一项丹麦的研

究显示，妊娠晚期基础率较妊娠早期约增加 1/3~1/2，最大增幅出现在 5∶00，较 17∶00 的增幅更大。妊娠早期的糖类系数是妊娠晚期的 4 倍。在妊娠早期平均每 1U 胰岛素可以平衡 12g 糖类，而妊娠晚期 1U 胰岛素仅可平衡 3g 糖类[6]。闭环研究发现在妊娠期基础胰岛素的改变相对较小[7]，在妊娠 3 个月以后空腹血糖的改变基本可以忽略不计。

为了得出妊娠期合适的胰岛素剂量，1 型糖尿病妇女在妊娠不同阶段预计的每日总胰岛素剂量约为：

- 妊娠早期 0.7U/（kg·d）。
- 妊娠中期 0.8U/（kg·d）。
- 妊娠晚期 0.9U/（kg·d）[4]。

在妊娠早期基础胰岛素占每日总胰岛素的比例略低于 50%，到妊娠晚期该比例降至约 35%。

升级胰岛素剂量过程中最大的障碍是增加餐前大剂量比例和基础率时过于保守。增加餐前大剂量所占比例可以大胆一些。对于一些妇女来说，餐前和基础的比例达到 4∶1 或 6∶1 也并不罕见。每天的不同时段餐前大剂量所占的比例也不同。特别需要指出的是，由于晨起胰岛素抵抗程度的加重，对于给定摄入量的糖类，早饭时需要的餐前大剂量胰岛素要高于一天中的其他时候，早餐时胰岛素与糖类的比值是午餐和晚餐时该比值的数倍（如在早餐时该比值为 2∶1，而在午餐和晚餐时该比值为 1∶5）。尽管基础率的增加没有餐时胰岛素增加那样显著，已经使用胰岛素泵治疗过的妇女妊娠期基础率一般增幅为 0.1U/h，到了妊娠晚期可能不足，妊娠妇女要准备好需要小幅度频繁地调整基础率，一般在 24 周以后每周调整 1~2 次；或需要做出更大的调整，增加的幅度为 0.2~0.4U/h。考虑到以上的胰岛素需求的变化，妊娠妇女需要通过远程或在产前糖尿病中心规律地回顾上传胰岛素泵的数据以便指导治疗。

在餐前大剂量输注方面需要考虑到在妊娠晚期胰岛素吸收是延迟的，因此大剂量需要在餐前 1h 注射[8]。我们建议妊娠妇女于妊娠早期餐前 15~20min 注射餐前胰岛素，在妊娠中期开始餐前 30min 注射胰岛素，而在妊娠晚期，如果可能应在餐前 45~60min 注射胰岛素。

另一个挑战是控制早餐后血糖峰值，尤其在妊娠晚期。尽管改变食物组成可以帮助改善早餐后血糖，但对于使用胰岛素泵的患者还有另外的选择，即"基础-大剂量"转换法，也被称为"超级大剂量"，这种转换法的操作方法是将早餐后数小时的基础率降低，将减少的基础胰岛素总量加到平时的早餐大剂量中（见表17.2）。

最后，一些妊娠妇女在妊娠晚期会有胃排空延迟，这种情况下复杂的大剂量波形就非常有帮助。通常在双波大剂量中一定比例的餐前大剂量在 4~6h 被均匀输注。在一些极端案例中，可以只使用方波大剂量输注。

与餐前大剂量比例同时需要调整的是胰岛素敏感指数。在妊娠晚期胰岛素敏感指数降低为之前的 1/3~1/4。因此，如果在妊娠早期 1U 的胰岛素可以降低血糖 3mmol/L，到了妊娠晚期 1U 的胰岛素只能降低血糖 1mmol/L。

在计算大剂量时还需要考虑活性胰岛素的持续时间。尽管可以通过在注射准确大剂量胰岛素后计算血糖恢复至基线值的时间来得到这个数值，但是一般都直接定为 3~4h。在妊娠晚期，随着胰岛素吸收变缓，活性胰岛素时间一般会延长。如果在使用过程中发现大剂量向导计算器在妊娠晚期高估了所需的胰岛素剂量，妊娠妇女可以将胰岛素活性时间设置为 5~6h。

使用糖皮质激素促胎肺成熟的情况

患糖尿病的女性可能会同时接受糖皮质激素治疗，可能是用来治疗自身免疫性疾病（如系统性红斑狼疮）的固定剂量的泼尼松或其他类似药物。如果患者发生了临床需要提前终止妊娠情况（如严重的先兆子痫或早产），这时需要糖皮质激素促进胎肺成熟，在这种情况下有许多激素可以选用，在我们的临床实践中会在间隔 12h 的时间里给予两次倍他米松治疗。糖皮质激素有明显的升高血糖的作用，因此应当对接受该治疗的妇女进行严密的血糖监测和管理。我们发现应用胰岛素泵可以有效地控制糖皮质激素对患糖尿病妊娠妇女的影响。在首剂使用糖皮质激素后 72h 内将临时基础率增加 50%（设置为平时基础率的 1.5 倍）。在首剂使用糖皮质激素 6h 后的 24h 内将餐前大剂量增加 50%。一些女性的胰岛素使用量可能会是她们平时使用量的 2 倍。对于这些患者来说，正确使用校正大剂量可以帮助控制血糖，但是要避免大剂量胰岛素之间的累加蓄积。需要提醒患者在胰岛素需要量增加的期间，大剂量向导可能会低估所需的胰岛素量，因此还需要手动输入大剂量。

妊娠期其他需要考虑的方面

胰岛素泵常用的输注位置在腹壁，一体式胰岛素泵也可以安装在上臂。随着妊娠期进展，患者会发现将腹壁作为输注位置越来越难，尤其是当腹部皮肤变得紧绷时，在这种情况下，塑料管路会容易打折阻碍胰岛素的输注。为了避免这些情况可以选择其他的备选输注位置，包括腰部、大腿、臀部甚至乳房，或使用其他不容易打折的管路，如不锈钢针头。

由于当胰岛素输注失败时，妊娠期酮症会更容易发展为糖尿病酮症酸中毒，因此使用泵的患者需要经常注意有无输注装置堵塞和其他故障。一些专家建议夜间注射长效基础胰岛素（胰岛素类似物和精蛋白锌胰岛素）来替代一部分基础胰岛素，以避免在妊娠期间出现的胰岛素泵失效的风险，但是这并不是常用的方法。我们向使用泵的患者强调频繁更换管路的重要性，每48h至少要更换一次管路，以降低堵塞的风险和减慢输注率。笔者还建议当血糖水平大于10mmol/L时要检测血酮水平。

在妊娠期胰岛素的使用量是不断增加的，要考虑到胰岛素泵的储药器容量是有限的。储药器比较小（1.5～1.8ml）的胰岛素泵可能需要每天重新更换储药器。因此，妊娠期的后半段开始就应该换为更大储药器（≥3ml）的胰岛素泵。在妊娠前和妊娠期一开始选用胰岛素泵时就应当考虑到这一点。

围产期

胰岛素泵在整个妊娠期都可以连续使用，包括围产期在内，不论分娩方式如何。但这需要糖尿病医师、助产士、产科医师、麻醉医师团队协同教育和密切配合。如果已经制订好治疗方案的情况下，没有必要常规让使用胰岛素泵的妊娠妇女在分娩时改为静脉注射胰岛素。不过当胰岛素泵治疗不能有效地将血糖控制在理想范围内时，可以改为静脉注射胰岛素。

目前国际上对于是否在分娩时使用胰岛素泵没有一致的看法。在英国和美国的许多中心更喜欢对所有的糖尿病患者都通过不同速率静脉输注胰岛素（VRII）方法控制血糖，不论她们之前的胰岛素用法如何。准备将胰岛素泵改变为 VRII 时，建议患者事先将基础率减为妊娠期的50%，并且相应地将胰岛素/糖类比值减至受孕前后的水平。这样在患者分娩后恢复进食后继续胰岛素泵治疗时就可以马上使用。如果患者选择在分娩时继续使用胰岛素泵治疗，所有的产科和其他产房医疗人员都需要熟悉胰岛素泵的使用，产房诊疗常规中也需要包括胰岛素泵的治疗常规，同时也需要告诉患者在分娩时需要注意的事项和准备工作。

我们给准备在分娩期间使用胰岛素泵治疗的患者一份需要带到医院的物品清单。

- 备用电池 2 套。
- 储药器 2 个。
- 短效胰岛素 1 支。
- 管路 5 套、助针器。
- 胰岛素注射器 10 支。
- 长效胰岛素 1 支。
- 低血糖的应急处理物品（葡萄糖片、葡萄糖凝胶等）。
- 糖类零食。

当患者出现先兆临产时，我们还建议患者需要检查以下情况：

- 胰岛素泵内放入新的电池。
- 胰岛素泵内放入注满胰岛素的新储药器。
- 更换管路。
- 将输注部位选在肋骨下，朝向后背方向，远离紧急情况时可能有操作的部位。
- 写下或者在胰岛素泵内输入妊娠之前的基础率作为第二基础率，这一步需要事先就设置好，以便在分娩后可以立即切换到该基础率。如果在此次妊娠前没有用过胰岛素泵，那么需要事先咨询糖尿病医师基础率需要减少多少。如果没有事先咨询，建议在糖尿病医师到来之前立即将基础率改为目前的 50%。

由于存在紧急剖宫产的可能性，输注装置在皮肤的位置要尽可能远离手术区域。

一般来说，患者维持已有的基础率就可以维持在分娩和剖宫产术中的血糖稳定。如果血糖超出目标范围，我们也提供了纠正血糖的方法。

我们对术中胰岛素调整的推荐如下：

· 如果血糖＞7mmol/L，给予校正大剂量时将目标血糖值设置为5mmol/L、1U 胰岛素降低 2.5mmol/L 血糖（除非糖尿病专家有其他的建议）。正如上文提到的，在妊娠的该阶段，一些妊娠妇女可能需要 1U 才能降低 1mmol/L 血糖。因此，建议使用更大的校正大剂量。

· 如果在给予第 1 次校正大剂量后 1h 后血糖控制仍然不满意，那么给予第 2 次校正大剂量。

· 如果在半小时后复查血糖在 7～10mmol/L，可予第 3 次校正大剂量；如果大于 10mmol/L 改为静脉注射胰岛素治疗。

· 如果在给予第 3 次大剂量后 1h 复查血糖仍＞7mmol/L，则改为静脉注射胰岛素治疗。

· 血糖在控制不佳的情况下都可以改为静脉注射胰岛素治疗。

· 发生低血糖事件时（血糖＜4mmol/L），按照医院的诊疗常规进行处置。

· 如果患者出现反复低血糖，建议将基础率降低 50% 直到胎儿娩出。

胎儿娩出后，患者和医疗人员需要尽快将基础率调低，以便和迅速降低的胰岛素需要量相匹配。理想状态下，患者应事先设置好分娩后的基础率。有许多设定分娩后基础率的方法，最简单的方法是在分娩后直接使用刚受孕时的基础率。如果患者准备母乳喂养，那么基础率要减少1/3。另一种方法是按照 0.3U/kg 体重计算每日基础胰岛素总量，如果母乳喂养则按照 0.2U/kg 体重计算[9]。

分娩后阶段和哺乳期

分娩后胰岛素的需要量立即变得很低，所以如果患者血糖持续下降时应该使用降低的临时基础率。如果患者基础率出现大幅降低，也需要注意餐前大剂量的剂量，可以考虑少量多次的大剂量注射方法。

母乳喂养时经过一夜血糖经常会有下降，因为产生乳汁时利用了葡萄糖，基础率可能需要做出相应调整。在产后阶段血糖控制情况常会恶化，但使用胰岛素泵的患者在这一阶段维持血糖稳定更容易些[10]，因为胰岛素泵在血糖升高需要补充大剂量时有更好的灵活性，这在一定程度弥补了患者产后将更多的注意力集中在新生儿身上而忽略了自身糖尿病管理的缺憾。

未来的方向

胰岛素泵治疗可以和连续动态血糖监测结合在一起，被称为传感器增强的胰岛素泵治疗（参见第十六章）。这项技术可以帮助妊娠期妇女优化血糖控制。最近的技术提供了低血糖暂停功能，在低血糖可能会出现时自动停止胰岛素输注，在血糖水平开始上升后重新开始工作。在不远的将来，治疗目标范围系统有可能做到在血糖超出目标范围时输注小剂量的胰岛素来纠正血糖。在不久的将来，闭环胰岛素输注系统可以自动调整基础和餐时胰岛素的输注来维持正常的血糖。

选择题

1. 下列陈述正确的是（　　）
   A. 随着孕程进展，胰岛素泵中基础胰岛素所占每日总剂量的比例逐渐增加
   B. 随着孕程进展，餐前大剂量的给药时间与就餐的间隔时间逐渐增加
   C. 在妊娠晚期解决早餐时需要胰岛素量增加的方法是大剂量向基础剂量转换
   D. 母乳喂养时基础率的计算方法是每天0.3U/kg体重
   E. 在围产期不能够使用胰岛素泵治疗

正确答案是B。在非妊娠期餐前大剂量一般在餐前15～20min注射，但在妊娠晚期，大剂量在饭前60min注射。A是错误的，餐时胰岛素占每日总胰岛素的比例在妊娠前为50%，到妊娠晚期升至65%。C是错误的，基础剂量向大剂量的转换增加了餐前的胰岛素剂量，同时不增加上

午的低血糖风险。D 是错误的，由于分泌乳汁需要消耗糖类，当母乳喂养时所需的基础率更低。最后 E 也是错误的，胰岛素泵治疗可以在围产期安全有效地使用，但是必须具体问题具体分析，并在使用时确保方案和操作过程正确。

2. 胰岛素泵治疗优于每日多次胰岛素注射治疗的优点是（　　）
A. 基础率可以每 15min 调节一次
B. 控制血糖达标同时降低低血糖风险
C. 当血糖水平大于 10mmol/L，自动给予校正大剂量
D. 大剂量胰岛素可以方波注射
E. 大剂量向导计算时会考虑上次大剂量注射剩余的活性胰岛素

正确答案是 B、D 和 E。B 选项：有许多随机对照实验和荟萃分析都证实胰岛素泵治疗在控制血糖达标同时可以降低低血糖风险。D 选项：目前市售的胰岛素泵可以在数小时内方波注射胰岛素（一般 1~6h），还可以同常规大剂量注射相结合，即双波注射。E 选项：大剂量向导通过使用者估计的活性胰岛素时间或者真实指尖血糖与期待血糖的差值得出算法计算出上次注射剩余的活性胰岛素。A 是错误的：因为目前市售的胰岛素泵基础率时间间隔在 30min 或 60min。C 是错误的：因为目前唯一有自动调节功能的 Medtronic Veo 和 640G systems 只能被用来暂停输注胰岛素以防止低血糖，将来的治疗目标范围系统有可能做到自动输注校正剂量的胰岛素来纠正高血糖。

（朱海清　译，王　冰　校）

参 考 文 献

1　Pickup JC & Sutton AJ. Severe hypoglycaemia and glycaemic control in type 1 diabetes: meta analysis of multiple daily injections compared with continuous subcutaneous insulin infusion. Diabet Med 2008;25:765–774.
2　NICE NG3. Diabetes in pregnancy: management of diabetes and its complications from preconception to postnatal period. February 2015. www.nice.org/guidance/ng3
3　Simmons D, Thompson CF, Conroy C, & Scott DJ. Use of insulin pumps in pregnancies complicated by type 2 diabetes and gestational diabetes. Diabetes Care 2001;24:2078–2082.
4　Castorino K, Paband R, Zisser H, & Jovanovic L. Insulin pumps in pregnancy: using technology to achieve normoglycemia in women with diabetes. Curr Diab Rep 2012;12:53–59.
5　Bernasko J. Insulin pump therapy for

pregnancy: a primer. J Maternal-Fetal & Neonat Med 2012;25:552–557.
6 Mathiesen JM, Secher AL, & Ringholm L. Changes in basal rates and bolus calculator settings in insulin pumps during pregnancy in women with type 1 diabetes. J Maternal-Fetal & Neonat Med 2014;27:724–728.
7 Murphy HR, Elleri D, Allen JM, et al. Closed-loop insulin delivery during pregnancy complicated by type 1 diabetes. Diabetes Care 2011;34:406–411.
8 Murphy HR, Elleri D, Allen JM, et al. Pathophysiology of postprandial hyperglycaemia in women with type 1 diabetes during pregnancy. Diabetologia 2012;55:282–293.
9 Riviello C, Mello G, & Jovanovic L. Breastfeeding and the basal insulin requirement in type 1 diabetic women. Endocrine Pract 2009;15:187–193.
10 Gabbe SG, Holing E, Temple P, et al. Benefits, risks, costs, and patient satisfaction associated with insulin pump therapy for the pregnancy complicated by type 1 diabetes mellitus. Am J Obstet Gynecol 2000;182(6):1283–1291.

第十八章 减肥手术后的妊娠、围产期和生育结局

Aubrey R. Raimondi[1] and Eyal Sheiner[2]

1 Ben-Gurion University of the Negev, Beer-Sheva, Israel
2 Department of Obstetrics and Gynecology, Faculty of Health Sciences, Soroka University Medical Center, Ben-Gurion; and University of the Negev, Beer-Sheva, Israel

实践要点
- 减肥手术史不是剖官产的独立指征。
- 全面的微量营养素缺乏筛查,包括铁、维生素 B_{12}、维生素 A、维生素 D、维生素 E、维生素 K、叶酸、钙和蛋白质,应作为产前常规检查。
- 减肥后妇女所生的孩子患 LGA 的风险降低,而患 SGA 和其他生长异常疾病的风险增加。
- 减肥后的状态与降低妊娠高血压疾病的风险有关。
- 在减肥以后,不孕可能会改善,但还需更多的研究。

需要避免的问题
- 减肥手术史从来不是剖官产的独立适应证。

病 例

一名25岁的女性,孕2产1,有长期肥胖史及3年糖尿病和高血压病史,第二次妊娠6周。一年前曾做过减肥手术,术后BMI从 $44kg/m^2$ 降至目前的 $36kg/m^2$。经检查,血压(125/85mmHg)和糖化血红蛋白(6.3%)较减肥前(156/92mmHg和7.6%)有所改善。她说,自从手术以来,已经停止服用降压药,只服用二甲双胍降糖。第一次妊娠,由于胎儿窘迫,在 35^{+4} 周时进行了剖官产。新生儿体重3500g(高于第90百分位),分娩时 Apgar 评分在 1min 和 5min 时分别为7分和9分。目前的妊娠状态还是理想的,但患者对减肥手术后的效果仍然存在担忧。
- 患者的减肥手术后的状态是否为剖官产的指征。
- 女性减肥后的状态是否会增加早产的风险。
- 患者是否因其减肥后的状态而降低妊娠高血压的风险。
- 患者的孩子是否会因为减肥后的状态而增加胎儿畸形或体重相关异常的风险。

这些是许多医师在治疗产后患者时可能遇到的一些问题。本章对这些问题进行了探讨,为临床医师提供了指导和参考。

引言

在美国的人口中，肥胖人群所占的比例高达30%，尤其是育龄妇女肥胖更为普遍[1-3]。BMI超过30kg/m²即被定义为肥胖，其与许多生殖健康问题相关，如不孕、流产、妊娠高血压、妊娠糖尿病（GDM）、子痫前期和剖宫产[4-11]。

肥胖的分级（以BMI为依据）

肥胖：BMI＞30kg/m²

Ⅰ级肥胖：BMI 30～34.9kg/m²

Ⅱ级肥胖：BMI 35～39.9kg/m²

Ⅲ级类肥胖：BMI＞40kg/m²

依据：世界卫生组织（WHO）[3]，美国国立卫生研究院（NIH）[4]

此外，肥胖患者的检查也很困难，这可能会使本已高危妊娠的管理更加困难。例如，肥胖妇女中少排卵/不排卵发生率的增加可能会干扰建立准确的末次月经时间（LMP）以确定妊娠年龄。此外，在超声诊断过程中对肥胖母亲胎儿的可视化降低，阻碍了对子宫内环境的准确评估[12]，突出了早期经阴道超声（TVUS）在肥胖患者中的重要性[13]。减肥手术是实现显著减肥的一种手段，因此可以减少妊娠期间与肥胖相关的共病风险[14-16]。本章查询和总结了记录在案的减肥手术后妊娠的结果，并为参与这些妇女术后生殖健康护理的临床医师提供指导。

减肥手术的分类

减肥手术使体重减轻的机制包括限制、吸收不良和（或）神经内分泌改变。这些机制根据生理反应的类型在不同的层面上起作用。目前最常用的手术是腹腔镜下支架行Roux-en-Y胃旁路术（RYGB）、袖状胃切除术（SG）、腹腔镜下可调胃束带术（LAGB）、胆胰分流/十二指肠转换术（BPD/DS）（图18.1）[17]。在过去的10年里，减肥手术方式的趋势发生了变化，RYGB在2013年仍然是一个非常流行的手术，从2008年的49%下降到45%。SG是第二常见的手术，比例从2008年的5.3%大幅上升至 2013 年的 37%[17-19]。然而，可调节胃束带术（AGB）和 BPD/DS 等手术的比例显著下降。AGB 手术率从 2008 年的 42.3%下降到 2013 年的 10%，BPD/DS 手术率从 2008 年的 4.9%下降到 2013 年的 1.5%。本章将回顾总结上述手术类型。

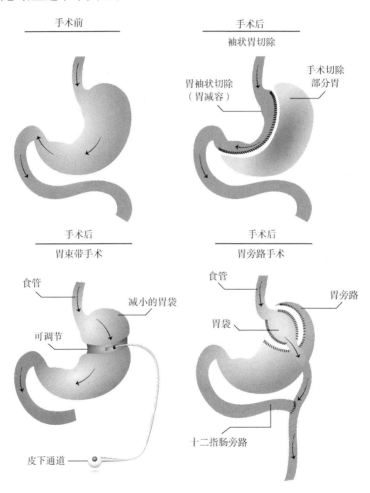

图 18.1 减肥手术常用的手术方式

资料来源：Adobe.com，经过允许使用

Roux-en-Y 胃旁路术和胆胰分流/十二指肠转换术

RYGB 手术包括通过缝合创建胃囊，这样胃囊的外侧边界就分别构成了胃的小曲率和切面。空肠从幽门切下 50~100cm 长，远端绕过十二指肠直接连接到胃囊。胃的大部分，包括胃大弯、幽门、十二指肠和空肠近端都在远端吻合，长 100~150cm[20]。体重减轻的比例从多余 BMI 的（56.2%±29.3%）（长期结果）到多余 BMI 的（88.0%±29.6%）（术后 2 年）[21]。RYGB 与微量营养素缺乏的风险增加有关，最常见的是铁、钙、维生素 B_{12} 和维生素 D，其他还有包括脂溶性维生素（维生素 A、维生素 E 和维生素 K）、叶酸和硫胺素的缺乏[22]。

BPD/DS 手术从幽门远端切口开始。在切口中插入一个法式弯刀，放置在胃小弯处，并结合线性吻合器的多种应用创造了套管式胃切除术。这个新的胃囊与回肠远端相连，形成消化道肢体。十二指肠、空肠和回肠近端保持完整，构成胆胰肢体，胆胰肢体与消化道肢体远端 100cm 部分相连，形成共同通道[23]。与 RYGB[24] 相比，BPD/DS 术后出现类似的微量营养素缺乏，以及其他与 BPD/DS 相关的术后问题，包括蛋白吸收不良和营养不良继发的低蛋白血症发生率增加，可能需要短期的肠外营养支持[25]。

研究表明，较长的肢体长度可以增加蛋白质吸收不良的发生率，但能提高减肥效果[26, 27]。一项研究报道称，BPD/DS 术后妊娠期间需要肠外营养的比例高达 20%，文献报道的比例是可变的[14, 28, 29]，因此建议 RYGB 和 BPD/DS 手术的患者补充钙、叶酸、铁、维生素 B_{12} 和维生素 D[21, 30, 31]。重要的是，RYGB 被发现可以降低 2 型糖尿病的发病率[32]。这个改善似乎在减肥成功之前就已经发生了，主要是由两大机制引起的：一是受热量限制的影响，肝胰岛素敏感性得到改善；二是与绕过十二指肠的营养转运改变有关的——细胞功能的改善，导致 GLP-1 的分泌增加[33]。

在妊娠并发症方面，BPD/DS 和 RYGB 很少导致宫内生长受限（IUGR）、小于胎龄儿（SGA）和胎儿畸形[34-36]。然而，在有文件记载的文献中还没有就这个问题达成共识。术后队列研究中 IUGR、SGA 和胎儿畸形的发生率已被证明与普通人群中的发生率相似[29]。事实上，研究表明,RYGB 和 BPD/DS 手术后妊娠的风险相当低。在一项对 RYGB 后妊娠的回顾性研究中,Wittgrove 等[37]发现,LGA、糖尿病、高血压疾病的发生率与患者自身术前比较有所增加。Wax 等[38]的另一项研究发现,RYGB 治疗后的患者与普通人群在新生儿出生体重或 IUGR 比率方面没有显著差异。在瑞典最近的一项研究中,近 98%的减肥手术是胃旁路手术,在减肥手术后妊娠(与未进行减肥手术的妊娠女性相比),SGA 婴儿的发生率更高(15.6% vs 7.6%;OR:2.20;95%CI:1.64~295;$P<0.001$)和死产或新生儿死亡风险的增加(1.7% vs 0.7%;OR:2.39;95%CI:0.98~5.85;$P=0.06$)[39]。同样的研究发现,胎儿畸形率没有增加,而 LGA 和 GDM 的发病率也有所下降。在 Sheiner 等[40]进行的一项回顾性研究中,作者比较了不同类型减肥手术的结果,发现低出生体重率或 LGA 率在不同类型的减肥术式中没有明显差异。总体而言,有证据表明,RYGB 和 BPD/DS 术后患者的结局比肥胖患者好,但比其他人群差。

可调节胃束带术

AGB 是一种限制性手术,其减肥效果不如 RYGB 和 BD,通常与营养缺乏或低蛋白血症无关[41, 42]。一项研究发现,AGB 在 72 个月时出现过度减肥的比率是 57%±15%[43]。妊娠期 AGB 合并的并发症包括与束带紧密相关的不适感,束带滑脱引起的常见但可能致命的并发症,以及罕见的维生素 K 缺乏导致的脑出血[44, 45]。LAGB 术后妇女所生婴儿的出生体重与非肥胖人群相似,低于严重或病态肥胖对照组[46, 47]。与肥胖对照组相比,LAGB 患者 GDM、低出生体重、子痫前期和 LGA 的发病率更低[48-50]。妊娠期间,如果出现严重恶心或呕吐,或体重有不适当的减轻或增加[51-53],则需进行束带的调节。关于是否应该常规考虑束带调整,目前还没有明确的指导方针,特别是考虑到妊娠期间过早的束带紧缩导致体重增加的风险可能超过根据需要进行束带调整所带来的风险。此外,还没有确定的是,母亲定期调整束带所生的孩子是否能够得到更好的结果。因此,必须仔细监测这些患者是否有过度恶心、呕吐和腹部不适的症状。如果出现这些症状,建议与专门治疗 LAGB 的合格的减肥外科医师进行适当的会诊以控制妊娠。医疗服务提供者应该认识到，AGB 术后妊娠妇女可能需要对过度恶心和呕吐、体重波动进行束带调整。

袖状胃切除术

SG 最初是在 1990 年作为 BPD/DS 的一种改进术式。当意识到患者在接受 SG 治疗体重减轻后，它作为一种单独的治疗方法受到了广泛的欢迎。这一手术是通过在 38 个 French bougie 上使用多个线性订书机垂直横切胃来完成的[54]。SG 的主要优点是手术技术简单，减肥效果显著，吸收不良的风险较低，避免了肠道手术及相关并发症的发生。一项对 SG 患者进行了 5 年跟踪调查的研究发现，患者的体重减轻了 $55\%\pm6.8\%$[55]。研究显示，减肥的主要机制与神经内分泌的变化有关，切除了产生胃饥饿素的胃部分。胃饥饿素是一种神经内分泌肽激素，主要作用是增加饥饿感信号、胃肠运动和胃酸分泌，所有这些都会增强食欲[56-58]。Ghrelin 与瘦素（一种在饱腹信号中起重要作用的肽）共享相同的中心受体，并且 Ghrelin 被认为在与该受体结合时阻碍了身体感到饱腹的能力[59]。在 SG 期间，切除胃中产生 Ghrelin 的部分可能会产生显著的减肥效果和长期的保持[60]。最近的研究表明 SG 的结果是值得期待的。目前已经进行了几项研究，检查 SG 术后的孕产妇和胎儿结局；然而，目前的数据还不足以得出明确的结论[61, 62]。尚需进一步研究以确定 SG[63]之后的生殖健康结果。

生育能力

肥胖与少食/闭经和不孕症的发病率增高有关，这一点已得到充分证实[64, 65]。此外，众所周知，减肥有助于恢复生育能力[66]。各种研究都试图确定减肥手术是否也有助于恢复生育能力[66-69]。然而，这一问题受到多种因素的干扰，如接受减肥手术的妇女不孕率增加（已发现术前高达 41.9%[69]），并且减肥术后患者的体重也有所增加。显然，在确定减肥手术是否会加重或改善不孕症之前，必须进行更广泛的前瞻性研究，特别是与肥胖人群和社区发病率相比较。

避孕

有证据表明，口服避孕药的有效性可能受减肥后状态的影响，因为口服避孕药的有效性依赖于充分的吸收[70,71]。在一项关于减肥手术后药物吸收的系统回顾中，发现关于减肥手术后状态对口服避孕药吸收影响的相互矛盾的证据。减少吸收的理论机制与口服避孕药的代谢有关，包括减少药物的崩解和溶解、延迟胃排空、大部分小肠的旁路形成，这可能对药物吸收很重要，并且口服避孕药对首过代谢和肠肝再循环有一定的依赖[72]。如果患者希望推迟或避免妊娠，ACOG 通常建议医疗服务提供者应该鼓励患者使用合适的非口服避孕药[73,74]。

手术-妊娠间隔

考虑到减肥后患者生育状况的良好改善，确定手术后的理想受孕时间具有重大意义。目前，ACOG 建议患者在减肥手术后等待 12~24 个月再尝试妊娠[75]。这一建议对快速减肥相关的潜在微量营养素缺乏和不良围产期结局有所关注。然而，一些研究表明，这些观点可能缺少依据。在一项大型研究中，并没有发现从手术到分娩的间隔时间的不同导致 SGA 或早产率的差异[76]。

在另一项研究中，104 名女性在手术后 1 年内妊娠，385 名女性在手术 1 年后妊娠，研究还显示手术间隔缩短与妊娠不良事件无关[77]。此外，在一项研究中，对 158 例 RYGB 术后 1 年内妊娠的妇女和 128 例在第 1 年之后的某个时候妊娠的妇女进行比较，没有发现在子痫前期、GDM、早产（37 周前）、引产、剖宫产、产后出血（>500ml）、出生体重、SGA、LGA、Apgar 评分（5min）低于 7 分或新生儿需要重症监护[78]方面存在显著差异。这些研究及越来越多的证据表明，理想的手术-受孕间隔可能不像以前认为的那么关键[79]。尽管如此，即使在术后第 1 年内妊娠的患者与在术后第 1 年后妊娠的患者的短期围产期结局相当，但似乎有理由建议妇女推迟一年妊娠，直到产科社区达成共识。然而，如果妊娠的间隔时间较短，现有的数据可能会有助于护理人员为这些患者提供建议。

在进行减肥手术后，医师应该为患者提供有关资料，并订定适合他们的生殖时间表。

流产

目前尚未有研究全面评估减肥手术和流产之间的关系。在一项大型回顾性调查研究中，流产率未受 BD 前后状态的影响，表明 BD 可能不会影响流产的发生率[29]。另一项研究发现，减肥后患者流产率降低；然而，这项研究被低估了[80]。总的来说，这些研究表明流产的发生率可能更多地与患者的术前状况有关，而不是术后状态。此外，重要的是要认识到，进行减肥手术的患者可能是为了恢复多次流产后的生殖能力。然而，由于研究数量不足，样本量较小，可能无法得出明确的结论。

早产

肥胖与早产风险增加有关。这是降低孕产妇/胎儿风险的关键组成部分，因此研究减肥手术对这一结果的影响是有意义的。在瑞典的一个大型队列研究中，减肥术后的女性与未接受过减肥手术的普通女性相比妊娠期更短（273.0d vs 277.5d；平均差：-4.5d；95% CI：-2.9～6.0；$P<0.001$），并且两组间有很多影响因素都是匹配的，如 BMI；值得注意的是，早产率没有显著差异（10.0% vs 7.5%；OR：1.28；95%CI：0.92～1.78；$P=0.15$）[39]。总的来说，目前的证据还不能确定在进行减肥手术后早产的发生率是否有明显的不同[39, 81-83]。

妊娠高血压

长期以来，肥胖与妊娠高血压和超高血压疾病的发病率增加有关[5]，这对胎儿和孕妇构成风险[65, 84]。因此，确定与减肥相关的减肥手术是否能降低妊娠高血压疾病是至关重要的。总的来说，减肥后的状态似乎与妊娠期间患高血压疾病的风险较低有关；与患者的术前状态和肥胖人群相比[15, 50, 52, 84]，这种风险均有所降低。Bennett 等[85]进行了一项回顾性队列研究，比较了减肥手术前后女性慢性高血压影响妊娠和妊娠高血压的发生率，发现术后这些疾病的发生率较低。一些研究没有发现在减肥手术后患者和肥胖人群中高血压发病率有任何显著差异[86, 87]。其他研究发现，与正常体重指数组相比，减肥手术后患者高血压发病率增加，但低于肥胖组[88]。现在许多研究致力于确定减肥手术后子痫前期的风险。一项研究发现，RYGB 手术后，子痫前期的发病率与正常的 BMI 队列[87]相比并无相关增加，但肥胖对照组子痫前期的风险增加，这表明子痫前期的减肥后状态可能有一定的益处。其他研究发现，与未做手术的肥胖女性相比，RYGB 和 AGB 手术后子痫前期风险也有类似的降低[10, 84, 89]。

妊娠糖尿病

GDM 与母亲肥胖密切相关，可导致多种不良妊娠结局，包括 LGA、肩难产和婴儿低血糖[90-92]。即使肥胖患者能够获得足够的血糖控制，与非肥胖人群相比，妊娠并发症的风险仍会增加 2~3 倍[93]。现有证据表明，体重减轻可能对 GDM 产生积极影响[93]。最初的研究表明，减肥手术可能会带来潜在的好处，这不仅是因为减肥带来的体重减轻，还因为潜在的相关神经内分泌变化[94]。在 Sheiner 等[67]进行的一项基于大人群的研究中，与普通人群相比，接受过减肥手术的女性 GDM 的发病率更高。然而，在考虑 BMI 等混杂因素后，术后母亲患 GDM 的风险没有明显增加[67]。事实上，GDM 患病率（17.3% vs 11.0；P=0.009）与肥胖患者相比有所下降[15, 50]；然而，如果将 GDM 的术后发生率与患者自身的术前 GDM 发生率或一般人群进行比较，证据就不那么直接了[52, 68, 95]。在最近的另一项研究中，包括瑞典医学出生登记处的产妇在内，670 例单胎妊娠发生在曾接受过减肥手术并记录了术前体重的妇女。与一般人群的对照组比较，减肥手术后患者 GDM（1.9% vs 6.8%；OR：0.25；95% CI：0.13~0.47；$P<0.001$）和 LGA 的风险降低（8.6% vs 22.4%；OR：0.33；95%CI：0.24~0.44；$P<0.001$）（BMI 等变量比较）[39]。因此，似乎减肥手术后患者的 GDM 率低于肥胖人群，尽管他们可能永远无法达到普通人群的正常水平。

剖宫产术

一些研究发现，减肥手术后剖宫产率并不高于社区剖宫产率[37]，而另一些研究表明，减肥手术后剖宫产率更高[15, 67]。尽管在减肥后的患者中，剖宫产率较高，但有几个因素可能混淆这一比例，包括研究者偏倚、既往剖宫产史和术后 BMI。例如，最近的一项大型前瞻性研究发现，选择减肥手术的患者中，既往剖宫产的比例很高，这突出了既往剖宫产史在混淆术后发生率方面的影响[88]。这项研究还发现，与对照组相比，术后患者的紧急剖宫产率更低[88]。并且研究主要比较了减肥后患者的剖宫产率和社区的剖宫产率，这使得在分析数据时很难考虑 BMI。此外，很难知道剖宫产的粗率是否受到提供者对患者术后肥胖状况的偏见的影响。根据 ACOG 关于减肥手术后妊娠的指南，减肥后的状态并不意味着剖宫产。在考虑改行剖宫产时，医疗服务提供者应仔细核对手术适应证，而不应受患者减肥后状态的影响[74]。

胎儿预后

考虑到与肥胖患者相比，减肥后患者的产科风险状况较好，因此推测减肥后患者是否也能改善围产期和胎儿预后是合乎逻辑的。Sheiner 等[67]在一份关于 159 210 例妊娠的报道中指出，298 例减肥后分娩患者与普通人群分娩的围产期结局没有显著差异。具体来说，围产儿并发症的发生率，如围产儿死亡率、胎粪染色的羊水，均没有显著变化。两组的 Apgar 评分在 1min 和 5min 时较低。另一项研究比较了减肥手术后妊娠患者和未行减肥手术肥胖患者的围产儿并发症发生率，没有显著差异，尽管与非肥胖者相比，两者的并发症发生率更高[79]。因此，在考虑 BMI 后，围手术期的风险率似乎不受减肥后状态的影响。

出生体重

母亲肥胖增加 LGA 的风险[96, 97]。减肥手术后，LGA 的风险降低，这一结果最有可能与母亲 BMI 的变化有关[15, 50, 52, 82]。然而，值得注意的是，在进行减肥手术后，与普通人群[39, 67]相比，肥胖女性发生 LGA 的风险仍然增加。尽管减肥后患者 LGA 出生的风险降低（与肥胖对照组相比），但胎儿体重相关异常的粗率仍在增加，尤其是 SGA 和 IUGR[98]。然而，这些关联往往不存在于多变量分析中，与一般群体相比，SGA 的发生率没有显著差异。一项大型回顾性研究表明，与正常 BMI 和肥胖对照组相比，减肥手术后患者 LGA 发病率降低，SGA 发病率升高[88]。与 SGA 相关的主要长期风险是认知和教育程度的降低。然而，几项研究发现，这些儿童的就业率、婚姻状况和生活满意度相当[99]，其中一项研究对患者进行了长达 26 年的跟踪调查。

胎儿畸形

医学界的另一个重要事项是确定减肥手术是否与胎儿畸形或其他先天性缺陷的增加有关。引起关注的理论机制可能与母体微量营养素缺乏及其对宫内环境的影响有关[100]。Josefsson 等[101]最近进行了一项基于人群的前瞻性研究，研究了 270 805 名初生婴儿，其中 341 名为减肥术后母亲分娩的，与普通产妇相比，减肥术后的状态并未改变先天畸形的风险。在 Weintraub 等[15]的另一项大型研究中，507 例减肥手术后母亲分娩的胎儿畸形粗率高于 301 例减肥手术前分娩的胎儿畸形粗率，然而，在控制早产和产妇年龄后，这种关系并没有持续。重要的是，在上述研究中进行的多变量分析中没有控制母亲的 BMI，这是已知的增加先天畸形的危险因素。Sheiner 等[67]对 159 210 例妊娠妇女的研究表明，胎儿畸形与减肥手术之间没有关联，这一结论得到了其他研究[39, 102]的支持。即使有强有力的证据，卫生保健提供者也应该继续检查母亲的微量营养素缺乏和胎儿畸形，并提供适当的医学治疗。这对于术后持续肥胖的患者尤为重要，因为肥胖是神经管缺陷的独立危险因素[100]。ACOG 指南目前建议对微量营养素缺乏进行全面筛查，包括铁、维生素 B_{12}、维生素 D、叶酸、钙和蛋白质，并每 3 个月进行一次随访筛查[74]。

总结

鉴于到目前为止文献记载的大量证据，我们可以就减肥手术对生殖健康结果的影响得出几个一般性结论。首先，减肥手术可能会提高生育能力，但还需要进一步的研究。在进行减肥手术后，建议患者在妊娠前等待一年，尽管以大量人群为基础的研究没有发现术后一年内或一年后妊娠的显著差异。因此，如果患者希望推迟或预防妊娠，临床医师应该推荐一种非口服避孕药，因为理论上口服避孕药存在吸收和有效性降低的风险，而且目前还没有进行结论性研究。有证据表明，减肥手术后患者妊娠高血压疾病和 GDM 的风险降低。此外，减肥手术后母亲所生的儿童患 LGA 的风险较低，但患 SGA 的风险较高。妇女在妊娠期间应监测微量营养素缺乏情况。最后，在妊娠期间，减肥后患者可能会出现手术并发症，如果出现并发症，除妇女保健者外，还应有减肥外科医师对其进行监测。

未来的方向

还需要进一步的研究来确定减肥手术对早产和流产率的影响。此外，研究肥胖手术后口服避孕药的疗效对于建立适当的避孕指南是必要的。由于 SG 在减肥外科医师中越来越受欢迎，因此有必要进行更多的研究以明确 SG 后的患者是否能像接受其他减重手术的患者一样，期望获得类似的母婴结局。最后，额外的以人群为基础的大型试验和随机对照试验应该解决微量营养素缺乏对发育中的胎儿可能造成的后果。

选择题

1. 一名孕 3 产 2 的女性在妊娠的前 3 个月来到你的办公室，她在 3 年前接受了减肥手术，她对自己在妊娠期间可能会因为减肥手术而出现的问题很清楚。她的前两个孩子是剖宫产的。除了之前的剖宫产手术，她的产科病史并不突出。下列陈述正确的是（　　）

A. 由于她的减肥手术后状态，这名妇女有极高的早产风险。她本应该推迟她的减肥手术，直到她确定自己不想再要孩子
B. 这名妇女有很高的流产风险，因为她有减肥手术史
C. 医疗服务者应该考虑剖宫产的必要性，因为她的减肥手术后状态，而不考虑患者以前剖宫产史
D. 以上都不是

正确答案是 D。

2. 一名 20 多岁的女士来到你的办公室，告诉你她正在考虑减肥手术。她对生殖健康有几个问题。下列陈述正确的是（   ）
A. 为了保证最好的母婴结局，该女士最好的妊娠时间是在术后的第 1 年
B. 减肥手术后，口服避孕药是最有效的避孕方式，比其他避孕方法更受欢迎
C. 减肥手术是不孕不育的主要原因
D. 口服避孕药在减肥手术后的有效性值得怀疑，尤其是在快速减肥的情况下，应该选择另一种避孕方法

正确答案是 D。

3. 一名妇女 3 周前错过了月经期，家庭妊娠测试呈阳性。她来你的办公室是为了确认测试结果，她对这个梦寐以求的妊娠感到非常兴奋。为了恢复生育能力，她在 9 个月前进行了减肥手术，期间她的体重指数从 $39kg/m^2$ 降到了 $28.5kg/m^2$。下列陈述正确的是（   ）
A. 这名妇女的孩子有更高的风险成为 LGA，尽管患者的体重在减肥手术后大幅下降
B. 由于患者在减肥手术后体重显著下降，胎儿宫内生长受限的风险降低
C. 由于减肥手术时间较近，该患者妊娠糖尿病和妊娠高血压的风险升高
D. 根据最近的 ACOG 公告，建议妊娠期追踪铁、维生素 B_{12}、维生素 D、钙、叶酸和蛋白质的水平在妊娠早期是否有不足

正确答案是 D。

（李晶晶　译，朱海清　校）

参 考 文 献

1. Ogden C, Carroll M, Kit B, Flegal K. Prevalence of childhood and adult obesity in the United States, 2011–2012. JAMA 2014;311:806–814.
2. Ogden C, Carroll M, Kit B, Flegal K. Prevalence of obesity among adults: United States, 2001–2012. NCHS Data Brief 2013;131(131):1–8.
3. Catalano P, Ehrenberg H. The short- and long-term implications or maternal obesity on the mother and her offspring. BJOG 2006;113:1126–1133.
4. CDC National Center for Health Statistics. Prevalence of overweight, obesity, and extreme obesity among adults: United States, 1960–1962 through 2011–20. NHANES data report. http://www.cdc.gov/nchs/data/hestat/obesity_adult_11_12/obesity_adult_11_12.pdf
5. Weiss JL, Malone FD, Emig D, Ball RH, Nyberg DA, Comstock CH, Saade G, Eddleman K, Carter SM, Craigo SD, Carr SR, D'Alton ME, FASTER Research Consortium. Obesity, obstetric complications and cesarean delivery rate – a population-based screening study. Amer J Obstetr Gynecol 2004;190(4):1091–1097.
6. Cnattingius S, Bergström R, Lipworth L, Kramer MS. Prepregnancy weight and the risk of adverse pregnancy outcomes. New Engl J Med 1998;338:147–152.
7. Liu Y, Dai W, Dai X, Li Z. Prepregnancy body mass index and gestational weight gain with the outcome of pregnancy: a 13-year study of 292,568 cases in China. Gynecol Obstetr 2012;286(4):905–911.
8. Sebire NJ, Jolly M, Harris JP, Wadsworth J, Joffe M, Beard RW, Regan L, Robinson S. Maternal obesity and pregnancy outcome: a study of 287,213 pregnancies in London. Intl J Obes Rel Metab Disord 2001;25(8):1175–1182.
9. Burstein E, Levy A, Mazor M, Wiznitzer A, Sheiner E. Pregnancy outcome among obese women: a prospective study. Am J Perinatol 2008;25(9):561–566.
10. Vrebosch L, Bel S, Vansant G, Guelinckx I, Devlieger R. Maternal and neonatal outcome after laparoscopic adjustable gastric banding: a systematic review. Obes Surg 2012;22(10):1568–1579.
11. Isaacs JD, Magann EF, Martin RW, Chauhan SP, Morrison JC. Obstetric challenges of massive obesity complicating pregnancy. J Perinatol 1994;14(1):10–14.
12. Hendler I, Blackwell SC, Bujold E, Treadwell MC, Wolfe HM, Sokol RJ, Sorokin Y. The impact of maternal obesity on midtrimester sonographic visualization of fetal cardiac and craniospinal structures. Intl J Obes 2004;28:1607–1611.
13. Paladini D. (2009). Sonography in obese and overweight pregnant women: clinical, medicolegal and technical issues. Ultrasound Obstetr Gynecol 2009;33(6):720–729.
14. Maggard MA, Yermilov I, Li Z, Maglione M, Newberry S, Suttorp M, et al. Pregnancy and fertility following bariatric surgery: a systematic review. JAMA 2008;300(19):2286–2296.
15. Weintraub AY, Levy A, Levi I, Mazor M, Wiznitzer A, Sheiner E. Effect of bariatric surgery on pregnancy outcome. Int J Gynaecol Obstet 2008;103(3):246–251.
16. Buchwald H, Estok R, Fahrbach K, Banel D, Sledge I. Trends in mortality in bariatric surgery: a systematic review and meta-analysis. Surgery 2007;142(4):621–635.
17. Buchwald H, Oien D. Metabolic/bariatric surgery worldwide 2011. Obes Surg 2013;23(4):427–436.
18. Santry HP, Gillen DL, Lauderdale DS. Trends in bariatric surgical procedures. JAMA 2005;294(15):1909–1917.
19. Angrisani L, Santonicola A, Iovino P, Formisano G, Buchwald H, & Scopinaro N. Bariatric surgery worldwide 2013. Obes Surg 2015;1–11.
20. Nguyen NT. The ASMBS Textbook of Bariatric Surgery, vol. 2. Springer: New York, 2014.

21. Himpens J, Verbrugghe A, Cadière GB, Everaerts W, & Greve JW. Long-term results of laparoscopic Roux-en-Y gastric bypass: evaluation after 9 years. Obes Surg 2012;22(10):1586–1593.
22. Bloomberg R, Fleishman A, Nalle J, Herron D, Kini S. Nutritional deficiencies following bariatric surgery: what have we learned? Obes Surg 2005;15(2):145–154.
23. Ren CJ, Patterson E, & Gagner M. Early results of laparoscopic biliopancreatic diversion with duodenal switch: a case series of 40 consecutive patients. Obes Surg 2000;10(6);514–523.
24. Skroubis G, Sakellaropoulos G, Pouggouras K, Mead N, Nikiforidis G, Kalfarentzos F. Comparison of nutritional deficiencies after Roux-en-Y gastric bypass and after biliopancreatic diversion with Roux-en-Y gastric bypass. Obes Surg 2002;12(4):551–558.
25. Skroubis, G., Sakellaropoulos, G., Pouggouras, K., Mead, N., Nikiforidis, G., & Kalfarentzos, F. Comparison of nutritional deficiencies after Roux-en-Y gastric bypass and after biliopancreatic diversion with Roux-en-Y gastric bypass. Obes Surg 2002;12(4):551–558.
26. Kalfarentzos F, Dimakopoulos A, Kehagias I, et al. Vertical banded gastroplasty versus standard or distal Roux-en-Y gastric bypass based on specific selection criteria in the morbidly obese: preliminary results. Obes Surg 1999;9:433–442.
27. Brolin RE, LaMarca LB, Kenler HA, et al. Malabsorptive gastric bypass in patients with superobesity. J Gastrointest Surg 2002;6:195–203, discussion 4–5.
28. Friedman D, Cuneo S, Valenzano M, Marinari GM, Adami GF, Gianetta E, et al. Pregnancies in an 18-year follow-up after biliopancreatic diversion. Obes Surg 1995;5(3):308–313.
29. Marceau P, Kaufman D, Biron S, Hould FS, Lebel S, Marceau S, et al. Outcome of pregnancies after biliopancreatic diversion. Obes Surg 2004;14(3):318–324.
30. Poitou BC, Ciangura C, Coupaye M, Czernichow S, Bouillot JL, Basdevant A. Nutritional deficiency after gastric bypass: diagnosis, prevention and treatment. Diabetes Metab 2007;33(1):13–24.
31. Wax JR, Pinette MG, Cartin A, Blackstone J. Female reproductive issues following bariatric surgery. Obstet Gynecol Surv 2007;62(9):595–604.
32. Schauer, P. R., Burguera, B., Ikramuddin, S., Cottam, D., Gourash, W., Hamad, G., ... & Kelley, D. Effect of laparoscopic Roux-en-Y gastric bypass on type 2 diabetes mellitus. Ann Surg 2003;238(4):467.
33. Dirksen, C., Jørgensen, N. B., Bojsen-Møller, K. N., Jacobsen, S. H., Hansen, D. L., Worm, D., ... & Madsbad, S. Mechanisms of improved glycaemic control after Roux-en-Y gastric bypass. Diabetologia 2012;55(7):1890–1901.
34. Huerta S, Rogers LM, Li Z, Heber D, Liu C, Livingston EH. Vitamin A deficiency in a newborn resulting from maternal hypovitaminosis A after biliopancreatic diversion for the treatment of morbid obesity. Am J Clin Nutr 2002;76(2):426–429.
35. Haddow JE, Hill LE, Kloza EM, Thanhauser D. Neural tube defects after gastric bypass. Lancet 1986;1(8493):1330.
36. Martin L, Chavez GF, Adams MJ, Jr., Mason EE, Hanson JW, Haddow JE, et al. Gastric bypass surgery as maternal risk factor for neural tube defects. Lancet 1988;1(8586):640–641.
37. Wittgrove AC, Jester L, Wittgrove P, Clark GW. Pregnancy following gastric bypass for morbid obesity. Obes Surg 1998 Aug;8(4):461–464.
38. Wax JR, Cartin A, Wolff R, Lepich S, Pinette MG, Blackstone J. Pregnancy following gastric bypass surgery for morbid obesity: maternal and neonatal outcomes. Obes Surg 2008;18(5):540–544.
39. Johansson K, Cnattingius S, Naslund I, Roos N, Trolle L, Granath F, Stephansson O, Neovius M. Outcomes of pregnancy after bariatric surgery. New Engl J Med 2015;372(9):814–824.
40. Sheiner E, Balaban E, Dreiher J, Levi I, Levy A. Pregnancy outcome in patients following different types of bariatric surgeries. Obes Surg 2009;19(9):1286–1292.

41 Buchwald H, Avidor Y, Braunwald E, et al. Bariatric surgery: a systematic review and meta-analysis. JAMA 2004;292(14):1724–1737. doi:10.1001/jama.292.14.1724
42 Tice J, Karliner L, Walsh J, Petersen A, Feldman M. Gastric banding or bypass? A systematic review comparing the two most popular bariatric procedures. Amer J Med 2008;121(10):885–893.
43 O'Brien, P. E., Dixon, J. B., Brown, W., Schachter, L. M., Chapman, L., Burn, A. J., ... & Baquie, P. The laparoscopic adjustable gastric band (Lap-Band®): a prospective study of medium-term effects on weight, health and quality of life. Obes Surg 2002;12(5):652–660.
44 Bar-Zohar D, Azem F, Klausner J, Abu-Abeid S. Pregnancy after laparoscopic adjustable gastric banding: perinatal outcome is favorable also for women with relatively high gestational weight gain. Surg Endosc 2006;20(10):1580–1583.
45 Eerdekens A, Debeer A, Van HG, De BC, Sachar V, Guelinckx I, et al. Maternal bariatric surgery: adverse outcomes in neonates. Eur J Pediatr 2010;169(2):191–196.
46 Patel JA, Patel NA, Thomas RL, Nelms JK, & Colella JJ. Pregnancy outcomes after laparoscopic Roux-en-Y gastric bypass. Surgery for Obesity and Related Diseases 2008;4(1):39–45.
47 Dixon JB, Dixon ME, & O'Brien PE. Birth outcomes in obese women after laparoscopic adjustable gastric banding. Obstetrics & Gynecology 2005;106(5 Pt 1):965–972.
48 Skull AJ, Slater GH, Duncombe JE, Fielding GA. Laparoscopic adjustable banding in pregnancy: safety, patient tolerance and effect on obesity-related pregnancy outcomes. Obes Surg 2004;14:230–235.
49 Lapolla A, Marangon M, Dalfrà MG, Segato G, De Luca M, Fedele D, Favretti F, et al. Pregnancy outcome in morbidly obese women before and after laparoscopic gastric banding. Obes Surg 2010;20:1251–1257.
50 Ducarme G, Revaux A, Rodrigues A, Aissaoui F, Pharisien I, Uzan M. Obstetric outcome following laparoscopic adjustable gastric banding. Int J Gynaecol Obstet 2007;98:244–247.
51 Ducarme G, Revaux A, Rodrigues A, Aissaoui F, Pharisien I, Uzan M. Obstetric outcome following laparoscopic adjustable gastric banding. Int J Gynaecol Obstet 2007;98(3):244–247.
52 Dixon JB, Dixon ME, O'Brien PE. Birth outcomes in obese women after laparoscopic adjustable gastric banding. Obstet Gynecol 2005;106(5 Pt 1):965–972.
53 Martin LF, Finigan KM, Nolan TE. Pregnancy after adjustable gastric banding. Obstet Gynecol 2000;95(6 Pt 1):927–930.
54 Alvarenga ES, Menzo EL, Szomstein S, & Rosenthal RJ. Safety and efficacy of 1020 consecutive laparoscopic sleeve gastrectomies performed as a primary treatment modality for morbid obesity. A single-center experience from the metabolic and bariatric surgical accreditation quality and improvement program. Surg Endosc 2015;1–6.
55 Bohdjalian, A., Langer, F. B., Shakeri-Leidenmühler, S., Gfrerer, L., Ludvik, B., Zacherl, J., & Prager, G. Sleeve gastrectomy as sole and definitive bariatric procedure: 5-year results for weight loss and ghrelin. Obes Surg 2010;20(5):535–540.
56 Chuang JC, Perello M, Sakata I, Osborne-Lawrence S, Savitt JM, Lutter M, & Zigman JM. Ghrelin mediates stress-induced food-reward behavior in mice. J Clin Invest 2011;121(7):2684.
57 Chuang JC, Perello M, Sakata I, Osborne-Lawrence S, Savitt JM, Lutter M, & Zigman JM. Ghrelin mediates stress-induced food-reward behavior in mice. J Clin Invest 2011;121(7):2684.
58 Perello M, Scott MM, Sakata I, Lee CE, Chuang JC, Osborne-Lawrence S, ... & Zigman JM. Functional implications of limited leptin receptor and ghrelin receptor coexpression in the brain. J Comparat Neurol 2012;520(2):281–294.

59 Meier U, & Gressner AM. Endocrine regulation of energy metabolism: review of pathobiochemical and clinical chemical aspects of leptin, ghrelin, adiponectin, and resistin. Clin Chem 2004;50(9):1511–1525.
60 Gumbs A, Gagner M, Dakin G, & Pomp A. Sleeve gastrectomy for morbid obesity. Obes Surg 2007;17(7):962–969.
61 Ducarme G, Chesnoy V, Lemarié P, Koumaré S, & Krawczykowski D. Pregnancy outcomes after laparoscopic sleeve gastrectomy among obese patients. Intl J Gynecol Obstetr 2015;130(2):127–131.
62 Han SM, Kim WW, Moon R, & Rosenthal RJ. Pregnancy outcomes after laparoscopic sleeve gastrectomy in morbidly obese Korean patients. Obes Surg 2013;23(6):756–759.
63 Shi X, Karmali S, Sharma A, Birch D. A review of laparoscopic sleeve gastrectomy for morbid obesity. Obes Surg 2010;20(8):1171–1177.
64 Crosignani PG, Colombo M, Vegetti W, Somigliana E, Gessati A, Ragni G. Overweight and obese anovulatory patients with polycystic ovaries: parallel improvements in anthropometric indices, ovarian physiology and fertility rate induced by diet. Hum Reprod 2003;18(9):1928–1932.
65 Pasquali R, Pelusi C, Genghini S, Cacciari M, Gambineri A. Obesity and reproductive disorders in women. Hum Reprod Update 2003;9(4):359–372.
66 Clark AM, Thornley B, Tomlinson L, Galletley C, Norman RJ. Weight loss in obese infertile women results in improvement in reproductive outcome for all forms of fertility treatment. Hum Reprod 1998;13(6):1502–1505.
67 Sheiner E, Levy A, Silverberg D, Menes TS, Levy I, Katz M, et al. Pregnancy after bariatric surgery is not associated with adverse perinatal outcome. Am J Obstet Gynecol 2004;190(5):1335–1340.
68 Sheiner E, Menes TS, Silverberg D, Abramowicz JS, Levy I, Katz M, et al. Pregnancy outcome of patients with gestational diabetes mellitus following bariatric surgery. Am J Obstet Gynecol 2006;194(2):431–435.
69 Gosman GG, King WC, Schrope B, Steffen KJ, Strain GW, Courcoulas AP, et al. Reproductive health of women electing bariatric surgery. Fertil Steril 2010;94(4):1426–1431.
70 Gerrits EG, Ceulemans R, van HR, Hendrickx L, Totte E. Contraceptive treatment after biliopancreatic diversion needs consensus. Obes Surg 2003;13(3):378–382.
71 Victor A, Odlind V, Kral JG. Oral contraceptive absorption and sex hormone binding globulins in obese women: effects of jejunoileal bypass. Gastroenterol Clin North Am 1987;16(3):483–491.
72 Padwal R, Brocks D, & Sharma AM. (2010). A systematic review of drug absorption following bariatric surgery and its theoretical implications. Obes Rev 2010;11(1):41–50.
73 Merhi ZO. Challenging oral contraception after weight loss by bariatric surgery. Gynecol Obstet Invest 2007;64(2):100–102.
74 Armstrong C. ACOG Guidelines on Pregnancy After Bariatric Surgery. Am Fam Physician 2010;81(7):905–906.
75 American College of Obstetricians and Gynecologists. ACOG practice bulletin no 105: bariatric surgery and pregnancy. Obstet Gynecol 2009;113:1405–1413.
76 Roos N, Neovius M, Cnattingius A, et al. Perinatal outcomes after bariatric surgery: nationwide population based matched cohort study. BMJ 2013;347:f6460.
77 Sheiner E, Edri A, Balaban E, et al. Pregnancy outcome of patients who conceive during or after the first year following bariatric surgery. Am J Obstet Gynecol 2011;204:50e1–6.
78 Kjaer M, Nilas L. Timing of pregnancy after gastric bypass – a national register-based cohort study. Obes Surg 2013;23(8):1281–1285.
79 Ducarme G, Parisio L, Santulli P, Carbillon

L, Mandelbrot L, Luton D. Neonatal outcomes in pregnancies after bariatric surgery: a retrospective multi-centric cohort study in three French referral centers. J Matern Fetal Neonat Med 2103;26(3):275-278.
80. Bilenka B, Ben-Shlomo I, Cozacov C, Gold CH, Zohar S. Fertility, miscarriage and pregnancy after vertical banded gastroplasty operation for morbid obesity. Acta Obstetric Gynecolog Scandinav 1995;74(1):44.
81. Marceau P, Kaufman D, Biron S, et al. Outcome of pregnancies after biliopancreatic diversion. Obes Surg 2004;14(3):318-324.
82. Patel JA, Patel NA, Thomas RL, Nelms JK, Colella JJ. Pregnancy outcomes after laparoscopic Roux-en-Y gastric bypass. Surg Obes Rel Dis 2008;4(1):39-45.
83. Ducarme G, Revaux A, Rodrigues A, Aissaoui F, Pharisien I, Uzan M. Obstetric outcome following laparoscopic adjustable gastric banding. Int J Gynaecol Obstet 2007;98(3):244-247.
84. Ananth CV, Basso O. Impact of pregnancy-induced hypertension on stillbirth and neonatal mortality. Epidemiology 2010;21(1):118-123.
85. Bennett WL, Gilson MM, Jamshidi R, Burke AE, Segal JB, Steele KE, et al. Impact of bariatric surgery on hypertensive disorders in pregnancy: retrospective analysis of insurance claims data. BMJ 2010;340:c1662.
86. Santulli P, Mandelbrot L, Facchiano E, Dussaux C, Ceccaldi PF, Ledoux S, et al. Obstetrical and neonatal outcomes of pregnancies following gastric bypass surgery: a retrospective cohort study in a French referral centre. Obes Surg 2010;20:1501-1508.
87. Josefsson A, Blomberg M, Bladh M, Frederiksen SG, Sydsjö G. Bariatric surgery in a national cohort of women: sociodemographics and obstetric outcomes. Am J Obstet Gynecol 2011;205:206.e1-8.
88. Berlac J, Skovlund C, Lidegaard O. Obstetrical and neonatal outcomes in women following gastric bypass: a Danish national cohort study. Acta Obstetric Gynecolog Scandinav 2014;93(5):447-453.
89. Lapolla A, Marangon M, Dalfrà MG, Segato G, De Luca M, Fedele D, et al. Pregnancy outcome in morbidly obese women before and after laparoscopic gastric banding. Obes Surg 2010;20:1251-1257.
90. Xiong X, Saunders LD, Wang FL, Demianczuk NN. Gestational diabetes mellitus: prevalence, risk factors, maternal and infant outcomes. Intl J Gynaecol Obstetr 2001;75(3):221-228.
91. Chu S, Callaghan W, Kim S, Schmid C, Lau J, England L, Dietz P. Maternal obesity and risk of gestational diabetes mellitus. Diabetes Care 2007;30(8):2070-2076.
92. Langer O, Yogev Y, Xenakis EM, Brustman L. Overweight and obese in gestational diabetes: the impact on pregnancy outcome. Am J Obstet Gynecol 2005;192(6):1768-1776.
93. Artal R, Catanzaro R, Gavard J, Mostello D, Friganza J. A lifestyle intervention of weight-gain restriction: diet and exercise in obese women with gestational diabetes mellitus. Appl Physiol Nutr Metab 2007;32:596-601.
94. Peterli R, Wolnerhanssen B, Peters T, Devaux N, Kern B, Christoffel-Courtin C, Drewe J, Von Flue M, Beglinger C. Improvement in glucose metabolism after bariatric surgery: comparison of laparoscopic Roux-en-Y gastric bypass and laparoscopic sleeve gastrectomy: a prospective randomized trial. Ann Surg 2009;250(2):234-241.
95. Aricha-Tamir B, Weintraub AY, Levi I, & Sheiner E. Downsizing pregnancy complications: a study of paired pregnancy outcomes before and after bariatric surgery. Surg Obes Relat Dis 2012;8(4):434-439.
96. Jensen DM, Damm P, Sorensen B, Molsted-Pedersen L, Westergaard JG, Ovesen P, et al. Pregnancy outcome and prepregnancy body mass index in 2459 glucose-tolerant Danish women. Am J Obstet Gynecol 2003;189(1):239-244.

97 Ehrenberg HM, Mercer BM, & Catalano PM. The influence of obesity and diabetes on the prevalence of macrosomia. Am J Obstet Gynecol 2004;191(3):964–968.

98 Guelinckx I, Devlieger R, & Vansant G. Reproductive outcome after bariatric surgery: a critical review. Human Reprod Update 2009;15(2):189–201.

99 Strauss RS. (2000). Adult functional outcome of those born small for gestational age: twenty-six–year follow-up of the 1970 British birth cohort. JAMA 2000;283(5):625–632.

100 Hezelgrave NL & Oteng-Ntim E. Pregnancy after bariatric surgery: a review. J Obes 2011;2011:501939.

101 Josefsson A, Bladh M, Wirehn A, & Sydsjo G. Risk for congenital malformations in offspring of women who have undergone bariatric surgery: a national cohort. BJOG 2013;120(12):1477–1482.

102 Willis K, Lieberman N, & Sheiner E. Pregnancy and neonatal outcome after bariatric surgery. Best Pract Res Clin Obstet Gynaecol 2015 Jan;29(1):133–144.

第十九章 胎儿监护

Dipanwita Kapoor1 and Nia Jones[1,2]

1 Department of Obstetrics and Gynaecology, Nottingham University Hospitals NHS Trust, Nottingham, UK

2 School of Medicine, University of Nottingham, Nottingham, UK

实践要点

- 糖尿病妇女妊娠与围产期发病率和死亡率增加有关。
- 在正常或加速生长的过程中发生的胎儿预后不良的机制尚不清楚,很可能是多因素造成的。
- 糖尿病合并血管病变或子痫前期孕妇的胎儿损害可能与胎盘血管疾病有关。
- 目前已有的胎儿监护技术尚未证明可以用来预测糖尿病妊娠妇女的胎儿风险或防止不良结局。
- 建议在妊娠后半期进行连续生长扫描,以检测胎儿的加速生长和(或)羊水过多或生长受限。
- 监测方法仅在糖尿病妊娠血管并发症或严重胎儿生长受限或妊娠期超过38周时才有价值。

病例

一名22岁先前未生育的1型糖尿病妇女在妊娠7周时到产前诊所进行登记,20周后进行常规的排查异常的扫描,28周开始连续进行生长扫描,显示胎儿生长加速,腹围大于95cm,羊水过多,脐动脉多普勒超声血流量正常。动脉多普勒每周查一次,每隔一周做一次生物计量学检查,虽然羊水过多的情况保持稳定,但胎儿生长继续加速,在妊娠35周时估算胎儿体重为3900g。

在妊娠38周时,因疑似巨大儿拟引产,但经阴道分娩出一名体重4200g的健康女婴,并发肩难产。新生儿因持续低血糖、黄疸而住院5d。母亲和婴儿8d后出院,但医师因担心婴儿臂丛神经损伤而随访。

- 糖尿病妊娠妇女和正常妊娠妇女的胎儿生长模式为何不同?
- 如何定义巨大儿?
- 为什么糖尿病与死产的风险增加有关,死产最有可能发生在什么时候?
- 有疑似胎儿过大的糖尿病妊娠妇女的最佳胎儿监测是什么?
- 分娩前对胎儿肺成熟是否能进行评估?如果可以评估,用的是什么方法?

背景

糖尿病妇女妊娠与围产期发病率和死亡率呈高相关，增加胎儿和新生儿风险的并发症包括以下方面。

与胎儿有关的

- 流产
- 先天畸形
——心脏畸形
——神经管缺陷
——小头畸形
——肾功能异常
——骶神经发育不全
- 羊水过多
- 早产
- 死产
- 巨大儿
- 子宫内生长迟滞（特别是胎盘功能不全而导致血管并发症的妇女）

与新生儿有关的

- 分娩创伤：肩部难产、骨折、臂丛损伤和窒息
- 心肌病
- 呼吸窘迫综合征
- 代谢紊乱
——低血糖
——低钙血症
——低镁血症
- 低体温

- 红细胞增多
- 黄疸病

在过去几十年中,糖尿病护理和孕前咨询的改善使围产期死亡率(PNM)下降[1],但不幸的是,更多最近的研究表明,1989年"圣文森特宣言"的目标尚未实现[2,3]。在英格兰和威尔士糖尿病妇女的死产率和新生儿死亡率在今后10年内将保持不变[3],死产率为12.8/1000,新生儿死亡率为7.6/1000。而2012年全国死产率和新生儿死亡率分别为4.9/1000和2.8/1000。然而,与10年前的CEMACH调查相比,不需要入院的新生儿重症监护病房的婴儿数量有了显著的改善(70.3% vs 33.3%)[3,4]。欧洲国家和其他英国区域研究的围产期死亡率相当,每1000名活产婴儿中有28~48名死产婴儿。胎儿监测包括胎儿生长监测和胎儿健康评估。确定有风险的胎儿,以便及时和适当地进行干预,降低围产期的发病率和死亡率。本章重点介绍目前可用的工具和未来在妊娠糖尿病的妊娠晚期对胎儿监测的方向。

妊娠糖尿病胎儿妥协的病理生理学研究

胎儿预后不良的病理生理学可能是多因素的,在此过程中胎儿在妊娠期是正常生长或过大生长的。大多数原因不明的死胎是由胎儿缺氧和(或)胎儿酸血症继发于母体/胎儿高血糖和胎儿高胰岛素血症引起的[5]。这可以用Pedersen假说[6]来解释,该假说指出,母体高血糖和由此产生的胎儿高血糖通过胎儿胰岛B细胞过度刺激引起明显的胎儿高胰岛素血症,进而导致胎儿生长加速,皮下脂肪沉积过多,肝糖原储存增加。与高血糖相关的胎儿代谢增加可能导致胎儿相对缺氧和代谢紊乱,这一假说目前已被普遍接受,也使医师在对糖尿病妊娠妇女的医疗护理中坚信对母亲进行更好的血糖控制可以延缓胎儿的生长,从而降低围产期的发病率和死亡率。

关于妊娠合并糖尿病妇女的胎儿损伤有几种假设的机制,即母体高血糖、高胰岛素血症和胎盘改变。第一种机制与组织缺氧有关。糖尿病妇女出现胎儿缺氧时,羊水中促红细胞生成素(EPO)水平通常升高[5]。妊娠晚期孕妇的HbA1c浓度与分娩时胎儿脐静脉EPO相关[7],表明产前孕妇高血糖是胎儿缺氧的一个重要因素。此外，胎儿羊水胰岛素水平与胎儿血浆 EPO 水平无关，提示胰岛素对胎儿氧合的影响超过母体血糖[7]。体重、脐带血胰岛素[8]和羊水 EPO 水平[5]提示，胎儿越大，导致胎儿缺氧的风险越大。髓外造血在糖尿病母亲的死胎婴儿中更常见[9]。在糖尿病妇女和无糖尿病妇女的配对死胎的尸检报道中发现，在组织学上胎儿胸腺出现了"星空"，表明糖尿病妇女的 50%以上的死胎具有严重的亚急性代谢紊乱[10]。此外，研究发现糖尿病妇女胎盘绒毛增厚[11]，这可能会减少氧转移。

另一种机制主张，胎儿心功能不全可能是妊娠糖尿病死胎的原因之一[12]。母/胎高血糖、胎儿高胰岛素血症和 EPO 浓度升高可能对胎儿宫内心脏产生负面影响[13]。研究人员发现妊娠初期血糖控制不良妇女的 B 型钠尿肽（BNP）、前 BNP 和肌钙蛋白 T 偏高，并有急性心肌损害的迹象[14]。此外，40%的糖尿病母亲的婴儿发现肥厚性心肌病，其原因尚不清楚[15-17]。这些变化是短暂的，通常在出生后的前 6 个月内消失，但也可能导致严重的发病率甚至死亡[17]。

对四项有关 1 型和 2 型糖尿病不良妊娠结局研究的系统评价发现，围产期死亡率增加与血糖控制不良有关（OR：3.23；95% CI：1.87～4.92）[18]，尽管这些研究有方法论上的局限性。产妇血糖控制的显著波动可以解释胎儿加速生长和胎儿受损的原因，这在一些明显控制糖尿病的妊娠中可以看到[19]。产妇低血糖似乎并没有对胎儿产生明显的影响，然而很少有研究涉及这个问题。

死产通常在妊娠 32 周后出现[3, 4]，并且经常发生在血糖控制不良、羊水过多和（或）胎儿加速生长[20]的情况下。相反，患有糖尿病和血管病变的妇女和（或）子痫前期妇女可能早在中期就会出现 IUGR 和胎儿死亡，可能与胎盘血管疾病有关。然而，50%的死胎原因仍无法解释，即临床检查或标准死后[12]无法确定明显的原因。

加速胎儿生长

目前正在使用各种加速胎儿生长的定义，包括超过 4000g 或 4500g 的出生体重，或第 90 百分位以上的出生体重，或高于胎龄和性别的平均体重的两个标准差。后者是首选的，因为它允许对胎儿过度生长的早产儿进行鉴别，但即便如此，糖尿病妇女婴儿的选择性器官肿大也不具有特征。患有糖尿病的母亲的新生儿巨大的特征是身体脂肪过多、肌肉质量增加、器官肿大，而大脑大小没有增加。新生儿体脂百分比、母亲血糖和胎儿胰岛素水平之间存在线性与持续性的关系[21]。CEMACH 的调查[4]报道称，21%的糖尿病妇女的独生子女体重超过 4000g，而在一般人口中这一比例为 11%。

生长加速可能早在妊娠 18 周就开始了[22]。然而，胎儿的生长潜力似乎取决于在此之前普遍存在的产妇血糖水平。尽管晚期妊娠期间血糖控制最佳[23]，但过度生长仍可继续。

在处理疑似胎儿巨大儿妊娠时的主要挑战之一是如何将疑似加速生长婴儿的肩难产、臂丛神经损伤和其他重大分娩创伤降到最低。肩难产在较大的婴儿中更常见，从小于 2500g 的婴儿的发生率为 1%到 4500g 以上的婴儿的发生率为 43%不等。此外，据报道，患有糖尿病的妇女所生的婴儿在每一特定体重类别中肩部难产的风险比没有糖尿病的妇女高出 3~7 倍[24]。这可以用患有糖尿病和没有糖尿病的母亲的婴儿之间的人体测量差异来解释[25]。在妊娠前糖尿病的报道中，臂丛神经损伤的发生率为每千个新生儿 4.5 次，比一般人群的 4 倍还多。

尽管如此，妊娠期间的最佳血糖控制与胎儿加速生长[26]的发生率降低有关，因此与围产期结局的改善有关。

妊娠糖尿病的胎儿监护

虽然许多评估胎儿风险和产前监测的数据与 1 型糖尿病有关，但不断发展的证据表明，2 型糖尿病的结果也同样差[4]。事实上，在 2 型糖尿病中，胎儿加速生长和围产期发病率/死亡率的风险可能更大，因为其他产科结局不良的危险因素经常出现，如孕产妇年龄过高、体重指数（BMI）升高、非白种人种族、社会贫困和妊娠准备不良（参见第十四章）。此外，2 型糖尿病的围产期死亡主要是由于死产、绒毛膜羊膜炎和出生窒息。新西兰一项单一中心的研究表明，在 20 年的时间里，75%的 1 型糖尿病死亡是继发于先天畸形或早产并发症[26a]。

胎儿监护问题在 GDM 中甚至比先天糖尿病更有争议，文献中很少有支持或反驳 GDM 产前胎儿监测的数据。GDM 胎儿监护的最佳方法、时机和频率尚不清楚，只有通过前瞻性随机对照试验才能解决。然而，控制不良的 GDM 妇女，其婴儿生长加速，需要胰岛素或有其他危险因素，如高血压或不良产科病史，应该和患有先天糖尿病的妇女一样进行胎儿监护[27]。超声测量腹围也可能有助于指导临床医师将胰岛素治疗的需求与家庭血糖监测的结果相结合[27]。

胎儿监护标准方法

考虑到糖尿病妊娠的病因和胎儿死亡时机的多因素性质，故很难知道哪些形式的胎儿监测是合适的。人们普遍认为，标准的临床评估需要辅之以其他的监测方法，尽管两项关于妊娠糖尿病[9, 28]的回顾分析显示，目前还没有任何技术证明可以预测胎儿的危险或防止不良结局。标准胎儿监测方法包括以下方面：
- 产前 CTG。
- 二维超声（2d USS）评估胎儿生长。
- 超声评估羊水体积。
- 脐动脉多普勒血流速度
- 胎儿生理活动评估
- 羊膜穿刺术——评估胎儿肺成熟度和胎儿胰岛素。

产前心电图

目前尚无随机对照试验评估产前 CTG 在糖尿病妊娠妇女胎儿监护中的价值。非随机研究表明，该工具是糖尿病胎儿妥协的一个很差的预测因子，在正常追踪数小时后报道胎儿死亡[29]。考虑到妊娠糖尿病胎儿死亡的可能机制，这并不令人惊讶。回顾七项产前 CTG 研究发现，在正常妊娠 7d 内，糖尿病妊娠的死胎率为 1.4%，与合并 IUGR 的妊娠相似（2%）[30]。

一项比较计算机化 CTG 与传统 CTG 的系统回顾研究发现，计算机化 CTG 能显著降低围产儿死亡率（RR：0.20；95%CI：0.04～0.88）[29]。然而，样本量很小（$n=496$），包括所有高危妇女。今后还需要对高危妊娠和糖尿病妇女的妊娠进行进一步的研究。

总之，现有证据不支持在通常适应证之外的糖尿病患者中常规使用产前 CTG，包括减少胎儿运动、胎儿生长受限、先兆子痫或产前出血[31]。

二维超声对胎儿生长发育的评价

用二维超声生物计量法预测糖尿病妊娠妇女的胎儿体重是不准确的，应该谨慎地解释结果。这是因为糖尿病通过对胰岛素敏感组织如肝脏（糖原储存）和腹壁脂肪组织的影响而影响腹围（AC），而不是骨骼测量。因此，USS 测量将预测 IUGR，但对胎儿加速生长的检测不太可靠，因此不能准确预测这些婴儿分娩时的创伤[24]。尽管如此，生物特征测量被纳入糖尿病妇女管理标准推荐治疗手段中[31-33]。

一项系统的关于将近两万名妊娠妇女的统计表明[34]，超声估计胎儿体重（EFW）和腹围在预测出生体重 4000g 以上的准确性没有差别。然而，这些研究是针对没有糖尿病的妇女，因此不能直接推断为糖尿病妇女，但后者的准确性可能更低。这一系统综述最近被更新，包括 2D USS 与 3D USS 和 MRI[35]的比较；仅 2D USS 腹围（>35cm）的敏感性[0.80（95%CI：0.69~0.87）]明显优于 2D USS 估计胎儿体重[0.56（95%CI：0.49~0.62）]，但特异性明显较低，表明仅测量腹围就有更多的假阳性结果（P=0.012）。对巨大儿有较高的敏感度（0.93%CI：0.76~0.98）和特异度（0.95%CI：0.92~0.97）。然而，在这项技术应用于临床实践之前，还需要更多的研究。在这一项分析中，3D USS 对巨大儿的诊断准确性评估是不可能的。

总之，妊娠糖尿病的连续生长扫描有助于识别胎儿生长受限。如果 USS 表明胎儿加速生长，那么胎儿在产前或分娩时的确切风险是不确定的，因此这些信息的价值是有限的。胎儿加速生长可能表明母亲血糖控制不良，因此可能有助于加强母亲血糖控制措施和给予生活方式建议。

羊水指数的超声评价

羊水测量有两种方法：羊水指数（AFI）和最大池深度（MPD）。AFI 计算为羊水深度垂直池（以厘米为单位）之和，不含脐带和胎儿部位，位于子宫的每一象限。MPD 只测量单个最大的垂直深度。对于哪种方法是确定羊水异常的最佳方法，还没有达成共识。AFI 耗时较长，MPD 同样能有效地测定羊水过少和羊水过少。在 27~42 周，糖尿病妊娠妇女的 AFI 测量值比没有糖尿病的妊娠妇女要大[36]。这可能反映了胎儿多尿继发于高血糖引起的渗透利尿。目前还没有前瞻性的研究来证明 AFI 测量在结构正常的足月妊娠合并糖尿病中预测胎儿结局的价值。一个提高的 AFI 本身似乎无助于预测产前胎儿结局，尽管它可能暗示需要加强血糖控制。

脐动脉多普勒测速

脐动脉多普勒测速是胎盘血流阻力的间接测量。Cochrane 系统回顾发现围产期死亡显著减少（RR：0.71；95%CI：0.52~0.98），在高危妊娠（包括糖尿病）中使用胎儿和脐动脉多普勒超声的产科干预较少[37]。

然而，在糖尿病中，胎儿血流动力学和母体高血糖的代谢反应是复杂的，并且取决于妊娠期的持续时间。胎儿氧化代谢增加，低氧血症加重。脑和肾脏的灌注甚至在胎儿胎盘灌注没有任何变化的情况下也会增加。在母体糖尿病中，尽管胎儿低氧血症（除非也有血管病变或胎盘功能不全和胎儿生长受限），脐动脉多普勒测速可能保持不变，而且正常多普勒指数的存在并不排除胎儿妥协[38, 39]。应保留脐动脉多普勒测速仪供有可能患 IUGR 的糖尿病孕妇使用[31, 32]。

胎儿生理评估

生物物理评分（BPP）包括四项超声评估（胎儿呼吸、胎儿音调、胎儿身体运动和 AFI）和 CTG 分析。它最初被用于没有重大先天异常的情况下的胎儿生长受限的妊娠。然而，妊娠糖尿病的 BPP 不是一个好的针对良性妊娠结局的预测因素[40]，因为在解释结果时存在一些问题；产妇高血糖可能与增加 AFI 和增加胎儿呼吸有关，因此糖尿病本身可以影响这五个参数中的两个。然而，一个正常的测试结果通常被认为是对胎儿健康的安慰[41]。BPP 在妊娠糖尿病中的作用仍然存在争议；在英国[31]，BPP 不是例行倡导的，而在美国却是所有妊娠糖尿病妇女标准护理的一部分[32, 33]。

羊膜穿刺术与胎儿肺成熟度的评估

从历史上看，对妊娠糖尿病胎儿肺成熟度（FLM）的评估有助于产科医师计划何时分娩早产儿，目的是减少呼吸窘迫综合征的风险，并避免死产。各种羊水分析已被用于评估 FLM，如卵磷脂/鞘磷脂（L∶S）值，磷脂酰甘油（PG）的存在，表面蛋白/白蛋白值，层状体计数（LBC），泡沫稳定性指数（FSI）和光密度[42]。

近年来，羊膜穿刺术对胎儿肺成熟度的影响最大，但与未成熟的结果一致[43, 44]，因此羊膜穿刺术的应用较少。后者可能导致不必要的类固醇的使用，这有医源性高血糖的风险，或不必要的延迟所指示的分娩，在这种情况下，测试结果会错误地预测胎儿肺发育不成熟。

羊水穿刺术预测巨大儿及用羊水胰岛素评价血糖控制

妊娠晚期高胰岛素水平与胎儿生长加速和胎儿酸血症[45]有关。从概念上讲，在分娩前对高胰岛素血症胎儿的识别可能有助于加强母体胰岛素治疗，从而降低糖尿病相关胎儿疾病的发病率和严重程度[46]。然而，目前还没有足够的数据来保证产前羊水胰岛素水平在常规临床实践中的测量。

胎儿监护方法：未来是什么？

三维超声估测胎儿体重及脏器体积

3D USS 可以对胎儿体重和器官体积（如肝脏）进行体积评估。据推测，体积法计算的 EFW 值更可靠，因为理想的生物特征值可以在体积范围内进行优化，胎儿皮下脂肪的评估也可以包括在内。然而，到目前为止，研究还没有显示出糖尿病妇女巨大儿检测敏感度的提高[47]，而且这项技术耗费时间[48]，除非经验丰富，否则执行起来并不容易。在将其纳入常规临床实践之前，还需要更多的研究。

静脉导管测速

静脉导管（DV）（图 19.1）是一种重要的胎儿血管，氧合血可通过脐静脉流向卵圆孔。20%～30%的脐静脉血流通过 DV[49]绕过肝循环。

在胎儿酸中毒和正向心功能下降的情况下，可以发现 DV 的血流异常。静脉峰值流速指数（PVIV）的评估是一种可靠而有用的静脉多普勒指数[50]。

妊娠糖尿病母亲的胎儿患先天性心脏病、心肌肥厚和胎儿酸血症的风险增加，导致心功能受损。此外，右心功能在控制不良的糖尿病（51 例）中可能会更严重地恶化[51]。研究[52]发现糖尿病妇女胎儿的 DV-PVIV 升高，且与 HbA1c 值有统计学意义的相关性，但预测胎儿不良结局的敏感性和特异性是不够的。

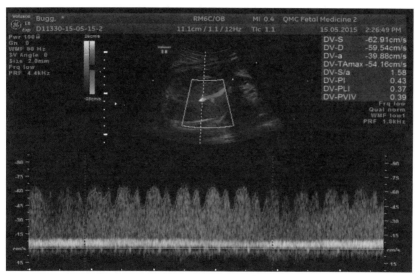

图 19.1　静脉导管多普勒的典型波形

胎儿心脏功能评价

许多研究使用了心肌性能指数（或 Tei 指数），这是一个整体心功能的预测指标。大多数人认为，母亲糖尿病与胎儿心脏功能的不同程度的损害有关，其中最常见的是舒张功能障碍。然而，有关胎儿超声心动图的最大一项研究（一项回顾性研究）涉及 2000 例，包括 140 例母亲糖尿病，发现糖尿病组的结果与其他受试者没有差异[53]。目前很少有关于心脏功能障碍与胎儿结局有关的研究，而这项研究目前仍然是一种研究工具，需要高水平的技术来完成。

羊水促红细胞生成素、氧化亚硝基应激标志物

组织缺氧是 EPO 合成的主要刺激,高羊水 EPO 水平是慢性胎儿缺氧的替代标志物。促红细胞生成素既不穿过胎盘也不在胎盘储存。因此胎儿血浆和羊水水平是胎儿 EPO 合成和消除的指示。重复羊水 EPO 测量显示在妊娠糖尿病胎儿缺氧和其他高危妊娠时呈指数增加[54]。从第 37 周起,每周对羊水 EPO 进行测量可能是管理这些复杂的高风险妊娠糖尿病的方法,但这仍然是一个需要在临床试验中被证实的理论。

MRI 研究

胎儿肥胖

患有糖尿病的母亲所产的婴儿往往随着皮下脂肪沉积的增加而变大。使用 MRI 测量胎儿肥胖是在其发展的早期阶段,可以量化皮下脂肪,并显示妊娠早期糖尿病妇女和第 3 个月妊娠妇女身体上的差异[55]。

胎儿肺成熟度预测

虽然羊膜穿刺术已经被用于近预产期妇女的胎儿肺成熟度的检查,但专家正在研究,试图以非侵入性的方式获得类似的信息。本文介绍了两种技术:第一,测量多种化合物的磁共振波谱,包括胆碱和卵磷脂;第二,肺-肝信号强度比较肺内液体与肝脏的比值,并被认为反映肺内细胞数量、磷脂含量及肺上皮和间质组织的发育。这两种技术都具有挑战性,处于发展的早期阶段,而且也没有应用于妊娠糖尿病妇女。

胎儿监护的实用方法

鉴于缺乏理想的胎儿监测测试,现有测试的局限性及缺乏严格的科学试验,包括随机对照试验,用于胎儿监测的所有程序都是经验性的,

而不是基于证据的,而且都有局限性(表19.1)。在制订地方协议时,必须考虑到对卫生资源的财政影响、产妇的焦虑及缺乏关于检测效果的证据。

表19.1 在妊娠糖尿病的情况下,妊娠中期胎儿健康检查在临床实践中的有用性摘要

胎儿监护试验	建议
二维超声连续生长扫描(USS)	建议例行
脐动脉多普勒测速	建议在特定情况下,如IUGR、子痫前期,减少调频
产前心电图	建议在美国妊娠前糖尿病妇女每周两次,但在英国针对具体情况,如IUGR、先兆子痫、FM降低等
胎儿生理评估	在美国的妊娠糖尿病患者中常规推荐,但在英国针对特定的病例,如IUGR、子痫前期、FM降低等
羊膜穿刺术与胎儿肺成熟度的评估	选择性使用
羊水胰岛素	在常规临床实践中不推荐
三维超声估测胎儿体重和器官体积*	在常规临床实践中不推荐
静脉导管测速法*	在常规临床实践中不推荐
胎儿心脏结构与功能的评估	在常规临床实践中不推荐
羊水促红细胞生成素*	在常规临床实践中不推荐
磁共振研究*	在常规临床实践中不推荐

*可能有用的测试,但需要更多的研究才能纳入常规的临床实践。FM,胎儿运动;IUGR,宫内生长受限

在英国,NICE准则[31]建议:

- 妊娠28~36周时应用超声每4周监测1次胎儿生长和液体量情况。
- 胎儿健康的额外监测(如胎儿脐动脉多普勒记录、CTG和BPP)只需要对有危险因素的妊娠进行监测。频率将取决于潜在共病的严重程度。
- 如果妊娠超过38周,每周进行胎儿健康检查。

相反,ACOG指南规定定期超声检查胎儿生长,以及每周两次的CTG和BPP的适当间隔,从妊娠32~34周开始,是监测已有糖尿病患者胎儿的一种有价值的方法。脐动脉多普勒测速应保留给妊娠伴有血管并发症和胎儿生长不良[32]。胎儿监护对血糖控制差的GDM妇女可能有好处——检查的方法和频率将取决于当地的做法[33]。

主要研究方向

- 了解妊娠合并糖尿病胎儿死亡的机制。
- 3D 超声和 MRI 在子宫中胎儿脂肪、身体成分和体重的测定中的应用。
- 3D 多普勒在胎盘体积、血管化、血流和结构评估中的作用。
- 羊水促红细胞生成素（EPO）的随机对照试验以检测"高危"胎儿。
- 无创性评估 FLM 和胎儿妥协的方法。
- 检测加速胎儿生长后最适当的管理策略。
- 随机对照试验，以确定最优监测试验和测试频率。

选择题

1. 在糖尿病妇女的死胎中，大多数死胎在死后发现的特点是（ ）
   A. 大胎盘　　　　　　　　　　B. 胎盘后出血
   C. "星空"在胎儿胸腺中的出现　　D. 胸腺肥大
   正确答案是 C。

2. 下列与妊娠合并母亲糖尿病胎儿的加速生长无关的是（ ）
   A. 急性胎儿缺氧　　　　　　　B. 臂丛神经损伤
   C. 宫内胎死　　　　　　　　　D. 肩难产
   正确答案是 A。糖尿病妇女胎儿生长加速通常导致慢性胎儿缺氧，而不是急性胎儿缺氧。

3. 目前，在糖尿病妇女胎儿监护的常规临床实践中，推荐进行的检查是（ ）
   A. 静脉导管测速
   B. 胎盘超声评价
   C. 二维超声连续生长扫描
   D. 胎儿体重和脏器体积的三维超声估计
   正确答案是 C。

致谢

感谢 George Bugg 先生对撰写这一章时提出的有益建议。

(赖 杰 译,王 冰 校)

参 考 文 献

1. McElvy SS, Miodovnik M, Rosenn B, Khoury JC, Siddiqi T, Dignan PS, et al. A focused preconceptional and early pregnancy program in women with type 1 diabetes reduces perinatal mortality and malformation rates to general population levels. J Matern Fetal Med 2000;9(1):14–20.
2. Diabetes care and research in Europe: the St Vincent's Declaration. Diabet Med 1990;34:655–661.
3. National Pregnancy in Diabetes Audit Report 2014. Health and Social Care Information Centre: Leeds, 2015.
4. Confidential Enquiry into Maternal and Child Health. Pregnancy in women with type 1 and type 2 diabetes in 2002–03, England, Wales and Northern Ireland. CEMACH: London, 2005.
5. Teramo KA. Obstetric problems in diabetic pregnancy – the role of fetal hypoxia. Best Pract Res Clin Endocrinol Metab 2010;24(4):663–671.
6. Pedersen J. Diabetes and pregnancy; blood sugar of newborn infants during fasting and glucose administration. Nord Med 1952;47(30):1049.
7. Widness JA, Teramo KA, Clemons GK, Voutilainen P, Stenman UH, McKinlay SM, et al. Direct relationship of antepartum glucose control and fetal erythropoietin in human type 1 (insulin-dependent) diabetic pregnancy. Diabetologia 1990;33(6):378–383.
8. Schwartz R, Gruppuso PA, Petzold K, Brambilla D, Hiilesmaa V, Teramo KA. Hyperinsulinemia and macrosomia in the fetus of the diabetic mother. Diabetes Care 1994;17(7):640–648.
9. Landon MB, Vickers S. Fetal surveillance in pregnancy complicated by diabetes mellitus: is it necessary? J Matern Fetal Neonatal Med 2002;12(6):413–416.
10. Edwards A, Springett A, Padfield J, Dorling J, Bugg G, Mansell P. Differences in post-mortem findings after stillbirth in women with and without diabetes. Diabet Med 2013;30(10):1219–1224.
11. Björk O, Persson B. Villous structure in different parts of the cotyledon in placentas of insulin-dependent diabetic women: a morphometric study. Acta Obstet Gynecol Scand 1984;63(1):37–43.
12. Mathiesen ER, Ringholm L, Damm P. Stillbirth in diabetic pregnancies. Best Pract Res Clin Obstet Gynaecol 2011;25(1):105–111.
13. Salvesen DR, Brudenell JM, Snijders RJ, Ireland RM, Nicolaides KH. Fetal plasma erythropoietin in pregnancies complicated by maternal diabetes mellitus. Am J Obstet Gynecol 1993;168(1 Pt 1):88–94.
14. Russell NE, Higgins MF, Amaruso M, Foley M, McAuliffe FM. Troponin T and pro-B-type natriuretic Peptide in fetuses of type 1 diabetic mothers. Diabetes Care 2009;32(11):2050–2055.
15. Evers IM, de Valk HW, Visser GH. Risk of complications of pregnancy in women with type 1 diabetes: nationwide prospective study in the Netherlands. BMJ 2004;328(7445):915.
16. Sheehan PQ, Rowland TW, Shah BL, McGravey VJ, Reiter EO. Maternal diabetic control and hypertrophic cardiomyopathy in infants of diabetic mothers. Clin Pediatr (Phila) 1986;25(5):266–271.
17. Abu-Sulaiman RM, Subaih B. Congenital

heart disease in infants of diabetic mothers: echocardiographic study. Pediatr Cardiol 2004;25(2):137–140.
18 Inkster ME, Fahey TP, Donnan PT, Leese GP, Mires GJ, Murphy DJ. Poor glycated haemoglobin control and adverse pregnancy outcomes in type 1 and type 2 diabetes mellitus: systematic review of observational studies. BMC Pregnancy Childbirth 2006;6:30.
19 Kyne-Grzebalski D, Wood L, Marshall SM, Taylor R. Episodic hyperglycaemia in pregnant women with well-controlled Type 1 diabetes mellitus: a major potential factor underlying macrosomia. Diabet Med 1999;16(8):702–706.
20 Mondestin MA, Ananth CV, Smulian JC, Vintzileos AM. Birth weight and fetal death in the United States: the effect of maternal diabetes during pregnancy. Am J Obstet Gynecol 2002;187(4):922–926.
21 Group HSCR. Hyperglycemia and Adverse Pregnancy Outcome (HAPO) study: associations with neonatal anthropometrics. Diabetes 2009;58(2):453–459.
22 Wong SF, Chan FY, Oats JJ, McIntyre DH. Fetal growth spurt and pregestational diabetic pregnancy. Diabetes Care 2002;25(10):1681–1684.
23 Raychaudhuri K, Maresh MJ. Glycemic control throughout pregnancy and fetal growth in insulin-dependent diabetes. Obstet Gynecol 2000;95(2):190–194.
24 Langer O, Berkus MD, Huff RW, Samueloff A. Shoulder dystocia: should the fetus weighing greater than or equal to 4000 grams be delivered by cesarean section? Am J Obstet Gynecol 1991;165(4 Pt 1):831–837.
25 McFarland MB, Trylovich CG, Langer O. Anthropometric differences in macrosomic infants of diabetic and nondiabetic mothers. J Matern Fetal Med 1998;7(6):292–295.
26 Page RC, Kirk BA, Fay T, Wilcox M, Hosking DJ, Jeffcoate WJ. Is macrosomia associated with poor glycaemic control in diabetic pregnancy? Diabet Med 1996;13(2):170–174.

26a Cundy T, Gamble G, Neale L, Elder R, McPherson P, Henley P, Rowan J. Differing causes of pregnancy loss in type 1 and type 2 diabetes. Diabetes Care 2007; 30(10):2603–2607.
27 Mitanchez D, Yzydorczyk C, Siddeek B, Boubred F, Benahmed M, Simeoni U. The offspring of the diabetic mother – short- and long-term implications. Best Pract Res Clin Obstet Gynaecol 2015;29(2):256–269.
28 Siddiqui F, James D. Fetal monitoring in type 1 diabetic pregnancies. Early Hum Dev 2003;72(1):1–13.
29 Grivell RM, Alfirevic Z, Gyte GM, Devane D. Antenatal cardiotocography for fetal assessment. Cochrane Database Syst Rev 2015;9:CD007863.
30 Barrett JM, Salyer SL, Boehm FH. The nonstress test: an evaluation of 1,000 patients. Am J Obstet Gynecol 1981;141(2):153–157.
31 National Institute of Health and Clinical Exellence. Diabetes in Pregnancy: Management of Diabetes and Its Complications from Preconception to the Postnatal Period. NICE: London, 2015.
32 American College of Obstetricians and Gynecologists. Pre-gestational diabetes mellitus. ACOG Practice Bulletin No. 60. Obstet Gynecol 2005;105:675–685.
33 American College of Obstetricians and Gynecologists. Gestational diabetes mellitus. ACOG Practice Bulletin No. 137. Obstet Gynecol 2013;122:406–416.
34 Coomarasamy A, Connock M, Thornton J, Khan KS. Accuracy of ultrasound biometry in the prediction of macrosomia: a systematic quantitative review. BJOG 2005;112(11):1461–1466.
35 Malin GL, Bugg GJ, Takwoingi Y, Thornton JG, Jones NW. Antenatal magnetic resonance imaging versus ultrasound for predicting neonatal macrosomia: a systematic review and meta-analysis. BJOG 2015;123:77–88.
36 Kofinas A, Kofinas G. Differences in amniotic fluid patterns and fetal biometric parameters in third trimester pregnancies with and without diabetes. J Matern Fetal

第十九章 胎儿监护

37 Alfirevic Z, Stampalija T, Gyte GM. Fetal and umbilical Doppler ultrasound in high-risk pregnancies. Cochrane Database Syst Rev 2013;11:CD007529.
38 Wong SF, Chan FY, Cincotta RB, McIntyre DH, Stone M. Use of umbilical artery Doppler velocimetry in the monitoring of pregnancy in women with pre-existing diabetes. Aust N Z J Obstet Gynaecol 2003;43(4):302–306.
39 Pietryga M, Brazert J, Wender-Ozegowska E, Dubiel M, Gudmundsson S. Placental Doppler velocimetry in gestational diabetes mellitus. J Perinat Med 2006;34(2):108–110.
40 Dicker D, Feldberg D, Yeshaya A, Peleg D, Karp M, Goldman JA. Fetal surveillance in insulin-dependent diabetic pregnancy: predictive value of the biophysical profile. Am J Obstet Gynecol 1988;159(4):800–804.
41 Johnson JM, Lange IR, Harman CR, Torchia MG, Manning FA. Biophysical profile scoring in the management of the diabetic pregnancy. Obstet Gynecol 1988;72(6):841–846.
42 Ventolini G, Neiger R, Hood D, Belcastro C. Update on assessment of fetal lung maturity. J Obstet Gynaecol 2005;25(6):535–538.
43 American College of Obstetricians and Gynecologists. ACOG committee opinion no 560: Medically indicated late-preterm and early-term deliveries. Obstet Gynecol 2013;121(4):908–910.
44 Towers CV, Freeman RK, Nageotte MP, Garite TJ, Lewis DF, Quilligan EJ. The case for amniocentesis for fetal lung maturity in late-preterm and early-term gestations. Am J Obstet Gynecol 2014;210(2):95–96.
45 Salvesen DR, Brudenell JM, Proudler AJ, Crook D, Nicolaides KH. Fetal pancreatic beta-cell function in pregnancies complicated by maternal diabetes mellitus: relationship to fetal acidemia and macrosomia. Am J Obstet Gynecol 1993;168(5):1363–1369.
46 Fraser RB, Bruce C. Amniotic fluid insulin levels identify the fetus at risk of neonatal hypoglycaemia. Diabet Med 1999;16(7):568–572.
47 Pagani G, Palai N, Zatti S, Fratelli N, Prefumo F, Frusca T. Fetal weight estimation in gestational diabetic pregnancies: comparison between conventional and three-dimensional fractional thigh volume methods using gestation-adjusted projection. Ultrasound Obstet Gynecol 2014;43(1):72–76.
48 Bennini JR, Marussi EF, Barini R, Faro C, Peralta CF. Birth-weight prediction by two- and three-dimensional ultrasound imaging. Ultrasound Obstet Gynecol 2010;35(4):426–433.
49 Kiserud T, Acharya G. The fetal circulation. Prenat Diagn 2004;24(13):1049–1059.
50 Hecher K, Campbell S, Snijders R, Nicolaides K. Reference ranges for fetal venous and atrioventricular blood flow parameters. Ultrasound Obstet Gynecol 1994;4(5):381–390.
51 Wong SF, Chan FY, Cincotta RB, McIntyre HD, Oats JJ. Cardiac function in fetuses of poorly-controlled pre-gestational diabetic pregnancies – a pilot study. Gynecol Obstet Invest 2003;56(2):113–116.
52 Stuart A, Amer-Wåhlin I, Gudmundsson S, Marsál K, Thuring A, Källen K. Ductus venosus blood flow velocity waveform in diabetic pregnancies. Ultrasound Obstet Gynecol 2010;36(3):344–349.
53 Ghawi H, Gendi S, Mallula K, Zghouzi M, Faza N, Awad S. Fetal left and right ventricle myocardial performance index: defining normal values for the second and third trimesters –single tertiary center experience. Pediatr Cardiol 2013;34(8):1808–1815.
54 Teramo K, Kari MA, Eronen M, Markkanen H, Hiilesmaa V. High amniotic fluid erythropoietin levels are associated with an increased frequency of fetal and neonatal morbidity in type 1 diabetic pregnancies. Diabetologia 2004;47(10):1695–1703.
55 Bulas D, Egloff A. Benefits and risks of MRI in pregnancy. Semin Perinatol 2013;37(5):301–304.

第二十章　妊娠并发症：高血压和糖尿病肾病

Elisabeth R. Mathiesen [1,2], *Lene Ringholm* [1,2,3] *and Peter Damm* [1,4]

1 Center for Pregnant Women with Diabetes, Rigshospitalet, Faculty of Health Sciences, University of Copenhagen, Copenhagen, Denmark

2 Department of Endocrinology, Rigshospitalet, Faculty of Health Sciences, University of Copenhagen, Copenhagen, Denmark

3 Steno Diabetes Center Copenhagen, Gentofte, Denmark

4 Department of Obstetrics, Rigshospitalet, Faculty of Health Sciences, University of Copenhagen, Copenhagen, Denmark

实践要点

- 与正常妊娠相比，糖尿病妊娠患慢性高血压、妊娠高血压、先兆子痫和并发先兆子痫的风险更高。
- 妊娠早期，应对慢性高血压、微量白蛋白尿和糖尿病肾病进行评估。
- 所有合并糖尿病的妊娠女性，达到并维持严格的血糖控制，密切监测先兆子痫的发展是非常重要的。
- 在预约和每隔1~2周的随访时要进行血压测量。
- 在合并糖尿病和慢性高血压的女性中，降压治疗的目标收缩压是110~139mmHg，舒张压是65~89mmHg。一些中心要求控制在135/85mmHg以下或130/80mmHg以下。当出现微量白蛋白尿和糖尿病肾病时，严格的降压治疗是非常重要的。
- 能够安全用于妊娠期的降压药应持续加量，直至血压控制达标。
- 妊娠期间可以应用甲基多巴、β肾上腺素能阻滞剂（如拉贝洛尔）和缓释钙通道阻滞剂。
- ACEI和ARB在妊娠时是禁忌的，因此在妊娠前或最晚也要在妊娠早期用安全的药物进行替代。
- 在哺乳期可以用甲基多巴、拉贝洛尔、卡托普利和依那普利。
- 大多数文献来自于合并1型糖尿病的女性，但是由于合并2型糖尿病女性的临床表现与此类似，因此这里的临床推荐适用于1型和2型糖尿病患者，或许也适用于妊娠糖尿病女性。

病 例

一名 28 岁的女性，1 型糖尿病病史 23 年，糖尿病肾病病史 2 年，第一次妊娠已 10 周。服用 ACEI 和呋塞米 2 次/天。查体时，她的血压是 114/75mmHg；血清肌酐是正常的，但尿白蛋白定量是 941mg/24h（正常＜30mg/24h）。将 ACEI 调整为甲基多巴 250mg，每天 2 次，继续呋塞米 40mg，每天 2 次。29 周时血压超过了 140/90mmHg，甲基多巴逐渐加量至 500mg，每天 4 次。不幸的是，她发展成子痫前期伴严重高血压和蛋白尿。用 2d 的时间应用倍他米松促进胎肺成熟，32 周时进行剖宫产。胎儿出生体重 1800g。

几年后，她又妊娠了。这次，她的血清肌酐水平已升至 120μmol/L，尿白蛋白升至 3000mg/24h。应用 ACEI 和利尿剂使她的血压（108/68mmHg）控制良好。ACEI 再次被停用，但这次用了更强化的降压策略，目的是将她的血压控制在 135/85mmHg 以下，尿白蛋白低于 300mg/24h。16 周时甲基多巴的剂量已达最大量（2000mg/d），利尿剂治疗没变，联用了拉贝洛尔，并逐渐加量至最大剂量。她的尿白蛋白排泄仍处于临床肾病阶段（＞2000mg/24h），但是血压保持在 130/80mmHg 以下。妊娠 36 周时，她没有子痫前期的症状，由于血清肌酐水平升高而进行分娩。胎儿的出生体重是 2584g。

问题：
- 在妊娠早期蛋白尿的出现影响妊娠结局吗？
- 在第二次妊娠为什么结局更好？
- 妊娠时可以应用什么类型的降压药？
- 妊娠时高血压的降压目标是什么？
- 哺乳时可以应用什么类型的降压药？

非妊娠糖尿病人群的高血压

非妊娠人群，合并糖尿病的女性与背景人群相比，高血压更常见。在合并 1 型糖尿病的非妊娠女性中，15～30 岁患者高血压（血压 140/90mmHg 以上）的患病率为 12%，30～44 岁为 22%，表明即使在肾脏未受累的患者高血压的患病率亦是升高的[1,2]。对于合并微量白蛋白尿和糖尿病肾病的患者，高血压的患病率和严重性均升高[2]。合并 2 型糖尿病的女性与 1 型糖尿病患者相比，高血压的患病率相当甚至更高[1,3]。

在合并糖尿病的患者中，高血压诊断的切点值是 140/90mmHg，但是在肾功能正常的患者中血压治疗的目标值是 135/85mmHg，当肾脏受累时，为了预防肾功能的恶化，血压治疗的目标值甚至降至 130/80mmHg[4]。有关治疗的一般指南请参阅"事实框"内容。

知 识 框

妊娠合并糖尿病和微量白蛋白尿或糖尿病肾病患者的治疗
- 严格的血糖控制目标：HbA1c＜6.0%
- 在妊娠前 12 周补充叶酸
- 从 10～12 周至分娩前 1 周应用小剂量阿司匹林
- 降压治疗目标：血压＜135/85mmHg 和尿白蛋白排泄＜300mg/24h
- 应用妊娠时可服用的降压药
- 检查妊娠时禁忌的药物清单（如降脂药）
- 密切进行产科监护
- 筛查糖尿病视网膜病变
- 哺乳期几种 ACEI 可以安全使用

在合并糖尿病的患者中，高血压的进展也许与尿白蛋白排泄增加、微量白蛋白尿或大量蛋白尿有关。微量白蛋白尿定义为次尿白蛋白/肌酐比值 30～300μg/mg，显性糖尿病肾病定义为尿白蛋白/肌酐比值＞300μg/mg，并且除外其他肾脏或泌尿道疾病，确定诊断至少需要进行两次尿检。糖尿病肾病是以蛋白尿、高血压、水肿及肾功能逐渐恶化直至终末期肾病为特征的。

在非妊娠的 1 型糖尿病患者中，高血压与心血管疾病发病风险升高密切相关。应用降压药尤其是应用影响肾素-血管紧张素系统的降压药所致的血压下降，对于合并糖尿病和微量白蛋白尿或糖尿病肾病的患者，预防肾脏疾病的进展、降低心血管疾病发病率和改善预后是非常重要的[4-6]。甚至对于合并糖尿病和微量白蛋白尿、显性糖尿病肾病早期血压仍正常的非妊娠患者，这些降压药也是适用的[7]。

妊娠高血压

10 位妊娠女性中会有 1 位患有高血压[8]。在合并糖尿病的女性中，高血压的患病率甚至更高，在妊娠期间甚至 40% 的女性血压超过

140/90mmHg[1, 9]。高血压不仅见于合并 1 型糖尿病和 2 型糖尿病的女性，也见于妊娠糖尿病女性。妊娠时有四类高血压疾病：①慢性高血压；②妊娠高血压；③先兆子痫；④合并高血压或糖尿病肾病的先兆子痫[10]。上述四种疾病均有其独特的病理生理特征，对于降压治疗有指导意义（表20.1）。合并糖尿病的女性与未合并糖尿病的女性相比，上述四种疾病均更常见[1]。在合并糖尿病的妊娠女性中，高血压的诊断标准同正常人群的诊断标准（≥140/90mmHg）；然而，在非妊娠糖尿病人群中，慢性高血压患者建议采用更低的控制目标[1, 9]。在哥本哈根，妊娠时慢性高血压的控制目标为 135/85mmHg[9]，Kitzmiller 教授建议糖尿病妊娠女性慢性高血压的控制目标为 130/80mmHg[1]。

表 20.1　妊娠期高血压疾病

慢性高血压	妊娠前或妊娠前 20 周收缩压≥140mmHg 或舒张压≥90mmHg，或妊娠期间第一次诊断高血压，并且分娩后未恢复正常[1]
	然而，在一些中心，对于合并糖尿病的女性，血压＞135/85mmHg 甚至血压＞130/80mmHg 亦需要考虑降压治疗[1, 9]
妊娠高血压	妊娠 20 周以后首次发现收缩压≥140mmHg 或舒张压≥90mmHg，无蛋白尿。如果产后 12 周前，升高的血压恢复至正常范围，可诊断为妊娠期一过性高血压。如果高血压持续存在，诊断为慢性高血压[8]
先兆子痫	在妊娠 20 周后，收缩压≥140mmHg 或舒张压≥90mmHg，合并蛋白尿（≥1+无菌尿试纸或≥300mg/24h）[8]
合并先兆子痫的慢性高血压	在妊娠早期合并高血压的女性，出现蛋白尿，符合先兆子痫诊断标准
	在妊娠早期合并糖尿病肾病的女性，如果伴随收缩压或舒张压突然上升≥15%，先兆子痫的定义同上[7]
	蛋白尿突然上升 2～3 倍和（或）血小板减少（血小板计数＜100×10^9/L）和（或）谷草转氨酶或谷丙转氨酶升高均表明先兆子痫[1]

慢性高血压（也就是在妊娠前或妊娠前 20 周出现的高血压）除与流产、并发先兆子痫、早产、胎儿宫内生长受限和新生儿发病率风险增加有关[11]外，合并慢性高血压的女性妊娠时有发生严重高血压（≥160/110mmHg）和卒中的风险。

妊娠高血压是妊娠 20 周后出现的高血压，在轻型病例中与妊娠并发症无关。然而，在相当大比例（10%～50%）的病例中，妊娠高血压可能进展成先兆子痫或严重高血压（≥160/110mmHg），与合并先兆子痫女性发生严重妊娠并发症的风险相当[11]。

先兆子痫传统定义为妊娠 20 周后出现高血压伴有蛋白尿≥1+，通过无菌尿试纸法检测或≥300mg/24h。近来，更广义的定义为高血压合并蛋白尿和（或）母亲靶器官并发症（血小板减少、肝脏氨基转移酶升高、血清肌酐升高、头痛或眼部症状、肺水肿）或累及胎儿[10,12]。先兆子痫与严重的母亲和胎儿并发症风险增加相关，如胎盘破裂、大脑损伤、子痫、凝血异常、肝功能异常甚至母亲死亡。终止妊娠是最有效的治疗手段，因此先兆子痫经常导致早产，以及由此造成的后果。7%～20%的 1 型糖尿病妊娠女性合并有先兆子痫，约是健康女性的 5 倍[1]。对于慢性高血压患者，在妊娠中更早并发先兆子痫，临床表现更重。

合并糖尿病的妊娠女性的正常血压

在合并高血压的妊娠糖尿病女性中，对于正常血压的了解与制订治疗靶目标值有关。甚至对于正常血压、正常白蛋白尿的女性，在妊娠期间，糖尿病本身就会导致血压轻度升高，但仍在正常范围内，见表 20.2[9,13]。

表 20.2 妊娠时健康女性对照组和 1 型糖尿病女性组的血压（mmHg）

作者	病例数	妊娠早期	妊娠中期	妊娠晚期	平均
Napoli 等[13]	对照 48 例	114/68	117/69	114/69	
	1 型糖尿病 71 例	118/71	116/72	115/72	
Nielsen 等[9]	对照 25 例				117/70
	1 型糖尿病 86 例				120/72

妊娠时高血压检测的实践

妊娠第一次随访时，应测量血压和尿白蛋白，应记录高血压、微量白蛋白尿或糖尿病肾病病史，以及降压治疗情况。患者可被分类为合并有高血压、微量白蛋白尿、糖尿病肾病或无上述疾病两种情况。此后，每次随访时应记录患者的血压。在妊娠期间，合并高血压的女性，家庭自测血压也许是有用的，但是 24h 动态血压监测通常是无用的。在每次随访时，正常血压、正常尿微量白蛋白女性应进行尿试纸检测确定是否存在蛋白尿；而对于合并高血压、微量白蛋白尿或糖尿病肾病的女性，在每次随访时，检测尿的白蛋白/肌酐值或蛋白/肌酐值来监测尿白蛋白排泄是否有进展。

血糖控制与高血压

在妊娠早期和晚期，先兆子痫与血糖控制不佳有关[14, 15]。因此，糖尿病患者妊娠时，妊娠前和妊娠期间的严格的血糖控制也许有助于降低高血压负担。推荐糖化血红蛋白的控制目标为6%以下[1]；哥本哈根的糖尿病妊娠妇女中心推荐糖化血红蛋白的控制目标为5.8%以下。由于先兆子痫的高发病率，推荐所有合并糖尿病的妊娠女性密切监测先兆子痫的发生发展。

妊娠时高血压的治疗原则

轻中度高血压

在临床试验中，对于合并慢性或妊娠期高血压的非糖尿病妊娠女性，血压轻-中度升高（140～160mmHg/90～110mmHg）的降压治疗是否获益未进行论证[16]。近来的一项综述显示降压治疗似乎降低了重度高血压的风险，但是并没有减少先兆子痫、新生儿死亡、早产和小于胎龄儿的发生率[17]。

妊娠时高血压治疗的国际指南[8, 18, 19]在起始治疗的时机和血压控制目标值等方面均存在差异，但是均高于全国委员会指南[8]制订的非妊娠高血压治疗的目标值。在合并糖尿病的女性中，广泛接受的目标值是140/90mmHg以下[3]，笔者所在中心推荐为135/85mmHg以下[9]。

重度高血压

大家普遍认同妊娠时重度高血压（血压≥160/110mmHg）需要治疗，因为母亲颅内出血的风险增加，并且治疗后降低了母亲死亡的风险[8, 11]。在高血压的治疗过程中避免出现低血压也是很重要的，因为胎盘自我血流调节功能是低下的，血压的降低也许会导致胎儿缺氧[1]。

糖尿病肾病和高血压

在合并糖尿病的妊娠女性中，糖尿病肾病的发病率是3%～15%，另外，5%～11%的糖尿病女性妊娠时会出现微量白蛋白尿[9, 20-22]。大多数文献来源于1型糖尿病的女性，但是合并2型糖尿病的女性的临床所见与此类似[20]。糖尿病肾病主要通过两种机制影响妊娠结局：①母亲重度高血压的发展要求终止妊娠，因此早产；②胎盘发育受损导致胎儿生长受限和死胎的风险。此外，在预约随访时如果血清肌酐水平在176μmol/L以上，妊娠期间母亲肾功能可以明显恶化[23-25]。在妊娠前或妊娠早期，1型糖尿病尿白蛋白排泄率正常的女性，先兆子痫的发病率是6%～10%；但是有微量白蛋白尿的女性升至42%，合并糖尿病肾病的女性升至64%[9]。一些临床医师认为在此之前已存在微量白蛋白尿或糖尿病肾病的女性，血压和白蛋白排泄的增加是由于肾脏疾病的恶化，而不是先兆子痫的发展。然而，由于大多数病例导致母亲出现其他靶器官疾病的表现如血小板减少或胎儿问题导致早产，因此在这些患者中，把血压的显著升高当作并发先兆子痫的征象是很重要的[22]。

在合并1型糖尿病和糖尿病肾病或微量白蛋白尿的女性中，导致先兆子痫发生发展的病理生理因素包括内皮功能紊乱、血管最大舒张能力受损[26]、肾素血管紧张素系统组分活化的增强[27]、心脏负荷过重[28]和抗血管生成因素[29-31]。上述大多数因素可由降压治疗调节。为防止血压和（或）尿白蛋白排泄的增加，在这些女性妊娠期间强化降压治疗从理论上来讲应该是有益处的。

所有合并1型糖尿病和2型糖尿病的女性在妊娠前和妊娠早期都应该进行微量白蛋白尿的筛查，以便发现微量白蛋白尿或显性糖尿病肾病。至少需要两次随机尿标本评估白蛋白/肌酐值或收集24h尿诊断微量白蛋白尿或糖尿病肾病。在所有合并糖尿病的妊娠女性中，达到并维持严格的血糖控制，密切监测先兆子痫的发生是很重要的。在潜在肾功能异常的女性中，尽早起始降压治疗是合理的，把白蛋白排泄水平作为治疗的关键[9, 32]。妊娠前即存在微量白蛋白尿或糖尿病肾病的女性，也许可以从降压治疗中获益，这其中是把尿白蛋白排泄水平作为靶目标而不考虑血压的水平[9, 32]。在妊娠前即存在微量白蛋白尿或糖尿病肾病的糖尿病女性中，我们团队的控制目标是尿白蛋白排泄水平在 300mg/24h 以下，血压控制在 135/85mmHg 以下[9]。在一项先前包含 1 型糖尿病女性的研究中，14%的尿白蛋白排泄正常的女性、50%的微量白蛋白尿的女性、100%的合并糖尿病肾病的女性在妊娠期间均接受了降压治疗[9]。与更早的研究系列[21, 24, 32]相比，早期、严格的降压治疗似乎与妊娠结局的改善和降低早产率相关[9]。在 2 型糖尿病女性中也观察到了类似的结果[20]。

总之，对于血清肌酐适度升高（＜124μmol/L）、尿蛋白不足 1g/24h 和妊娠早期血压正常的女性，如果积极进行降压治疗，妊娠结局相对来说是较好的。在妊娠期间，这些女性患者的肾功能通常没有恶化。相比之下，血清肌酐在 176μmol/L 以上、重度高血压或尿蛋白在 3g/24h 以上和（或）已合并心血管疾病与母亲和胎儿不良结局的高风险是相关的[33]。而且，妊娠早期血清肌酐在 176μmol/L 以上母亲的妊娠肾功能可能进一步恶化，甚至肾衰竭[34-36]。然而，这些长期的结果仅见于小样本研究[34, 36]。

糖尿病肾病女性的产科监护

约妊娠 20 周时这些女性应进行超声检查筛查先天畸形。在妊娠 23～24 周时，母亲子宫动脉血流下降与先兆子痫的风险增加相关，因此可以考虑进行血流的测量。在妊娠晚期，密切的产科监护包括反复对胎儿的生长发育情况进行超声检查和无应激试验，对于诊断并发症和计划分娩的时间及方式是非常重要的，目的是预防死胎和降低早产的发病率。

高血压和重度视网膜病变

妊娠时高血压与视网膜病变的恶化相关[37]。妊娠期间合适的降压治疗的目的是将血压稳定地控制在正常范围，此有可能对糖尿病女性的眼睛具有保护作用。然而，血压突然大幅度下降有可能导致视网膜病变恶化，因此降压治疗要逐渐强化。因此，对于合并糖尿病和高血压的女性应至少筛查两次威胁视力的糖尿病视网膜病变，特定病例需更频繁的筛查，这对于病情评估是很重要的。

妊娠前和妊娠期降压药的选择

在年轻的非妊娠糖尿病女性中，ACEI 和 ARB 均经常被用来治疗高血压和微量白蛋白尿。这些药物的致畸性和胎儿毒性已有报道[19,38,39]。最常见的畸形在心血管或中枢神经系统[38]。除了先天畸形，在服用这些降压药的女性中，也观察到了胎儿和新生儿的肾衰竭及羊水过少[19,39]。因此，推荐在计划妊娠前将降压药从肾素-血管紧张素受体阻滞剂转换为其他类型[1]。然而，在合并糖尿病肾病的女性中，有必要对每个病例进行个体化分析，尤其是要对直至确定妊娠才停用抑制肾素-血管紧张素系统的药物的获益与停用药物后妊娠前疾病恶化的风险进行权衡，特别是对于那些妊娠推迟导致肾素-血管紧张素受体阻滞剂撤退期延长的患者。

妊娠前，利尿剂是治疗原发性高血压的处方药物，考虑到它们的安全性，美国国家高血压教育项目妊娠高血压工作组认为这些药物在整个妊娠期间可以继续使用，可以尝试减少剂量或与其他降压药联用[8]。合并微量白蛋白尿的糖尿病女性或糖尿病肾病的高血压通常是盐敏感的。鉴于此，为了避免停药后反跳性高血压，继续应用这些药物是适合的[9,32]。然而，先兆子痫的女性应用利尿剂治疗也许降低了胎盘的血流，从而导致胎儿缺氧[17]。因此，应避免妊娠晚期开始利尿剂治疗，除非一些特定的病例，而且要对胎儿生长、羊水和多普勒血流谱进行密切的超声监测。

甲基多巴仍是妊娠期高血压治疗时最广泛应用的药物之一。它是作用于中枢的 α 肾上腺素能激动剂，基于有限的研究证实其没有致畸性，已用于妊娠高血压的治疗 40 多年。在一些试验中，妊娠女性已进行了其与安慰剂和其他降压药的对比[17]。它似乎对子宫-胎盘或胎儿血流动力学或胎儿健康没有不良影响。在一项子代的随访研究中，这些子代的年龄为 7 岁，胎儿时期暴露于甲基多巴环境中，这些孩子的智力和认知发育与对照组相似[17]。

β 受体阻滞剂已广泛用于妊娠，没有致畸的报道，但是妊娠时的长期使用也许导致了更低的出生体重[36]。静脉应用 β 受体阻滞剂与胎儿心动过缓和新生儿低血糖相关[36]。此外，在妊娠期间应用 β 受体阻滞剂降低了母亲低血糖的肾上腺症状,因此也许增加了糖尿病患者低血糖性意识障碍和重度低血糖的风险。然而,非选择性β受体阻滞剂拉贝洛尔具有血管α受体阻滞剂作用,在妊娠期间已被广泛地研究,也已被广泛接受用于合并糖尿病的妊娠女性。在美国,如果舒张压在105～110mmHg的水平,推荐静脉用肼屈嗪和拉贝洛尔[40]。

钙通道阻滞剂也较常用于治疗慢性高血压和先兆子痫。硝苯地平、维拉帕米或其他钙通道阻滞剂无致畸性。硝苯地平是被广泛研究的用于妊娠高血压治疗的钙通道阻滞剂,似乎没有引起子宫血流的下降[41]。短效硝苯地平应用时要谨慎,因为它可以导致血压急剧下降,这种血压的急剧下降与母亲发生心肌梗死及胎儿心动过缓和缺氧有关。硝苯地平缓释剂型没有这种不良反应,广泛用于妊娠时的高血压治疗[12];钙通道阻滞剂和其他降压药可以和硫酸镁一起使用,在先兆子痫时用硫酸镁预防癫痫发作,此没有增加严重不良反应的风险[41]。

肼屈嗪选择性地扩张小动脉平滑肌,在妊娠晚期,已广泛应用肼屈嗪的口服和静脉剂型治疗重度高血压,但是已被更少不良反应的药物替代[12,41]。然而,它可能在对其他降压药抵抗的女性患者中占有一席之地。其余的降压药极少用于妊娠。

降脂药如他汀类药物在妊娠时禁用,因为它们可能影响大脑和神经的发育[42]。

小剂量阿司匹林

小剂量阿司匹林(75～150mg)广泛用于合并糖尿病的非妊娠女性,以便降低心血管事件的发生率。在妊娠16周前开始小剂量使用阿司匹林可以降低高危女性先兆子痫的发病率[43]。虽然阿司匹林已广泛应用于妊娠早期,但是小剂量阿司匹林是否会引起畸形风险的轻度增加仍是一个存在争议的问题[44]。因此,在器官形成过程中应用小剂量阿司匹林不是常规的,而是要基于个体的风险-获益评估。如果一个女性在妊娠前由于心血管事件的风险增加已经应用了小剂量阿司匹林,在器官发生过程中可以继续应用。总之,我们在妊娠10周时起始小剂量阿司匹林治疗。在妊娠36～37周停用小剂量阿司匹林。

抗氧化剂

合并 1 型糖尿病的女性补充抗氧化剂（维生素 C 和维生素 E）似乎并没有降低先兆子痫的发病率[45]，因此不推荐使用。

母乳喂养期间的抗高血压药物

在甲基多巴治疗过程中母乳喂养是安全的。然而，不同于妊娠期间，由甲基多巴所致的乏力和产后抑郁状态恶化等不良反应，在母乳喂养期间，甲基多巴不是降压治疗的首选[46]。在母乳喂养期间，硝苯地平、拉贝洛尔、美托洛尔、卡托普利和依那普利都被认为是安全的[47-49]。

未来的方向

对于合并糖尿病和高血压的妊娠女性来说，需要随机对照试验来确定血压的治疗目标，尤其是要关注慢性高血压、微量白蛋白尿或糖尿病肾病的患者。在妊娠期间也需要试验对比不同类型降压药（如甲基多巴对比钙通道阻滞剂）有益的影响和不良反应。

选择题

1. 在妊娠期间，降压药为禁忌的是（　　　）（选两个）
   A. 甲基多巴
   B. β 肾上腺素能受体阻滞剂（如拉贝洛尔）
   C. 血管紧张素转换酶抑制剂
   D. 血管紧张素受体阻滞剂
   E. 钙通道阻滞剂（如缓释硝苯地平）
   F. 以上皆不是

正确答案是 C 和 D。

2. 糖尿病妊娠与正常妊娠相比，下面疾病更常见的是（ ）
   A. 妊娠高血压
   B. 慢性高血压
   C. 先兆子痫
   D. 并发先兆子痫
   E. 以上皆是

正确答案是 E。

3. 下面陈述正确的是（ ）
   A. 先兆子痫临床上表现为妊娠 20 周后出现高血压伴随高血糖
   B. 妊娠时先兆子痫的发生发展与血糖控制不佳有关
   C. 先兆子痫很少导致早产
   D. 以上皆对

正确答案是 B。

（张雪冰　译，朱海清　校）

参 考 文 献

1. Kitzmiller JL, Block JM, Brown FM, Catalano PM, Conway DL, Coustan DR, et al. Managing preexisting diabetes for pregnancy: summary of evidence and consensus recommendations for care. Diabetes Care 2008;31(5):1060–1079.

2. Norgaard K, Feldt-Rasmussen B, Borch-Johnsen K, Saelan H, Deckert T. Prevalence of hypertension in type 1 (insulin-dependent) diabetes mellitus. Diabetologia 1990;33(7):407–410.

3. Cundy T, Slee F, Gamble G, Neale L. Hypertensive disorders of pregnancy in women with type 1 and type 2 diabetes. Diabetic Med 2002;19:482–489.

4. Standards of medical care in diabetes – summary of revisions. Diabetes Care 2017;38(Suppl):S4.

5. Efficacy of atenolol and captopril in reducing risk of macrovascular and microvascular complications in type 2 diabetes: UKPDS 39. UK Prospective Diabetes Study Group. BMJ 1998;317(7160):713–720.

6. Hansson L, Zanchetti A, Carruthers SG, Dahlof B, Elmfeldt D, Julius S, et al. Effects of intensive blood-pressure lowering and low-dose aspirin in patients with hypertension: principal results of the Hypertension Optimal Treatment (HOT) randomised trial. HOT Study Group. Lancet 1998;351(9118):1755–1762.

7. Mathiesen ER, Hommel E, Hansen HP, Parving H-H. Preservation of normal GFR with long term captopril treatment in normotensive IDDM patients with microalbuminuria. BMJ 1999;319:24–25.

8. Report of the National High Blood Pressure Education Program Working Group on High Blood Pressure in Pregnancy. Am J Obstet Gynecol 2000;183(1):S1–S22.

9. Nielsen LR, Damm P, Mathiesen ER. Improved pregnancy outcome in type 1 diabetic women with microalbuminuria or diabetic nephropathy: effect of intensified antihypertensive therapy? Diabetes Care 2009;32(1):38–44.

10. American College of Obstetrics and Gynecology. Recommendationa on hypertenion in pregnancy. http://www.acog.org/Resources-And-Publications/

Task-Force-and-Work-Group-Reports/Hypertension-in-Pregnancy

11 Sibai BM. Chronic hypertension in pregnancy. Obstet Gynecol 2002;100(2):369-377.

12 Magee LA, Abalos E, Dadelszen Pv, Sibai B, Easterling T, Walkinshaw S, for the CHIPS study group. How to manage hypertension in pregnancy effectively. Brit J Clin Pharmacol 2011;72(3):394–401.

13 Napoli A, Sabbatini A, Di BN, Marceca M, Colatrella A, Fallucca F. Twenty-four-hour blood pressure monitoring in normoalbuminuric normotensive type 1 diabetic women during pregnancy. J Diabetes Complications 2003;17(5):292-296.

14 Hiilesmaa V, Suhonen L, Teramo K. Glycaemic control is associated with pre-eclampsia but not with pregnancy-induced hypertension in women with type I diabetes mellitus. Diabetologia 2000;43(12):1534-1539.

15 Maresh MJ, Holmes VA, Patterson CC, Young IS, Pearson DW, Walker JD, et al. Glycemic targets in the second and third trimester of pregnancy for women with type 1 diabetes. Diabetes Care 2015;38(1):34-42.

16 Magee LA, von DP, Rey E, Ross S, Asztalos E, Murphy KE, et al. Less-tight versus tight control of hypertension in pregnancy. N Engl J Med 2015;372(5):407-417.

17 Abalos E, Duley L, Steyn DW, Henderson-Smart DJ. Antihypertensive drug therapy for mild to moderate hypertension during pregnancy. Cochrane Database Syst Rev 2001;(2):CD002252.

18 Helewa ME, Burrows RF, Smith J, Williams K, Brain P, Rabkin SW. Report of the Canadian Hypertension Society Consensus Conference: 1. Definitions, evaluation and classification of hypertensive disorders in pregnancy. CMAJ 1997;157(6):715-725.

19 Brown MA, Hague WM, Higgins J, Lowe S, McCowan L, Oats J, et al. The detection, investigation and management of hypertension in pregnancy: full consensus statement. Aust N Z J Obstet Gynaecol 2000;40(2):139-155.

20 Damm JA, Asbjornsdottir B, Callesen NF, Mathiesen JM, Ringholm L, Pedersen BW, et al. Diabetic nephropathy and microalbuminuria in pregnant women with type 1 and type 2 diabetes: prevalence, antihypertensive strategy, and pregnancy outcome. Diabetes Care 2013;36(11):3489-3494.

21 Ekbom P, Damm P, Feldt-Rasmussen B, Feldt-Rasmussen U, Molvig J, Mathiesen ER. Pregnancy outcome in type 1 diabetic women with microalbuminuria. Diabetes Care 2001;24(10):1739-1744.

22 Klemetti MM, Laivuori H, Tikkanen M, Nuutila M, Hiilesmaa V, Teramo K. Obstetric and perinatal outcome in type 1 diabetes patients with diabetic nephropathy during 1988-2011. Diabetologia 2015;58(4):678-686.

23 Biesenbach G, Stoger H, Zazgornik J. Influence of pregnancy on progression of diabetic nephropathy and subsequent requirement of renal replacement therapy in female type I diabetic patients with impaired renal function. Nephrol Dial Transplant 1992;7(2):105-109.

24 Carr DB, Koontz GL, Gardella C, Holing EV, Brateng DA, Brown ZA, et al. Diabetic nephropathy in pregnancy: suboptimal hypertensive control associated with preterm delivery. Am J Hypertens 2006;19(5):513-519.

25 Purdy LP, Hantsch CE, Molitch ME, Metzger BE, Phelps RL, Dooley SL, et al. Effect of pregnancy on renal function in patients with moderate-to-severe diabetic renal insufficiency. Diabetes Care 1996;19(10):1067-1074.

26 Clausen P, Ekbom P, Damm P, Feldt-Rasmussen U, Nielsen B, Mathiesen ER, et al. Signs of maternal vascular dysfunction precede preeclampsia in women with type 1 diabetes. J Diabetes Complications 2007;21(5):288-293.

27 Ringholm L, Pedersen-Bjergaard U, Thorsteinsson B, Boomsma F, Damm P, Mathiesen ER. A high concentration of

prorenin in early pregnancy is associated with development of pre-eclampsia in women with type 1 diabetes. Diabetologia 2011;54(7):1615–1619.
28 Ringholm L, Pedersen-Bjergaard U, Thorsteinsson B, Boomsma F, Damm P, Mathiesen ER. Atrial Natriuretic Peptide (ANP) in early pregnancy is associated with development of preeclampsia in type 1 diabetes. Diabetes Res Clin Pract 2011;93(3):e106–e109.
29 Holmes VA, Young IS, Patterson CC, Maresh MJ, Pearson DW, Walker JD, et al. The role of angiogenic and antiangiogenic factors in the second trimester in the prediction of preeclampsia in pregnant women with type 1 diabetes. Diabetes Care 2013;36(11):3671–3677.
30 Maynard SE, Karumanchi SA. Angiogenic factors and preeclampsia. Semin Nephrol 2011;31(1):33–46.
31 Yu Y, Jenkins AJ, Nankervis AJ, Hanssen KF, Scholz H, Henriksen T, et al. Anti-angiogenic factors and pre-eclampsia in type 1 diabetic women. Diabetologia 2009;52(1):160–168.
32 Nielsen LR, Muller C, Damm P, Mathiesen ER. Reduced prevalence of early preterm delivery in women with Type 1 diabetes and microalbuminuria – possible effect of early antihypertensive treatment during pregnancy. Diabet Med 2006;23(4):426–431.
33 Sibai. Diabetic Nephropathy in Pregnancy: A Practical Manual of Diabetes in Pregnancy. Blackwell Publishing: Oxford, 2008, 153–156.
34 Cooper WO, Hernandez-Diaz S, Arbogast PG, Dudley JA, Dyer S, Gideon PS, et al. Major congenital malformations after first-trimester exposure to ACE inhibitors. N Engl J Med 2006;354(23):2443–2451.
35 Hod M, van Dijk DJ, Karp M, Weintraub N, Rabinerson D, Bar J, et al. Diabetic nephropathy and pregnancy: the effect of ACE inhibitors prior to pregnancy on fetomaternal outcome. Nephrol Dial Transplant 1995;10(12):2328–2333.
36 Magee LA, Duley L. Oral beta-blockers for mild to moderate hypertension during pregnancy. Cochrane Database Syst Rev 2000;(4):CD002863.
37 Vestgaard M, Ringholm L, Laugesen CS, Rasmussen KL, Damm P, Mathiesen ER. Pregnancy-induced sight-threatening diabetic retinopathy in women with Type 1 diabetes. Diabet Med 2010;27(4):431–435.
38 Alwan S, Polifka JE, Friedman JM. Angiotensin II receptor antagonist treatment during pregnancy. Birth Defects Res A Clin Mol Teratol 2005;73(2):123–130.
39 Shotan A, Widerhorn J, Hurst A, Elkayam U. Risks of angiotensin-converting enzyme inhibition during pregnancy: experimental and clinical evidence, potential mechanisms, and recommendations for use. Am J Med 1994;96(5):451–456.
40 American College of Obstetricians and Gynecologists practice bulletin. Diagnosis and management of preeclampsia and eclampsia. Number 33, January 2002. American College of Obstetricians and Gynecologists. Int J Gynaecol Obstet 2002;77(1):67–75.
41 Podymow T, August P. Hypertension in pregnancy. Adv Chronic Kidney Dis 2007;14(2):178–190.
42 Kazmin A, Garcia-Bournissen F, Koren G. Risks of statin use during pregnancy: a systematic review. J Obstet Gynaecol Can 2007;29(11):906–908.
43 Ruano R, Fontes RS, Zugaib M. Prevention of preeclampsia with low-dose aspirin – a systematic review and meta-analysis of the main randomized controlled trials. Clinics (Sao Paulo) 2005;60(5):407–414.
44 Norgard B, Puho E, Czeizel AE, Skriver MV, Sorensen HT. Aspirin use during early pregnancy and the risk of congenital abnormalities: a population-based case-control study. Am J Obstet Gynecol 2005;192(3):922–923.
45 McCance DR, Holmes VA, Maresh MJ, Patterson CC, Walker JD, Pearson DW, et al. Vitamins C and E for prevention of pre-eclampsia in women with type 1

46 Ringholm L, Mathiesen ER, Kelstrup L, Damm P. Managing type 1 diabetes mellitus in pregnancy – from planning to breastfeeding. Nat Rev Endocrinol 2012;8(11):659–667.
47 Devlin RG, Fleiss PM. Captopril in human blood and breast milk. J Clin Pharmacol 1981;21(2):110–113.
48 Rush JE, Snyder DL, Barrish A, Hichens M. Comment on Huttunen K, Gronhagen-Riska C and Fyhrquist F, 1989. Enalapril treatment of a nursing mother with slightly impaired renal function: Clin Nephrol 31: 278. Clin Nephrol 1991;35(5):234.
49 American Academy of Pediatrics Committee on Drugs. The transfer of drugs and other chemicals into human milk. Pediatrics 1994;93(1):137–150.

第二十一章　妊娠糖尿病视网膜病变

Jesia Hasan[1] and Emily Y. Chew[2]

1 Department of Ophthalmology，University of Montreal，Montreal，Canada
2 National Eye Institute of National Institutes of Health，Bethesda，Maryland，USA

实践要点

- 在年轻人和中年人群中，糖尿病微血管并发症糖尿病视网膜病变仍是导致后天失明的主要原因之一。
- 妊娠、激素、血流动力学、代谢和免疫的改变是引发糖尿病性视网膜病变的危险因素。
- 妊娠期视网膜病变加速的病因尚不清楚，尽管提出的机制涉及快速血糖控制、改变血流动力学特性和免疫炎症成分。
- 如果患者在妊娠前和妊娠期间有最佳的系统性眼部管理，那么导致视力丧失的糖尿病性视网膜病变在妊娠期加重是可以预防的。
- 在妊娠期应该加强眼部检查，之后至少每3个月复查1次（通常取决于眼科医师，根据视网膜病变基线状态和之前的糖尿病性视网膜病变的病史）。

问题

- 因为糖尿病患者不报告任何视觉症状，所以未能向妊娠妇女推荐眼科筛查。糖尿病妊娠妇女虽然视力良好，但糖尿病视网膜病变仍可发生。
- 未能向糖尿病女性推荐提前进行眼科筛查。妊娠前稳定糖尿病视网膜病变可减缓妊娠期进展。

病　例

一位27岁的妇女，有20年1型糖尿病病史，在妊娠期间接受眼科检查。在妊娠的前3个月，她的双眼视力为20/20，并在散瞳检查中发现轻微的非增生性糖尿病视网膜病变（图21.1A）。在加强代谢控制后，妊娠早期HbA1C由8.6%降至7.0%。妊娠中期检查时双眼视力为20/25，视网膜病变进展为重度非增生性糖尿病视网膜病变（图21.1B）。妊娠晚期，由于黄斑水肿明显，右眼视力下降至20/60，左眼视力下降至20/80（图21.1C）。激光治疗后，黄斑水肿消退，双眼视力部分恢复至20/40。

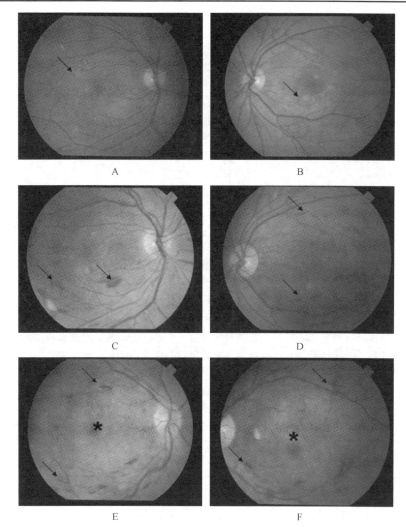

图 21.1 妊娠早期（A）右眼和（B）左眼散瞳检查偶见视网膜腔内出血（箭头所示），符合最小限度的非增生性糖尿病视网膜病变。C、D. 在进行快速血糖控制后，患者出现越来越多的视网膜内出血（箭头所示），妊娠中期严重非增殖性糖尿病视网膜病变。E、F. 在妊娠晚期，检查显示视网膜病变进一步发展（箭头所示），并发展为显著的黄斑水肿（*所示）

> **本章要回答的问题**
> - 什么是妊娠期间的视网膜病变进展的危险因素及公认的机制?
> - 强化血糖控制与视网膜病变进展相关吗?这是暂时现象吗?
> - 妊娠期间应该多久检查一次视力?
> - 妊娠期间该如何治疗威胁视力的糖尿病性视网膜病变?
>
> 首先,我们需简要回顾糖尿病视网膜病变的一般情况,然后重点关注妊娠的独特状态如何影响视网膜病变的进展。

概述

糖尿病视网膜病变基线患病率

糖尿病视网膜病变是糖尿病的微血管并发症,是中青年人获得性失明的主要原因[1]。目前估计美国视网膜病变和威胁视力的视网膜病变的一般人群患病率分别为 3.4%(410 万人)和 0.75%(89.9 万人)[2]。这些汇总的数据几乎全部集中在 2 型糖尿病患者人群中。一项关于 1 型糖尿病的流行病学研究估计,视网膜病变和威胁视力的视网膜病变的患病率分别为每 300 名年龄在 18 岁及以上的患者中有 1 人,每 600 名患者中有 1 人[3]。确切地说,估计美国 30 岁前诊断出 1 型糖尿病的人有 88.9 万人,其中 76.7 万人(86.3%)患有糖尿病视网膜病变和 37.6 万人(42.3%)有威胁视力的视网膜病变[3]。这些数据令人担忧,因为糖尿病的患病率在不断上升[1]。

妊娠是视网膜病变恶化的危险因素

妊娠时患者的激素、血流动力学、代谢和免疫变化是导致糖尿病视网膜病变加速发展的危险因素。而具有里程碑意义的研究则集中于 1 型糖尿病妊娠妇女视网膜病变的恶化[4-6],这些研究结果可以推及 2 型糖尿病妊娠妇女,两组视网膜病变本质相似。然而,妊娠糖尿病不是妊娠期视网膜病变发展的危险因素,但可能提示继发糖尿病的遗传风险[7]。

糖尿病视网膜病变分类综述

1型和2型糖尿病的视网膜病变一般分为非增生性或增生性（表21.1）。非增生性糖尿病视网膜病变（NPDR）仅发生于视网膜管微血管病变，如微动脉瘤和视网膜出血（图21.2）。在晚期NPDR中，视网膜进行性毛细血管无灌注可能发展并导致缺血增加，从而导致更严重的增殖期。增生性糖尿病视网膜病变（图21.3）的特征是视网膜表面或视盘上的新血管会出血，并导致玻璃体积血、纤维化瘢痕和牵拉性视网

表21.1 糖尿病视网膜病变的分类

分类	病变表现
无视网膜病变	无损害表现
非增生性视网膜病变	仅视网膜内微血管改变
轻度	轻度微动脉瘤及视网膜内出血
中度	中度微动脉瘤和视网膜内出血
重度	有下列特征之一（4：2：1规则）
	·视网膜内出血出现在所有4个象限
	·在两个或两个以上的象限出现静脉瘤
	·中度视网膜内微血管异常（IRMA）至少一个象限
增生性视网膜病变	视网膜表面新生血管形成

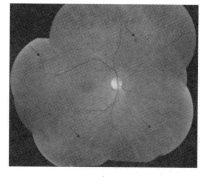 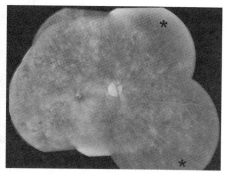

A　　　　　　　　　　　　　　B

图21.2　A. 右眼眼底照片显示4个象限（箭头所示）均有多处视网膜内出血，符合严重的非增生性糖尿病视网膜病变；B. 荧光素造影显示视网膜周围未灌注斑块（*所示），提示视网膜非增生改变的严重程度

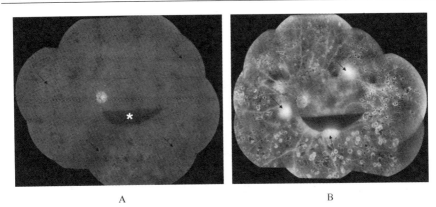

图 21.3　A. 左眼眼底照片显示视网膜前出血覆盖黄斑（*所示）。视网膜周边有许多激光光凝治疗后瘢痕（箭头所示），提示以前曾治疗过增殖性糖尿病视网膜病变；B. 荧光血管造影显示斑块呈明亮的强荧光（箭头所示）对应着增生性糖尿病视网膜病变的新生血管渗漏区域

膜脱离等视觉威胁并发症。无论是非增生性糖尿病视网膜病变还是增生性糖尿病视网膜病变，视网膜血管通透性的增加都会导致液体在视网膜中央区域积聚，而这里是产生视力的主要区域。这种视网膜增厚称为黄斑水肿（图 21.4），是糖尿病患者失明的主要原因。

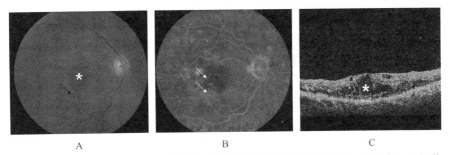

图 21.4　A. 右眼眼底照片可见黄斑液（*所示）和脂质（箭头所示），与临床明显的黄斑水肿一致。B. 荧光素血管造影显示多个渗漏的小动脉瘤（箭头所示）。C. 光学相干断层扫描证实黄斑内存在囊性液体改变（*所示）

糖尿病视网膜病变进展的危险因素

糖尿病视网膜病变是微血管并发症，是终末器官对系统性疾病的反

映。因此，伴随的系统性问题影响糖尿病视网膜病变的发展和进展[8]。深入了解糖尿病性视网膜病变是探讨糖尿病妊娠妇女视网膜病变的必要条件。在大规模的流行病学研究中，发现了许多危险因素。虽然它们在妊娠的动态生理状态中的作用是独特的，但它们与妊娠和非妊娠状态都相关。

血糖控制

慢性高血糖可引起糖尿病微血管并发症的一系列事件。糖尿病控制和并发症试验（DCCT）与英国前瞻性糖尿病研究（UKPDS）都证明了强化血糖控制在降低视网膜病变进展方面的有益作用。

糖尿病控制和并发症试验（DCCT）

DCCT 试验是一项随机、多中心、前瞻性的试验，旨在确定以接近正常糖化血红蛋白水平为目标的强化血糖控制是否会减缓 1 型糖尿病并发症的发展。1441 名参与者被随机分配到常规或强化治疗的血糖控制组中，平均随访 6.5 年[9-11]。强化治疗组平均 HbA1c 为 7.2%，常规对照组平均 HbA1c 为 9.1%。DCCT 研究中的强化治疗降低了 1 型糖尿病患者糖尿病视网膜病变的发生和发展。强化治疗的不良反应之一是视网膜病变的初期恶化；然而，18 个月后情况发生了逆转。没有任何可见视网膜病变的患者加入 DCCT 时，与标准治疗组相比，强化治疗组视网膜病变 3 年的风险降低了 75%。严格控制血糖对现有视网膜病变患者的益处很明显。与对照组相比，视网膜病变的进展率降低了 50%。当将 DCCT 结果按 Hb1Ac 水平分层时，结果为每减少 10% 的 Hb1Ac（如从 8% 降至 7.2%），视网膜病变进展的风险就会降低 35%～40%。

英国前瞻性糖尿病研究（UKPDS）

UKPDS 是对 2 型糖尿病患者进行的规模最大、时间最长的研究，对 3867 例新诊断的糖尿病患者进行了常规和强化血糖管理对糖尿病并发症的影响评估[12]。本研究证实，严格控制血糖对糖尿病视网膜病变的发生和发展的有益作用也适用于 2 型糖尿病。具体来说，与常规治疗组相比，强化治疗组的 UKPDS 显示"任何与糖尿病相关的微血管终点"的风险降低了 25%,,包括需要视网膜光凝术治疗。在 UKPDS 中,HbA1c 每降低一个百分点(如 9%到 8%),微血管并发症的风险就会降低 35%。同样,2 型糖尿病控制糖尿病心血管风险的作用(ACCORD)的研究显示,在强化血糖控制下,糖尿病视网膜病变进展的风险降低了 1/3。

伴发高血压

多项研究表明,尽管存在相互矛盾的数据,但糖尿病伴发高血压的患者糖尿病视网膜病变的发展和进展风险增加。高血压被认为是通过内皮细胞的机械拉伸加重糖尿病视网膜病变,导致血管内皮细胞增加生长因子(VEGF)释放[13]。

威斯康星糖尿病视网膜病变流行病学研究(WESDR)

WESDR 是一项基于 14 年人群的队列研究,评估了 30 岁前诊断的 634 名 1 型糖尿病患者中糖尿病视网膜病变的患病率和风险[14]。除了基线时 HbA1c 升高和视网膜病变加重外,高血压被证明是增生性糖尿病视网膜病变发展的危险因素之一。此外,参与者中 1/4 收缩压和舒张压均比较低的患者同 1/4 收缩压和舒张压均比较高的患者相比,血压偏低组进展为增生性糖尿病视网膜病变的比率明显较低。这些发现与糖化血红蛋白无关[14]。

英国前瞻性糖尿病研究

包含 3867 名 2 型糖尿病受试者的研究中,评估 1148 名高血压患者,758 名患者随机分配到严格控制血压组(ACEI 或 β 受体阻滞剂)和 390 名患者分配到非严格控制组,随访时间长达 8.4 年[12]。严格控制血压为低于 150/85mmHg。严格控制组相对非严格控制组有 34%的患者减少了两步视网膜病变的进展,中度视力丧失的风险减少 47%(≥15 个字母)。视力数据虽然没有控制糖化血红蛋白,但表明严格的血压控制降低了糖尿病黄斑水肿的风险,而黄斑水肿是 2 型糖尿病患者失明的主要原因。

糖尿病患者适当血压控制（ABCD）试验

ABCD 试验也显示了严格控制血压降低视网膜病变的风险[15-17]。在 480 例 2 型糖尿病患者的正常血压队列中，随机分配到强化或中度降压治疗组的患者的糖化血红蛋白水平无显著差异。在过去 4 年的随访中，平均血压为 128/75mmHg 为严格控制组，中度组平均血压水平为 137/81mmHg[15]。在 5 年的随访期内，强化组视网膜病变进展率为 34%，而中度对照组为 46%，$P=0.019$。

血脂水平升高

在 WESDR 和早期治疗糖尿病视网膜病变的研究（ETDRS）中均发现血脂升高与糖尿病视网膜病变有关。血脂水平升高与视网膜硬性渗出的严重程度增加有关[18, 19]。ETDRS 患者血清总胆固醇为 6.21mmol/L（240mg/dl）或以上的人，有硬渗出物的可能性是胆固醇低于 5.17mmol/L（200mg/dl）的人的两倍。低密度脂蛋白（LDL）水平与血清总胆固醇水平相当，与低于 3.36mmol/L（130mg/dl）的患者相比，血清 LDL 水平为 4.14mmol/L（160mg/dl）或更高的患者发生硬性渗出物的风险几乎是后者的两倍。硬性渗出物很重要，因为它们在基线时的严重程度与 ETDRS 的视力下降有关，这种视力下降与黄斑水肿无关。事实上，ETDRS 糖尿病黄斑水肿患者视网膜下纤维化对视力发展的最大危险因素是存在严重的硬性渗出物[20]。264 只眼睛在基线或随访期间有多个硬性渗出物，其中 30.7% 的眼睛发生视网膜下纤维化。相比之下，在 5498 只眼睛中，有临床意义的黄斑水肿只占 0.05%，但无严重硬性渗出物[20]。

随机对照试验表明，血脂可能在糖尿病视网膜病变的发病机制中发挥重要作用，非诺贝特（可降低三酰甘油水平，增加高密度脂蛋白含量）可降低糖尿病视网膜病变进展的风险及激光光凝固的需要[21, 22]。在 ACCORD 研究中，非诺贝特疗法与安慰剂相比降低了糖尿病视网膜病变的进展率（调整优势比：0.60；95%CI：0.42～0.87；$P=0.006$）[21]。在实地研究中，非诺贝特组视网膜病变、黄斑水肿或激光治疗的复合终点显著低于安慰剂组（危险比：0.66；95%CI：0.47～0.94；$P=0.022$）[22]。

在妊娠期间糖尿病视网膜病变进展的危险因素

早期病例对照研究显示，妊娠是糖尿病视网膜病变进展的危险因素[23, 24]，尽管这些变化往往在产后进展较快[23]。一些更大的研究已经证实，妊娠期间糖尿病视网膜病变的短暂进展不会增加长期风险[5, 6]。

视网膜病变的进展与 1 型糖尿病的关系比 2 型糖尿病更密切[25]。视网膜病变加速的机制尚不清楚，目前多种多样的现有理论开始考虑与妊娠期间激素、血流动力学、代谢和免疫学的变化有关。已报道的糖尿病妊娠妇女视网膜病变进展的危险因素包括血糖控制、高血压和高脂血症。

血糖控制

妊娠早期糖尿病（DIEP）研究

DIEP 研究是前瞻性队列研究，纳入 155 名糖尿病妇女从围产期观察到产后 1 个月[4]。在 10.3% 的没有视网膜病变的患者中观察到视网膜病变的发展；在 21.1% 的微动脉瘤，18.8% 的轻度 NPDR 患者中观察到视网膜病变进展。然而在基线时，中度至重度 NPDR 患者进展最大，其中 54.8% 的患者视网膜病变恶化。增生性糖尿病视网膜病变在轻度和重度糖尿病患者中占 6.3% 和 29%。与早期的研究不同[23]，DIEP 发现代谢控制的变化在预测视网膜病变加速方面比糖尿病持续时间更重要。在本研究中，妊娠前血糖控制最差，妊娠前 3 个月 HbA1c 水平下降幅度最大的女性视网膜病变进展风险较高。虽然 DIEP 的研究并没有阐明视网膜病变恶化的机制，但它是一种有效的治疗方法，提示优化妊娠前代谢控制以降低视网膜病变进展风险的临床重要性。

糖尿病控制和并发症研究（DCCT 研究）

DCCT 的一项辅助研究评估了妊娠在糖尿病视网膜病变进展中的作用[5]。与 DIEP 的研究类似，DCCT 也强调了妊娠前最佳的血糖控制。在这项对 680 名女性糖尿病患者的研究中，有 180 名女性妊娠。与 500 名未妊娠的研究参与者相比，这些妊娠妇女视网膜病变进展的风险更高。此外，在传统治疗组中，妊娠前没有严格控制的妇女患视网膜病变的风险是正常对照组的 2.48 倍。在强化治疗组中，与未妊娠的妇女相比，妊娠前有更严格控制的妇女在妊娠期间视网膜病变进展的风险只有 1.63 倍（95%CI：1.01～2.64）。因此，在受孕前严格控制代谢是最理想的。

高血压

妊娠期高血压是视网膜病变进展的危险因素之一。一项对 154 名糖尿病妇女的前瞻性研究发现，55%的慢性或妊娠期高血压妇女有视网膜病变进展，相比之下，只有 25%的没有高血压的妊娠糖尿病妇女有视网膜进展，$P<0.05$[26]。另一项前瞻性研究表明，舒张压升高是视网膜病变进展的危险因素，尽管同血糖控制相比危险性没有那么大[24]。

血脂

虽然在一般糖尿病研究中，血脂异常与黄斑渗出物增多有关，黄斑渗出物增多可导致视网膜下纤维化并发症发生，威胁视力[18, 19]，但是血脂升高在妊娠糖尿病妇女中的作用尚未得到广泛研究。然而，由于脂质控制对健康的普遍益处，建议在妊娠前优化胆固醇和脂质，因为这可以降低黄斑渗出物的风险。

妊娠期糖尿病视网膜病变进展的可能机制

代谢理论

简单地说，在妊娠期间血糖迅速正常化会加速糖尿病视网膜病变发生。妊娠是一种长期尝试积极控制血糖的状态[4, 9, 26]。快速血糖控制导致视网膜病变的短暂恶化的概念以前在妊娠期外就已经被注意到了[27-29]。一些研究表明，即使在调整了 HbA1c 水平后，妊娠本身也可能是视网膜病变进展的一个危险因素，但在妊娠初期实施严格控制的常见做法令我们不能够断定妊娠本身就是视网膜病变加速的原因[24]。

激素理论

激素的变化也被怀疑是糖尿病视网膜病变恶化的原因。妊娠期黄体酮的特征性升高可上调眼内 VEGF[30]，导致视网膜毛细血管渗漏增加和新生血管形成。此外，胎盘激素会产生一种生理上适应性的胰岛素抵抗状态，以确保母体葡萄糖能充分供应给胎儿，以优化宫内生长。其中一个关键因素是人胎盘生长激素，它似乎可以调节胎盘的生长及母体胰岛素样生长因子-1（IGF1）水平。和人胎盘生长因子一样，IGF1 在妊娠 20 周后会增加。转基因小鼠研究表明，人类胎盘生长激素可导致胰岛素抵抗状态，尽管确切机制尚不清楚[31]。此外，血清 IGF1 水平升高可能通过支持 VEGF 诱导内皮细胞增殖促进视网膜新生血管形成[32]。在一项对 88 名 1 型糖尿病患者进展的观察研究中发现，循环 IGF1 水平升高同妊娠期糖尿病视网膜病变的进展相关[33]。

血流动力学理论

妊娠时血容量和心输出量的增加与周围血管阻力降低有关[31]。这种血流增加及糖尿病患者视网膜血管自身调节反应受损，可能通过增加血管内皮细胞和离开毛细血管的液体净增加，导致视网膜毛细血管血流过度活跃[34]。一些研究表明，与非糖尿病妊娠妇女相比，所有糖尿病妊娠妇女的视网膜循环和高灌注都有所增加[35]，而其他人只有在妊娠时[34]才显示视网膜血流量增加的前驱症状[36]。另一项小型研究显示，与非糖尿病妊娠妇女相比，糖尿病妊娠妇女视网膜容积血流量下降，视网膜静脉直径下降更为严重[37]。这些研究的矛盾结果可能与不同的患者群体或视网膜循环评估技术有关。也有学者提出，血糖控制的突然改善可能导致视网膜血流减少，继发性缺氧和视网膜病变可能恶化[25]。

免疫炎症理论

糖尿病视网膜病变被认为是一种低级别炎症性疾病，白细胞黏附在视网膜血管上可能导致视网膜血管功能障碍[38, 39]。在妊娠期间发展成妊娠糖尿病患者的炎症增加[40]。前瞻性研究母体细胞因子水平与糖尿病视网膜病变的关系表明，尽管促炎因子 IL-6、C 反应蛋白和血管细胞黏附分子 1 在妊娠糖尿病患者和非糖尿病患者中水平相当，但 C 反应蛋白水平在视网膜病变进展和血糖控制欠佳的妊娠妇女体内水平明显高于稳定的视网膜病变及更严格的代谢控制的妊娠妇女。另一项研究检测了妊娠期子宫内膜腺体分泌的抗炎血清标志物糖皮质激素，发现低水平的糖皮质激素与妊娠糖尿病妇女视网膜病变的进展有关[41]。

妊娠前、妊娠中、妊娠后视网膜病变的临床处理

妊娠前的系统性和眼部管理对于降低妊娠期和产后视网膜病变进展的风险至关重要。

系统管理

从系统的角度来说，妊娠前的最佳代谢控制是至关重要的。妊娠前逐渐严格控制避免了妊娠期伴随视网膜病变进展的 HbA1c 迅速下降。

此外，应控制高血压和血脂升高，以减少视网膜病变的风险。这样的处理不仅降低了视网膜病变进展的风险，而且对母亲和胎儿的全身健康也很重要。

扩张性检查的目视管理和安排

所有糖尿病妇女在妊娠前和妊娠前 3 个月都应该接受眼科医师或验光师的扩张性眼科检查。根据个别发现，额外的成像如视网膜摄影、光相干断层摄影和荧光血管摄影可由审查员自行决定。美国眼科学会制定的 1 型和 2 型糖尿病妊娠妇女视网膜护理的官方指南如下[42]：

1. 计划妊娠的糖尿病患者应在妊娠前进行眼科检查。
2. 妊娠早期应重复眼部检查，并根据视网膜病变的严重程度进行随访评估。

（1）轻度或中度 NPDR，无视网膜病变：每 3～12 个月随访一次。

（2）严重 NPDR 或更严重：每 1~3 个月随访一次。

3. 妊娠糖尿病患者的视网膜病变风险不增加，不需要额外的眼科检查。

NICE 也制定了指导糖尿病妊娠妇女眼科治疗的指导方针，具体如下[43, 44]：

1. 糖尿病前期的妊娠妇女在第一次产前门诊预约后，如果第一次评估正常，应在第 28 周再次进行视网膜评估，并使用带有散瞳的数字成像技术。

2. 如果有糖尿病视网膜病变，应在第 16~20 周进行额外的视网膜评估。

3. 妊娠期诊断为增生性糖尿病视网膜病变的妇女，当孩子出生后应至少进行 6 个月的眼科随访。

4. 妊娠早期糖化血红蛋白含量高的女性，糖尿病视网膜病变不应被认为是血糖控制优化的禁忌证。

5. 糖尿病视网膜病变不应被认为是经阴道分娩的禁忌证。

这些指南仅仅是对实践模式的一般性建议，而不是对个别患者的护理。因此，后续的随访检查要看视网膜的表现而异，但通常在妊娠期间每 3 个月进行一次。考虑到妊娠后期激素的变化会加剧或诱发视网膜病变，即使没有视网膜病变出现在第 1 或第 2、3 个月，第 3 个月妊娠检查也是必要的。有时，患者需要荧光血管造影来评估视网膜的灌注状态和血管模式。虽然荧光素染料在妊娠期间是安全使用的[7]，但它会透过胎盘，大多数视网膜专家依赖扩张型检查和无创成像/摄影的结果来确定视网膜病变的阶段，指导患者的治疗。例如，临床表现如出血增加、静脉畸形、视网膜内微血管异常表明病情恶化到严重的 NPDR 阶段，而明显的视网膜表面或视神经的新生血管证实增生阶段的存在。

糖尿病视网膜病变、糖尿病性黄斑水肿和增生性糖尿病性视网膜病变是威胁视力的并发症，可能在妊娠期间发展和（或）恶化。

如果妇女在妊娠前有严重的 NPDR 或增生性视网膜病变的迹象，应根据《糖尿病视网膜病变研究指南》[45]进行分散或泛视网膜光凝。同样，对于临床上显著的黄斑水肿，也应开始激光治疗[46]。妊娠前稳定糖尿病视网膜病变可减缓妊娠期进展。

如果在妊娠期间视网膜发生新的变化，符合激光的标准治疗，应该这样做，因为这样的治疗对妊娠妇女与非妊娠妇女同样有效和安全[47]。考虑到产后自发回归的可能性，对于激光光凝的作用众说纷纭。然而，尽管在许多情况下，公认的产后视力下降，保守治疗可能是有害的，因为在妊娠期间，由于增生性变化或严重黄斑水肿的并发症，视力可能会丧失。激光光凝治疗黄斑水肿和增生性糖尿病视网膜病变尚未有报道在妊娠期间对妊娠妇女或胎儿造成伤害。

激光光凝治疗曾经是糖尿病黄斑水肿和增生性糖尿病视网膜病变的一线治疗方法，而现在眼内注射 VEGF 抗体已成为治疗这些糖尿病视网膜病变并发症的重要手段。大量的试验已经证明眼内抗 VEGF 治疗糖尿病黄斑水肿的疗效[48-50]，但关于其在妊娠期应用的数据很少。与传统激光治疗黄斑水肿相比，抗 VEGF 注射与更好的视力结果和减少中央黄斑厚度有关。这可能需要多次注射才能获得并维持这些收益[48-50]。眼内抗 VEGF 在增生性糖尿病视网膜病变的视网膜新生血管形成中也起着重要作用[50]。

贝伐珠单抗和雷珠单抗是目前美国最常使用的两种眼内使用的抗 VEGF 药物。

近年来一些病例报道，或无意或故意在妊娠期间使用抗 VEGF[51-55]。一份在妊娠晚期发生特发性脉络膜新生血管膜使用单一雷珠单抗玻璃体腔内注射的病例报道描述了在产后 12 个月内没有母婴损害[53]。4 例妊娠妇女在 5 个不同妊娠周的妊娠期间共接受了 13 次玻璃体腔内贝伐珠单抗注射，在平均随访 14 个月（56 个月）后，均未报道母亲或胎儿发生不良事件[56]。有报道称，玻璃体腔注射贝伐珠单抗 1 周后发生 2 例早期自然流产，但自然发生的妊娠前期流产率较高，难以建立因果关系[52]。

目前尚不清楚两种最常用的抗 VEGF 药物，即雷珠单抗或贝伐昔单抗，在妊娠期是否安全。尽管大多数报道的病例令人放心，但妊娠期间使用抗 VEGF 药物仍存在一些理论上的担忧。抗 VEGF 药物可能对胎儿血管生成产生有害影响。子痫前期与血管生成因子不足有关，因此进一步的医源性血管内皮生长因子阻滞可加重子痫前期[57]。鉴于大多数关于妊娠期玻璃体内抗 VEGF 使用的研究都是回顾性的，患者数量较少，随访时间有限，对孕产妇和胎儿健康的风险仍然未知。

在某些情况下，对妊娠期间患者的增生性视网膜病变行手术干预是必要的。最常见的手术指征是玻璃体积血不清除、视网膜牵张性脱离和新生血管性青光眼。关于妊娠期眼内手术的文献非常有限[25]。

幸运的是，妊娠糖尿病视网膜病变的视力威胁进展并不常见。需要详细讨论每种治疗方式的可能风险和获益。此外，有报道称，妊娠对糖尿病视网膜病变的不良影响持续到产后第一年，在此期间应继续进行视网膜监测。

未来的方向

随着糖尿病的系统性和眼部管理的不断发展，糖尿病的治疗也取得了长足的进步，妊娠糖尿病视网膜病变的研究也在不断深入，妊娠糖尿病视网膜病变加重视力损失通常是可以预防的。妊娠前对血糖、高血压和血脂进行最佳的全身管理是必要的。同样，在妊娠前或妊娠期间及时适当地干预视网膜病变的进展对预防视力丧失至关重要。随着医师和患者越来越多地认识到系统性和眼部护理的重要性，糖尿病妊娠妇女的视觉前景是乐观的。

选择题

1. 在妊娠期间不需要进行眼科检查的人群是（　　）
    A. 有 5 年病史的 1 型糖尿病患者
    B. 新诊断为妊娠糖尿病的患者
    C. 有 5 年 2 型糖尿病病史的患者
正确答案是 B。
2. 下列因素与妊娠期间糖尿病视网膜病变恶化有关的是（　　）
    A. 血糖控制差　　　　　　B. 高血压
    C. 糖化血红蛋白水平迅速提高　D. 所有这些
正确答案是 D。
3. 下列陈述错误的是（　　）
    A. 妊娠糖尿病视网膜病变的进展与 1 型糖尿病的相关性大于 2 型糖尿病

B. 糖尿病视网膜病变是阴道分娩的禁忌证
C. 激光光凝术可在妊娠期安全进行

正确答案是 B。

（王　冰　译，朱海清　校）

参 考 文 献

1 Klein BE. Overview of epidemiologic studies of diabetic retinopathy. Ophthalm Epidemiol 2007;14(4):179-183.
2 Kempen JH, O'Colmain BJ, Leske MC, Haffner SM, Klein R, Moss SE, et al. The prevalence of diabetic retinopathy among adults in the United States. Arch Ophthalm 2004;122(4):552-563.
3 Roy MS, Klein R, O'Colmain BJ, Klein BE, Moss SE, Kempen JH. The prevalence of diabetic retinopathy among adult type 1 diabetic persons in the United States. Arch Ophthalm 2004;122(4):546-551.
4 Chew EY, Mills JL, Metzger BE, Remaley NA, Jovanovic-Peterson L, Knopp RH, et al. Metabolic control and progression of retinopathy: the Diabetes in Early Pregnancy Study. National Institute of Child Health and Human Development Diabetes in Early Pregnancy Study. Diabetes Care 1995;18(5):631-637.
5 Diabetes C, Complications Trial Research G. Effect of pregnancy on microvascular complications in the diabetes control and complications trial. The Diabetes Control and Complications Trial Research Group. Diabetes Care 2000;23(8):1084-1091.
6 Verier-Mine O, Chaturvedi N, Webb D, Fuller JH. Is pregnancy a risk factor for microvascular complications? The EURODIAB Prospective Complications Study. Diabetic Med 2005;22(11):1503-1509.
7 Soubrane G, Canivet J, Coscas G. Influence of pregnancy on the evolution of background retinopathy. Preliminary results of a prospective fluorescein angiography study. Intl Ophthalm 1985;8(4):249-255.
8 Aiello LP, Cahill MT, Wong JS. Systemic considerations in the management of diabetic retinopathy. Amer J Ophthalm 2001;132(5):760-776.
9 Diabetes Control and Complications Trial Research Group. The effect of intensive treatment of diabetes on the development and progression of long-term complications in insulin-dependent diabetes mellitus. New Engl J Med 1993;329(14):977-986.
10 Reichard P, Nilsson BY, Rosenqvist U. The effect of long-term intensified insulin treatment on the development of microvascular complications of diabetes mellitus. New Engl J Med 1993;329(5):304-309.
11 Pregnancy outcomes in the Diabetes Control and Complications Trial. Amer J Obstet Gynecol 1996;174(4):1343-1353.
12 UK Prospective Diabetes Study Group. Tight blood pressure control and risk of macrovascular and microvascular complications in type 2 diabetes: UKPDS 38. BMJ 1998;317(7160):703-713.
13 Suzuma I, Hata Y, Clermont A, Pokras F, Rook SL, Suzuma K, et al. Cyclic stretch and hypertension induce retinal expression of vascular endothelial growth factor and vascular endothelial growth factor receptor-2: potential mechanisms for exacerbation of diabetic retinopathy by hypertension. Diabetes 2001;50(2):444-454.
14 Klein R, Klein BE, Moss SE, Cruickshanks KJ. The Wisconsin Epidemiologic Study of Diabetic Retinopathy: XVII. The 14-year

incidence and progression of diabetic retinopathy and associated risk factors in type 1 diabetes. Ophthalmology 1998;105(10):1801-1815.
15 Schrier RW, Estacio RO, Esler A, Mehler P. Effects of aggressive blood pressure control in normotensive type 2 diabetic patients on albuminuria, retinopathy and strokes. Kidney Intl 2002;61(3):1086-1097.
16 Schrier RW, Estacio RO, Mehler PS, Hiatt WR. Appropriate blood pressure control in hypertensive and normotensive type 2 diabetes mellitus: a summary of the ABCD trial. Nature Clin Pract Nephrol 2007;3(8):428-438.
17 Yam JC, Kwok AK. Update on the treatment of diabetic retinopathy. Hong Kong Med J 2007;13(1):46-60.
18 Klein BE, Moss SE, Klein R, Surawicz TS. The Wisconsin Epidemiologic Study of Diabetic Retinopathy. XIII. Relationship of serum cholesterol to retinopathy and hard exudate. Ophthalmology 1991;98(8):1261-1265.
19 Chew EY, Klein ML, Ferris FL, 3rd, Remaley NA, Murphy RP, Chantry K, et al. Association of elevated serum lipid levels with retinal hard exudate in diabetic retinopathy. Early Treatment Diabetic Retinopathy Study (ETDRS) Report 22. Arch Ophthalm 1996;114(9):1079-1084.
20 Fong DS, Segal PP, Myers F, Ferris FL, Hubbard LD, Davis MD. Subretinal fibrosis in diabetic macular edema. ETDRS Report 23. Early Treatment Diabetic Retinopathy Study Research Group. Arch Ophthalm 1997;115(7):873-877.
21 Chew EY, Ambrosius WT, Davis MD, Danis RP, Gangaputra S, Greven CM, et al. Effects of medical therapies on retinopathy progression in type 2 diabetes. New Engl J Med 2010;363(3):233-244. Epub 2010/07/01.
22 Keech AC, Mitchell P, Summanen PA, O'Day J, Davis TM, Moffitt MS, et al. Effect of fenofibrate on the need for laser treatment for diabetic retinopathy (FIELD study): a randomised controlled trial. Lancet 2007;370(9600):1687-1697.

23 Moloney JB, Drury MI. The effect of pregnancy on the natural course of diabetic retinopathy. Amer J Ophthalm 1982;93(6):745-756.
24 Klein BE, Moss SE, Klein R. Effect of pregnancy on progression of diabetic retinopathy. Diabetes Care 1990;13(1):34-40.
25 Errera MH, Kohly RP, da Cruz L. Pregnancy-associated retinal diseases and their management. Surv Ophthalm 2013;58(2):127-142.
26 Rosenn B, Miodovnik M, Kranias G, Khoury J, Combs CA, Mimouni F, et al. Progression of diabetic retinopathy in pregnancy: association with hypertension in pregnancy. Amer J Obstet Gynecol 1992;166(4):1214-1218.
27 Lauritzen T, Frost-Larsen K, Larsen HW, Deckert T. Effect of 1 year of near-normal blood glucose levels on retinopathy in insulin-dependent diabetics. Lancet 1983;1(8318):200-204.
28 Kroc Collaborative Study Group. Blood glucose control and the evolution of diabetic retinopathy and albuminuria: a preliminary multicenter trial. New Engl J Med 1984;311(6):365-372.
29 Dahl-Jorgensen K, Brinchmann-Hansen O, Hanssen KF, Sandvik L, Aagenaes O. Rapid tightening of blood glucose control leads to transient deterioration of retinopathy in insulin dependent diabetes mellitus: the Oslo study. Brit Med J 1985;290(6471):811-815.
30 Sone H, Okuda Y, Kawakami Y, Kondo S, Hanatani M, Matsuo K, et al. Progesterone induces vascular endothelial growth factor on retinal pigment epithelial cells in culture. Life Sci 1996;59(1):21-25.
31 Barbour LA, Shao J, Qiao L, Pulawa LK, Jensen DR, Bartke A, et al. Human placental growth hormone causes severe insulin resistance in transgenic mice. Amer J Obstet Gynecol 2002;186(3):512-517.
32 Smith LE, Shen W, Perruzzi C, Soker S, Kinose F, Xu X, et al. Regulation of vascular endothelial growth factor-dependent retinal neovascularization by insulin-like

growth factor-1 receptor. Nature Med 1999;5(12):1390-1395.
33 Ringholm L, Vestgaard M, Laugesen CS, Juul A, Damm P, Mathiesen ER. Pregnancy-induced increase in circulating IGF-I is associated with progression of diabetic retinopathy in women with type 1 diabetes. Growth Horm IGF Res 2011;21(1):25-30.
34 Patel V, Rassam S, Newsom R, Wiek J, Kohner E. Retinal blood flow in diabetic retinopathy. BMJ 1992;305(6855):678-683.
35 Loukovaara S, Harju M, Kaaja R, Immonen I. Retinal capillary blood flow in diabetic and nondiabetic women during pregnancy and postpartum period. Invest Ophthalm Visual Sci 2003;44(4):1486-1491.
36 Chen HC, Newsom RS, Patel V, Cassar J, Mather H, Kohner EM. Retinal blood flow changes during pregnancy in women with diabetes. Invest Ophthalm Vis Sci 1994;35(8):3199-3208.
37 Schocket LS, Grunwald JE, Tsang AF, DuPont J. The effect of pregnancy on retinal hemodynamics in diabetic versus nondiabetic mothers. Amer J Ophthalm 1999;128(4):477-484.
38 Adamis AP. Is diabetic retinopathy an inflammatory disease? Brit J Opthalm 2002;86(4):363-365.
39 Gardner TW, Antonetti DA, Barber AJ, LaNoue KF, Levison SW. Diabetic retinopathy: more than meets the eye. Surv Ophthalmol 2002;47(Suppl 2):S253-S262.
40 Wolf M, Sandler L, Hsu K, Vossen-Smirnakis K, Ecker JL, Thadhani R. First-trimester C-reactive protein and subsequent gestational diabetes. Diabetes Care 2003;26(3):819-824.
41 Loukovaara S, Immonen IR, Loukovaara MJ, Koistinen R, Kaaja RJ. Glycodelin: a novel serum anti-inflammatory marker in type 1 diabetic retinopathy during pregnancy. Acta Ophthalm Scandinav 2007;85(1):46-49.
42 Remaury A, Vita N, Gendreau S, Jung M, Arnone M, Poncelet M, et al. Targeted inactivation of the neurotensin type 1 receptor reveals its role in body temperature control and feeding behavior but not in analgesia. Brain Res 2002;953(1-2):63-72.
43 Walker JD. NICE guidance on diabetes in pregnancy: management of diabetes and its complications from preconception to the postnatal period. NICE Clinical Guideline 63, March 2008. Diabetic Med 2008;25(9):1025-1027.
44 National Institute for Health and Clinical Excellence (NICE). Diabetes in Pregnancy: Management from Preconception to the Postnatal Period. 2015. http://www.nice.org.uk/guidance/ng3/chapter/1-Recommendations
45 Diabetic Retinopathy Study Research Group. Four risk factors for severe visual loss in diabetic retinopathy: the third report from the Diabetic Retinopathy Study. Arch Ophthalm 1979;97(4):654-655.
46 Early Treatment Diabetic Retinopathy Study Research Group. Photocoagulation for diabetic macular edema. Early Treatment Diabetic Retinopathy Study Report No. 1. Arch Ophthalm 1985;103(12):1796-1806.
47 Horvat M, Maclean H, Goldberg L, Crock GW. Diabetic retinopathy in pregnancy: a 12-year prospective survey. Brit J Optalm 1980;64(6):398-403.
48 Diabetic Retinopathy Clinical Research N, Elman MJ, Aiello LP, Beck RW, Bressler NM, Bressler SB, et al. Randomized trial evaluating ranibizumab plus prompt or deferred laser or triamcinolone plus prompt laser for diabetic macular edema. Ophthalmology 2010;117(6):1064-1077 e35.
49 Mitchell P, Bandello F, Schmidt-Erfurth U, Lang GE, Massin P, Schlingemann RO, et al. The RESTORE study: ranibizumab monotherapy or combined with laser versus laser monotherapy for diabetic macular edema. Ophthalmology 2011;118(4):615-625.
50 Nguyen QD, Brown DM, Marcus DM, Boyer DS, Patel S, Feiner L, et al. Ranibizumab for diabetic macular edema: results from 2 phase III randomized trials: RISE and RIDE. Ophthalmology

2012;119(4):789-801.
51 Spaide RF, Laud K, Fine HF, Klancnik JM, Jr., Meyerle CB, Yannuzzi LA, et al. Intravitreal bevacizumab treatment of choroidal neovascularization secondary to age-related macular degeneration. Retina 2006;26(4):383-390.
52 Petrou P, Georgalas I, Giavaras G, Anastasiou E, Ntana Z, Petrou C. Early loss of pregnancy after intravitreal bevacizumab injection. Acta Ophthalm 2010;88(4):e136.
53 Wu Z, Huang J, Sadda S. Inadvertent use of bevacizumab to treat choroidal neovascularisation during pregnancy: a case report. Annals Acad Med (Singapore) 2010;39(2):143-145.
54 Introini U, Casalino G, Cardani A, Scotti F, Finardi A, Candiani M, et al. Intravitreal bevacizumab for a subfoveal myopic choroidal neovascularization in the first trimester of pregnancy. J Ocular Pharmacol Therap 2012;28(5):553-555.
55 Sullivan L, Kelly SP, Glenn A, Williams CP, McKibbin M. Intravitreal bevacizumab injection in unrecognised early pregnancy. Eye 2014;28(4):492-494.
56 Tarantola RM, Folk JC, Boldt HC, Mahajan VB. Intravitreal bevacizumab during pregnancy. Retina 2010;30(9):1405-1411.
57 Cross SN, Ratner E, Rutherford TJ, Schwartz PE, Norwitz ER. Bevacizumab-mediated interference with VEGF signaling is sufficient to induce a preeclampsia-like syndrome in nonpregnant women. Rev Obstet Gynecol 2012;5(1):2-8.

第四篇 分娩与产后护理

第二十二章 分娩和产后护理：1型、2型或妊娠期糖尿病妇女的分娩及分娩和产后的产科管理

Jacques Lepercq

Maternité Port Royal，Université Paris Descartes，Paris，France

实践要点

- 患有1型或2型糖尿病的妇女，分娩应在适当的围产期环境中进行。
- 分娩时间：
  ——1型或2型糖尿病妇女在妊娠37～39周。
  ——妊娠糖尿病妇女不超过40周+6天。
- 分娩方式将取决于过去的产科病史、可疑巨大儿、骨盆的充分性、胎儿的表现和当地情况。在分娩过程中，毛细血管血糖应维持在4～7mmol/L。
- 1型糖尿病妇女分娩时应考虑静脉注射葡萄糖和胰岛素。
- 产程管理要遵循规范的做法。
- 建议在产程中行连续胎儿监测。

病 例

一名40岁的高加索妇女，第二次妊娠，有一次活产，现妊娠37周，无人工流产产前护理的情况。她的体重是120kg，血压是130/80mmHg，子宫长度为38cm。患者过去的产科病史为8年前有一名4.2kg重的男婴在妊娠40周自发阴道分娩。患者介绍说这个孩子的健康状况很好。

妊娠糖尿病是在本次妊娠的26周被诊断出来的（75g OGTT：空腹血糖为6.4mmol/L；1h血糖为10.7mmol/L；2h血糖为9.1mmol/L）。经饮食不能控制血糖；

于妊娠 32 周时开始使用胰岛素，现在用量为门冬胰岛素 10U/d、15U/d、15U/d 和甘精胰岛素 0U/d、0U/d、20U/d。上周平均毛细血管血糖（42 次测量）为 6.9mmol/L。胎头处于子宫颈位置，估计胎儿体重为 3950g。子宫颈闭合。

背景

有 1 型或 2 型糖尿病病史的女性，分娩时应注意要在适当的围产期环境并通过预先制订的糖尿病和麻醉方案进行管理（参见第二十三章）。分娩通常建议在妊娠 37~39 周进行，以减少死胎和胎儿并发症的风险[1]。

1 型糖尿病妇女的新生儿巨大儿率增加：49%~63%的新生儿体重大于胎龄，20%~25%为巨大儿（即出生体重超过4000g）[2-4]。巨大儿的发生率在患有 2 型糖尿病妇女的新生儿中是相似的[5]。巨大儿与肩难产和臂丛神经损伤的风险增加有关[6]。

加拿大的一项研究发现，患有糖尿病的女性比没有糖尿病的女性更有可能发生剖宫产或引产。患有糖尿病的妊娠妇女更容易发生难产和肩难产[7]。剖宫产应该能消除臂丛神经损伤的风险。因此，1 型糖尿病妇女的剖宫产率是普通人群的 2~4 倍，为 45%~73%[2, 4, 8-10]。在荟萃分析中，2 型糖尿病患者的剖宫产率低于 1 型糖尿病患者（OR：0.80；95%CI：0.59~0.94），其他结果无差异[5]。

剖宫产与产妇发病率增加有关[11]。此外，子宫瘢痕对许多产科医师来说是引产的禁忌，使妇女面临子宫破裂、前置胎盘、胎盘植入等风险或所有这些风险增加，并且增加了第二次剖宫产后子宫切除的风险[12]。因此，避免不必要的初次剖宫产对未来妊娠有重要影响。

分娩时间

分娩的时间和方式应该在妊娠妇女产前预约期间，特别是在妊娠晚期要与患者讨论。

目前的各个国家指导方针差别很小：

- 英国：NICE 指南建议，1 型或 2 型糖尿病患者应该在妊娠 $37^{+0} \sim 38^{+6}$ 周[13]接受选择性分娩，假设在此之前没有其他重要因素发生；如果有代谢改变或任何其他母体或胎儿并发症，应考虑 37^{+0} 周前出生。患有妊娠糖尿病的妇女最迟应在 40^{+6} 周内分娩，如果有母体或胎儿并发症，应在此之前分娩。
- 美国：美国糖尿病协会的指导方针指出，一个正在形成的共识表明，在没有产科并发症的情况下，受到良好监控的糖尿病妇女可以等待妊娠 39～40 周自然分娩[14]。
- 法国：目前法国的指导方针建议，在没有并发症的情况下，如果糖尿病得到很好的控制，应该允许妊娠至 38～39 周[15]。

尽管有一般的指导方针要遵循，但对分娩的时间和方式采取个性化的方法是至关重要的。许多因素需要考虑，包括血糖控制、糖尿病并发症、产科病史、胎儿生长和医疗资源的可用性。

早产

患有糖尿病的女性早产率（小于 37 周）很高。在过去 10 年内发表的 12 项基本人群的研究中（14 099 名 1 型糖尿病妇女），自发或有指征的早产发生率为 25.2%（13.0～41.7），而正常组为 6.0%（4.7～7.1）（RR 为 4.2）。早孕时 HbA1c 阳性与不良妊娠结局包括早产呈正相关[16]。在 2014 年英国全国糖尿病妊娠报告中，42.6%的 1 型糖尿病妊娠妇女早产，而 2 型糖尿病妊娠妇女早产率为 23.6%[17]。

先前的研究表明，糖尿病患者早产占了所有早产的 2/3。肾病的进展、先兆子痫的发生和血糖控制不良与早产有显著关联[18]。

如果显示要早产，并且当地没有设施，那么应该将产妇转移到有这些设施的产科病房。

足月分娩

从长远来看，分娩时间反映了产科医师对胎龄的看法，在这个胎龄下，胎儿可能有过度生长的风险，加上意外死产的风险，会被引产和（或）剖宫产的风险所平衡。

在决定分娩时间时，有必要考虑到母亲和胎儿的一些因素，将护理个性化。

• 母亲血糖控制不良时——由于母亲高血糖发作可能导致胎儿酸血症，胎儿在子宫内可能有意外死亡的风险。

• 母体糖尿病并发症的发展——母体肾损害、高血压、神经病变或视网膜病变都可能引起对母体健康的密切关注（参见第二十章）。

• 胎儿生长异常（限制或过度）或损害——通过超声波和其他胎儿监测方法评估（参见第十九章）。

• 产妇意愿，尤其是在产科病史不佳的情况下。

1 型糖尿病与妊娠期间死产风险增加 3～5 倍有关。不明原因的死产与血糖控制不良、糖尿病肾病、吸烟和低社会经济地位有关[19]。

目前正在努力识别死产风险胎儿，但还没有取得共识。回顾性研究报道称，频繁的应力测试可以识别死产的高危胎儿，一些学者[20, 21]建议选择性分娩这些新生儿以降低死产率，尽管其他学者[22]对此提出质疑。许多中心每周进行 1～2 次应力测试，从妊娠 32～34 周直到分娩。英国现行指南不建议在 38 周前对胎儿健康状况进行常规监测，除非存在胎儿生长受限的风险[13]。据报道，当血糖控制良好时，在没有肾病、先兆子痫和异常胎儿生长的情况下，胎儿不太可能受到损害[22]。主要问题在于定义血糖控制不良并决定胎儿死亡风险与出生风险平衡的最佳胎龄。在一项嵌套病例对照研究中，479 名患有 1 型糖尿病和单胎妊娠的前瞻性队列中，通过标准化方案进行管理，异常应力测试的即刻或紧急剖宫产率为 4%。死产率是每 1000 人中有 2 人。分娩时 HbA1c 为 47mmol/mol（6.4%）或更高，是与胎儿危害即刻或紧急剖宫产相关的唯一独立因素（敏感度、特异度、阳性似然比和阴性似然比分别为 70.6%、66.7%、2.1 和 0.4）[23]。如果血糖不稳定，尽管给予住院治疗和强化胰岛素治疗仍会发生早产[24]。

需要大规模研究来证明 38～39 周分娩的风险和益处。少数相关研究全部或主要由患有 GDM 的妇女组成，因此他们的结论可能不适用于患有 1 型或 2 型糖尿病的妇女。美国的一项研究[25]将 187 名需要胰岛素治疗的 GDM 妇女和 13 名妊娠前患有糖尿病的妇女随机分为 38 周干预组和期待治疗组。干预与较低的 LGA 率相关（孕龄超过第 90 百分位）（10% vs 23%；$P=0.02$）和肩难产减少的趋势（0% vs 3%；差异无统计学意义）。同样，一项来自以色列的需要胰岛素治疗的 GDM 病例对照研究（$n=260$）[26] 显示，与 40 周或超过 40 周分娩的妇女相比，38～39 周分娩的妇女肩部难产的发病率降低（1.4% vs 10.2%；$P<0.05$）。虽然预计 38～39 周的引产会降低围产期死亡的风险，但目前还没有证据支持这一观点。

生产方式

分娩方式的选择将取决于产科病史（如子宫瘢痕和肩难产史）、可疑巨大儿、骨盆的充分性、胎儿的表现和局部情况。糖尿病妇女剖宫产率的增加主要与对疑似巨大儿肩难产风险增加的预期有关[27]。生殖器创伤和产后出血的风险也增加了，产后出血包括剖宫产和阴道分娩。

肩难产是一种严重的并发症，在婴儿体重为 4000～4500g 的糖尿病妇女中，有 8.4%～16.7% 的会发生，相比之下，在背景人群中，这一比例为 1.4%。当出生体重超过 4500g 时，糖尿病患者的比例为 20%～50%，非糖尿病患者的比例为 9.2%～24%[28]。此外，据报道，84% 患有糖尿病的母亲所生的婴儿肩难产体重超过 4000g[29]。因此，避免先前患有糖尿病的女性阴道分娩巨大儿应该可以消除大多数肩难产的情况。在一项研究中，估计体重阈值为 4250g，作为剖宫产指征，可以降低肩难产的发生率，而不会增加剖宫产率[30]。在该研究中，大多数女性患有 GDM，对于患有 1 型或 2 型糖尿病的女性，还不能得出明确的结论。

在出现肩难产的情况下，臂丛神经损伤的风险随着每次必要的拔除动作而增加。在工业化国家，臂丛神经损伤的发生率为 0.5%～3%[31]，肩难产的发生率为 4%～40%[28]。然而，绝大多数臂丛神经损伤是暂时性的，严重后遗症的发生率为 1.5%。

这种风险突出了产前检测巨大儿的重要性，但这仍然很困难，体格检查和超声的阳性预测值也很差[32]。足月时，超声估计胎儿体重的平均误差约为 15%[33]。在糖尿病女性中，确认体重超过 4000g 的新生儿的测试后概率超过 60%[34]。

目前还没有随机试验来检验糖尿病患者中可疑巨大儿妊娠的最佳分

娩方式。不同来源有不同的阈值，范围从 4000g 到大于 4500g，以估计胎儿过度生长为主要指征[13, 30, 35, 36]。

在缺乏共识的情况下，患有糖尿病的妊娠妇女如果有超声诊断的巨大儿，应该被告知阴道分娩、引产和剖宫产的风险与益处[13]。

剖宫产史

关于糖尿病妇女剖宫产后阴道分娩（VBAC）结果的数据很少。在对 19 个中心进行的一项观察性研究的二次分析中，约一半患有 GDM 的女性尝试了 VBAC，成功率约为 60%，母亲和新生儿并发症很少。由于妊娠前患有糖尿病的女性人数相对较少，作者无法得出强有力的结论[37]。糖尿病本身并不是尝试 VBAC 的禁忌证[13]。尝试 VBAC 的决定应该在个案基础上由该妇女及其医师共同做出。

计划剖宫产——实际问题

除了胰岛素疗法之外，患有糖尿病的女性和没有糖尿病的女性的管理方式相同（参见第二十三章）。由于这些妇女中有许多人身体肥胖或有其他糖尿病并发症，通常需要进行术前麻醉检查。局部麻醉比全身麻醉更受欢迎，这一点与非糖尿病妇女类似。应该防止可能与局部麻醉相关的血流动力学影响和低血压。计划内和紧急剖宫产都推荐预防性使用抗生素。输卵管结扎术的问题应该事先向所有患有糖尿病并发症的妇女和多胞胎妇女提出。

产程诱导——实际问题

除了几个具体的方面，产程管理有糖尿病与没有糖尿病的妇女类似。产程诱导应该在分娩室或其他人员充足的环境中进行，在那里可以使用 CTG 监测胎儿状况。在使用前列腺素使宫颈成熟过程中，如果妇女没有明显疼痛，并且分娩还没有开始，她应该被允许继续她通常的胰岛素治疗方案，同时进行常规葡萄糖测量。分娩时，通常每小时监测毛细血管血糖。本章将进一步讨论胰岛素方案。

分娩第一阶段的具体产科问题

催产素的生产和使用进展

产程管理遵循标准惯例，主要的担忧是胎儿和母亲之间意外的比例失调，以及可能的创伤性分娩。对分娩过程的仔细监控是必要的，可以通过使用产程图或 Friedman 分娩曲线来实现。虽然分娩困难可能发生在相对快速的第一产程之后，但是产程活跃期的缓慢进展（即≥5cm 宫颈扩张）需要有经验的产科医师仔细检查。在第一次分娩的妇女中，如果宫缩从未非常频繁或强烈，可以考虑用催产素刺激子宫。然而，在分娩取得良好进展，宫颈扩张停止后，必须谨慎使用催产素。宫内压力导管虽然没有广泛使用，但可能有助于量化子宫对催产素的反应。

分娩中胎儿状况的监测

糖尿病母亲的胎儿可能比没有糖尿病的妇女的胎儿有更高的产时窒息风险，因此建议分娩时持续胎儿电子监护[38]。在早期分娩中，如果产妇血糖正常（4～7mmol/L），可以间歇地进行 CTG 监测；产程一旦建立，就应该持续进行。如果 CTG 显示可疑或病理模式，第一步应该检查母体血压、改变母体位置、给氧及检查母体血糖是否正常。如果存在高糖血症，那么应该通过静脉注射胰岛素来纠正（参见第二十三章），因此 CTG 模式可能会得到很好的改善。如果母亲血糖正常，或者测得血糖正常，仍不能纠正 CTG 异常，那么应该使用其他评估胎儿状况和（或）加速分娩（如剖宫产）的方法。如果宫颈扩张允许，可以采集胎儿血样。

分娩镇痛

使用阿片类药物或硬膜外镇痛没有禁忌证。鉴于 GDM 剖宫产风险增加，如果需要剖宫产，分娩早期硬膜外麻醉通常就足够了（有合适的剂量方案）。

分娩期间血糖控制

分娩期间每小时应监测毛细血管血糖，确保血糖维持在 4～7mmol/L。

对于患有1型糖尿病的妇女及从分娩开始血糖未保持在 4～7mmol/L 的其他糖尿病妇女，应考虑静脉注射葡萄糖和胰岛素。

分娩第二阶段的具体产科问题

第二阶段的主要问题与第一阶段类似，即对胎儿状况和延迟的担忧。鉴于糖尿病妇女分娩中肩难产的风险增加，无论是自然分娩还是低产钳分娩或真空分娩，护理人员都必须经历并准备应对潜在的肩难产。任何肩难产的早期迹象都应该用标准的动作来应对，如 McRorbert 位置和耻骨上压力。如果需要手术分娩（除了低产钳/真空吸引器），那么有经验的产科医师需要在麻醉良好的手术室里进行评估。相对困难的胎头分娩后可能会出现肩部难产的极端情况。除非在将妇女送入手术室并获得有效麻醉所需的时间内，头部有显著下降和旋转，否则应认真考虑采用剖宫产。

出生后的具体问题

• 应该鼓励 GDM 妇女母乳喂养（参见第二十六章）。有些具体问题需要医疗投入。
• 第二十三章详细讨论了降低胰岛素用量和血糖的控制。
• 患有糖尿病的女性应该被告知产后低血糖风险增加，尤其是母乳喂养时，并鼓励她们在进食前或进食过程中加餐或零食。
• 患有2型糖尿病的女性可能会再次使用口服降糖药，如二甲双胍和格列本脲，即使她们是母乳喂养（参见第十五章和第二十六章）。
• 被诊断 GDM 的妇女应该在婴儿出生后立即停止降糖治疗，并检查毛细血管血糖水平，以排除持续高血糖症[13]。

- 可能需要修改抗高血压方案，包括重新推荐血管紧张素转换酶抑制剂。后者虽然在妊娠期间禁用，但在哺乳期间可以合理使用。
- 必须注意剖宫产术后伤口感染的风险增加。
- 剖宫产后建议产后至少 5d 进行血栓预防。
- 关于避孕和可能的计划生育的讨论应该在出院前开始（参见第二十五章）。

随诊管理

出院时，必须为妊娠期间患有糖尿病的所有女性（无论是妊娠前存在的糖尿病还是妊娠期糖尿病）做出安排，以便进行后续检查，通常在 6 周后，但如果从糖尿病的角度来看有必要，可以提前进行。对于那些已经患有糖尿病的患者来说，这可能是需要由妊娠团队中的糖尿病专家或普通糖尿病医师决定的。患有 2 型糖尿病的妇女特别有可能得不到最佳护理[39]。对于那些在妊娠期间需要进行详细眼科或肾脏检查的妇女来说，有必要安排在产后继续检查（参见第二十一章）。对于没有持续高血糖的 GDM 女性，在产后 6 周的检查中提供生活方式建议（包括体重控制、饮食和锻炼）和空腹血糖测试[13]。

提醒患有糖尿病妇女避孕的重要性，以及在计划未来妊娠时需要妊娠前护理。

结论

所有患有任何形式糖尿病的妇女都应该评估分娩的时间和方式，并且该妇女在和她的临床医师讨论后应该做出个性化的决定，同时应考虑到母亲和胎儿因素。糖尿病妇女常规剖宫产是不合适的。

在分娩时，必须特别注意监测胎儿状况，维持母亲正常血糖并注意潜在的不均衡迹象。

选择题

1. 在本章的病例病史中产程管理正确的是（　　）
    A. 等待自发分娩
    B. 在 38 周左右引产
    C. 如果未按期限分娩，则引产
    D. 在 39 周左右进行选择性剖宫产

正确答案是 B。考虑到先前一个巨大婴儿的自然分娩，估计胎儿体重<4.5kg，血糖控制不佳。

2. 分娩期间血糖控制应该采取的措施是（　　）
    A. 维持胰岛素治疗
    B. 停止胰岛素治疗
    C. 静脉内葡萄糖和胰岛素输注
    D. 每小时毛细血管血糖监测
    E. 血糖目标在 4～7mmol/L

正确答案是 B、D 和 E。

（孙　焱　译，朱海清　校）

参 考 文 献

1　Sacks DA, Sacks A. Induction of labor versus conservative management of pregnant diabetic women. J Matern Fetal Neonatal Med 2002;12:438–441.

2　Evers IM, de Valk HW, Visser GH. Risk of complications of pregnancy in women with type 1 diabetes: nationwide prospective study in the Netherlands. BMJ 2004;328:915–918.

3　Macintosh MC, Fleming KM, Bailey JA, Doyle P, Modder J, Acolet D, et al. Perinatal mortality and congenital anomalies in babies of women with type 1 or type 2 diabetes in England, Wales, and Northern Ireland: population based study. BMJ 2006;333:177–182.

4　Jensen DM, Damm P, Moelsted-Pedersen L, Ovesen P, Westergaard JG, Moeller M, et al. Outcomes in type 1 diabetic pregnancies: a nationwide, population-based study. Diabetes Care 2004;27:2819–2823.

5　Balsells M, García-Patterson A, Gich I, Corcoy R. Maternal and fetal outcome in women with type 2 versus type 1 diabetes mellitus: a systematic review and meta-analysis. J Clin Endocrinol Metab 2009;94:4284–4291.

6　Nesbitt TS, Gilbert WM, Herrchen B. Shoulder dystocia and associated risk factors with macrosomic infants born in California. Am J Obstet Gynecol 1998;179:476–480.

7　Feig DS, Razzaq A, Sykora K, et al. Trends in deliveries, prenatal care, and obstetrical complications in women with

pregestational diabetes: a population-based study in Ontario, Canada, 1996–2001. Diabetes Care 2006;29:232–235.
8. Wylie BR, Kong J, Kozak SE, Marshall CJ, Tong SO, Thompson DM. Normal perinatal mortality in type 1 diabetes mellitus in a series of 300 consecutive pregnancy outcomes. Am J Perinatol 2002;19:169–176.
9. Diabetes and Pregnancy Group, France. French multicentric survey of outcome of pregnancy in women with pregestational diabetes. Diabetes Care 2003;26:2990–2993.
10. Kjos SL, Berkowitz K, Xiang A. Independent predictors of cesarean delivery in women with diabetes. J Matern Fetal Neonatal Med 2004;15:61–67.
11. Takoudes TC, Weitzen S, Slocum J, Malee M. Risk of cesarean wound complications in diabetic gestations. Am J Obstet Gynecol 2004;191:958–963.
12. Silver RM, Landon MB, Rouse DJ, Leveno KJ, Spong CY, Thom EA, et al., for the National Institute of Child Health and Human Development Maternal-Fetal Medicine Units Network. Maternal morbidity associated with multiple repeat cesarean deliveries. Obstet Gynecol 2006;107:1226–1232.
13. National Collaborating Centre for Women's and Children's Health. Diabetes in Pregnancy: Management of Diabetes and its Complications from Preconception to the Postnatal Period. National Collaborating Centre for Women's and Children's Health: London, 2015.
14. Kitzmiller JL, Jovanovic L, Brown F, Coustan D, Reader DM. Managing preexisting diabetes and pregnancy: technical reviews and consensus recommendations for care. American Diabetes Association: Alexandria, VA, 2008.
15. Bismuth E, Bouche C, Caliman C, Lepercq J, Lubin V, Rouge D, Timsit J, Vambergue A. Management of pregnancy in women with type 1 diabetes mellitus: guidelines of the French-Speaking Diabetes Society. Diabetes Metab 2012;38:205–216.
16. Colstrup M, Mathiesen ER, Damm P, Jensen DM, Ringholm L. Pregnancy in women with type 1 diabetes: have the goals of St. Vincent declaration been met concerning foetal and neonatal complications? J Matern Fetal Neonatal Med 2013;26:1682–1686.
17. Health and Social Care Information Centre. National Pregnancy in Diabetes Audit Report 2014. England, Wales and the Isle of Man. Health and Social Care Information Centre: London, 2015.
18. Lepercq J, Coste J, Theau A, Dubois-Laforgue D, Timsit J. Factors associated with preterm delivery in women with type 1 diabetes: a cohort study. Diabetes Care 2004;27:2824–2828.
19. Tennant PW, Glinianaia SV, Bilous RW, Rankin J, Bell R. Pre-existing diabetes, maternal glycated haemoglobin, and the risks of fetal and infant death: a population-based study. Diabetologia 2014;57:285–294.
20. Kjos SL, Leung A, Henry OA, Victor MR, Paul RH, Medearis AL. Antepartum surveillance in diabetic pregnancies: predictors of fetal distress in labor. Am J Obstet Gynecol 1995;173:1532–1539.
21. Brecher A, Tharakan T, Williams A, Baxi L. Perinatal mortality in diabetic patients undergoing antepartum fetal evaluation: a case-control study. J Matern Fetal Neonatal Med 2002;12:423–437.
22. Landon MB, Vickers S. Fetal surveillance in pregnancy complicated by diabetes mellitus: is it necessary? J Matern Fetal Neonatal Med 2002;12:413–416.
23. Miailhe G, Le Ray C, Timsit J, Lepercq J. Factors associated with urgent cesarean delivery in women with type 1 diabetes mellitus. Obstet Gynecol 2013;121:983–989.
24. Spong CY, Mercer BM, D'alton M, Kilpatrick S, Blackwell S, Saade G. Timing of indicated late-preterm and early-term birth. Obstet Gynecol 2011;118(2 Pt 1):323–333.
25. Kjos SL, Henry OA, Montoro M, Buchanan TA, Mestman JH. Insulin-requiring diabetes in pregnancy: a randomized trial

of active induction of labor and expectant management. Am J Obstet Gynecol 1993;169:611–615.
26 Yogev Y, Ben-Haroush A, Chen R, Glickman H, Kaplan B, Hod M. Active induction management of labor for diabetic pregnancies at term: mode of delivery and fetal outcome – a single center experience. Eur J Obstet Gynecol Reprod Biol 2004;114:166–170.
27 Rouse DJ, Owen J, Goldenberg RL, Cliver SP. The effectiveness and costs of elective cesarean delivery for fetal macrosomia diagnosed by ultrasound. JAMA 1996;276:1480–1486.
28 Dildy GA, Clark SL. Shoulder dystocia: risk identification. Clin Obstet Gynecol 2000;43:265–282.
29 Langer O, Berkus MD, Huff RW, Samueloff A. Shoulder dystocia: should the fetus weighing greater than or equal to 4000 grams be delivered by cesarean section? Am J Obstet Gynecol 1991;165:831–837.
30 Conway DL, Langer O. Elective delivery of infants with macrosomia in diabetic women: reduced shoulder dystocia versus increased cesarean deliveries. Am J Obstet Gynecol 1998;178:922–925.
31 Gilbert WM, Nesbitt TS, Danielsen B. Associated factors in 1611 cases of brachial plexus injury. Obstet Gynecol 1999;93:536–540.
32 Johnstone FD, Prescott RJ, Steel JM, Mao JH, Chambers S, Muir N. Clinical and ultrasound prediction of macrosomia in diabetic pregnancy. Br J Obstet Gynaecol 1996;103:747–754.
33 Lee W, Comstock CH, Kirk JS, Smith RS, Monck JW, Deenadayalu R, et al. Birthweight prediction by three-dimensional ultrasonographic volumes of the fetal thigh and abdomen. J Ultrasound Med 1997;16:799–805.
34 Chauhan SP, Grobman WA, Gherman RA, Chauhan VB, Chang G, Magann EF, Hendrix NW. Suspicion and treatment of the macrosomic fetus: a review. Am J Obstet Gynecol 2005;193:332–346.
35 Gonen R, Bader D, Ajami M. Effects of a policy of elective cesarean delivery in cases of suspected fetal macrosomia on the incidence of brachial plexus injury and the rate of cesarean delivery. Am J Obstet Gynecol 2000;183:1296–1300.
36 ACOG Practice Bulletin. Clinical Management Guidelines for Obstetrician – Gynecologists. Number 60, March 2005. Pregestational diabetes mellitus. Obstet Gynecol 2005;105:675–685.
37 Cormier CM, Landon MB, Lai Y, Spong CY, Rouse DJ, Leveno KJ, Varner MW, SimhanHN, Wapner RJ, Sorokin Y, Miodovnik M, Carpenter M, Peaceman AM, O'Sullivan MJ, Sibai BM, Langer O, Thorp JM, Mercer BM, Eunice Kennedy Shriver National Institute of Child Health and Human Development Maternal-Fetal Medicine Units (NICHD MFMU) Network. White's classification of maternal diabetes and vaginal birth after cesarean delivery success in women undergoing a trial of labor. Obstet Gynecol 2010;115:60–64.
38 Clinical Effectiveness Support Unit. The Royal College of Obstetricians and Gynaecologists. The Use of Electronic Fetal Monitoring. RCOG Press: London, 2001. www.rcog.org.uk
39 Confidential Enquiry into Maternal and Child Health. Diabetes in Pregnancy. Are We Providing the Best Care? Findings of a National Enquiry. England, Wales and Northern Ireland. CEMACH: London, 2007. www.cemach.org.uk

第二十三章　临产后、产时和产后的饮食管理

Una M. Graham and David R. McCance

Regional Centre for Endocrinology and Diabetes, Royal Victoria Hospital, Belfast, Northern Ireland, UK

实践要点

- 临产后、产时和产后的饮食管理应该有一个量化的指南。
- 分娩应该在具备新生儿重症监护设施的中心进行。
- 早产应用肾上腺皮质激素的同时应根据确定的指南补充胰岛素。
- 维持母亲血糖正常对预防新生儿低血糖至关重要。
- 除非有医学指征，新生儿的血糖测试应该延迟到第一次喂养后，以免不必要地治疗低血糖或不必要地收入新生儿重症监护病房。
- 分娩后，应该鼓励所有母亲进行母乳喂养，并予以恰当的支持。

病例

一名有20年1型糖尿病史的32岁妇女，在第二次妊娠12周时见到她的家庭医师。她最近一次入院检查是在3个月前，没有发现并发症。此次为非计划妊娠。预约登记时HbA1c升高到8.5%。除了胰岛素治疗（餐前可溶性超短效胰岛素和睡前中效胰岛素），她没有用其他药物。她被紧急转诊到当地的糖尿病联合产前诊所。尽管医师反复建议，但她仍没有按时随访，她在家检测的末梢血血糖值总是高于目标值，HbA1c没有降到7%以下。妊娠34周时因为阴道出血入院，给予肌内注射倍他米松（12mg×2）。还根据当地的指南给予了补充的胰岛素，以避免引起高血糖。妊娠持续到38周行引产术，分娩过程中，通过静脉应用胰岛素-葡萄糖，每小时监测末梢血的血糖水平，血糖维持在5.2～7.1mmol/L。她分娩了一个体重4500g的男婴。分娩后的4h内，婴儿表现易激惹、觅食反射迟钝。实验室血清血糖检测1.9mmol/L，婴儿被送到重症监护病房，予以静脉注射葡萄糖，随后要求24h内予以食管喂养，直至建立正常的觅食反射。婴儿使用奶瓶喂养。母亲持续应用静脉胰岛素-葡萄糖治疗，直至可以进食，同时开始皮下注射胰岛素。

- 产前应用肾上腺皮质激素的患者应该如何控制血糖？
- 分娩时血糖控制与新生儿低糖血症之间有什么关系？
- 分娩过程中母亲血糖水平的标准是什么？

- 这一标准对于 1 型糖尿病、2 型糖尿病和妊娠糖尿病患者分别如何达到?
- 关于产后母亲的胰岛素需要量有哪些问题?
- 是否鼓励 1 型糖尿病患者母乳喂养?
- 应该对糖尿病患者的母乳喂养给予什么建议?

研究背景

CEMACH 发现,糖尿病患者所生婴儿的围产期死亡率风险增加了 3.8 倍[1]。糖尿病母亲的早产率很高,自发早产为 9.4%(普通人群为 7.4%),医源性早产为 26.4%[1]。剖宫产率也升高到了 67%(急诊剖宫产为 37.6%,择期剖宫产为 29.8%),而普通人群是 22%[1]。因此,分娩对于糖尿病母亲和她的孩子来说是一个高风险事件。从出生前严密监护到顺利分娩需要无缝对接。这需要通过产前、产时和产后多学科合作来获得。本章将围绕糖尿病母亲在这三个时期的护理展开。

分娩前,医师必须确保母亲对于产时血糖的控制有一个清晰的计划。尽管对于更复杂的患者来说需要个体化的计划,但还是应该有一个量化的指导方法。因为患者早产的风险高,所以应该在妊娠晚期或妊娠中期的后期之前就谨慎地讨论与胰岛素管理相关的分娩计划。

产时,医师首先应该为糖尿病母亲考虑的是维持正常血糖。这可以避免母亲发生酮症酸中毒、胎儿酸中毒和新生儿低血糖。产后阶段,胰岛素需要量迅速改变,医师应该继续提供进一步的支持,保证稳定的血糖。对于多学科联合的糖尿病团队来说,这是一个独特的机遇,为糖尿病母亲提供支持和教育,将会对于她本人及婴儿的健康产生潜在的长期影响。

分娩前

对于糖尿病母亲来说,在产程中有计划地管理血糖是非常重要的。这不仅能确保第一产程的母亲血糖在正常范围,而且有助于进一步确保母亲有计划地管理她的糖尿病。

确定分娩医院

早孕期或妊娠期一旦确诊为 GDM，应确保妊娠妇女在合适的医疗机构定点管理。糖尿病妇女应该在有妊娠妇女和新生儿监护条件的诊疗机构就诊与分娩[1,2]。应将有明确指征的婴儿收入新生儿病房，如严重的低血糖，但要避免不必要的母婴分离。这点较英国先前的临床实践是有变化的，约 1/3 的机构常规将糖尿病母亲的婴儿收入新生儿病房[3]。

产前肾上腺皮质激素

NICE 建议，妊娠 34^{+6} 周前有早产风险的妇女接受肾上腺皮质激素[4]。同样的，美国国立卫生研究所建议妊娠 24^{+0}～34^{+0} 周时应用肾上腺皮质激素促进胎儿肺成熟[5]。经典的用法是倍他米松 12mg 间隔 24h，肌内注射两次（或偶尔可以间隔 12h 以限制激素引起的高血糖持续时间），或倍他米松 6mg 肌内注射，每 12h 一次，共 4 次[4]。产前肾上腺皮质激素的应用与母亲高血糖风险显著相关，并可能导致糖尿病酮症酸中毒。这对于糖尿病合并妊娠的妇女来说是公认的，偶尔在 GDM 妇女中也有报道[6-8]。因此，应用肾上腺皮质激素应严密监测血糖和预先增加胰岛素用量。由于个体对肾上腺皮质激素反应的不可预测性，只能应用于住院患者。

饮食或口服药物控制的妊娠糖尿病

饮食或口服降糖药物治疗的 GDM 女性在应用肾上腺皮质激素治疗时经常需要胰岛素，至少是暂时性应用。一个小样本的针对妊娠妇女（9 例饮食控制的 GDM，3 例非糖尿病）的观察研究发现，GDM 患者血糖升高 33%～48%，没有糖尿病的患者血糖升高 16%～33%[9]。因此，50%的 GDM 患者需要在应用肾上腺皮质激素后开始降糖治疗[10]。

预测哪个妊娠妇女需要胰岛素治疗是很困难的，因此所有饮食控制的 GDM 产妇应严密监测睡前血糖，至少 2～4h 一次，如果血糖水平高于目标值应快速给予适量胰岛素治疗。

胰岛素治疗患者

胰岛素治疗的妊娠妇女给予激素治疗后和治疗期间需要额外增加胰岛素用量。好几个指南都曾提出要在激素应用过程中管理血糖。我们成功研究出一种运算法则，通过这种方法，胰岛素用量逐步增加，以维持血糖＜6.0mmol/L 而不会发生低血糖[11]。这种运算法则应用于住院患者，包括 GDM 和潜在的 GDM 患者，具体如下：

第一天（第一次肾上腺皮质激素应用）：夜间的胰岛素用量增加 30%。

第二天：所有胰岛素用量增加 50%。

第三天：所有胰岛素用量增加 50%。

第四天：所有胰岛素用量增加 30%。

第五天：所有胰岛素用量增加 20%。

第六天和第七天：胰岛素用量逐渐降至使用肾上腺皮质激素之前水平。

这种算法与 Scandinavian 研究组提出的一种非激进性的算法相类似。最近 Scandinavian 研究组提出的非激进性的算法被英国 NICE 所采用，作为糖尿病患者妊娠期接受肾上腺皮质激素治疗的管理方法[2, 12]。还有一些中心应用静脉注射胰岛素，从第一次肾上腺皮质激素使用开始追加至患者日常胰岛素使用剂量。在一个包括 8 名糖尿病患者（3 名 GDM 和 5 名妊娠前糖尿病）的小样本研究中，需要 1.3～3.7U/h 静脉注射胰岛素来维持 75%的血糖测量值在 4～10mmol/L[13]。

根据肾上腺皮质激素用量逐步增加胰岛素用量，与发生高血糖以后再增加胰岛素用量相比高血糖事件发生非常少，也没有严重的低血糖事件发生[12]。因此，无论是参照哪种指南，应用肾上腺皮质激素后应随即积极增加胰岛素用量。

应用胰岛素泵治疗的患者

随着应用胰岛素泵治疗 1 型糖尿病的增加，此类患者也会妊娠。胰岛素泵治疗者应用肾上腺皮质激素后的治疗指导也是根据本章提到的运算法则来推算的。非常重要的一点是，除了确定基础率和推注比率，高血糖矫正率也需要确定。因为胰岛素使用量会增加，因此有必要保证在使用肾上腺皮质激素前泵里充满胰岛素。由于有肾上腺皮质激素治疗相关的糖尿病酮症酸中毒风险，在肾上腺皮质激素使用前使用新的胰岛素注入装置也很重要，同时传统的胰岛素笔可以应用于任何泵治疗的补充（参见第十七章）。

早产和宫缩抑制剂

宫缩抑制剂应用于早产妇女以提供没有禁忌证的延长妊娠的作用[14]。主要的益处是抑制分娩，使得肾上腺皮质激素有足够的时间来显效或使早产妇女有机会转运到有新生儿病房的机构。本药包括硝苯吡啶、阿托西班或β受体激动剂。拟交感激动剂可能导致血糖快速升高，还有报道称酮症酸中毒提前发生[15]，妊娠糖尿病妇女目前不建议使用[2]。

产时

分娩过程中血糖控制的主要目的是避免母亲高血糖，以及因此而导致的胎儿贫血风险和新生儿低血糖。

新生儿低血糖

新生儿低血糖率是变化的，由下列因素决定：所使用的低血糖的定义、母亲糖尿病的类型、妊娠期血糖控制和婴儿出生体重[16]。总的来说，30%~50%的糖尿病母亲分娩的婴儿出生后早期用常规方法检测会发现低血糖[16-19]。

定义新生儿低血糖是很困难的。非糖尿病妊娠妇女，新生儿血糖下限是 3.0mmol/L，出生后 2h 会下降到 2.8mmol/L[20, 21]。即使是没有给予喂食，出生后 3h 血糖也会回升。病理性低血糖是持续性的，超过出生后的数小时。到目前为止，还没有关于临床新生儿低血糖数值的统一意见[22]。指南建议监测高危婴儿，保证血糖维持在 2.6mmol/L 或以上[23]。高危新生儿包括糖尿病患儿、小于或大于胎龄儿和过期妊娠儿[23]。

血糖是胎儿的主要能量物质，胎儿血糖水平与 60%~80%的母体血糖水平有关[24]。对于糖尿病母亲，新生儿低血糖还与胎儿高胰岛素血症有关，胎儿高胰岛素血症是对母亲妊娠高血糖及随之而来的胎儿高血糖的反应[25-27]。分娩导致母亲血糖供应的突然中断，这在胎儿胰高血糖血症的情况下会引起新生儿低血糖。关于母亲分娩时血糖对新生儿低血糖的影响的评估总结在表23.1中。

胎儿酸中毒

母亲高血糖也与胎儿酸中毒风险增加有关。两个1型糖尿病母亲的观察研究显示，分娩过程中血糖的控制与胎儿窘迫有关。在一个有149例观察对象的研究中，27%（$n=40$）发生了围产期窒息。围产期窒息的临床定义是分娩时胎儿窘迫（妊娠晚期减速、持续胎心减慢或两者共存），1min Apgar评分小于等于6分或胎死宫内。发生围产期窒息婴儿的母亲分娩时血糖最高值高于那些没有发生的[9.5mmol/L±3.7mmol/L vs 7.0mmol/L±3.0mmol/L；$P \leq 0.0001$]。第二个研究有65例，持续皮下胰岛素输注（CSII）者28例分娩时平均血糖水平为4.8mmol/L±0.6mmol/L，37例持续静脉胰岛素输注者为7.2mmol/L±1.1mmol/L，两组比较$P<0.025$。[30]。

急性胎儿窘迫（用胎儿头皮血气pH定义）在静脉注射胰岛素组的发生率是27%，而CSII组是14.3%（$P<0.001$），剖宫产率分别是38%和25%（$P<0.05$）[30]。

这些数据表明，在临产后和分娩时维持母亲血糖水平4～7mmol/L（72～126mg/dl）可以降低新生儿低血糖和胎儿窘迫的发生[2]。

临产后和分娩时血糖的控制

临产后的主要目标是维持稳定的血糖水平和避免母亲高血糖。这个可以通过用标准化的指南依据产程和分娩方式来实现。除了分娩方式不同外，还有糖尿病类型和治疗方法不同。

表 23.1 不同研究时毛细血管血糖和新生儿低血糖之间的关系

作者（年份）	研究对象	方法/定义	研究结果
Andersen 等 (1985)[28]	53 例 1 型糖尿病	分娩时和产后 2h 监测血清血糖；NH（血糖<1.7mmol/L）	母亲分娩时血糖和新生儿血糖呈正相关（r=0.82，P<0.001），和出生后 2h 新生儿血糖呈负相关（r=-0.46，P<0.001。母亲分娩时血糖≥7.1mmol/L（11/30）和母亲血糖<7.1mmol/L 相比，新生儿低血糖发生率为 37% vs 0%
Miodovnik 等 (1987)[29]	122 例 1 型糖尿病	静脉输注葡萄糖±胰岛素维持 CBG 为 3.9~5.6mmol/L；NH（血糖<1.7mmol/L）	母亲 CBG>5mmol/L（90mg/dl），47%的婴儿发生 NH，而母亲 CBG<5mmol/L 则为 14%
Feldberg 1998[30]	65 例 1 型糖尿病	比较 CSII（n=28）和持续静脉胰岛素输注	持续静脉胰岛素输注组 8 例发生新 NH，而 CSII 组没有（P<0.05）
Lean 等 (1990)[31]	29 例胰岛素治疗母亲	调整静脉注 10%右旋葡萄糖和胰岛素以维持 CBG 为 4~7mmol/L NH（血糖<1.7mmol/L）	11 例发生了 NH（37.9%），新生儿 CBG 与母亲分娩时血糖呈负相关（r=-0.58，P<0.01）
Cure 等 (1997)[32]	233 需要胰岛素患者（77 例 1 型，156 例 2 型）	分娩日：10%葡萄糖-果糖输注；静脉注射胰岛素 1~4U/h 以维持 CBG 为 3.3~5.0mmol/L NH（血糖<1.7mmol/L）	NH 发生率为 16.5%。产时 BG 平均水平显著低于没有发生低血糖婴儿的母亲（P<0.005）
CarronBrown 等 (1999)[33]	80 例 1 型糖尿病	静脉注射 10%右旋葡萄糖和加入变化的短效胰岛素量以维持 CBG 为 4~7mmol/L NH-CBG<2.2mmol/L	23.8%的婴儿（19/80）发生 NH。如果母亲血糖维持在目标范围，没有升高至 8mmol/L，没有发现对新生儿有副作用
Balsells 等 (2000)[34]	54 例胰岛素治疗	静脉注射葡萄糖（8.3g/h）；使用注射泵静脉注射胰岛素	5 名婴儿发生 NH；分娩后 2h 母血糖与 NH 有关
Rosenberg 等 (2006)[35]	35 例妇女，妊娠期糖尿病 28 例，妊娠前糖尿病 7 例	胰岛素输注或混合液维持 CBG 为 5.6mmol/L。具体方案见表 23.2 NH-出生后 24h 血糖<1.9mmol/L	5 名婴儿发生 NH：1 名（6.7%）使用混合液；4 名（19.0%）腹岛素输注（生理盐水）

BG，血糖；CBG，毛细血管血糖；NH，新生儿低血糖

分娩方式

选择性剖宫产

- 应该安排使用胰岛素的妇女先手术,并在手术前一天或当日早上早些入院。
- 在清淡易消化的晚餐前,正常使用长效胰岛素。
- 手术前一天 22:00 后应禁食,安排第二天第一台手术;短效胰岛素应停用。
- 术前 1~2h 开始每小时监测一次血糖,必要时建议输葡萄糖-胰岛素,维持血糖 4~7mmol/L。
- 胰岛素用量和速度应根据母亲毛细血管血糖调整。

引产

- 应该继续目前的胰岛素方案直到确定临产。
- 常规的胰岛素用量,提前早餐。
- 一旦确定临产,母亲禁食,建议将输入葡萄糖-胰岛素作为常规,直到分娩结束。
- 每小时监测母亲血糖。
- 血糖水平应当维持在 4~7mmol/L。
- 根据母亲血糖调整胰岛素用量和速度。

自然临产

- 自然临产入院后,患者禁食。
- 入院时和此后每小时监测血糖水平。
- 饮食控制的产妇普遍不需要输注葡萄糖-胰岛素,除非毛细血管血糖>7mmol/L 或直到确定临产。
- 一旦确定临产,建议将葡萄糖-胰岛素输注作为常规。
- 毛细血管血糖应维持在 4~7mmol/L。
- 胰岛素用量和速度根据母亲血糖及当地的指南进行调整。

糖尿病类型

临产后饮食调整的 GDM 妇女应当每 1～2h 监测毛细血管血糖，目的是维持血糖<7.0mmol/L。如果不能达到该标准，应当常规静脉注射胰岛素-右旋葡萄糖。妊娠期需要应用胰岛素治疗的 GDM 妇女应当和妊娠前使用胰岛素治疗的产妇一样对待。

应用 CSII 的 1 型糖尿病妇女在分娩前应当找机会和主管医师讨论血糖的管理。个性化的方案应当在病历中保存。关于产程中 CSII 的效果的数据局限于一个有 65 例 1 型糖尿病患者的标准化研究，其中 CSII 28 例，持续静脉输注胰岛素 37 例。产程中 CSII 组平均血糖水平显著低于另一组（4.8mmol/L±0.6mmol/L vs 7.2mmol/L±1.1mmol/L；$P<0.025$）[30]。因此，产程中 CSII 是控制血糖的高效有利的方法，特别是临产前讨论了基础调整方法的病例。重要的一点是，要清楚麻醉师和产房工作人员可能对 CSII 都不熟悉，或当血糖高于目标值时更喜欢静脉注射胰岛素，所以产程中需要额外的医学支持和建议。妊娠后 CSII 应用在第十七章具体讨论。

胰岛素注射方法

英国 NICE 指南建议，1 型糖尿病分娩发动时，以及所有的糖尿病妊娠妇女如果血糖不能维持在 4～7mmol/L 时，应静脉输注右旋葡萄糖和胰岛素[2]。无论应用什么方法维持正常血糖，执行的医师、助产士和护士应该熟悉静脉输注的开始与管理。

根据个人经验设计，有不同的方法可以用。在 Belfast，最近用静脉注射右旋葡萄糖和可变的胰岛素方法（表 23.2，方法 1）。这个变化的方法是 Lepercq 等描述的，229 例妊娠妇女中 174 例是 1 型糖尿病，采取了可变速率的静脉注射胰岛素和 10%葡萄糖的治疗（表 23.2，方法 2）[37]。应用这种方法，母亲产程中的血糖为 6.1mmol/L±1.6mmol/L，新生儿低血糖发生率为 13%[37]。在一个"混合液体"（$n=15$）和"胰岛素滴注"（$n=20$）的对比研究中，母亲血糖分别是 5.8mmol/L±0.5mmol/L 和 5.7mmol/L±

1.0mmol/L，新生儿低血糖发生率没有显著性差异（6.7% vs 19.0%；P=0.9）。新生儿低血糖的定义是出生后 24h 内毛细血管血糖<1.9mmol/L[35]。这两个方法见表 23.2（方法 3 和方法 4）。

表 23.2 糖尿病母亲产时胰岛素输注治疗方案

方案 1：分娩发动或剖宫产前开始的方案						
母亲毛细血管血糖（mmol/L）	10%葡萄糖输注	胰岛素输注速度（ml/h=U/h）	10%葡萄糖输注时间	10%葡萄糖输注速度（ml/h）	血糖监测	
<2.0	150ml	0	10min	900	15min 后复测	
2.0～3.9	500ml	0	5h	100	30min 后复测	
4.0～5.9	500ml	1.0	6h	83	每小时	
6.0～7.9	500ml	2.0	6h	83	每小时	
8.0～9.9	500ml	2.5	6h	83	每小时	
10.0～11.9	500ml	3.0	6h	83	每小时	
>12	500ml	4.0	6h	83	每小时	
>16	电话联系内分泌医师（或者在周末电话咨询）					
方案 2（Lepercq 等，2008[37]）：分娩日早晨或自然临产入院后立即开始方案						
• 静脉注射 10%右旋葡萄糖溶液，80ml/h • 静脉注射短效胰岛素，用泵，起始剂量 1U/h • 每小时测量 CBG 直到分娩 • 通过调整胰岛素用量，达到目标 CBG 为 3.4～7.8mmol/L 　-1U/h，如果 CBG 为 3.4～7.8mmol/L 　-1.5U/h，如果 CBG 为 7.8～10.0mmol/L 　-2U/h，如果 CBG 为 10.0～12.2mmol/L 　-3U/h，如果 CBG 超过 12.2mmol/L • 在低血糖（CBG≤3.3mmol/L）病例中，停止胰岛素输注 30min 后，如果 CBG 持续不升，给予 30%葡萄糖静注						
方案 3（Rosenberg 等，2006[35]）：混合液体						
每小时测 CBG 值，目标值是 5.6mmol/L • CBG<5.6mmol/L：静脉注射 5%葡萄糖 125ml/h • CBG 为 5.6～7.8mmol/L：乳酸林格液 125ml/h • CBG>7.8mmol/L：开始调整胰岛素滴注（参见方案 4）						
方案 4（Rosenberg 等，2006[35]）：胰岛素滴注						
• 维持 125ml/h 静脉输注 5%葡萄糖和持续的胰岛素输注 • 当 CBG>4.5mmol/L 开始应用胰岛素 • 每小时监测 CBG 如下所示调整胰岛素，维持目标值 5.6mmol/L						

续表

CBG	速度（U/h）
<4.4mmol/L	停用
4.5~5.6mmol/L	0.5
5.6~7.8mmol/L	1.0
7.8~10.0mmol/L	1.5
10.0~12.2mmol/L	2.0
>12.2mmol/L	2.5

产后母亲血糖控制

产后胰岛素敏感性迅速增加，在接下来的两周内恢复正常[38]。一旦断脐，胰岛素输入应该减少50%，常规测量毛细血管血糖和静脉输液直到母亲开始正常进食。在一个有36例1型糖尿病的队列研究中，血糖值和胰岛素需要量在产后第一周显著低于预期[39]。这种效果在母乳喂养和非母乳喂养的母亲中都发现了[39]。因此，1型糖尿病的母亲常规皮下胰岛素减量继续使用，通常使用妊娠前一半的量。这是在糖尿病团队的密切监督下进行的，并根据需要进行滴定。

2型糖尿病的母亲产后胰岛素需要量也有类似的减少。如果妊娠期加了胰岛素，分娩时在严密血糖监测下应停止使用。妊娠前就应用胰岛素治疗的母亲，应该继续她们妊娠前的剂量，在产后早期阶段进行调整。妊娠前应用口服降糖药的母亲，如果产后不进行母乳喂养可以继续。母乳喂养者应用口服降糖药在第十五章具体讨论。

母乳喂养

糖尿病母亲建议哺乳前少量进食以免低血糖，通常容易发生在喂奶后1h。白天，由于热量摄入增加，对胰岛素的需求可能会增加，而夜间，由于葡萄糖虹吸入母乳，导致胰岛素需求量下降。因此，经常建议哺乳期妇女减少长效胰岛素。在一个有30例1型糖尿病的队列研究中，哺乳妇女产后6周时空腹血浆血糖水平显著低于已停止母乳喂养或仅仅人工喂养的妇女[40]。母亲血糖应尽可能保持正常以避免乳汁中糖含量升高和母亲低血糖。这个可以依靠糖尿病专家团队的指导通过规律进食和仔细调整胰岛素用量来实现。

总结和未来研究方向

妊娠前或妊娠糖尿病妇女应在能提供妊娠晚期和新生儿护理的机构中分娩。文献中很清楚,优化母亲围产期血糖能将新生儿低血糖和胎儿窘迫风险降至最低。应该进行 CSII 和传统的胰岛素-葡萄糖输注的随机对照研究,已经初步显示出 1 型糖尿病妇女妊娠后应尽早使用 CSII。

选择题

1. 一名 28 岁第一次妊娠的孕妇,患有 1 型糖尿病,37 周临产入院,宫颈开 4～5cm。她的常规胰岛素是餐前门冬胰岛素和夜间 30U 地特胰岛素。妊娠期血糖控制较好。她的糖尿病控制措施正确的是（　　）
   A. 继续给予她日常的胰岛素使用
   B. 继续地特胰岛素 30U 和保持门冬胰岛素直到可以正常进食
   C. 开始胰岛素-右旋葡萄糖输注,每小时调整速度维持毛细血管血糖 4～7mmol/L
   D. 每小时监测毛细血管血糖并以此为依据按比例增减皮下门冬胰岛素用量
   E. 继续常规皮下给予胰岛素,减少 50%的门冬胰岛素和地特胰岛素用量

正确答案是 C。开始胰岛素-右旋葡萄糖输注,每小时调整速度维持毛细血管血糖 4～7mmol/L

当临产妇女入院后并禁食,她需要立即开始执行胰岛素-右旋葡萄糖输注方案,每小时检测和调整胰岛素速度以维持毛细血管血糖为 4～7mmol/L。皮下注射胰岛素作为常规调整方法不够灵活,容易导致母亲低血糖。

2. 分娩了一个健康男孩后，患者 19：00 转入产后病房，进食两片面包。毛细血管血糖为 6.0mmol/L。分娩前，胰岛素用量是门冬胰岛素（早餐前 22U、午餐前 14U、晚餐前 20U）和地特胰岛素（夜间 30U）。妊娠前胰岛素用量是门冬胰岛素（早餐前 8U、午餐前 6U、晚餐前 8U）和地特胰岛素（夜间 16U）。她计划母乳喂养。她的糖尿病管理措施正确的是（　　）

　　A. 继续皮下使用胰岛素，用量是妊娠期的一半（如门冬胰岛素，早餐前 11U，午餐前 7U，晚餐前 10U）和地特胰岛素（夜间 15U），必要时监测血糖和调整胰岛素用量

　　B. 继续皮下使用胰岛素，用量是妊娠前的一半（如门冬胰岛素，早餐前 4U，午餐前 3U，晚餐前 4U）和地特胰岛素（夜间 8U），必要时监测血糖和调整胰岛素用量

　　C. 开始以妊娠前常规皮下胰岛素用量为基础，规律地监测血糖，必要时调整一定使用量

　　D. 继续皮下使用胰岛素，用量同妊娠前（早餐前 22U、午餐前 14U、晚餐前 20U）和地特胰岛素（夜间 30U），计算因为母乳喂养增加的热量摄入，规律地监测血糖和调整胰岛素用量

　　E. 继续皮下使用胰岛素，同妊娠期餐前的用量（早餐前 22U、午餐前 14U、晚餐前 20U），计算因为母乳喂养增加的热量摄入。减少夜间地特胰岛素用量为 20U

　　正确答案是 B。继续皮下使用胰岛素，用量是妊娠前的一半（如门冬胰岛素，早餐前 4U，午餐前 3U，晚餐前 4U）和地特胰岛素（夜间 8U），必要时监测血糖和调整胰岛素用量。

　　产后胰岛素敏感性立即增加，大约 2 周后趋于正常。因此，必须减少胰岛素用量至妊娠前的 50%，母乳喂养需要增加母亲热量摄入，并且可能会与夜间低血糖有关，因为糖分分泌到了乳汁中。这时关注点是避免母亲低血糖。随后密切监测血糖和调整胰岛素用量，加上糖尿病专家团队的支持，是维持满意血糖的控制基础。

（杨　蓉　译，王　冰　校）

参 考 文 献

1. Confidential Enquiry into Maternal and Child Health. Diabetes in Pregnancy: Are We Providing the Best Care: Findings of a National Enquiry: England, Wales and Northern Ireland. CEMACH: London, 2007.
2. National Institute for Clinical Excellence. Diabetes in Pregnancy: Management of Diabetes and Its Complications from Pre-conception to the Postnatal Period. NICE: London, 2015. www.nice.org.uk/guidance/ng3/evidence/full-guideline-3784285
3. Confidential Enquiry into Maternal and Child Health, Maternity Services in 2002 for Women with Type 1 and Type 2 Diabetes, England, Wales and Northern Ireland. CEMACH: London, 2004.
4. Royal College of Obstetricians and Gynaecologists. Antenatal corticosteroids to reduce neonatal morbidity and mortality. Green-top Guidance No. 7. 2010. www.rcog.org.uk/en/guidelines-research-services/guidelines/gtg7
5. NIH Consensus Statement. Antenatal corticosteroids revisited: repeat courses. National Institutes of Health 2000;17(2):1–18.
6. Betalov A & Balasubramanyam A. Glucocorticoid induced ketoacidosis in gestational diabetes: sequela of the acute treatment of preterm labour. Diab Care 1997;20:922–924.
7. Alexandre L, Shipman KE, Brahma A, et al. Diabetic ketoacidosis following steroid treatment in a patient with gestational diabetes mellitus. Practical Diab Int 2011;28:21–23.
8. Graham UM, Cooke IE, & McCance DR. A case of euglycaemic diabetic ketoacidosis in a patient with gestational diabetes mellitus. Obstet Med 2014;7:174–176.
9. Refuerzo JS, Garg A, Rech B, et al. Continuous glucose monitoring in diabetic women following antenatal corticosteroid therapy: a pilot study. Amer J Perinatol 2012;29:335–338.
10. Kreiner A, Gil K, & Lavin J. The effect of antenatal corticosteroids on maternal serum glucose in women with diabetes. Open J Obs Gynae 2012;2:112–115.
11. Kennedy A, Hadden DR, Ritchie CM, Gray O, McCance DR. Insulin algorithm for glycaemic control following corticosteroids in type 1 diabetic pregnancy. Irish J Med Sci 2003;172:40.
12. Mathiesen ER, Christiensen AB, Hellmuth E, et al. Insulin dose during glucocorticoid treatment for fetal lung maturation in diabetic pregnancy: test of an algorithm. Acta Obstet Gynecol Scand 2002;81:835–839.
13. Kaushal K, Gibson JM, Railton A, et al. A protocol for improved glycaemic control following corticosteroid therapy in diabetic pregnancies. Diabetic Med 2003;20:73–75.
14. Royal College of Obstetricians and Gynaecologists. Tocolysis for women in preterm labour. Green-top Guideline No. 1b. 2011. www.rcog.org.uk/globalassets/documents/guidelines/gtg1b26072011.pdf
15. Tibaldl JM, Lorber DR, Nerenberg A. Diabetic ketoacidosis and insulin resistance with subcutaneous terbutaline infusion: a case report. American J Obs Gynae 1990;163:509–510.
16. VanHaltren K, Malhotra A. Characteristics of infants at risk of hypoglycaemia secondary to being "infant of a diabetic mother". J Pediatr Endocrinol Metab 2013;26:861–865.
17. Harris DL, Weston PJ, Harding JE. Incidence of neonatal hypoglycaemia in babies identified as at risk. J Pediatrics 2012;161:787–791.
18. Harris DL, Weston PJ, Signal M, et al. Dextrose gel for neonatal hypoglycaemia (the Sugar Babies Study): a randomised, double blind, placebo-controlled trial. Lancet 2013;382:2077–2083.

19 Klemetti M, Nuutila M, Tikkanen M, et al. Trends in maternal BMI, glycaemic control and perinatal outcome among type 1 diabetic pregnant women in 1989–2008. Diabetologia 2012;55:2327–2334.
20 Kalhan SC. Metabolism of glucose and methods of investigation in the fetus and newborn. In: Polin RA, Fox WW, Abman SH, editors. Fetal and Neonatal Physiology. Saunders/Elsevier: Philadelphia, 2004, 449–464.
21 Cowett RM, Farrag HM. Selected principles of perinatal-neonatal glucose metabolism. Semin Neonatol 2004;9:37–47.
22 Hay W, Raju TK, Higgins RD, Kalhan SC, Devaskar SU. Knowledge gaps and research needs for understanding and treating neonatal hypoglycaemia: workshop report from Eunice Kennedy Shriver National Institute of Child Health and Human Development. J Pediatr 2009;155:612–617.
23 Adamkin DH and Committee of Fetus and Newborn. Clinical report – postnatal glucose homeostasis in late-preterm and term infants. Pediatrics 2011;127:575–579.
24 Chandran S, Rajadurai VS, Haium AAA, et al. Current perspectives on neonatal hypoglycaemia, its management, and cerebral injury risk. Res Rep Neonatology 2015;5:17–30.
25 Pederson J. Weight and length at birth of infants of diabetic mothers. Acta Endocrinol 1954;16:330–342.
26 Taylor R, Lee C, Kyne-grzebalski D, Marshall SM, Davison JM. Clinical outcomes of pregnancy in women with Type 1 diabetes. Obstet Gynaecol 2002;99:537–541.
27 Nold JL, Georgieff MK. Infants of diabetic mothers. Pediatr Clin North Am 2004;51:619–637.
28 Anderson O, Hertel J, Schmolker L, et al. Influence of the maternal plasma glucose concentration at delivery on the risk of hypoglycaemia in infants of insulin-dependent diabetic mothers. Acta Paediatr Scand 1985;74:268–273.
29 Miodovnik M, Mimouni F, Tsang RC. Management of the insulin-dependent diabetic during labor and delivery. Influences on neonatal outcome. Am J Perinatol 1987;4:106–114.
30 Feldberg D, Dicker D, Samuel N, et al. Intrapartum management of insulin-dependent diabetes mellitus (IDDM) gestants. A comparative study of constant intravenous insulin infusion and continuous subcutaneous insulin infusion pump (CSIIP). Acta Obstetric Gynecolog Scandinav 1988;67(4):333–338.
31 Lean ME, Pearson DW, Sutherland HW. Insulin management during labour and delivery in mothers with diabetes. Diabet Med 1990;7:162–164.
32 Curet LB, Izquierdo LA, Gilson GJ, et al. Relative effects of antepartum and intrapartum maternal blood glucose levels on incidence of neonatal hypoglycaemia. J Perinatol 1997;17:113–115.
33 Carron Brown S, Kyne-Grzebalski D, Mwangi B, et al. Effect of management policy upon 120 Type 1 diabetic pregnancies: policy decisions in practice. Diabet Med 1999;16:573–578.
34 Balsells M, Corcoy R, Adelantado JM, et al. Gestational diabetes mellitus: metabolic control during labour. Diabetes Nutr Metab 2000;13:257–262.
35 Rosenberg VA, Eglinton GS, Rauch ER, Skupski DW. Intrapartum maternal glycaemic control in women with insulin requiring diabetes: a randomized clinical trial of rotating fluids versus insulin drip. Am J Obs Gynae 2006;195:1095–1099.
36 Mimouni F, Miodovnic K, Siddiqi TA, et al. Perinatal asphyxia in infants of diabetic mothers is associated with maternal vasculopathy and hyperglycaemia in labour. J Paediatr 1988;113:345–353.
37 Lepercq J, Abbou H, Agostini C, et al. A standardised protocol to achieve normoglycaemia during labour and delivery in women with type 1 diabetes. Diabet Metab 2008;34:33–37.
38 American Diabetes Association Guidelines.

Management of diabetes in pregnancy. Diabetes Care 2015;38:S77–S79.

39 Saez-de-Ibarra L, Gaspar R, Obesso A, et al. Glycaemic behaviour during lactation: postpartum practical guidelines for women with type 1 diabetes. Pract Diabetes Intl 2003;20:271–275.

40 Ferris AM, Dalidowitz CK, Ingardia CM, et al. Insulin requirements of diabetic women who breast feed. BMJ 1989;298:1357–1358.

第二十四章　分娩和分娩后护理：新生儿护理

Jane M. Hawdon

Women's and Children's Health Clinical Academic Group, Barts Health NHS Trust, London, UK

实践要点

- 与妊娠前糖尿病相关的新生儿死亡率比普通人群高2倍。
- 与妊娠前糖尿病相关的早产和其相关的新生儿患病率是普通人群的5倍，并且通常可避免。
- 在妊娠前糖尿病中重大先天异常是普通人群的3~5倍。
- 其他已识别的妊娠糖尿病相关的新生儿并发症包括巨大儿、产伤、新生儿缺血缺氧性脑病和低血糖。
- 大多数糖尿病母亲的婴儿没有并发症，也不需要特殊护理。
- 母婴分离和人工喂养应该是有临床指征的偶发事件，而不是常规。

应当注意避免的陷阱

- 意外的心肺损害在出生时比一般情况更常见，而拥有先进的新生儿生命支持技能的医护人员延迟出诊可能会影响结果。
- 想当然地认为婴儿会发生临床严重低血糖会造成常规母婴分离和人工喂养，进而影响母乳喂养。
- 出生后巨大儿体重增加的大幅下降（绘制在百分位图中）不应该引起不必要的关注。

病　例

AB夫人，26岁，从10岁左右就发现患有1型糖尿病。她是计划妊娠，并去了一个妊娠前诊所，讨论在这个关键时期血糖最好的控制方法。她很羡慕自己的好朋友在家分娩，也计划在家分娩自己的第一个孩子，但是经过评估，医师认为即使是能很好地控制糖尿病，孩子还是有很多危险因素的，建议院内分娩。早期超声提示正常生长，胎儿解剖结构正常。

AB夫人在28周时还出现早产风险。她住进了医院，给予肌内注射倍他米松以降低早产后新生儿呼吸窘迫综合征的风险。倍他米松给药后的36h，给予最高到10U/h的胰岛素注射将血糖维持在可以接受的范围。幸运的是，宫缩抑制了，妊娠持续到了接近足月。少数产科医师建议 AB 夫人剖宫产，因为她有糖尿病。她咨询了会诊医师，医师认为没有危险因素，可以考虑正常分娩。当她知道关于剖宫产婴儿呼吸问题的风险增加时，AB 夫人感到很宽慰。

婴儿 Tom 是 38 周自然分娩的。他的出生体重是 3.6kg（第 91 百分位数）。出生后 Tom 立即趴在妈妈胸部和妈妈进行了皮肤接触，30min 内进行了母乳喂养，含乳和吸吮反射都很好。出生后 4h，测血糖（使用新生儿实验室的机器）为 1.5mmol/L（27mg/dl）。助产士考虑到 Tom 哭声、肤色和生命体征都正常，鼓励母亲再喂喂他。他初乳吃得不错，依然保持活力和正常哭声。间歇的皮肤接触喂养，但每次都很好地含乳和吸吮。到出生后 8h，他的血糖是 2.2mmol/L（40mg/dl），而且临床状态很好，没有给予额外的人工喂养来补充。Tom 持续喂养情况良好，血糖水平保持在 2.0mmol/L 以上（>36mg/dl）。24h 以后没有继续监测血糖，第 2 天 Tom 就回家了。

Tom 的健康观察师开始很关注他的 6 周随访，担心他的体重降到第 50 百分位以下。但是，健康观察师回顾了母亲妊娠期的糖尿病史，认为 Tom 表现的是他的正常体重。

- 为什么母亲被建议不要在家分娩？
- 为什么 Tom 出生后并发症极少？
- 为什么没有给 Tom 人工喂养？
- 为什么 Tom 的体重降到了较低的百分位数？

研究背景

母亲妊娠前和妊娠糖尿病对胎儿和新生儿产生的不良后果包括几个方面：直接的有害的代谢环境，母亲血糖控制不好时需要的产科干预和不恰当的"常规"处理。优化糖尿病的控制，特别是怀孕前，能将母亲和胎儿的风险降低到最低，并减少产后并发症的风险[1-5]。在许多母亲和婴儿获得健康结局的病例中，能够提前意识到会发生什么并发症是非常重要的。

随着 2 型糖尿病女性人群的年轻化，特别是某些种族，2 型糖尿病合并妊娠的比例接近糖尿病合并妊娠的一半[6, 7]。2 型糖尿病妇女所产婴儿发生并发症的比例接近或甚于 1 型糖尿病[8-10]。

最终，发展成妊娠糖尿病的母亲的胎儿和新生儿也有并发症的危险[11-17]。有证据表明，筛查和治疗妊娠糖尿病能够减少一些围产期并发症[14, 18, 19]。但是，最近国际糖尿病和妊娠研究组对妊娠糖尿病筛查的建议[19a]，以及随后 WHO 的建议[19b]导致了关于这方面的医疗花费和临床效果及在实践中变化的一场论战[14, 20-23]。

妊娠糖尿病控制良好的健康婴儿的护理

对许多妇女来说，特别是那些获得产前咨询和加强糖尿病护理的妇女，在妊娠期间血糖得到良好的控制，不太可能在妊娠期间发生与糖尿病有关的胎儿和新生儿并发症。重要的是要认识到，一个并发症风险非常低的婴儿应该按照健康新生儿的正常标准来管理[24, 25]。尤其重要的是，避免不必要的母婴分离，为有母乳喂养的母亲提供成功母乳喂养的便利。近期英国的一项审计显示了这方面的成功[7]。不能按照这些规则和所导致的医源性并发症也有所提及。

新生儿并发症——病因学和处理

尽管人们希望改善母婴糖尿病护理将围产期发病率和死亡率降到最低，但最近的资料表明所取得的进展还是不明显的（表 24.1）[6, 8, 10-12, 16, 26-33]。有一些新生儿并发症是由于早产或剖宫产，而其他的是继发于宫内或产时缺血缺氧或胎儿妊娠期所暴露的异常糖尿病代谢环境。最后，还有一些新生儿问题是医源性的（表 24.2）。

围产期死亡率

队列研究资料显示，从 20 世纪 90 年代开始，妊娠前糖尿病母亲分娩的婴儿的围产期死亡率（死产和出生后 1 周内的新生儿死亡）高于同一研究背景人群 2.3～3.8 倍[6-8, 12, 26, 28-30, 32, 33]，死产和新生儿死亡的数据分别表明，随着时间的推移，差异的幅度相同，没有任何改善。然而，妊娠糖尿病妇女的围产期死亡率并无明显上升的迹象[25]。

来自 CEMACH 的婴儿的队列研究显示，最常见的死因与先天异常和分娩并发症有关（表 24.3）[29]。

表 24.1 最近发表的文献中糖尿病妊娠和妊娠糖尿病与普通人群相比存在统计学显著差异的比值比（OR）和相对危险度（RR）

糖尿病类型	CEMACH(2005)[8] 妊娠前	Lai等(2014)[16] 妊娠前	Lai等(2014)[16] GDM	Vinceti等(2014)[10] 妊娠前	Feig等(2014)[12] 妊娠前	Feig等(2014)[12] GDM	Colstrup等(2013)[28] 妊娠前	Dunne等(2012)[30] 妊娠前	Al-Agha等(2012)[26] 妊娠前	Balsells等(2012)[11] 妊娠前	Balsells等(2012)[11] GDM	Eidem等(2010)[31] GDM
死产		3.7										
新生儿死亡	2.6	2										
围生期死亡率	3.8											
自发性早产		4.2	1.7		2.3		3.7	3.5	3.7			
引产早产		3.8	2									
早产	5						4.2	5				
剖宫产		2.5	1.6									
先天异常	2.6	1.6	1.2	1.8	1.8	1.3	2.4	2		2.7~4.7	1.2~1.4	
出生体重大于第90百分位	5.2	2.1	1.3				4.5		1.8			2.1
肩难产	2.6	1.5	1.32									
臂丛神经损伤	11											
5min Apgar评分<7分	3.4											
收入新生儿病房	5.6	3.8	1.6									
收入特护病房	3.3											

表 24.2　妊娠糖尿病后新生儿并发症

直接和妊娠糖尿病相关
- 先天异常
- 宫内生长受限
- 产时缺血缺氧
- 巨大儿、梗阻性分娩、产伤
- 新生儿死亡
- 红细胞增多症/黄疸
- 低酮血症性低血糖症
- 低钙血症、低镁血症
- 肥厚型心肌病

必要或不必要的产科干预的并发症
- 早产有关的并发症
- 剖宫产有关的并发症——呼吸窘迫，影响母乳喂养

医源性
- 不恰当的母婴分离
- 不恰当的人工喂养——影响母乳喂养

表 24.3　英国引起围产期死亡的原因[n（%）][8]

死亡原因	调查表（n=98）中的例数和占比	普通人群（n=5756）中的例数和占比	P 值
不明原因	58（59）	2516（44）	0.002
先天异常	18（18）	1087（19）	0.68
产时原因	10（10）	429（8）	0.30
早熟	4（4）	1027（18）	<0.001
感染	1（1）	252（4）	0.10

早产

早产（<37 周）率，无论是自发还是引产妊娠糖尿病妇女均显著高于同背景人群或没有糖尿病的妇女（表 24.1）[7, 8, 15, 16, 28, 32]。

早产原因在第二十二章已经讲述。和其他影响妊娠的母亲条件一样，在持续妊娠直到妊娠和缩短胎儿与母亲暴露在有害环境中的时间之间总是有一种平衡。但是，对于 CEMACH 队列研究中的妇女，19%的早产是非自发的或可以用母儿问题解释的，因此是可以避免的[8]。这个研究

期间阻止了 235 例因为新生儿护理而入院的患者。

如果是计划早产,必须在能提供新生儿重症监护的医院,这可能需要母亲转运到合适的机构,最好是在围产期网络系统内的机构。现在已经广泛认识到,如果早产可以预料,糖尿病母亲应当接受肾上腺皮质激素注射,这样糖尿病母亲分娩的婴儿不会普遍存在比同一孕周的婴儿更严重的呼吸窘迫。肾上腺皮质激素治疗的基本原理和随后的母亲管理也已经在第二十三章讨论了。

糖尿病母亲的早产婴儿应当依据标准方案管理。特别是,应当鼓励母亲吸出和储存母乳。糖尿病母亲的婴儿其他的特殊问题是可能会入院和需要额外护理(本章进一步讨论)。

剖宫产分娩的影响

妊娠糖尿病妇女的剖宫产率显著高于同样背景下没有糖尿病的妇女[8, 16, 32]。在英国的妊娠前糖尿病的研究中发现,9%的剖宫产不能用影响母儿安危的情况来解释,4%是"糖尿病的常规"或"母亲要求的"[8]。如前所述,一些这种"常规的"剖宫产还会造成早产(第二十二章也提到过)。

避开产程和阴道分娩虽然能够保护婴儿避免缺血缺氧性脑损伤,但是非必需的剖宫产的潜在副作用如母乳喂养延迟和中断及呼吸系统发病率(新生儿短暂性呼吸增快或表面活性剂缺乏)却是加倍的[34-36]。如果非必需的剖宫产过早,这种影响还会更大,也会因此经常导致一些不可避免的入住新生儿病房和母婴分离。

产前和产时缺血缺氧的影响

缺血缺氧是血液氧化不足和灌注不足(继发于缺氧对心脏功能的影响)的混合病理现象。对所有的器官系统都有潜在损害,特别是大脑。宫内缺血缺氧和继发于缺血缺氧的新生儿并发症的机制还没有完全清楚(参见第三章和第十九章)。但是,巨大儿和产程阻滞会导致产时缺血缺氧,增加新生儿并发症的危险。

糖尿病母亲的婴儿比非糖尿病母亲的婴儿可能更需要专业的新生儿

复苏。这也是为什么糖尿病母亲的婴儿分娩要求必须在能提供先进的新生儿生命支持的机构进行的原因之一。如果新生儿发生了不可预料的和严重的缺血缺氧的并发症,如果出生医院不能提供能严密观察的新生儿病房,包括必要时进行全身降温治疗,患儿将被要求转运到能提供的医院。

相关细胞缺氧会增加红细胞生成素分泌,因而增加胎儿红细胞生成[37]。所致的新生儿红细胞增多症可能导致新生儿黄疸加重(由于红细胞溶解)和偶发的高黏滞度综合征。肾静脉血栓或其他脏器栓塞比较罕见,但是糖尿病母亲的新生儿比其他非糖尿病母亲的新生儿发生更频繁。

对于这些婴儿的临床护理必须针对这些并发症做出改变,如果有异常临床征象,如易怒、昏睡和厌食,需要进行试验检查。就减少葡萄糖向大脑转运来说,红细胞增多和低血糖作用会叠加,红细胞增多相关的临床症状,如易怒和昏睡,根据标准的新生儿指南,必须进行部分换血治疗。

先天异常

人们很早就认识到,在妊娠期合并糖尿病的患者有比较高的先天畸形发生率[38]。自20世纪90年代以来,发生率比背景人群高1.6~2.7倍,而且至今也没有发生变化。引起先天畸形的因素包括妊娠早期进行治疗前的高血糖的致畸作用(表24.1)[7, 8, 10-12, 16, 27, 28, 30-33]。妊娠糖尿病的发生率低于妊娠前糖尿病的发生率,但仍然高于背景研究人群的发生率,可能与母亲2型糖尿病未诊断的病例或独立的肥胖因素对于先天异常发生率的影响有关[11, 12, 16]。

最普遍的异常是先天性心脏疾病和肢体、肌肉骨骼系统或结缔组织异常(发生率为0.7%)[8]。神经管缺陷,尽管从数字上来说比较少,但是比普通人群高3.4倍[8]。这些异常可能的病因学和预防应对措施在第十章和第十一章中阐述。

产科医师和新生儿科医师必须保证与新生儿父母有足够的交流,包括新生儿出生后负责护理的专家团队,要保证在一个恰当的中心(取决于异常的性质)进行分娩,能够在早期开始进行专家护理。并不提倡常规的产后心脏超声筛选先天心脏异常，除非产前超声筛查怀疑有异常或婴儿有先天心脏疾病的临床征象[25]。

巨大儿——分娩梗阻、产伤和器官巨大症

巨大儿和大于胎龄儿并不是刻意互换的术语。严格讲，巨大儿（器官大）描述的是一个婴儿重于他的由基因决定的出生体重，临床上表现为婴儿的躯干生长超过了头的生长，可能表现的是"正常的"出生体重。归因于胎儿胰高血糖素的巨大儿和巨器官有一个很好识别的特点就是妊娠期并发糖尿病[13, 39]。妊娠糖尿病婴儿出生体重超过第 90 百分位的可能性是普通背景人群的 1.8～5.2 倍[8, 16, 26, 28]。最近英国的研究治疗表明还有一些升高（表 24.1）[7]。

巨大儿的临床意义是分娩一个巨大儿的相关的危险并发症，如肩难产、分娩梗阻、围产儿缺血缺氧性脑病和产伤（如臂丛神经损伤、锁骨或肱骨骨折）。一些并发症不会引起长期的发病率，如骨折，显著的长期神经发育障碍可能与 Erb 瘫痪和继发于难产的缺氧缺血有关。

父母和专业的医疗人士必须对巨大儿出生后体重增长的减少有所准备，特别是母乳喂养者。这是正常的和健康的适应，提供给婴儿恰当的喂养，看起来是健康的，不必关注出生后早期体重增加少和体重曲线到了百分位线以下。过度喂养和持续超重有长期的健康后果（如远期的心血管疾病和糖尿病风险）。这是提倡和支持母乳喂养的一个进一步的原因，能保护预防远期的代谢性障碍[40, 41]。

肥厚型心肌病

肥厚型心肌病的特点是肥厚的隔膜肌肉阻挡了左心室流出道，严重者可导致胎儿和新生儿死亡[37]。在一些轻微的病例中，通常表现为出生后最初几周内发生心肺窘迫和充血性心力衰竭。大部分婴儿仅仅需要支持治疗，症状可能在随后的 2～4 周解决。隔膜肥厚在 2～12 个月退化。不需要常规进行出生后的超声心动检查，除非有心功能异常的临床表现[25]。

宫内生长受限

宫内胎儿生长受限通常与严重的糖尿病血管病变有关，可能导致出生后进一步的问题。糖尿病母亲的小于胎龄儿显然有更严重不良预后的风险，特别是相关的神经发育后遗症[42]。通常还会因为要求提前终止妊娠而进一步恶化。分娩必须有计划性的在合适的机构进行，还可能需要专业的新生儿护理。

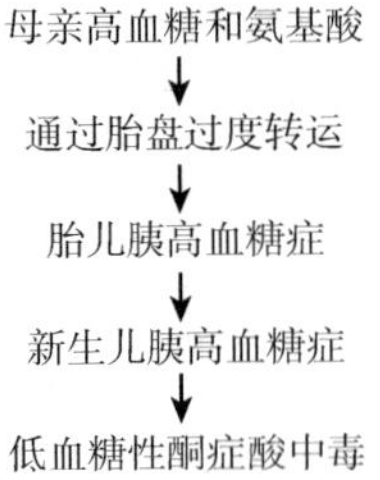

随着出生时胎盘营养的中断，健康的新生儿经历了代谢适应以保证重要脏器的能量供给。糖尿病母亲的婴儿会有暂时的高胰岛素血症的风险，会导致血糖吸收和转换成脂肪的比例增加，减少肝糖产生，减少脂代谢，因此减少酮体产生，这是血糖的代用能量（图24.1）[37,43]。极端的情况下还会导致低血糖性酮症酸中毒，脑部和其他重要脏器可获得的能量显著减少。

母亲高血糖和氨基酸
↓
通过胎盘过度转运
↓
胎儿胰高血糖症
↓
新生儿胰高血糖症
↓
低血糖性酮症酸中毒

图24.1 受损的新生儿代谢适应

最令人关注的是脑损伤和远期的神经发育后遗症，回顾已发表的一些研究都暗示新生儿低血糖和神经发育不良预后之间存在联系，但是没有一篇能够排除母亲糖尿病的其他的潜在的并发症[37,43]。尽管已经很明确，未经治疗的低血糖如果足够严重且持续足够久能够引起脑损伤，但是没有证据证明无临床症状的低血糖会引起脑损伤。临床症状提示（但是不是特异性的）低血糖的表现有以下方面：
- 异常的语气。
- 异常的意识水平。
- 不良口服给药。
- 非典型的表现（如表现为呼吸暂停）。

临床监测（见下文）的目的是在早期发现低血糖，使它变得有临床意义和给予合适的处理[25,44]。

幸运的是，很少有婴儿发展到具有临床症状的严重低血糖。原因可能包括标准化的母亲妊娠期和分娩期的糖尿病控制（参见第二十三章），因此严重的产后高胰岛素血症并不普遍，因为短暂的自然高胰岛素血症和早期预防性管理（本章下文进一步讨论）。

由于缺乏稳健的证据基础，本章由临床专家写的参考文献与英国NICE的指南都来自于经验，这要求临床医师能对每个婴儿进行个体化的治疗，强调认真临床评估的重要性（表24.4）[25, 37, 43-46]。

表 24.4　新生儿低血糖管理的问题

- 母亲血糖控制不良，特别是分娩前，增加危险
- CEMACH 观察——准确的新生儿血糖监测方法只应用在 1/4 的病例中
- 增加配方奶可能会抑制代谢适应
- 配方奶喂养可能会增加后期肥胖和代谢障碍的风险
- 必须避免不必要的母婴分离

临床监测

除非婴儿有足够严重的临床并发症要求入住新生儿病房，否则应当母婴同室[25, 47]。

那些照顾婴儿的人必须规律监测婴儿的喂养表现和异常的神经学体征，并记录他们的发现。除非有其他并发症（如感染）的危险因子，只要婴儿表现良好，不必要监测生命体征（体温、脉搏和呼吸速度）或筛查其他潜在的并发症（如红细胞增多症）[25]。如果任何时候出现了异常的临床症状，必须检测血糖水平，紧急安排儿科会诊。

能够普遍接受的是糖尿病母亲的婴儿应当规律地监测血糖[25]。血糖监测必须用一种准确的、有实验基础的方法。还没有仪表测量的试纸能够提供足够准确的测量以诊断或排除新生儿低血糖症[45]。推荐的标准是能够快速获得准确、定量的分析[25, 29, 43-45, 48, 49]。但是，英国的资料显示，只有约25%的婴儿用准确的方法监测了血糖[8]。

血糖监测建议在出生后 3～4h，早于这个的研究尚不详实，出生后1h 婴儿的血糖会经历生理性的暂时性下降，即使是健康婴儿也会低于2.0mmol/L。另外，健康婴儿在出生后3～4h 血糖水平偏低，也无助于区分婴儿是低血糖还是暂时性胰高血糖症。

血糖监测应当在喂养之前发现血糖水平的最低点。没有临床症状

的婴儿，检测喂养后的血糖水平是没有用的，还会使婴儿过多扎脚后跟。

如果发生胰高血糖症，通常发生在出生后最开始的 1~2 天，而且是暂时性的，最多持续数天。因此，如果婴儿临床表现平稳，没有任何严重的临床低血糖的证据，当实验室测量的血糖水平持续高于 2.0mmol/L 应当停止监测血糖，如果一切都好（表 24.5），出生后 24h 转到社区进行护理是恰当的[25]。

显然，早产的，不是很满意的及收入到新生儿病房的婴儿将会经历血糖监测，这也是临床护理的一部分。

表 24.5　新生儿血糖监测的实践方面

- 用一种准确的试验基础的方法
- 出生后 3~4h 开始
- 建议：大约 4h
- 有需要干预的临床症状（不考虑血糖水平）或连续两次血糖水平低于 2.0mmol/L（＜36mg/dl）
- 当连续两次血糖水平高于 2.0mmol/L（＞36mg/dl）停止监测

喂养

母乳喂养是所有婴儿的适用喂养方式（除非罕见的个例，如母亲 HIV 感染）。但是，英国的一个队列研究显示，只有 53% 的糖尿病母亲想要母乳喂养，到分娩后 28d，只有 27% 的足月分娩的婴儿进行母乳喂养[8]。一项加拿大的研究显示，相比没有糖尿病的母亲，即便是已经控制了混杂因子的影响，妊娠前糖尿病的母亲在院内可能只有不到 50% 进行了母乳喂养[50]。

应该在产前就鼓励妊娠妇女考虑母乳喂养，接受足够的关于母乳喂养的益处的信息以做出选择。分娩后，健康婴儿应该立即和母亲肌肤接触，尽早开始母乳喂养，帮助并保证有效的吸吮。母乳喂养应每 3~4h 一次（如果婴儿有要求可以更频繁），如果需要可以给予帮助。

只有临床指征时，包括干预低血糖（见后文"需要管理的血糖阈值"），才要求人工喂养辅助母乳喂养。人工喂养经常会导致母乳喂养的频率降低，因此会减少母乳分泌和抑制正常的新生儿代谢适应的建立。

因此，如果需要人工喂养，必须只给需要量，不要给更多。如果一个母亲选择人工喂养，需要量通常每天不能超过 100ml 每公斤体重，但是量应该根据临床监测调整。最后，也必须考虑潜在的远期的过度喂养和肥胖的代谢风险。

如果母婴分离或婴儿需要人工喂养辅助，应该鼓励母亲吸奶，这可以维持泌乳，并将母乳喂给婴儿。

需要管理的血糖阈值

低血糖相关的临床症状（如本章讨论的）必须治疗。没有异常临床症状，建议需要进行干预的血糖阈值必须注重实际，必须在发展为严重的临床低血糖和影响母乳喂养及造成母婴分离之间找到平衡点。英国指南建议，分娩后至少 3~4h，如果没有临床症状，两次连续的血糖测量（通常间隔 2~4h）低于 2.0mmol/L 时需要进行干预以升高血糖[25]。

临床严重低血糖的管理

对伴有异常临床体征的低血糖水平的管理（如这里所讨论的）是一种医疗紧急情况，需要对其进行全面的临床评估，并将其转到新生儿病房。如果临床症状不严重（如精神好但是吸吮差），间隔合适的间隔评估滴管喂养的效果是合理的。但是，如果滴管喂养后血糖水平没有升高或婴儿出现了严重的临床症状（如意识水平降低或惊厥），必须立刻静脉给予葡萄糖输注，5mg/（kg·min）[相当于 10%葡萄糖 3ml/（kg·h）]开始，但是应当注意的是，通过频繁的血糖监测，必要时可能需要增加用量[51]。如果有临床症状并且静脉给药延迟了，肌内注射胰高血糖素（200μg/kg）也是有用的，在它的作用下，糖原可以降解释放出葡萄糖，但是作用是短暂的，持续在 1h 内。

低钙和低镁血症

糖尿病合并妊娠的随访中，短暂的新生儿低钙血症曾有报道，发生率和严重程度都与母亲糖尿病的控制情况有关[37]。通常和高磷血症有关，偶尔与低镁血症有关。病因学尚不明确，但是发现有新生儿甲状旁腺功能减退，可能部分继发于母亲镁缺乏。已发表的研究和临床实践显示低钙血症和低镁血症没有明显的临床表现，除非合并其他并发症（如围产期缺血-缺氧）。因此，健康婴儿没有监测的指征。如果有临床症状，必须按照新生儿教科书上的标准进行纠正。

医源性并发症

分娩时机和分娩方式都会影响新生儿的发病率。偶尔是由于胎儿情况做出的决定，大多数是和母亲的并发症有关。但是在一些情况下，早产或剖宫产都没有明确的母儿原因，因此将新生儿置于危险的境地。

即使是没有严重的母亲或胎儿的并发症，妊娠到足月或接近足月仍有证据显示婴儿被暴露于潜在的医源性伤害中（表24.6）。CEMACH问卷调查显示，医学和产科学护理的频繁失误影响了婴儿出生后的过程，特别是喂养的建立[8, 29, 44]。这些包括以下方面：

- "常规"将婴儿纳入新生儿病房。
- "常规"人工辅助喂养补充或替代母乳喂养。
- 延迟皮肤接触和最早的喂养。
- 不良的温度控制管理。
- 分娩后过早开始测血糖和对此做处理。
- 除了这些问题对于母亲和婴儿的不良影响，它们还会占用可以避免使用的新生儿病房资源。

表24.6 潜在的可以避免的婴儿不良后果[8, 29, 44]

- 16%早产——没有明确指征的引产和剖宫产
- 30%早产儿——没有给予母亲肾上腺皮质激素
- 5%婴儿在没有严密监护的情况下分娩
- 25%的住院足月儿——给出的原因是"常规"
- 9%接受了人工喂养——给出的原因是"常规"

远期预后

关于糖尿病母亲妊娠期血糖控制不好的婴儿，潜在的远期神经发育后遗症的研究是前后矛盾的[37, 43]。但是，母亲妊娠期血糖控制好的婴儿的研究表明神经发育预后良好[15]。这些在第二十八章详细讨论。作为糖尿病母亲的后代，到 20 岁发展为 1 型糖尿病的概率至少是非糖尿病母亲的 7 倍（如果父亲是 1 型糖尿病则低于这个风险）[37]。但是，关于妊娠前糖尿病和妊娠糖尿病的远期代谢后遗症的病因学还存在争议[52-55]。

总结——最小化风险

许多已发表的研究结果强调了推荐的实践方案，这些与减少新生儿并发症和医源性伤害有关（表 24.7）[25]。所有医院必须书面化临床指南，包括预防和管理潜在的新生儿并发症，以及收入新生儿病房，将临床风险和医源性伤害最小化。

表 24.7　临床实践中预防新生儿并发症的关键点

- 如果预期并发症发生，产前咨询有经验的临床医师
- 分娩和产后管理的书面政策和指导方针
- 避免不必要的早产和（或）剖宫产
- 如果预期会早产，给予母亲肾上腺皮质激素，并需密切观察和管理母体血糖控制
- 安排在有恰当的新生儿专家的医院分娩
- 鼓励母乳喂养；除非有临床指征，否则不要给母乳喂养的婴儿提高人工辅助喂养
- 尽早开始母乳喂养和皮肤接触
- 用准确的方法进行常规血糖监测，出生后 3～4h 进行
- 除非连续两次血糖＜2.0mmol/L 或有低血糖的临床体征，否则不要进行低血糖的治疗
- 除非有临床体征，否则不要进行其他潜在并发症的筛查
- 除非有临床指征需要将婴儿纳入新生儿病房，否则要保证母婴同室
- 给母亲和护理人员讲解巨大儿体重增长的正常模式

选择题

1. 关于妊娠糖尿病的围产期死亡率的说法正确的是（　　）
    A. 随着糖尿病管理的提高，已经降到了正常人群水平
    B. 尚未改善，因为死产和新生儿死亡仍高于普通人群

C. 产时并发症是重要的基础原因
D. 有先天异常是重要的基础原因
E. 受妊娠前护理情况的影响

正确答案是 B、C、D 和 E。

2. 关于妊娠糖尿病婴儿足月分娩的说法正确的是（   ）
   A. 出生时必须具有高级复苏技能的人员在场
   B. 婴儿必须纳入新生儿病房
   C. 应当出生后 3～4h 开始监测血糖
   D. 禁忌只给予母乳喂养
   E. 出生后应当进行超声心动图检查

正确答案是 A 和 C。

3. 胎儿缺血缺氧的并发症包括（   ）
   A. 红细胞增多症   B. 巨大儿
   C. 低钙血症   D. 脑病
   E. 死产

正确答案是 A、D 和 E。

（杨 蓉 译，王 冰 校）

参 考 文 献

1 Owens LA, et al. ATLANTIC DIP: closing the loop: a change in clinical practice can improve outcomes for women with pregestational diabetes. Diabetes Care 2012;35:1669–1671.
2 Peterson C, et al. Preventable health and cost burden of adverse birth outcomes associated with pregestational diabetes in the United States. Am J Obstet Gynecol 2015;212(1):74.e1–9.
3 Shannon GD, et al. Preconception health care and congenital disorders: mathematical modelling of the impact of a preconception care programme on congenital disorders. BJOG 2013;120:555–566.
4 Simeone RM, et al. Diabetes and congenital heart defects: a systematic review, metaanalysis and modelling project. Am J Prev Med 2015;48(2):195–204.
5 Wahabi HA, et al. Preconception care for diabetic women for improving maternal and fetal outcomes: a systematic review and meta-analysis. BMC Preg Childbirth 2010;10:63.
6 Bell R, Bailey K, Creswell T, et al. Trends in prevalence and outcomes of pregnancy in women with pre-existing type I and type II diabetes. BJOG 2008;115:445–452.
7 Health and Social Care Information Centre. National Diabetes in Pregnancy Audit, 2014. Health and Social Care Information Centre: London, 2015.
8 Confidential Enquiry into Maternal and Child Health. Pregnancy in Women with Type 1 and Type 2 Diabetes in 2002–2003. CEMACH: London, 2007.

9 Temple R, Murphy H. Type 2 diabetes in pregnancy – an increasing problem. Best Pract res Clin Endocrinol Metab 2010;24:591–603.
10 Vinceti M, et al. Risk of birth defects associated with maternal pregestational diabetes. Eur J Epidemiol 2014;29:411–418.
11 Balsells M, et al. Major congenital malformations in women with gestational diabetes mellitus: a systematic review and meta-analysis. Diabetes Metab Res Rev 2012;28:252–257.
12 Feig DS, et al. Trends in incidence of diabetes in pregnancy and serious perinatal outcomes: a large, population-based study in Ontario, Canada, 1996–2010. Diabetes Care 2014;37:1590–1596.
13 HAPO Study Cooperative Research Group, Metzger BE, Lowe LP, et al. Hyperglycemia and adverse pregnancy outcomes. N Engl J Med 2008;358:1991–2002.
14 Hartling L, et al. Benefits and harms of treating gestational diabetes mellitus: a systematic review and meta-analysis for the US Preventive Services Task Force and the National Institutes of Health Office of Medical Applications of Research. Ann Intern Med 2013;159:123–129.
15 Kock K, et al. Diabetes mellitus and the risk of preterm birth with regard to the risk of spontaneous preterm birth. J Matern Fetal Noenatal Med 2010;23:1004–1008.
16 Lai FY, et al. Outcomes of singleton and twin pregnancies complicated by pre-existing diabetes and gestational diabetes: a population-based study in Alberta, Canada, 2005–2011. J Diabetes 2016;8(1):45–55.
17 Ovesen P, et al. Maternal and neonatal outcomes in pregnancies complicated by gestational diabetes: a nation-wide study. J Matern Fetal Neonatal Med 2014;17:1–14.
18 Farrar D, et al. Evaluation of the impact of universal testing for gestational diabetes mellitus on maternal and neonatal health outcomes: a retrospective analysis. BMC Preg Childbirth 2014;14:317.

19 Horvath K, et al. Effects of treatment in women with gestational diabetes mellitus: systematic review and meta-analysis. BMJ 2010;340:c1395.
19a International Association of Diabetes and Pregnancy Study Groups Consensus Panel. International Association of Diabetes and Pregnancy Study Groups Recommendations on the diagnosis and classification of hyperglycemia in pregnancy. Diabetes Care 2010;33:676–682.
19b World Health Organization (WHO). Diagnostic Criteria and Classification of Hyperglycaemia First Detected in Pregnancy. WHO: Geneva, 2013.
20 Bodmer-Roy S, et al. Pregnancy outcomes in women with and without gestational diabetes mellitus according to the International Association of the Diabetes and pregnancy Study groups criteria. Obstet Gynecol 2012;120:746–752.
21 Langer O, et al. The proposed GDM diagnostic criteria: a difference, to be a difference, must make a difference. J Matern Fetal Neonatal Med 2013;26:111–115.
22 Tieu J, et al. Screening and subsequent management for gestational diabetes for improving maternal and infant health. Cochrane Database Syst Rev 2014;2:CD007222.
23 Wilmot EG, Mansell P. Diabetes and pregnancy. Clin Med 2014;14:677080.
24 National Collaborating Centre for Primary Care. Postnatal Care: Routine Postnatal Care of Women and Their Babies. NICE: London, 2006. http://www.nice.org.uk/Guidance/CG37
25 National Institute for Health and Clinical Excellence. Diabetes in Pregnancy. NICE: London, 2008. http://www.nice.org.uk/Guidance/CG63
26 Al-Agha R, et al. Outcome of pregnancy in type 1 diabetes mellitus (T1DMP): results from combined diabetes-obstetrical clinics in Dublin in three university teaching hospitals (1995–2006). Irish J Med Sci 2012;181:105–109.

27. Casson IF, Clarke CA, Howard CV, et al. Outcomes of pregnancy in insulin dependent diabetic women: results of a five year population cohort study. BMJ 1997;315:275–278.
28. Colstrup M, et al. Pregnancy in women with type 1 diabetes: have the goals of St Vincent declaration been met concerning foetal and neonatal complications? J Matern Fetal Neonatal Med 2013;26:1682–1686.
29. Confidential Enquiry into Maternal and Child Health. Diabetes in Pregnancy: Are We Providing the Best Care? Findings of a National Enquiry. CEMACH: London, 2007.
30. Dunne FP, et al. ATLANTIC DIP: pregnancy outcomes for women with type 1 and type 2 diabetes. Irish Med J 2012;105(5 Suppl):6–9.
31. Eidem I, et al. Congenital anomalies in newborns of women with type 1 diabetes: nationwide population-based study in Norway, 1999–2004. Acta Obstet Gynecol Scand 2010;89(11):1403–1411.
32. Evers IM, de Valk HW, Visser GH. Risk of complications of pregnancy in women with type 1 diabetes: nationwide prospective study in the Netherlands. BMJ 2004;328:915–918.
33. Penney GC, Mair G, Pearson DW. Outcomes of pregnancies in women with type 1 diabetes in Scotland: a national population based study. BJOG 2003;110:315–318.
34. Gawlick S, et al. Timing of elective repeat caesarean section does matter: Importance of avoiding early-term delivery especially in diabetic patients. J Obstet Gynaecol 2015;35(5):455–460.
35. Evans KC, Evans RG, Royal R, Esterman AJ, James SL. Effect of cesarean section on breast milk transfer to the normal term newborn over the first week of life. Arch Dis Child Fetal Neonatal Ed 2003;88:F380–F382.
36. Hansen AK, Wisborg K, Uldbjerg N, Henriksen TB. Risk of respiratory morbidity in term infants delivered by elective cesarean section: cohort study. BMJ 2008;336:85–87.
37. Hawdon JM. Neonatal complications after diabetes in pregnancy. In: Rennie JM (ed), Textbook of Neonatology, 5th ed. Churchill Livingstone: Edinburgh, 2012.
38. Molsted-Pedersen L, Tygstrup I, Pedersen J. Congenital malformations in newborn infants of diabetic women. Lancet 1964;i:1124–1126.
39. Mello G, Parretti E, Mecacci F, et al. What degree of maternal metabolic control in women with type 1 diabetes is associated with normal body size and proportions in full term infants? Diabetes Care 2000;23:1494–1498.
40. Owen CG, Martin RM, Whincup PH, Smith GD, Cook DG. Does breastfeeding influence risk of Type 2 diabetes in later life? A quantitative analysis of published evidence. Am J Clin Nutr 2006;84:1043–1054.
41. Owen CG, Whincup PH, Kaye SJ, et al. Does initial breastfeeding lead to lower blood cholesterol in adult life? A quantitative review of the evidence. Am J Clin Nutr 2008;88:305–314.
42. Petersen MB, Pedersen SA, Greisen G, Pedersen JF, Molsted-Pedersen L. Early growth delay in diabetic pregnancy: relation to psychomotor development at age 4. BMJ 1988;296:598–600.
43. Hawdon JM. Hypoglycemia and brain injury – when neonatal metabolic adaptation fails. In: Levene MI, Chervenak FA (eds), Fetal and Neonatal Neurology and Neurosurgery, 4th ed. Churchill Livingstone: Edinburgh, 2009.
44. Confidential Enquiry into Maternal and Child Health. Diabetes in Pregnancy: Caring for the Baby after Birth. Findings of a National Enquiry. CEMACH: London, 2007.
45. Cornblath M, Hawdon JM, Williams AF, et al. Controversies regarding definition of neonatal hypoglycemia: Suggested operational thresholds. Pediatrics 2000;105:1141–1145.
46. Rozance PJ, Hay WW. Hypoglycemia in

newborn infants: Features associated with adverse outcomes. Biol Neonate 2006;90:74–86.
47 Stage E, et al. Diabetic mothers and their newborn infants – rooming-in and neonatal morbidity. Acta Paediatr 2010;99:997–999.
48 Williams AF. Neonatal hypoglycemia: Clinical and legal aspects. Semin Fetal Neonatal Med 2005;10:363–368.
49 Deshpande S, Ward Platt MP. The investigation and management of neonatal hypoglycemia. Semin Fetal Neonatal Med 2005;10:351–361.
50 Finkelstein SA, et al. Breastfeeding in women with diabetes: lower rates despite greater rewards. A population-based study. Diabet Med 2013;30:1094–1101.
51 Hawdon JM. Disorders of metabolic homeostasis in the neonate. In: Rennie JM (ed), Textbook of Neonatology, 5th ed. Churchill Livingstone: Edinburgh, 2012.
52 Burquet A. Long-term outcome in children of mothers with gestational diabetes. Diabetes Med 2010;36:682–694.
53 Donavan LE, Cundy T. Does exposure to hyperglycaemia in utero increase the risk of obesity and diabetes in the offspring? A critical reappraisal. Diabet Med 2015;32;295–304.
54 Fraser A, Lawlor DA. Long-term health outcomes in offspring born to women with diabetes in pregnancy. Curr Diab Rep 2014;14:489.
55 Yessoufou A, Moutairou K. Maternal diabetes in pregnancy: early and long-term outcomes on the offspring and the concept of "metabolic memory." Exp Diab Res 2011;2011:218598.

其他参考文献

56 CESDI – Confidential Enquiry into Stillbirths and Deaths in Infancy: 8th Annual Report. Maternal and Child Health Research Consortium: London, 2001.

第二十五章 女性糖尿病患者的产后避孕

Anita L. Nelson

David Geffen School of Medicine at UCLA, University of California, Los Angeles, California, USA

实践要点

- 对于女性糖尿病患者而言，在 2 次妊娠间留出适当的时间间隔非常重要。这种方法使患有 GDM 的女性有机会减少妊娠中复发的风险因素。妊娠前患糖尿病的妇女需要时间进行严格的血糖控制，以降低先天异常和死产的风险。
- 母乳喂养对母亲和新生儿都有益，也有利于产后减轻体重。鉴于相对较少的妇女能继续母乳喂养较长时间，为母乳喂养的妇女提供最有效的避孕方法又不会影响哺乳非常重要。
- 患有妊娠前糖尿病或有 GDM 病史的女性需要安全有效的避孕措施，将对体重、血压、胰岛素抵抗或脂质的不良影响降到最小。植入物和宫内节育器（IUD）是首选，因为它们是最有效的且符合标准。
- WHO 和美国疾病控制和预防中心（CDC）医疗资格标准（MEC）均同意 GDM 本身不应影响避孕方法的选择；所有方法均被评为 1 类，但产后应避免立刻使用含雌激素的避孕方法。从安全的角度来说，需要考虑并发症（如肥胖、高血压、心血管疾病和抑郁症）的存在。
- 排卵通常在产后 25～39 天恢复，并且性冲动通常在产后 6 周的传统访视之前恢复。产后及时提供安全有效的避孕方法已成为金标准，因此必须在产前护理期间讨论避孕措施，并在分娩后和出院前加强避孕宣教。女性在选择分娩医院时应考虑的事项，如需要的新生儿设施和可用的分娩麻醉，实施输卵管结扎，宫内节育器和产后植入物的可能性。

病 例

一名 26 岁的 33 周龄妊娠妇女在 29 周时被诊断出患有 GDM。她的妊娠前 BMI 为 $34 kg/m^2$；直到她妊娠的这一时间点，她已经增加了约 16kg。她有曾妊娠 7 周时流产的病史。一系列超声测量结果提示胎儿有向巨大儿发展的趋势。目前正在接受药物治疗，在家自行监测指尖血糖，在节食和锻炼的情况下血糖值仍然居高不下。在使用口服避孕药时妊娠了一次，在依靠男用避孕套时妊娠了一次。她确信，在分娩后的数个月内，她不必考虑计划生育，因为她和她的丈夫将忙于新生儿。

- 何时是为糖尿病或 GDM 女性提供避孕建议的最佳时机？
- 何时是产后避孕的最佳时间？
- 产后哪些避孕方法是禁忌？
- 对于 GDM 女性，任何方法都会对 6 周后的葡萄糖检测产生不良影响吗？
- 对于 BMI>30kg/m^2 的女性，某些方法的效果不佳吗？
- 纯母乳喂养婴儿的女性应该避免采取哪些避孕方法？这些避孕方法在多长时间内应避免使用？
- 如果她认为家庭还不完整，我们的患者下次妊娠的最佳时间是什么时候？
- 她下次妊娠前应该达到什么目标？
- 什么方法（如果有的话）可能会使实现这些目标更加困难？
- 对这名年轻女性的健康更危险的是再次妊娠还是没有医学认可的避孕方式？
- 如果她已经生育子女怎么办？你会给她哪些选择？
- 如果她有妊娠前糖尿病，您会推荐哪种避孕方法？

背景

一般人群中妊娠的最佳间隔传统上被认为是 18～24 个月[1]。然而，美国 1/3 的再次妊娠是在孩子出生后 18 个月内发生的[2]。短暂的妊娠间隔可能对现有婴儿和新胎儿的生长产生负面影响。对于患有妊娠前糖尿病和妊娠期糖尿病的女性，妊娠间隔短则风险更大。在患有 GDM 的女性中，如果妊娠间隔小于 12 个月，则 GDM 复发率可高达 85%[3]。

尽管引入了安全有效的避孕措施，但在过去的 20 年中，美国的意外妊娠率一直保持在较高水平；最近的评估显示，美国 45% 的妊娠是非计划的[4]。低收入或受教育程度较低的女性和单身女性的比率最高，其中大多数也存在 GDM 的危险因素。

虽然在美国其余 55% 的妊娠被归类为"预期"，但这并不意味着他们是有计划和准备的，只是在那些女性妊娠的时候，她们并不反对妊娠。本章前面已经阐明了妊娠前糖尿病患者受孕前严格控制葡萄糖及使即将受孕女性的 GDM 危险因素最小化的重要性。2.2% 的分娩是针对妊娠前糖尿病（1 型或 2 型）的女性，包括最佳血糖控制在内的妊娠前保健，可避免每年 8397 例早产，3725 例新生儿出生缺陷，1872 例的产前死亡。减少的寿命成本总计 43 亿美元[5]。通过妊娠前护理确定以前未确诊的糖尿病将额外节省 12 亿美元[5]。为了准备妊娠，性活跃的女性必须有能力控制自己的生育。因此，提供有效和安全的控制措施应该是首要任务。

妊娠前糖尿病妇女和妊娠期糖尿病妇女在选择产后避孕方法时需要考虑许多重要因素。

- 这种方法必须是有效的；在这个患者群体中的意外妊娠与妊娠妇女和胎儿预后不良结局的风险增加数倍相关。
- 避孕方法不应对胰岛素敏感性或葡萄糖代谢造成显著影响。重要的是，在产后时期，患有 GDM 的女性必须避免可能对产后葡萄糖代谢测试产生不利影响的任何事情。
- 避孕药不应干扰母乳喂养或增加产后抑郁症的风险。
- 避孕方法应该方便实用。
- 在存在合并症的情况下，该避孕方法也必须是安全的（如肥胖、高血压和抑郁症）。
- 避孕方法不应增加长期心血管危险因素，如与代谢综合征或糖尿病并发症有关的因素。

糖尿病妇女的重要安全避孕注意事项

WHO 和美国 CDC 的医疗资格标准（表 25.1）一致认为，几乎所有避孕方法都可以用于患有 GDM 或妊娠前糖尿病的女性[6, 7]。对于患有糖尿病并发症的女性，包括视网膜病变、肾病或心血管疾病，应重点避免使用含有雌激素的避孕方法。糖尿病妇女还需要确保所提供的避孕方法都不会加速这些疾病的发展[8]。对于患有 GDM 的女性来说，考虑到避孕方式可能对其病情进展为显性糖尿病的影响也很重要。

通常，患有妊娠前糖尿病或 GDM 的女性患有合并症，如肥胖、代谢综合征或高血压，在开具避孕方法时必须考虑这些合并症[9, 10]。优选使用不会导致体重增加，已不会增加高 BMI 引起的任何风险（如静脉或动脉血栓形成）的方法。迄今为止，还没有确凿的证据表明联合口服激素避孕药（COC）可以诱导女性产生任何明显的代谢变化[11-13]。对于有 GDM 史的女性来说，重复妊娠比使用 COC 更容易引起随后的显性糖尿病[14]。

表 25.1 2016 年美国糖尿病和合并症的避孕药选择标准

疾病	合并疾病	Cu-IUD	LNG-IUD	移植	DMPA	POP	CHC
糖尿病	（1）妊娠期疾病病史	1	1	1	1	1	1
	（2）无血管疾病						
	1）非胰岛素依赖	1	2	2	2	2	2
	2）胰岛素依赖	1	2	2	2	2	2
	（3）肾病、视网膜病变或神经病变*	1	2	2	3	2	3/4**
	（4）其他血管疾病或糖尿病病史超过20年*	1	2	2	3	2	3/4**
高血压	（1）高血压充分控制	1**	1**	1**	2**	1**	3**
	（2）血压升高（正确测量）						
	1）收缩压 140~159mmHg 或舒张压 90~99mmHg	1**	1**	1**	2**	1**	3**
	2）收缩压≥160mmHg 或舒张压≥100mmHg*	1**	2**	2**	3**	2**	4**
	（3）血管疾病	1**	2**	2**	3**	2**	4**
心血管疾病的多种危险因素	如老年、吸烟、糖尿病、高血压、低 HDL、高低密度脂蛋白或高三酰甘油水平	1	2	2**	3**	2**	
肥胖	（1）体重指数（BMI）≥30kg/m²	1	1	1	1	1	2
	（2）初潮年龄 <18岁和BMI≥30 kg/m²	1	1	1	2	1	2

1，无限制（可使用方法）；2，优势通常大于理论或已证实的风险；3，理论或已证实的风险通常大于优势；4，不可接受的健康风险（不使用的方法）

CHC，激素联合避孕（药丸、贴片和环）；Cu-IUD，含铜宫内节育器；DMPA，长效醋酸甲羟孕酮；LNG-IUD，左炔诺孕酮释放宫内节育器；POP，仅孕激素片

*使妇女妊娠风险增加的情况；**请参阅完整的指南以了解对该分类的说明，www.cdc.gov/reproductivehealth/unintendedpregnancy/USMEC.htm. 完整摘要可查阅：https://www.cdc.gov/reproductivehealth/unintendedpregnancy/pdf/legal_summary-chart_english_final_tag508.pdf

功效

要考虑的第二个事项是如何对女性进行生育控制。避孕效果有三种不同的衡量标准：正确和持续避孕方式的第一年失败率，临床试验的总失败率，以及典型避孕方式的第一年失败率（表 25.2）。在美国，典型避

孕方式失败率的评估来自被称为全国家庭成长调查的周期性调查。正确和持续避孕方式使用的失败率评估与典型避孕方式失败率之间的差距（表25.2）表明人为因素和系统障碍可以导致避孕失败[15]。例如，如果每次性行为都正确使用男用安全套，应该只有2%的失败率，但在现实生活中，第一年的妊娠率为13%。在为女性提供咨询时，临床医师应该告知典型避孕方式的失败率，让患者知道通过理想的避孕可以更有效避孕，以激发女性正确使用避孕方式。唯一可逆、可靠且相当于永久避孕的避孕方式是宫内节育器和植入物。对于自信家庭完整的女性，提供永久性避孕（如输精管结扎术或输卵管切除术）是合理的。

表25.2 第一年避孕失败率

方法	第一年内意外妊娠的妇女的妊娠率（%）	
	完整使用	常规使用
不避孕	85	85
杀精剂	16	21
安全期避孕		15
体外射精	4	20
避孕海绵	12	17
避孕套		
女性	5	21
男性	2	13
带杀精剂的隔膜	16	17
联合避孕药和仅孕激素的避孕药	0.3	7
Evra贴，NuvaRing	0.3	7
长效醋酸甲羟孕酮	0.2	4
子宫内节育器		
ParaGard（铜T）	0.6	0.8
Mirena（LNG）	0.5	0.5
ENG植入	0.01	0.01
女性绝育	0.5	0.5
男性绝育	0.10	0.15

资料来源：节选自 Sundaram A, Vaughan B, Kost K, et al. Contraceptive failure in the United States: estimates from the 2006-2010 national survey of family growth. Perspect Sex Reprod Health 2017; 49 (1): 7-16

提倡母乳喂养

母乳喂养有许多好处，包括产后产妇体重的减少和葡萄糖代谢的适度改善[16, 17]。一些证据表明，母乳喂养至少 3 个月可降低 GDM 女性未来患 2 型糖尿病的风险[18, 19]。哺乳期闭经本身可以为产后前 6 个月的意外妊娠提供良好的保护（2%失败率）。在 6 个月之后，需要第二种方法避孕，因为这段时期排卵通常在第一次月经之前没有任何预兆地恢复。然而，大多数妇女在分娩后数周内停止母乳喂养[20]，因此必须为母乳喂养的妇女提供早期避孕。

传统上，当新妈妈正进入哺乳期时，激素疗法确实让人担忧。理论上讲，由于产后循环黄体酮水平的下降刺激了产奶量，因此分娩后过早给予黄体酮的方法可以减少产奶量。幸运的是，一些大规模研究对于早期使用黄体酮避孕对母乳产量、母乳喂养的持续和婴儿生长都是中性的推荐[20-23]。

避孕启动的时机

CDC 和 WHO 推广的首选避孕方法是为妇女提供她所希望的最有效的方法，并且只要临床医师有理由判断她没有妊娠，此方法就是合格的[24]。在产后期间需要有同样的紧迫性。有几个因素导致越来越多的学者认为，应该在妇女从医院回家之前进行起始避孕。首先是认识到排卵和性活动的恢复比先前估计的要早得多。总体而言，25%的女性在产后 25~39 天排卵[25]。年轻的女性比年长女性生育能力恢复更快[26]。其次是许多女性没有保留产后的医疗预约，即使她们保留了，但由于许多经济或医院原因，许多女性无法获得最有效的避孕方法。在新墨西哥州的一项研究中，实际只有 60%的需要宫内节育器女性在她们离开医院之前获得了一个节育器；没有得到宫内节育器的最常见原因之一是重复妊娠[27]。产后立即开始避孕需要在产前护理期间提供咨询，并且可以在分娩前获得所有相关的同意。

ACOG 发出警告及提示，许多女性在产后都没有提供所寻求的避孕措施。当分娩医院不提供这些服务时，就造成了未能提供永久性避孕的结果。获得知情同意[28]和将其交付给医院的外科医师也很困难。其他问题，如无法获得外科手术资源、缺乏选择程序的优先权，都与延误有关。在一项研究中，89名需要输卵管结扎的女性中，只有45名实际上按计划接受了这些手术[29]。没有接受产后输卵管结扎的女性在12个月内妊娠的可能性是产后就诊对照组的两倍（46.7% vs 22.3%）[30]。ACOG建议产后输卵管结扎术应考虑紧急外科手术[31]。

一些研究已经证明了产后即刻安装宫内节育器[32-35]（胎盘娩出后10min内）的安全性和有效性。排除这种方式的唯一标准是产后出血、绒毛膜炎/子宫内膜炎或此类感染的危险因素[7]。阴道分娩后的放置需要可以延伸到子宫内膜腔内的器械，可能是在超声引导下。剖宫产时宫内节育器的放置更为直接[36]。另外，在宫内节育器尾部应绑一条单丝缝合材料，以确保在任何时候需要取出宫内节育器时，阴道内有可用的尾部[37]。与产后6~8周子宫完全退化后放置宫内节育器相比，阴道分娩时放置宫内节育器的排斥率更高，为3%~24%，但在选择性剖宫产时放置率较低[33]。1年的延续率一般平均为75%[33]。

荷尔蒙避孕植入物是出院前放置的最佳选择，技术上比宫内节育器更简单。在分娩时没有立即植入种植体的紧迫性，这意味着未经避孕治疗的女性有更多机会考虑这一选择。产后种植体植入不会增加植入物的排斥率（如宫内节育器所示）或提前出血的风险[38]。第一年的持续率超过85%[39]，并且在快速重复意外妊娠风险最高的女性中最高[38, 40]。母乳喂养的女性在产后3~4d随机接受依托孕烯植入，与种植6~8周的女性相比，母乳喂养失败，乳汁成分、量或婴儿生长没有差异[23, 41]。

避孕方法的选择

永久避孕

输精管结扎术是最安全的，也是最有效的永久性避孕方法之一。在世界范围内，不到3%的已婚妇女（总共3300万）生育年龄依赖于伴侣的输精管切除术。但这些比率存在很大差异：加拿大、美国、中国和欧洲部分国家已婚夫妇中有10%~15%使用输精管切除术，但世界其他地区的比率较低[42,43]。在许多情况下，如无手术刀，输精管切除术简单到允许局部麻醉下在办公室环境中进行。在最近发表的研究总结中提到，切口长度为5.0～8.4mm，平均手术时间为8～20min，并发症发生率为0.67%～5%，最常见的并发症是血肿和感染[44]。

糖尿病妊娠妇女的伴侣通常希望等到分娩后进行输精管切除术。鉴于夫妇在手术后至少3个月不能依赖输精管切除术，应该给予该妇女一种短期桥接方法，如仅用孕激素注射或仅用孕激素药丸，以便在此期间使用。

另外，女性的永久性避孕（子宫切除术或输卵管结扎术）是美国年龄偏大的女性（>30岁）最常用的方法。有许多方法可用于中断输卵管。产后使用的最常用技术包括用无创伤夹钳抬高输卵管的一部分，在基部周围快速吸收缝合线并切断管的固定部分。该过程有各种变化，分别将管的两个切割端系在一起或将中断管的一端置于与另一端不同的隔室（腹膜后或子宫浆膜下方）。输卵管结扎术可在剖宫产时或阴道分娩后不久通过脐下小切口进行。当女性未妊娠时，其他程序作为间隔程序进行。一般而言，所使用的两种不同方法通过到达输卵管的方式分为腹腔镜检查和宫腔镜检查。通过腹腔镜手术，患者接受区域麻醉或全身麻醉；通过小的腹部切口，用缝合线或各种夹子中断每个管。这些方法立即提供避孕，但确实带来了与麻醉相关的风险和支出。在宫腔镜手术中，患者通常只需要静脉注射镇痛药。在每个输卵管的近端部分中填充有引起炎症反应的刺激性聚对苯二甲酸乙二醇酯（PET）流体的线圈。随着时间的推移，PET纤维诱导纤维化，这会使管闭塞。在闭塞完成之前，这对夫妇需要使用其他避孕措施。通常，在3个月时进行第二次测试（超声或荧光透视）以记录完全输卵管阻塞。

最新的认识认为，最具侵袭性的上皮性卵巢癌——浆液性腺癌来自输卵管内，许多学者认为输卵管切除术优于输卵管中断手术，特别是对于有卵巢癌风险的女性。如果在简单的剖宫产分娩时进行手术，这种建议最容易采用。随着有关可行性、安全性及长期利益和风险的更多证据的积累，使用这些不同技术的应用频率可能会发生变化[45,46]。

重要的是要记住，大量女性（>10%）后来对他们永久性避孕的决定感到遗憾。既然可以通过可逆方法提供等效的妊娠保护，其中许多方法提供了其他重要的非感染性益处，那么寻求输卵管手术的女性可能会更少。

避孕植入物

避孕植入物是糖尿病或先前 GDM 患者的最佳选择[47]。在美国，只有单杆 3 年系统的依托孕烯（ENG）植入物（Nexplanon）可用，但国际上有其他植入系统可用，包括单杆、3 年系统（埋植剂）和双杆，左炔诺孕酮 5 年系统（Jadelle/Norplant II 和 Sino II）。第一年失败率非常低(0～0.38%)，并且几乎没有医疗禁忌证。肥胖不会降低该方法的效率[48]。尽管所有提供植入物的美国提供者必须在 FDA 批准的公司赞助的培训课程中获得认证，但放置时需要很少的特殊培训。移除正确放置的植入物也很容易，但移除深植入物可能需要额外的支持或培训。植入物是繁忙实践的结果，就像初级保健临床医师；放置植入物本身需要 30s。ENG 植入物的作用机制吸引了许多不愿意接受可能具有受精后作用方法的女性，因为植入物抑制了 100% 的女性 30 个月的排卵[49]。在整个有效作用的过程中，宫颈黏液增厚可防止精子进入上生殖道。小规模的研究表明在植入物使用的第 4 年没有妊娠[50]。当与通过细胞色素 P450 系统诱导孕激素代谢增加的药物一起使用时，植入物具有更高的避孕失败率，这些药物包括一些抗癫痫药物、利福平和圣约翰草。作为仅含孕激素的方法，植入物可以减缓子宫复旧并且通常延长恶露的持续时间。如上所述，植入物对母乳成分或母乳喂养模式没有不利影响，对胰岛素抵抗、葡萄糖代谢、止血或血脂水平只有轻微的影响[51]。约 1/3 的女性在前 3 个月中月经周期令人满意；另外 1/3 将在 6 个月内完成。在美国的临床试验中，只有 14% 的女性因为月经紊乱而要求移除植入物[52]。

宫内节育器

美国目前有两大类宫内节育器可供使用：释放左炔诺孕酮（LNG）宫内节育器和铜制宫内节育器。在世界其他地方，还有其他的铜制（200～380mm^2 含铜 T 形装置）宫内节育器和一些未加药物的塑料装置（Lippes Loops，Safe-T-coil 等）。在铜制宫内节育器中，铜 T-380A 是最有效的，可以在产后立即放置[53]。然而，LNG-IUD 的产品标签建议至少延迟到产后 6 周放置。最近的研究表明，放置宫内节育器穿孔的风险为 1/（800～1000）个；而母乳喂养妇女的风险高出 6 倍[54]。

铜 T-380A 和 LNG-IUS 的第一年失效率均低于 1%；疗效不受女性 BMI 的影响。宫内节育器的选择取决于患者月经出血模式的倾向。LNG-IUS 20μg/24h 宫内节育器在点状出血和出血增加的过渡期后，随着时间的推移可能增加闭经的风险。8μg LNG-IUS 具有较低的黄体酮循环水平，并且具有更低的闭经率（3 年时为 13%）。LNG-IUS 12μg 是中等剂量，有 5 年的妊娠保护，并且 5 年时的闭经率为 23%。铜制宫内节育器通常会使月经失血量增加 30%～50%，对于希望保持每月月经轻度增加至正常量的女性及不能或不想使用任何外用激素的女性来说尤其具有吸引力。

在一项随机试验中，较高剂量的 LNG-IUS 对 1 型糖尿病女性的葡萄糖代谢没有不良影响[55]。同样，在一项研究中，对于近期给予 LNG-IUS 的 GDM 妇女与使用非激素方法的妇女进行比较，未观察到对葡萄糖耐量的不利影响[56]。使用 LNG-IUS 的女性（86.7%）在 12 个月时的持续率与使用铜制宫内节育器的女性（90.3%）相同。鉴于其安全性和有效性，宫内节育器被认为是糖尿病妇女和患有 GDM 患者的最佳避孕方法之一[47]，但它们应仅由熟练进行骨盆检查和骨盆手术的从业者安置。

仅含黄体酮的注射剂

在世界范围内，两种最常见的黄体酮注射剂是每 11～13 周肌内注射 1 次 150mg 的醋酸甲酯（DMPA）和每 60 天肌内注射 1 次 200mg 的醋酸炔诺酮（NETA）。每 12～14 周也可以使用较低剂量的皮下注射（DMPA-SQ 104mg），但很少使用。目前在美国只有 6% 的女性使用避孕药，但是在撒哈拉以南的一些国家，超过 1/3 的使用避孕药的女性依赖于孕激素注射。在所有避孕方法中，由于其高剂量，DMPA 对葡萄糖代谢和胰岛素抵抗具有最深远的影响。在一些女性中，DMPA 可能会增加体重或躯干脂肪沉积[57]。在一些高风险人群的研究中，如有 GDM 病史的西班牙裔女性，仅使用孕激素的方法与随后发生糖尿病的风险略增加有关，特别是在母乳喂养和体重增加的妇女中[58]。然而，在采用更有效的方法之前，仅使用孕激素注射可以作为产后避孕的一种有效方法。一些研究表明其对哺乳有轻微的不利影响，但证据并不一致。DMPA 不会增加产后抑郁的风险[59]。早先报道的骨矿化的不良影响现在已知是可逆的，不应影响注射避孕的开始或长期使用[60]。事实上，仅有孕激素的避孕措施可以预防产后母乳喂养妇女的骨质流失[61]。

激素组合方法

口服避孕药仍然是美国最常用的可逆方法。已经引入了长期导入系统（透皮贴剂和阴道环）以增加便利性。在国际上，每月一次含雌激素的注射剂也可用于月经周期规律时。在最近的一篇综述中报道，虽然数据稀少，但结果显示口服避孕药对糖尿病控制或糖尿病患者的微血管病变并没有恶化[62]。然而，由于血栓栓塞的风险，在患有心血管疾病或严重微血管疾病（肾病伴蛋白尿或增生性视网膜病变）的糖尿病女性中应该完全避免含雌激素的方法。

对于没有高凝危险因素的女性，如肥胖、剖宫产、先兆子痫、失血过多、反式融合或活动受限，含有雌激素的避孕方法可以在产后 21d 开始。有这些风险因素的妇女应该延迟到分娩后 42d 进行注射，而其他符合条件的产后妇女应使用复方激素避孕药[30]。最近的研究表明，早在产后 3 周开始使用低剂量复方激素方法的母乳喂养的女性对其泌乳没有不良影响[63]。

对于有多种医学问题的女性，谨慎地咨询 WHO 和美国 CDC 的医疗资格标准，以排除任何第 4 类病症，并在其他避孕选择的背景下考虑其第 3 类病症的总体情况（表 25.1）。早先的观察结果显示，BMI＞30kg/m^2 的女性口服避孕药和阴道环的失败率高于 BMI 较低的女性。最近的研究发现，那些较高的失败率可能是因为肥胖女性可能不会持续使用它们；与肥胖的关联可能是由社会经济因素引起的，如贫困，而不是生物学原因[64]。

障碍物和行为方法

从历史上看，这些方法通常被推荐为有医疗问题女性的一线选择，因为它们没有明显的风险，有些提供了重要的非避孕益处（如避孕套降低了性传播感染的风险）。然而，鉴于它们在典型避孕方式中具有较高的失败率（表25.2），今天这些方法仅适用于不能或不会使用其他更有效方法的妇女。因此，几乎所有其他疾病包括艾滋病和其他性传播疾病都可以使用障碍物（特别是避孕套）来预防。

这些方法的好处就是可以在柜台上买到。在欧洲，与精子素一起使用的单一尺寸隔膜无须处方即可使用。女性避孕帽（Femcap®）很容易根据女性的产科史（从未妊娠，没有阴道分娩或阴道分娩）来确定尺寸，并且在帽子的碗中使用少量杀精剂凝胶。世界各地的女用避孕套有各种材料和形状。通常情况下，女性安全套的失败率高于男用安全套，但是当伴侣不能或不会使用男用安全套时，它们提供了重要的好处。杀精子泡沫和海绵立即有效，但杀精子膜和栓剂需要10～15min才能融化并涂在子宫颈上。

如果一对夫妇没有其他保护措施，体外射精总是可用的，并且在典型避孕方式中它只比女性屏障方法稍微有效。生育意识方法帮助女性计算他们的风险日，以便他们在此期间可以使用禁欲或其他方法。老式的"节奏方法"已被计算机应用程序和产品（循环珠和生育日历）所取代，这些应用程序和产品更容易计算风险天数，并采用低技术方法（如2d方法）。在最后一种方法中，女性要做的就是每天触摸她的阴道口，确认是否干燥（即没有分泌物）。如果连续2d干燥，妊娠的风险很低，允许性交。

紧急避孕

最有效的紧急避孕（EC）形式是在无保护性交的5d内放置铜制宫内节育器。这将妊娠的风险降低到1/（800～1000）。EC所用的激素可通过柜台或1.5mg LNG的处方购买到，最多3d用完。如果在最初的12h内服用LNG-EC片剂是最有效的（妊娠概率为0.5%）；此后，临时风险迅速上升，在第72h上升至4%。BMI较高的女性效果明显较差。埃拉醋酸（UPA）30mg EC片剂在每个时间点比LNG-EC更有效，并且在超重和肥胖女性中更有效[65]。UPA可在暴露后5d内随时使用，随着时间的推移不会降低效果。使用UPA后激素避孕的开始应延迟至无保护性交的最后一次发生后5d，以造成所有精子死亡。

随访案例

在本章回到我们的上面提到的病例中,假设这名女性没有采用其他避孕方法,没有妊娠期间的并发症,那么最好在分娩之前与她讨论避孕问题。应该强烈建议她专门进行母乳喂养。虽然承认她禁欲的意图,但应该告诉她,多数时候难以实现禁欲计划。根据以前的经验,重要的是告诉她口服避孕药的失败率比植入物或宫内节育器的失败率高21倍[66]。

植入物对她来说也是一个很好的选择,可以在住院期间随时提供。如果她对巨大儿进行选择性剖宫产,可以很容易在手术中放置宫内节育器,但稍微增加较低风险的排斥反应。如果预计阴道分娩,可以娩出胎盘后置入。在拥有保险制度的国家,如果她的保险费不包括住院费用,她可以在医院门诊就诊,在出院后和离开医院场地之前植入(而不是宫内节育器)。如果这些选项都不可用,则应为她提供桥接方法。直到她产后,短期使用含黄体酮的药片是一种非常安全的桥接方法。DMPA注射对于忙碌的新妈妈来说更方便,但对于患有GDM的女性,如果进行为期6周的葡萄糖耐量测试,结果可能会受到影响,特别是对于接近显性糖尿病阈值的女性。在该患者分娩后至少6周内,复方口服避孕药不是一种选择,因为她的BMI超过$30kg/m^2$。障碍物方法是糟糕的第三选择,并应始终伴随着EC的提议。因为她还没有完整的家庭,永久的避孕方法是不合适的。为了她的长期健康,需要通过饮食减肥和定期运动。她还应该为下次妊娠做更充分的准备,并且妊娠不应该早于18个月。

未来的方向

许多新的避孕方法正在开发中,包括新的长效植入物,出血少的铜制宫内节育器,雌激素暴露较少的避孕贴片,新的易于使用的男用和女用避孕套,新的杀精子剂,以及可能长期提供的植入式芯片——荷尔蒙避孕。然而,即使能够获得最有效和最安全的避孕方法,女性仍然需要有动力去使用它们。今天,许多妇女并未意识到妊娠对健康的危害及在妊娠前需要优化健康。我们需要将普遍的信念从"妊娠刚刚发生"转变为"我们真的准备好了"。后者可能比开发新的避孕方法本身更具挑战性。

选择题

1. 对于糖尿病妇女而言，避孕方法最有效且医疗禁忌证最少的是（ ）
   A. 铜宫内节育器　　　　　B. 左炔诺孕酮宫内节育系统
   C. 植入物　　　　　　　　D. 长效醋酸甲孕酮注射
   正确答案是 C。

2. 孕激素可能引起糖尿病妇女的关注，因为它们可能（ ）
   A. 增加静脉血栓栓塞的风险　B. 增加子宫内膜癌的风险
   C. 增加贫血的风险　　　　　D. 增加胰岛素抵抗
   正确答案是 D。

3. 宫内节育器主要通过以下哪种机制起作用（ ）
   A. 阻塞植入　　　　　　　B. 防止受精
   C. 破坏受精卵　　　　　　D. 抑制排卵
   正确答案是 B。

4. 对于希望母乳喂养新生儿的女性，在出院前开始使用仅含孕激素的方法（ ）
   A. 是不必要的，因为哺乳期闭经，前 6 个月的妊娠率约为 2%
   B. 是不鼓励的，因为它会降低母亲建立泌乳的机会
   C. 是不鼓励的，因为女性对母乳喂养的动机较小
   D. 应该提供，因为许多妇女停止母乳喂养或不返回产后护理
   正确答案是 D。

（赖　杰　译，王　冰　校）

参 考 文 献

1　Zhu BP. Effect of interpregnancy interval on birth outcomes: findings from three recent US studies. Int J Gynaecol Obstet 2005;89(Suppl 1): S25–S33.

2　Gemmill A & Lindberg LD. Short interpregnancy intervals in the United States. Obstet Gynecol 2013;122(1):64–71.

3　Farrell J, Forrest JM, Storey GN, *et al.*

Gestational diabetes – infant malformations and subsequent maternal glucose tolerance. N Engl J Med 2016;374:843–852.
4 Finer LB & Zolna MR. Declines in unintended pregnancy in the United States, 2008–2011. Am J Public Health 2014;104(Suppl 1):S43–S48.
5 Peterson C, Grosse SD, Li R, et al. Preventable health and cost burden of adverse birth outcomes associated with pregestational diabetes in the United States. Am J Obstet Gynecol 2015;212:74.e1–e9.
6 World Health Organization (WHO). Medical Eligibility Criteria for Contraceptive Use, 5th ed. 2015. http://www.who.int/reproductivehealth/publications/family_planning/MEC-5/en/
7 US Centers for Disease Control and Prevention (CDC). US medical eligibility criteria (US MEC) for contraceptive use. 2016. https://www.cdc.gov/mmwr/volumes/65/rr/rr6503a1.htm?s_cid=rr6503a1_w
8 Kjos SL. After pregnancy complicated by diabetes: postpartum care and education. Obstet Gynecol Clin North Am 2007;34:335–349.
9 Kerlan V. Postpartum and contraception in women after gestational diabetes. Diabetes Metab 2010;36:566–574.
10 Garg SK, Chase PH, Guillermo M. et al. Oral contraceptives and renal and retinal complications in young women with insulin-dependent diabetes mellitus. JAMA 1994;271:1099–1102.
11 Ahmed SB, Hovind P, Parving HH, et al. Oral contraceptives, angiotensin-dependent renal vasoconstriction, and risk of diabetic nephropathy. Diabetes Care 2005;28:1988–1994.
12 ACOG Committee on Practice Bulletins – Gynecology. Use of hormonal contraception in women with coexisting medical conditions. ACOG Practice Bulletin No. 73. Obstet Gynecol 2006;107:1453–1472.
13 Grigoryan OR, Grodnitskaya EE, Andreeva EN, et al. Use of the NuvaRing hormone-releasing system in late reproductive-age women with type 1 diabetes mellitus. Gynecol Endocrinol 2008;24:99–104.
14 England L, Kotelchuck M, Wilson HG, Diop H, Oppedisano P, Kim SY, Cui X, & Shapiro-Mendoza CK. Estimating the recurrence rate of gestational diabetes mellitus (GDM) in Massachusetts 1998–2007: methods and findings. Matern Child Health J 2015;19:2303–2313.
15 Sundaram A, Vaughan B, Kost K, et al. Contraceptive failure in the United States: estimates from the 2006–2010 National Survey of Family Growth. Perspect Sex Reprod Health 2017;49:7–16.
16 Kramer MS & Kakuma R. Optimal duration of exclusive breastfeeding. Cochrane Database Syst Rev 2012;8:CD003517.
17 Gunderson EP, Crites Y, Chiang V, et al. Influence of breastfeeding during the postpartum oral glucose tolerance test on plasma glucose and insulin. Obstet Gynecol 2012;120:136–143.
18 Much D, Beyerlein A, Roßbauer M, et al. Beneficial effects of breastfeeding in women with gestational diabetes mellitus. Mol Metab 2014;3:284–292.
19 Kitzmiller JL, Dang-Kilduff L, & Taslimi MM. Gestational diabetes after delivery. Short-term management and long-term risks. Diabetes Care 2007;30:S225–S235.
20 Halderman LD & Nelson AL. Impact of early postpartum administration of progestin-only hormonal contraceptives compared with nonhormonal contraceptives on short-term breast-feeding patterns. Am J Obstet Gynecol 2002;186:1250–1256.
21 Kapp N, Curtis K, & Nanda K. Progestogen-only contraceptive use among breastfeeding women: a systematic review. Contraception 2010;82:17–37.
22 Reinprayoon D, Taneepanichskul S, Bunyavejchevin S, et al. Effects of the etonogestrel-releasing contraceptive implant (Implanon on parameters of breastfeeding compared to those of an

intrauterine device. Contraception 2000;62:239–246.
23 Braga GC, Ferriolli E, Quintana SM, Ferriani RA, Pfrimer K, & Vieira CS. Immediate postpartum initiation of etonogestrel-releasing implant: a randomized controlled trial on breastfeeding impact. Contraception 2015;92(6):536–542.
24 US Centers for Disease Control and Prevention. U.S. Selected Practice Recommendations for Contraceptive Use, 2013: Adapted from the World Health Organization Selected Practice Recommendations for Contraceptive Use, 2nd ed. http://www.cdc.gov/mmwr/preview/mmwrhtml/rr6205a1.htm
25 Jackson E & Glasier A. Return of ovulation and menses in postpartum nonlactating women: a systematic review. Obstet Gynecol 2011;117:657–662.
26 Morán C, Alcázar LS, Carranza-Lira S, *et al.* Recovery of ovarian function after childbirth, lactation and sexual activity with relation to age of women. Contraception 1994;50:401–407.
27 Ogburn JA, Espey E, & Stonehocker J. Barriers to intrauterine device insertion in postpartum women. Contraception 2005;72:426–429.
28 Zite NB, Philipson SJ, & Wallace LS. Consent to sterilization section of the Medicaid–Title XIX form: is it understandable? Contraception 2007;75:256–260.
29 Boardman LA, DeSimone M, & Allen RH. Barriers to completion of desired postpartum sterilization. R I Med J 2013;96:32–34.
30 Thurman AR & Janecek T. One-year follow-up of women with unfulfilled postpartum sterilization requests. Obstet Gynecol 2010;116:1071–1077.
31 Committee on Health Care for Underserved Women. Access to contraception. Committee Opinion No. 615. Obstet Gynecol 2015;125:250–255.
32 Washington CI, Jamshidi R, Thung SF, *et al.* Timing of postpartum intrauterine device placement: a cost-effectiveness analysis. Fertil Steril 2015;103:131–137.
33 Celen S, Möröy P, Sucak A, *et al.* Clinical outcomes of early postplacental insertion of intrauterine contraceptive devices. Contraception 2004;69:279–282.
34 Sonalkar S & Kapp N. Intrauterine device insertion in the postpartum period: a systematic review. Eur J Contracept Reprod Health Care 2015;20:4–18.
35 Grimes DA, Lopez LM, Schulz KF, *et al.* Immediate post-partum insertion of intrauterine devices. Cochrane Database Syst Rev 2010;12:CD003036 pub2.
36 Lester F, Kakaire O, Byamugisha J, *et al.* Intracesarean insertion of the Copper T380A versus 6 weeks postcesarean: a randomized clinical trial. Contraception 2015;91:198–203.
37 Nelson AL, Chen S, & Eden R. Intraoperative placement of the Copper T-380 intrauterine devices in women undergoing elective cesarean delivery: a pilot study. Contraception 2009;80:81–83.
38 Ireland LD, Goyal V, Raker CA, *et al.* The effect of immediate postpartum compared to delayed postpartum and interval etonogestrel contraceptive implant insertion on removal rates for bleeding. Contraception 2014;90:253–258.
39 Tocce KM, Sheeder JL, & Teal SB. Rapid repeat pregnancy in adolescents: do immediate postpartum contraceptive implants make a difference? Am J Obstet Gynecol 2012;206:481.e1–e7.
40 Han L, Teal SB, Sheeder J, & Tocce K. Preventing repeat pregnancy in adolescents: is immediate postpartum insertion of the contraceptive implant cost effective? Am J Obstet Gynecol 2014;211:24.e1–e7.
41 Gurtcheff SE, Turok DK, Stoddard G, *et al.* Lactogenesis after early postpartum use of the contraceptive implant: a randomized controlled trial. Obstet Gynecol 2011;117:1114–1121.

42 Pile JM & Barone MA. Demographics of vasectomy – USA and international. Urol Clin North Am 2009;36(3):295–305.
43 Shih G, Turok DK, & Parker WJ. Vasectomy: the other (better) form of sterilization. Contraception 2011;83(4):310–315.
44 Li L, Shao J, & Wang X. Percutaneous no-scalpel vasectomy via one puncture in China. Urol J 20146;11(2):1452–1456.
45 Kwon JS. Ovarian cancer risk reduction through opportunistic salpingectomy. J Gynecol Oncol 2015;26(2):83–86.
46 Committee on Gynecologic Practice. Salpingectomy for ovarian cancer prevention. Committee opinion no. 620. Obstet Gynecol 2015;125(1):279–281.
47 American College of Obstetricians and Gynecologists. Long-acting reversible contraception: implants and intrauterine devices. ACOG Practice Bulletin No. 121. Obstet Gynecol 2011;118:184–196.
48 Xu H, Wade JA, Peipert JF, et al. Contraceptive failure rates of etonogestrel subdermal implants in overweight and obese women. Obstet Gynecol 2012;120:21–26.
49 Mäkäräinen L, van Beek A, Tuomivaara L, et al. Ovarian function during the use of a single contraceptive implant: Implanon compared with Norplant. Fertil Steril 1998;69:714–721.
50 McNicholas C, Maddipati R, Zhao Q, et al. Use of the etonogestrel implant and levonorgestrel intrauterine device beyond the U.S. Food and Drug Administration-approved duration. Obstet Gynecol 2015;125:599–604.
51 Oderich CL, Wender MC, Lubianca JN, et al. Impact of etonogestrel-releasing implant and copper intrauterine device on carbohydrate metabolism: a comparative study. Contraception 2012;85:173–176.
52 Merck. Nexplanon: FDA-approved patient labeling. https://www.merck.com/product/usa/pi_circulars/n/nexplanon/nexplanon_ppi.pdf

53 Kulier R, O'Brien PA, Helmerhorst FM, et al. Copper containing, framed intra-uterine devices for contraception. Cochrane Database Syst Rev 2007;4:CD005347.
54 Heinemann K, Reed S, Moehner S, & Minh TD. Comparative contraceptive effectiveness of levonorgestrel-releasing and copper intrauterine devices: the European Active Surveillance Study for Intrauterine Devices. Contraception 2015;91(4):280–283.
55 Rogovskaya S, Rivera R, Grimes DA, Chen PL, Pierre-Louis B, Prilepskaya V, & Kulakov V. Effect of a levonorgestrel intrauterine system on women with type 1 diabetes: a randomized trial. Obstet Gynecol 2005;105(4):811–815.
56 Kiley JW, Hammond C, Niznik C, et al. Postpartum glucose tolerance in women with gestational diabetes using levonorgestrel intrauterine contraception. Contraception 2015;91:67–70.
57 Kim C. Managing women with gestational diabetes mellitus in the postnatal period. Diabetes Obes Metab 2010;12:20–25.
58 Xiang AH, Kjos SL, Takayanagi M, et al. Detailed physiological characterization of the development of type 2 diabetes in Hispanic women with prior gestational diabetes mellitus. Diabetes 2010;59:2625–2630.
59 Tsai R & Schaffir J. Effect of depot medroxyprogesterone acetate on postpartum depression. Contraception 2010;82:174–177.
60 American College of Obstetricians and Gynecologists. Depot medroxyprogesterone acetate and bone effects. ACOG Committee Opinion No. 602. Obstet Gynecol 2014;123:1398–1402.
61 Costa ML, Cecatti JG, Krupa FG, et al. Progestin-only contraception prevents bone loss in postpartum breastfeeding women. Contraception 2012;85:374–380.
62 Gourdy P. Diabetes and oral contraception. Best Pract Res Clin Endocrinol Metab 2013;27:67–76.

63 Espey E, Ogburn T, Leeman L, *et al*. Effect of progestin compared with combined oral contraceptive pills on lactation: a randomized controlled trial. Obstet Gynecol 2012;119:5–13.

64 Westhoff CL, Torgal AH, Mayeda ER, *et al*. Ovarian suppression in normal-weight and obese women during oral contraceptive use: a randomized controlled trial. Obstet Gynecol 2010;116:275–283.

65 Glasier A, Cameron ST, Blithe D, Scherrer B, Mathe H, Levy D, Gainer E, & Ulmann A. Can we identify women at risk of pregnancy despite using emergency contraception? Data from randomized trials of ulipristal acetate and levonorgestrel. Contraception 2011;84(4):363–367.

66 Winner B, Peipert JF, Zhao Q, *et al*. Effectiveness of long-acting reversible contraception. N Engl J Med 2012;366:1998–2007.

第二十六章　母乳喂养与糖尿病

Elizabeth Stenhouse

School of Nursing and Midwifery, Faculty of Health and Human Science, Plymouth University, Plymouth, UK

实践要点

- 在妊娠前患1型糖尿病和2型糖尿病及妊娠期糖尿病的妇女中，需要确定母乳喂养的流行率。
- 糖尿病妊娠妇女在开始和建立母乳喂养时应了解她们及其新生儿/婴儿可能遇到的特殊挑战。
- 卫生保健专业人员应了解糖尿病对乳汁生成的影响，因此由经过适当培训的卫生保健专业人员向妇女及其家庭提供适当的建议和保证。
- 如果不能母乳喂养新生儿，则应向打算母乳喂养的妇女传授产前采集初乳以治疗新生儿低血糖。
- 应鼓励在出生后1h内进行皮肤接触。
- 尽可能避免母婴分离。
- 应说明糖尿病母亲及其新生儿的短期受益。
- 在整个妊娠期和分娩后，应强调糖尿病母亲及其子女的长期受益。

问题

- 产前时期：未能向妇女及其家庭提供与母乳喂养的益处有关的基于公正信息的证据。对于那些决定母乳喂养的女性，未能指导她们如何表达和储存初乳。
- 分娩护理：母婴分离，未尽早进行皮肤接触至少1h。
- 出生后：未在出生后1h内开始母乳喂养。如果需要治疗新生儿低血糖，可补充配方奶而不是母乳，如果可以，也可补充产前收获的初乳。

病　例

　　Sally和她的伴侣在妊娠测试呈阳性后去了产前诊所,结果证实她已妊娠8周。莎丽今年21岁,有5年的1型糖尿病史。

　　研究人员记录了完整的医学和生殖史,并进行了生化检查。就莎丽打算如何喂养她的婴儿进行了简短的讨论。莎丽告诉助产士,如果可能她打算母

> 乳喂养。
> 　　Sally 随后参与了 20 周的胎儿排畸检查，结果是正常的。此时，她得到了关于母乳喂养对她和孩子有益的书面和口头信息。讨论了初乳在产前合成的可能性，Sally 和她的伴侣同意在妊娠 36 周时回来听取详细介绍及实践指导。
> 　　妊娠进展顺利。36 周时，Sally 和她的伴侣与助产士约好见面，在那里接受指导和学习设备使用方法，开始产前收集和储存初乳。
> 　　在妊娠 39 周时，根据当地的妊娠指南，Sally 经引产后，自然分娩一 4300g 男婴。
> 　　出生时，婴儿接受皮肤接触 1h。当婴儿与母亲接受皮肤与皮肤接触时，进行血糖检测。婴儿在出生后 1h 内母乳喂养，吮吸得很好。
> 　　随后，Sally 和她的婴儿被转移到产后病房，在那里她继续按需进行母乳喂养。她定期监测血糖水平，Sally 在喂奶前或期间会吃一些糖类点心，特别是在晚上。
> 　　根据新生儿低血糖检测指南监测婴儿的血糖，其处于正常范围内。
> 　　在第 3 天出院时，Sally 在家人的支持和社区内继续探望她的医护专业人员的持续支持下建立了母乳喂养。
> 　　出生后 6 个月，Sally 一直纯母乳喂养婴儿。

母乳喂养与糖尿病

　　母乳喂养是一个主要的公共卫生问题，因为它在短期和长期内影响母亲与婴儿的健康。鼓励母亲在前 6 个月纯母乳喂养婴儿，并继续母乳喂养直到其子女达到 2 岁[1, 2]。大量文献研究表明，母乳喂养或给婴儿提供母乳对母婴、社会、经济和环境有多样化及引人注目的优势[3]。对母亲来说，好处包括减少产后阴道出血，更快地恢复产前体重，增加骨密度，预防骨质疏松，以及降低乳腺癌和卵巢癌的风险[4]。对于婴儿，母乳喂养会降低感染性疾病、婴儿猝死综合征、淋巴瘤和白血病的发病率，提高认知发展测试的表现[3]。

　　对于患有糖尿病的妇女及其后代来说，已经确定了额外的好处。这些因素包括产后更好的母体血糖控制[5]，所需胰岛素的量减少[6]，胆固醇谱的改善[7]，以及更短的时间恢复到出生前体重，这对于患有 2 型糖尿病（T_2DM）的妇女尤其重要，在这一人群中肥胖发生率较高[4]。还有学者提出，婴儿期接触牛奶可引发 1 型糖尿病（T_1DM）发病前的免疫应答[8-10]，婴儿营养长期以来被认为是 T_2DM 发病的危险因素[11, 12]。

糖尿病对乳腺炎的影响

乳汁生成发生在整个妊娠期和出生后。这一过程包括乳腺的准备、母乳的生产和分泌（泌乳Ⅰ期），以及在产后胎盘娩出和随后黄体酮撤退，开始和维持乳汁供应（泌乳Ⅱ期）[13]。研究表明，乳腺已做好准备，有能力产生和分泌乳汁（泌乳Ⅰ期）不受糖尿病的影响[14]。然而，在先前患有糖尿病[15-21]的妇女中，泌乳Ⅱ期可能会延迟，这也发生在妊娠期糖尿病的母亲身上[22]。Hartmann 和 Cregan（2001）评估了与 T_1DM 母亲的泌乳Ⅱ期的四个标志物（乳汁柠檬酸盐、乳糖、钠和总蛋白）相关的证据，与非糖尿病母亲相比，乳糖和总蛋白的浓度降低，这与泌乳Ⅱ期延迟一致[14]。研究认为，母亲在产后所经历的母体葡萄糖和乳糖水平的波动也导致奶量减少[17,23]，动物研究表明母亲高血糖可减少产奶量[24]。

糖尿病对母乳成分的影响

乳汁生产发生在出生后 24h 内，初乳中乳糖、免疫球蛋白和蛋白质含量高，脂肪含量低。从出生后的 5～14d，母乳的组成发生变化，从初乳到过渡乳。过渡乳的组成与初乳相似，但脂肪含量较高。进一步的变化发生在出生后 4～6 周，母乳逐渐成熟，并具有满足生长中的婴儿需要的营养。在喂养过程中母乳也会随着婴儿营养平衡的需要和要求而改变其组成。例如，在母乳喂养开始时，脂肪含量低，乳糖高，为生长提供脂肪和乳糖能量的平衡。随着哺乳的发展，这会转化为高脂肪和低乳糖。

一旦确定了哺乳期，一些研究表明 T_1DM 妇女和非糖尿病母亲的母乳成分[25]与母亲的葡萄糖水平之间没有差异，而母亲的葡萄糖水平不影响母乳中的葡萄糖浓度[26]。然而，其他研究人员发现患有 T_1DM 母亲的母乳中平均脂肪和胆固醇含量较低，葡萄糖含量升高，提示母亲代谢控制的波动影响母乳组成[19,27]。糖尿病对泌乳Ⅱ期含量的影响，以及母乳产量的改变，可能导致新生儿出生后母乳供应减少，这可能增加新生儿低血糖的已知风险。

新生儿低血糖症

新生儿低血糖可发生在新生儿作为正常生理适应宫外生活。它通常是短暂的和无症状的，新生儿利用脂肪调节血糖。然而，低血糖是有妊娠前和妊娠期糖尿病的母亲所生新生儿的常见并发症，其原因是胎儿宫内高血糖和母亲高血糖导致的高胰岛素血症。因为关于确定新生儿低血糖的特定浓度的葡萄糖共识有限，新生儿低血糖的治疗是按照当地指南进行的[28]。低血糖可影响35%~64%的糖尿病妇女所生的婴儿，并且是进入婴儿特别护理室（SCBU）和新生儿重症监护病房（NICU）及母婴分离的主要原因[29]。为了尽量减少有糖尿病和无糖尿病母亲所生婴儿的低血糖，应鼓励早期和频繁的母乳喂养。

糖尿病妇女的母乳喂养率、持续时间和排他性

现有报道的母乳喂养率在糖尿病妇女与非糖尿病人群中是矛盾的。例如，一项研究报道，90%的患有 T_1DM 的母亲开始母乳喂养；然而，在6个月时，该比率显著下降，只有50%患有糖尿病的母亲在坚持母乳喂养，而70%非糖尿病母亲仍然母乳喂养[30]。然而，另一项研究发现，有糖尿病和没有糖尿病的母亲在出生后 2h 内的喂养率分别为 55%和87%，在产后阶段急剧下降。据报道，在2个月时，患有糖尿病的母亲与没有糖尿病的母亲采用部分或完全母乳喂养的比例为 OR：0.42（95%CI：0.18~0.96），$P=0.041$，6个月时，这一比例进一步降低[OR：0.50（95%CI：0.27~0.90），$P=0.022$）][31]。已经证明，母亲母乳喂养的意义是早期糖尿病妇女开始和维持母乳喂养的最有力的预测因素。

对于患有 GDM 的母亲，母乳喂养开始和持续排他性母乳喂养率与没有 GDM 的母亲相似[32]，而对需要胰岛素治疗的 GDM 的妇女的研究报道与未接受胰岛素治疗的 GDM 母亲相比，母乳喂养率更低[33]。一项研究报道指出，当患有 GDM 的妇女决定母乳喂养时，她们预期失败，并接受这种失败[34]。对患有糖尿病和 GDM 的妇女的进一步研究表明，这些母亲比普通人群喂养的时间短。这是由于糖尿病妇女母乳喂养障碍

因素增加（即手术分娩和母婴分离）[35-37]。GDM 与肥胖有关，并且已经表明 BMI＞30kg/m^2 与低母乳喂养开始率和持续率有关。这一观察归因于婴儿吸吮困难[38]。

鼓励和促进母乳喂养的干预措施

为了促进和加强在糖尿病人群中开始母乳喂养，可通过实施 WHO 亲婴倡议（BFI）[1, 2]采取具体步骤。BFI 主张，在产前阶段，所有妊娠妇女，包括糖尿病妇女，都应该有机会与卫生保健专业人员讨论她们打算的喂养选择。这个讨论应该包括无偏见的、基于证据的信息，这些信息由妊娠 34 周及住院或出生前给出。信息应该包括促进母乳喂养的益处和实践[39]。然而，一些研究显示，母乳/婴儿喂养问题并不作为其产前护理和教育的一部分，与 1 型和 2 型糖尿病或 GDM 妇女进行例行讨论，因为重点在于糖尿病的具体问题[34, 40]。

支持性医院实践，如产前阶段提供的母乳喂养信息文献，已显示出可提高一般人群的起始率。应向所有参加产前预约的妇女提供与糖尿病妇女母乳喂养特别有关的当地或国家制作的信息传单，因为这已表明可增加母乳喂养的开始和继续。妇女可能对母乳喂养和糖尿病感到焦虑，小组讨论可以解决这些具体问题[41-43]。此外，同伴支持通过面对面或电话向母亲提供信息、帮助和情感关怀，并已显示增加母乳喂养的持续性和排他性[44]。

BFI 进一步提倡产后人工收取母乳，以帮助解决诸如产后早期母乳供应不足的问题，并为接受 SCBU/NICU[1, 2, 45]的新生儿提供母乳。人工收取母乳也可以在产前期进行。

初乳的产前储存与收获

初乳可在出生前出现，收集和储存初乳用作治疗新生儿低血糖的补充喂养[46]。如果发生母婴分离，新生儿在 SCBU/NICU 中护理时无法吸吮喂养和（或）如果需要补充喂养，也可以使用储存的初乳。有学者提出,从妊娠34周到出生,糖尿病妇女每天人工收取初乳两次,持续数分钟[47],或从妊娠36周每天人工收取初乳两次,持续10min,直到出生[46]。在一项研究[47]中,引用了由妇女收取的初乳的总报告量为2.8~322ml,在另一项研究[46]中,引用数据为0.21~14.1ml。收取的初乳被收集到带有日期和识别细节的婴儿杯或注射器中,并存储在家用冰箱[47,48]的密封塑料袋中。入院分娩时,冷冻收集的初乳并将其装入冷袋储存在医院的冷藏库中。如果早期母乳喂养不足以治疗新生儿低血糖,给予初乳会减少补充配方奶粉或静脉注射葡萄糖的使用。而女性糖尿病患者对过程有高度的满意度[47,48],实践的安全性和有效性综述结论是,虽然该程序显然是有益的,但需要通过随机对照试验进行更彻底的评估[48]。

建立和维持泌乳的有利条件和障碍

由于母乳是所有婴儿特别是低血糖风险新生儿的最佳营养,因此应当采用促进早期和专属的母乳喂养政策与做法。在其他机构中,CEMACH建议患有糖尿病的母亲应在出生后尽可能快地进行母乳喂养[49,50]。

皮肤接触促进早期喂养

母亲和新生儿接受的直接产后护理对于帮助母乳喂养非常重要。有助于成功的早期母乳喂养的策略是母亲和新生儿之间的皮肤接触。SSC被定义为将赤裸的婴儿俯卧、头上盖着干帽、背上盖着暖毯、出生时或出生后不久放在母亲裸露的胸部[51]。SSC的益处包括促进乳汁产生和供应,通过提高出生后75~90min的血糖水平来改善新生儿葡萄糖水平[52],加强新生儿体温调节,以及早期母乳喂养[51]。BFI[2]主张所有母亲应该在生后至少一个小时或第一次母乳喂养后立即进行SSC。然而,SSC的实践可能会受到如分娩方式等因素的影响。

糖尿病妇女有更高的手术分娩发生率,包括剖宫产(CS)。进一步的证据显示,在CS分娩的妇女中[53],母乳喂养的开始和建立减少了。一般还发现,CS可影响第一次母乳喂养前的时间,减少排他性母乳喂养的发生率,并增加用配方奶[54]补充喂养的可能性。由于患有糖尿病的母亲 CS 所生的新生儿可能具有更大的低血糖风险，卫生保健专业人员应该对这种不利的新生儿结局更加警惕[55]。

另一个可能破坏出生时 SSC 的因素是母婴的分离。婴儿由于低血糖和呼吸问题需要在 SSBU/NICU 中进行葡萄糖监测，患有糖尿病母亲的新生儿更容易被分开。母婴分离已显示延迟和减少喂养频率，并增加补充喂养的可能性[53]。一项对患有 GDM 母亲所生婴儿的研究表明，那些在分娩室母乳喂养的婴儿比那些用配方奶喂养的婴儿低血糖的发生率低[56]。进一步的研究发现，当在分娩室开始母乳喂养时，新生儿的血糖稳定性增加[33]。当新生儿已经接受 SCBU/NICU 时，母亲可以通过手动或机械式母乳收集来启动和保持充足的母乳供应[45]。

母乳喂养及其对产妇血糖控制的影响

已经表明母乳喂养可以积极地影响糖尿病母亲的血糖控制。产后母亲葡萄糖水平的波动可能延迟乳汁生成，因为乳糖水平较低，导致乳汁量减少[17, 23]。在母乳喂养建立后的第一周内，母亲可能经历低血糖发作。因此，建议 T_1DM 妇女在出生后立即降低胰岛素剂量至其妊娠前剂量或更低，经常监测血糖水平并相应地自我调整胰岛素[57, 58]。妊娠期接受胰岛素治疗的 T_2DM 和 GDM 的母亲应该在出生后立即停止胰岛素治疗，因为他们的胰岛素需求将显著减少[57]。

母亲在母乳喂养期间也可能经历低血糖，因为已经建议 T_1DM 和 GDM 的母亲成功泌乳需要 50g 葡萄糖[58]。因此，需要 40~50g 额外的糖类来维持充足的乳汁供应。对于糖尿病母亲来说，在哺乳前或哺乳期间，特别是在晚上，吃正餐或吃零食是明智的。据报道，母乳喂养的糖尿病妇女在生后第 1 个月和第 2 个月[59]，胰岛素需求仍然显著降低。一项研究调查了 T_1DM 母乳喂养母亲的基础胰岛素需求，由于哺乳期间葡萄糖利用的增加，基础胰岛素的需求减少[58]。其他研究发现，母乳喂养的糖尿病妇女[5]母体血糖控制较好，而其他研究发现母乳喂养的 T_1DM[18]母亲高血糖。有学者提出，连续皮下胰岛素注射（CSII）对正在母乳喂养的 T_1DM 妇女是有用的，因为 CSII 降低了低血糖发作的频率，并改善了血糖控制。后者可以改善乳酸生成和促进母乳喂养[59]。

母乳喂养与药物治疗

一项对 T_1DM 和 T_2DM 母亲母乳中胰岛素水平的小型研究显示，内源性和外源性胰岛素从母亲血液中积极地转运到母乳中。提示母乳中的胰岛素可能对婴儿具有功能性或发育性作用[60]。

口服降糖药如二甲双胍和格列本脲，对哺乳期妇女已被认为是安全的。有 T_2DM 的妇女产后可以恢复或继续服用这些药[57]。用于治疗糖尿病并发症的药物，如血管紧张素转换酶抑制剂（ACEI）、血管紧张素Ⅱ受体阻滞剂（ARB）、他汀类药物、钙通道阻滞剂和治疗肥胖药物应避免使用，因为它们对新生儿和进入到母乳中的安全性尚未明确[57]。

母乳喂养 6 个月或以上的好处

大多数患有糖尿病的母亲无法纯母乳喂养婴儿。这可能是由于在新生儿不能母乳喂养或无法获得收集母乳的情况下使用配方奶补充喂养治疗新生儿低血糖有所增加。研究得出结论，婴儿发生 T_1DM 的风险更高，尤其是如果配方奶粉的使用比推荐的 6 个月提前。这种风险在婴儿中甚至更大，婴儿被认为是高风险的 T_1DM 和具有易感因素，如 T_1DM 的直系家庭成员[9]。虽然这一机制尚未完全了解，但也有学者提出，纯母乳喂养可以防止婴儿日后发生 T_2DM[61]。

母乳喂养对母婴的长期益处

在一般人群中，有证据表明，纯母乳喂养降低了母亲及其后代患 T_2DM 的风险。还有证据表明，在妊娠合并糖尿病的妇女中，母乳喂养与降低 T_2DM 的发病率有关。进一步的证据表明，母乳喂养时间越长，先前患有 GDM 的妇女中代谢综合征的发生率越低[61, 62]。

关于母乳喂养对儿童肥胖症的保护作用已有很多讨论。最近对每项研究使用调整 OR 和 95%CI 的荟萃分析结果表明，母乳喂养是预防儿童肥胖的重要保护因素，特别是如果母乳喂养持续超过 7 个月[63]。一些研究报道说，超重的母乳喂养儿童可能不会在青春期和成年期肥胖。母乳喂养如何降低肥胖患病率的原因和机制是复杂的，包括许多混杂可变因素[62]。

结论

患有糖尿病的女性可能会选择与没有糖尿病的女性一样母乳喂养。卫生保健专业人员应提供对促进、启动和持续适合女性及其家庭的专属母乳喂养提供支持的护理。产前准备、住院护理支持、SSC、早期和频繁的母乳喂养，以及保持母亲和婴儿在一起是可以采取的步骤之一，以促进糖尿病妇女成功与纯母乳喂养。

> **摘要**
>
> 母乳喂养和（或）母乳是所有婴儿的最佳营养。
> 母乳喂养对糖尿病母亲和婴儿都有很多好处。
> 对于患有糖尿病的母亲来说，在开始、建立和继续纯母乳喂养方面还有更多的挑战。
> 卫生保健专业人员应意识到这些挑战，支持母亲、婴儿和家庭克服这些挑战，并协助和促进母亲和婴儿顺利进行母乳喂养。

选择题

1. 妊娠合并糖尿病的妇女应该接受产前教育，了解母乳喂养的益处的时间是（   ）
   A. 妊娠 18 周　　　　　B. 妊娠 34 周
   C. 妊娠 28 周　　　　　D. 直到出生的时间
   正确答案是 B。

2. 新生儿出生后，应与母亲进行皮肤-皮肤接触（   ）
   A. 最少 45min　　　　　B. 仅次于儿科评估和血糖监测
   C. 最少 30min　　　　　D. 最少 1h

正确答案是 D。

(刘雅静 译,王 冰 校)

参 考 文 献

1 World Health Organization. Media Centre: WHO statements. 2009. http://www.who.int/mediacentre/news/statements
2 UNICEF. UK Baby Friendly Initiative: improving the health of the UK. 2009. http://www.unicef.org.uk/publications
3 American Academy of Pediatrics Work Group on Breastfeeding. Breastfeeding and the use of human milk. Pediatrics 2005;115:496–506.
4 Ip S, Chung M, Raman G, et al. Breastfeeding and Maternal and Infant Health Outcomes in Developed Countries. Evidence Report/Technology Assessment No. 153. Agency for Healthcare Research and Quality: Rockville, MD, 2007.
5 Saez-de-Ibarra L, Gaspar R, Obesso A, et al. Glycaemic behaviour during lactation: postpartum practical guidelines for women with type 1 diabetes. Pract Diabetes Intl 2003;20:271–275.
6 Sorkio S, Cuthbertson D, Bärlund S, et al. TRIGR Study Group. Breastfeeding patterns of mothers with type 1 diabetes: results from an infant feeding trial. Diabetes/Metab Res Rev 2010;26:206–211.
7 Oyer D & Stone N. Cholesterol levels and the breastfeeding mom. JAMA 1989;262:2092.
8 Luopajärvi K, Savilahti E, Virtanen SM, et al. Enhanced levels of cow's milk antibodies in infancy in children who develop type 1 diabetes later in childhood. Pediat Diabetes 2008;9:434–441.
9 Ziegler AG, Schmid S, Huber D, et al. Early infant feeding and risk of developing type 1 diabetes-associated autoantibodies. JAMA 2003;290:1721–1728.
10 Pérez-Bravo F, Oyarzún A, Carrasco E, et al. Duration of breast feeding and bovine serum albumin antibody levels in type 1 diabetes: a case-control study. Pediat Diabetes 2003;4:157–161.
11 Villegas R, Gao YT, Yang G, et al. Duration of breast-feeding and the incidence of type 2 diabetes mellitus in the Shanghai Women's Health Study. Diabetologia 2008;51:258–266.
12 Taylor JS, Kacmar JE, Nothnagle M, et al. A systematic review of the literature associating breastfeeding with type 2 diabetes and gestational diabetes. J Am Coll Nutr 2005;24:320–326.
13 Neville MC, Morton J, & Umemura S. Lactogenesis: the transition from pregnancy to lactation. Pediat Clin N Am 2001;48:35–52.
14 Hartmann P & Cregan M. Lactogenesis and the effects of insulin-dependent diabetes mellitus and prematurity. J Nutr 2001;131:3016S–3020.
15 Ferris AM, Dalidowitz CK, Ingardia CM, et al. Lactation outcome in insulin-dependent diabetic women. J Am Diet Assoc 1988;88:317–322.
16 Arthur PG, Kent JC, & Hartmann PE. Metabolites of lactose synthesis in milk from diabetic and nondiabetic women during lactogenesis II. J Pediat Gastroent Nutr 1994;19:100–108.
17 Neubauer SH, Ferris AM, Chase CG, et al. Delayed lactogenesis in women with insulin-dependent diabetes mellitus. Am J Clin Nutr 1993;58;54–60.
18 Murtaugh MA, Ferris AM, Capacchione CM, et al. Energy intake and glycemia in lactating women with type 1 diabetes. J Am Diet Assoc 1998;98:642–648.
19 Bitman J, Hamosh M, Hamosh P, et al. Milk composition and volume during the onset of lactation in a diabetic mother. Am J Clin Nutr 1989;50:1364–1369.
20 Arthur P & Kent J. Metabolites of lactose synthesis in milk from diabetic and

nondiabetic women during lactogenesis II. J Pediat Gastroent Nutr 1994;19:100–108.
21 Miyake A, Tahara M, Koike K, et al. Decrease in neonatal suckled milk volume in diabetic women. Euro J Obstet Gynaecol Reprod Biol 1989;33:49–53.
22 Matias SL, Dewey KG, Quesenberry CP Jr, et al. Maternal prepregnancy obesity and insulin treatment during pregnancy are independently associated with delayed lactogenesis in women with recent gestational diabetes mellitus. Am J Clin Nutr 2013;99:115–121.
23 Stage E, Nørgård H, Damm P, et al. Long-term breastfeeding in women with type 1 diabetes. Diabetes Care 2006;29:771–774.
24 Frohlich A & Dzialoszynski LM. Insulin dependence of milk formation and lactose biosynthesis. Clin Chim Acta 1973;47:33–38.
25 van Beusekom CM, Zeegers TA, Martini IA, et al. Milk of patients with tightly controlled insulin-dependent diabetes mellitus has normal macronutrient and fatty acid composition. Am J Clin Nutr 1993;57:938–943.
26 Ratzmann KP Steindel E, Hildebrandt R, et al. Is there a relationship between metabolic control and glucose concentration in breast milk of type 1 (insulin-dependent) diabetic mothers? Exper Clin Endocrin 1988;92:32–36.
27 Butte NF, Garza C, Burr R, et al. Milk composition of insulin-dependent diabetic women. J Pediat Gastroent Nutr 1987;6:936–941.
28 Adamkin DH & Committee on Fetus and Newborn. Clinical report – postnatal glucose homeostasis in late-preterm and term infants. Pediatrics 2011;127:575–579.
29 Sparud-Lundin C, Wennergren M, Elfvin A, et al. Breastfeeding in women with type 1 diabetes exploration of predictive factors. Diabetes Care 2011;34:296–230.
30 Sorkio S., Cuthbertson D., Brlund S, et al. Breastfeeding patterns of mothers with type 1 diabetes: results from an infant feeding trial. Diabetes Metab Res Rev 2010;26:206–221.
31 Cordero L, Thung S, Landon MB, et al. Breast-feeding initiation in women with pregestational diabetes mellitus. Clin Pediatr 2014;53:18–25.
32 Oza-Frank R, Chertok I, & Bartley A. Differences in breast-feeding initiation and continuation by maternal diabetes status. Public Health Nutr 2014;8:1–9.
33 Finkelstein SA, Keely E, Feig DS, et al. Breastfeeding in women with diabetes: lower rates despite greater rewards: a population-based study. Diabetic Med 2013;30:1094–1101.
34 Stenhouse E, Stephen N, Millward A, et al. Infant feeding: choices and experiences of pregnant women with pre-existing diabetes. Diabetic Med 2009;26:175–176.
35 Lavender T, Baker L, Smyth R, et al. Breastfeeding expectations versus reality: a cluster randomised controlled trial. Br J Obstet Gynaecol 2005;112:1047–1053.
36 Sikorski J, Renfrew MJ, Pindoria S, et al. Support for breastfeeding mothers: a systematic review. Paediat Perin Epidemiol 2003;17:407–417.
37 Soltani H & Arden M. Factors associated with breastfeeding up to 6 months postpartum in mothers with diabetes. J Obstet Gynaecol Neonat Nurs 2009;38:586–594.
38 Lovelady CA. Is maternal obesity a cause of poor lactation performance? Nutr Rev 2005;63:352–355.
39 Saadeh RJ. The Baby-friendly Hospital Initiative 20 years on: facts, progress, and the way forward. J Human Lact 2012;28:272–275.
40 Stenhouse E, Millward A, & Wylie J. An exploration of infant feeding choices for women whose pregnancy is complicated by gestational diabetes mellitus. Diabetic Med 2011;28:175.
41 Berg M, Erlandsson LK, & Sparud-Lundin C. Breastfeeding and its impact on daily life in women with type 1 diabetes during the first six months after childbirth: a prospective cohort study. Intl Breastfeed J 2012;7:20.
42 Letherby G, Stephen N, & Stenhouse E. Pregnant women with pre-existing diabetes: managing the pregnancy process. Human Fertil 2012;15:200–204.

43 Jolly K, Ingram L, Khan KS, et al. Systematic review of peer support for breastfeeding continuation: meta regression analysis of the effect of setting, intensity, and timing. BMJ 2012;344:1–18.
44 Kaunonen M, Hannula L, & Marja-Terttu T. A systematic review of peer support interventions for breastfeeding. J Clin Nurs 2012;21(13–14):1943–1954.
45 Renfrew M, Craig D, Dyson L, et al. Breastfeeding promotion in special care and neonatal intensive care units: an evidence synthesis. Health Tech Assess 2009;13(40):1–146.
46 Forster DA, McEgan K, Ford R, et al. Diabetes and antenatal milk expressing: a pilot project to inform the development of a randomised controlled trial. Midwifery 2011;27:209–214.
47 Rietveld C & Canterbury Breastfeeding Advocacy Service. Canterbury breastfeeding update and consultation hui report. 2012. http://www.cbnet.org.nz
48 East CE, Dolan WJ, & Forster DA. Antenatal breast milk expression by women with diabetes for improving infant outcomes. Cochrane Database Syst Rev 2014;7:1–20.
49 Confidential Enquiry into Maternal and Child Health (CEMACH). Diabetes in Pregnancy: Are We Providing the Best Care? Findings of a National Enquiry: England, Wales and Northern Ireland. CEMACH: London, 2007.
50 Confidential Enquiry into Maternal and Child Health (CEMACH). Diabetes in Pregnancy: Caring for the Baby after Birth. Findings of a National Enquiry, England. Wales and Northern Ireland. CEMACH: London, 2007.
51 Moore ER, Anderson GC, Bergman N, et al. Early skin-to-skin contact for mothers and their healthy newborn infants. Cochrane Database Syst Rev 2012;5:1–112.
52 Durand R, Hodges S, LaRock S, et al. The effect of skin-to-skin breastfeeding in the immediate recovery period on newborn thermoregulation and blood glucose values. Neonat Intens Care 1997;4:23–29.
53 Hauck YL, Fenwick J, Dhaliwal SS, et al. A western Australian survey of breastfeeding initiation, prevalence and early cessation patterns. Matern Child Health J 2011;15:260–268.
54 Stevens J, Schmied V, Burns E, et al. Immediate or early skin-to-skin contact after a Caesarean section: a review of the literature. Matern Child Nutr 2014;10:456–473.
55 Karlstrom A, Lindgren H, & Hildingsson I. Maternal and infant outcome after caesarean section without recorded medical indication: findings from a Swedish case-control study. Br J Obstet Gynaecol 2013;120:479–486.
56 Chertok IRA, Raz I, Shoham I, et al. Effects of early breastfeeding on neonatal glucose levels of term infants born to women with gestational diabetes. J Human Nutr Diet 2009;22:166–169.
57 National Institute for Health and Care Excellence. Diabetes in pregnancy: management of diabetes and its complications from pre-conception to the postnatal period. https://www.nice.org.uk/guidance/cg63
58 Riviello C, Mello G, & Jovanovic LG. Breastfeeding and the basal insulin requirement in type 1 diabetic women. Endocrine Pract 2009;3:187–193.
59 Abayomi J, Morrison G, McFadden K, et al. Can CSII assist women with type 1 diabetes in breastfeeding? J Diabetes Nurs 2005;9:346–351.
60 Whitmore TJ, Trengove NJ, Graham DF, et al. Analysis of insulin in human breast milk in mothers with type 1 and type 2 diabetes mellitus. Intl J Endocrinol 2012;1–9.
61 Jäger S, Jacobs S, Kröger J, et al. Breast-feeding and maternal risk of type 2 diabetes: a prospective study and meta-analysis. Diabetologia 2014;57:1355–1365.

62 Gunderson EP, Jacobs D Jr, Chiang V, et al. Duration of lactation and incidence of the metabolic syndrome in women of reproductive age according to gestational diabetes mellitus status: a 20-year prospective study in CARDIA (Coronary Artery Risk Development in Young Adults). Diabetes 2010;59:495–504.

63 Yan J, Liu L, Zhu Y, Huang G, & Wang P. The association between breastfeeding and childhood obesity: a meta-analysis. BMC Public Health 2014;14:1267.

: 第五篇 对未来的影响

第二十七章 妊娠对糖尿病母亲的影响

Ewa Wender-Ozegowska [1] and David A. Sacks [2,3]

1 Department of Obstetrics and Women's Diseases, Poznań University of Medical Sciences, Poznań, Poland

2 Associate Investigator, Department of Research and Evaluation, Kaiser Permanente Southern California, Pasadena, California, USA

3 Adjunct Clinical Professor, Division of Maternal-Fetal Medicine, Department of Obstetrics and Gynecology, Keck School of Medicine, University of Southern California, Los Angeles, California, USA

实践要点

- 1 型和 2 型糖尿病的微血管与大血管并发症可能在妊娠后持续或复发。
- 大量证据表明，妊娠本身不会导致或促进糖尿病血管病变的进展。
- 患有糖尿病的女性的代谢异常改善能延缓早期肾病的出现，也有可能降低癌症发生和进展的风险。
- 妊娠期间及分娩后社会心理学的健康对母亲和婴儿的良好分娩结局均是积极的。

病 例

一位 28 岁的孕 1 产 0 的女性，从 7 岁开始就患有 1 型糖尿病。她的记录显示，在妊娠前饮食和胰岛素治疗的依从性很差。她在 22 岁时被诊断出患有糖尿病性视网膜病变，由于视网膜病变恶化，她在妊娠期间接受了两次激光光凝手术治疗。26 岁时，她在急性心肌梗死后接受了右冠状动脉支架置入手术治疗。妊娠之前存在的其他问题还包括需要治疗的高血压和表现为 376mg/24h 的蛋白尿及最初的血清肌酐 1.2mg/dl（106μmol/L）的肾脏病变。由于不确定她在妊娠晚期尿蛋白定量的增加和高血压的加重是先兆子痫或者既往慢性高血压的恶化，还是两者都有，她在 32 周时进行了剖宫产。产后 3 个月的随访中，她的血压恢复到妊娠前水平，体重比妊娠前增加了 3kg。在那次随访中植入了一个含有左炔诺孕酮的节育器。

- 这次妊娠会如何影响这名女性以后的 1 型糖尿病和（或）并发症？
- 妊娠会如何影响一个妊娠前即患有 2 型糖尿病的女性？
- 如果有的话，何种治疗模式可能适用于患有 1 型或 2 型糖尿病的女性，以预防糖尿病和并发症的进展？

背景

近年来，妊娠期 1 型和 2 型糖尿病的患病率均有所上升[1]。正如第二十二章和第二十三章所讨论的，这对妊娠前患有糖尿病的妇女的护理提出了独特的挑战和关注点。本章将重点讨论在妊娠前患有 1 型和 2 型糖尿病的妇女在妊娠后可能发生的潜在问题。对这些妇女的短期和长期挑战的关注点及可能延缓或减轻不良后果的干预措施也将被讨论。

即时的产后期

就本讨论而言，即时的产后期定义为分娩生产后 1 年内。

1 型糖尿病

对于患有 T_1DM 的妇女，产后血糖控制可能会有所不同，这取决于妊娠前血糖控制的质量、孕妇体重和母乳喂养。妊娠的特点是胰岛素抵抗，主要的激素来源是胎盘产生的激素。在胎盘娩出后，胰岛素抵抗就会急剧下降，这通常会导致持续时间不等的胰岛素需求下降。与分娩后恢复外源性胰岛素的时间较短（小于 4h）相关的因素包括产时停用胰岛素的间隔时间较长、足月时 BMI 增加、足月时血清肌酐降低，但与足月时 HbA1c 无关[2]。在一份关于妊娠前 BMI 正常（平均 $24.6kg/m^2$）且 HbA1c 中位数为 6.4% 的妇女的报道中，我们注意到，与妊娠前相比，产后每日总胰岛素需求下降了 34%。胰岛素剂量不受母乳喂养或胰岛素给药途径（持续或间断）的影响[3]。在妊娠前进行干预会使产后血糖得到更好的控制已经被证实，与未参与该项目的妊娠妇女相比，参加受孕前规划项目的妇女的妊娠前和产后 1 年 HbA1c 值较低[4]。

除了第二十六章中提到的对孕产妇和新生儿的益处，母乳喂养被发现对产后 6 个月内 T_1DM 妇女在改善血糖调节方面有积极作用。在一项对产后 1 型糖尿病妇女的研究中，与单纯用奶瓶喂养的人相比，那些完全或主要母乳喂养（定义为每天至少 6 次喂奶）的妇女血糖指数较低，在持续监测血糖时血糖波动较少。与牛奶合成对葡萄糖需求的增加相一致，母乳喂养的妇女比奶瓶喂养的妇女有更高的糖类摄入量。虽然各组间整体低血糖指数无显著差异，但在哺乳的妇女中，有少数人的血糖在开始吮吸后 2~3h 低于 4.0mmol/L。然而，血糖过低与上次进餐时间之间存在正相关关系，与上次胰岛素注射时间存在负相关关系[5]。

过高的产后体重和产后体重滞留与炎症和胰岛素抵抗有关。在 T_1DM 患者中，血糖控制不良[6]和产后体重过多滞留可能会增加她们患糖尿病导致血管疾病的风险。研究人员对 136 名 T_1DM 患者进行了研究，这些患者从妊娠前到产后 12 个月一直被跟踪研究，以明确血糖控制不良是否与母亲体重和产后体重保持有关。在整个队列中，平均 HbA1c 水平从产后 6 周的 6.6%上升到产后 10 个月的 7.5%。总的来说，产后体重滞留率呈下降趋势（定义为产后体重与妊娠前体重的差异）。然而，产后 30 周内体重滞留超过 5kg 以上的妇女比体重滞留低于 5kg 的妇女的 HbA1c 水平平均高出 0.34%。那些妊娠前 $BMI \geqslant 25kg/m^2$ 与那些妊娠前 $BMI < 25kg/m^2$ 的女性相比，在分娩 1 年后存在类似的 HbA1c 差异（0.31%）[7]。从这些数据来看，减轻体重滞留可能有助于改善血糖控制。然而，没有长期的数据跟踪这两种结果的演变。

2 型糖尿病

虽然在产后发现的许多问题对于 T_1DM 或 T_2DM 的妇女来说是相似的，但对于最近妊娠的 T_2DM 妇女来说，有些挑战是独一无二的。考虑到 T_2DM 的病理生理学（升高的胰岛素抵抗和胰岛 B 细胞无力产生足够的胰岛素来克服它），考虑到在妊娠期间胰岛素抵抗被大大放大，有些 T_2DM 的孕妇可能会在产后恢复正常血糖。虽然研究这种可能性的文献很少，但一项研究发现，在根据妊娠期间葡萄糖耐量试验诊断为显性糖尿病的女性中，37%的人在分娩后 6~8 周恢复正常葡萄糖耐量[8]。首次发现于妊娠期间的程度符合显性糖尿病定义的血糖不耐受，在妊娠之前可能存在，也可能不存在。由于没有专门针对妊娠前患 T_2DM 的妊娠妇女实施干预措施以减少产后葡萄糖耐受不良的研究，从对 GDM 患者实施干预措施的研究结果进行推理可能是合理的。目前已经研究了两种预防 T_2DM 的主要干预措施，即母乳喂养和生活方式的改变。

与患有 T_1DM 的女性一样，患有 T_2DM 的女性也从母乳喂养中受益。尽管没有证据表明母乳喂养有助于患 T_2DM 女性的产后血糖恢复为正常水平，但不同持续时间的母乳喂养都可以证明母乳喂养可以改善患 T_2DM 女性的糖耐量，并在妊娠期间改善血脂水平[9, 10]。加强减重力度可能会进一步增强母乳喂养降低血糖的作用。在至少一项研究中，与没有减轻体重的同龄人相比，患有 GDM 且体重减轻超过 2kg 的产后母乳喂养妇女的空腹血糖和餐后 2h 血糖减少幅度更大，血浆胰岛素水平更低[11]。

对于患有 T_2DM 的产后母乳喂养的妇女而言，特别需要关注的是恢复使用口服降糖药。但关于母乳喂养时使用这些药物的明确结论，目前的可用数据量不足。一份报道表明母乳和哺乳婴儿的血液中未检出格列本脲[12]。两项关于母乳喂养的妇女的研究发现，母亲二甲双胍的乳浆比分别为 0.35[13]和 0.63[14]。母乳中获得的相应婴儿剂量是母亲体重调整剂量的 0.28%和 0.65%。在后者的研究中，3 名母乳喂养 4h 后的婴儿血糖浓度正常。没有其他类型的口服降血糖药的母乳喂养数据，如西他列汀等 DPP4 抑制剂、吡格列酮等噻唑烷二酮类、阿卡洛尔等 α-葡萄糖苷酶抑制剂及 exenetide 和 liraglutide 等 GLP1 激动剂。有关将药物用于哺乳期糖尿病妇女的其他适应证的讨论详见第二十六章。

妊娠对患有糖尿病的妇女长期的影响

糖尿病的最终器官效应主要是由疾病相关的大血管和小血管的病变引起的。尽管在不同的器官中发生的频率不同，但不论 T_1DM 还是 T_2DM 均会发生小血管和大血管病变，因此对于这两种类型的糖尿病，我们将共同讨论妊娠前和妊娠后进展结局之间的关系。妊娠对血管并发症发生和发展的影响是 20 多年来医学界研究的热点。研究小组的异质性包括不同的代谢控制，不同的血管病变严重程度的评估，以及新的血管并发症的监测和治疗,可能导致文献中发表结果的差异。记住了这些注意事项,我们将回顾一些糖尿病妇女妊娠后出现的主要并发症。

妊娠和糖尿病性视网膜病变

第二十一章讨论了妊娠糖尿病性视网膜病变的话题。妊娠期视网膜病变发生或发现的某些长期后果具有重要意义。糖尿病视网膜病变的流行与疾病的持续时间、高血糖[15]、血脂异常[16]、高血压[17]和肾病[18]呈正相关。由于这些并发症经常同时发生在同一个人身上,因此很难区分每个并发症对视网膜病变的发展和持续的相对贡献。由于妊娠妇女年龄、糖尿病持续时间、妊娠前和妊娠期间血糖控制及妊娠并发症的发生等方面的差异,在确定妊娠本身对糖尿病视网膜病变的发展和(或)恶化的独立影响方面遇到了进一步的困难。在妊娠前患有糖尿病的妇女中,糖尿病视网膜病变在妊娠期和妊娠后的流行与恶化情况已经被记录。然而,目前尚不清楚妊娠是否单独导致这些不良变化。一份报道发现,10%的T_1DM妇女在妊娠早期的眼科检查中发现有中度至重度的视网膜病变。在后者中,近50%的患者出现进展。有进展的人比没有进展的人患糖尿病的时间更长。发生视网膜病变进展的妇女,有较高的初始糖化血红蛋白浓度,从最初检查到第24周时糖化血红蛋白下降幅度更大,但这些差异无统计学意义[19]。糖尿病控制和并发症试验(DCCT)研究了最初没有妊娠的育龄妇女。在研究期间,未妊娠的500人与妊娠的180人之间的基线糖化血红蛋白差异不显著。在研究开始时,53%的经历妊娠的妇女和47%的未经历妊娠的妇女有一定程度的视网膜病变(P=NS)。在强化降糖组和常规控制组中,经历妊娠的女性视网膜病变恶化程度明显高于未妊娠女性。妊娠期间糖化血红蛋白水平减低与妊娠期间视网膜病变进展呈正相关。然而,在随后的6.5年的随访试验中,那些在试验中妊娠和没有妊娠的妇女的残余视网膜病变没有明显的区别[20]。在另一项研究中,妊娠的妇女更容易患增生性视网膜病变。然而,妊娠的女性年龄更大,而且在更年轻时就患上了糖尿病[21]。在EURODIAB(欧洲糖尿病并发症)多中心研究中也得到了类似的观察结果,长期的糖尿病病史和不良的代谢控制,是与妊娠后视网膜病变进展相关的因素[22],而不是妊娠。最后,在一项纳入

185 名妊娠妇女的研究中，研究人员研究了 T_1DM 或 T_2DM 视网膜病变进展的频率。在 T_1DM 患者中糖尿病视网膜病变进展（31%）明显大于 T_2DM 患者（12%）（$P=0.001$）。与其他报道一样，视网膜病变的进展与初期较高的 HbA1c 水平有关，而且与从妊娠早期到妊娠晚期 HbA1c 下降幅度较大有关[23]。

产后，糖尿病视网膜病变的严重程度可能会消退或完全缓解，尤其是在妊娠前没有视网膜病变的情况下[24]。增生性视网膜病变可能不会消退，应由有治疗糖尿病视网膜病变经验的专家随访至少 1 年。

妊娠和糖尿病肾病

糖尿病肾病是另一种长期糖尿病的血管并发症，据估计在 20%～30% 的 T_1DM 和 T_2DM 患者中发生，是发达国家终末期肾病的主要原因[25]。两种慢性肾病的标志物正在使用中。第一个指标是尿液白蛋白/肌酐值（UACR），如果≥30mg/gCr 被认为是异常的。然而，除了肾病外，当出现明显的高血糖、明显的高血压、发热、感染、充血性心力衰竭或月经期，UACR 均可能会升高[26]。第二个指标是肾小球滤过率（eGFR），是由慢性肾病流行病学合作研究得出的公式计算出来的。该公式基于血清肌酐、年龄、种族和性别，可在以下网址 http://www.niddk.nih.gov/health-information/health-communication-programs/nkdep/lab-evaluation/gfr-calculators/adults-conventional-unit-ckd-epi 找到。UACR 是慢性肾病严重程度的标志，而 eGFR 作为肾脏功能的一种标志物，也可用于对疾病严重程度进行分类，评估疾病进展并管理并发症[27]。然而，必须指出的是，eGFR 在妊娠期的有效性尚不清楚。因此，建议在缺乏妊娠特异性数据的情况下可以使用肌酐清除率或血清肌酐作为妊娠期间肾功能的检测指标[28]。

UACR 从 30～299mg/gCr 的升高是 T_1DM 和 T_2DM 患者中糖尿病肾病及心血管疾病（CVD）的标志物[29, 30]。然而，这种测量方法可能会自发减少，而且不应专门用于定义糖尿病肾病的存在[31]。持续的 UACR＞300mg/gCr 表明终末期肾病风险增加[32]。在存在糖尿病视网膜病变的患者中，UACR 为＞300mg/gCr 强烈提示存在糖尿病肾脏病变。然而，如果 UACR 小于 300mg/gCr，eGFR 降低但糖尿病视网膜病变不存在，则应寻找慢性肾病的非糖尿病原因[33]。

妊娠本身是否增加了糖尿病肾病发展或进展的可能性已经经过研究。在一项研究中，肾病（微量白蛋白尿）在 445 名 T_1DM 妇女中的患病率为 2.5%，在 220 名 T_2DM 妇女中为 2.3%（P=NS）。虽然 T_1DM 患者比 T_2DM 患者更频繁地服用抗高血压药物，但妊娠期和婴儿出生体重在各组间并无显著差异。血清肌酐在妊娠期间保持稳定，且无终末期肾病发生[34]。在另一项从妊娠前至产后 1 年研究中，将 T_1DM 和 T_2DM 合并肾病的妇女肾功能与无肾病的糖尿病妇女肾功能进行比较。从妊娠前到产后 1 年的测量数据表明，各组尿白蛋白排泄或肌酐无明显变化，提示妊娠与糖尿病肾病的发展和进展之间没有联系[35]。

一项早期随访 T_1DM 妊娠妇女的从妊娠前到分娩后 3 年或更长时间的研究表明，在没有肾病的妊娠妇女中，约有 10% 的在分娩后 18 年以内患上肾病。那些最终发展成肾病的妇女相比那些没有发展成肾病的妇女有更高的平均 HbA1c 水平和更多的妊娠合并高血压疾病。然而，对那些开始妊娠时伴有肾病的妇女的分析发现，在没有进展为终末阶段肾病和进展为终末阶段肾病的患者中，HbA1c 水平或高血压疾病没有差别。这两项研究均与肾脏疾病的发展或进展无关。因为随着时间的推移，糖尿病肾病的发展和进展比那些非妊娠人群少，作者得出结论，妊娠本身对这些并发症没有独立的影响[36]。

先兆子痫在妊娠合并糖尿病时更为常见[37]。除了增加患慢性高血压和慢性肾病的风险外，子痫前期的发生还与心脏并发症和妊娠后代谢综合征的高风险有关[38-40]。

对于患有糖尿病的妇女来说，慢性肾病的进展可能通过某些干预措施得以预防或延迟。将总蛋白摄入量限制在 0.8g/（kg·d）可以减缓肾小球滤过率的下降和蛋白尿的进展[33]。在 T_1DM 和 T_2DM 中，血糖的控制正常化已经被证明可以延迟蛋白尿和 eGFR 降低的发生与进展[32,41]。最后，对于患有糖尿病且 eGFR<60ml/（min·1.73m^2）和 UACR>300mg/gCr 的妇女，通过 ACEI 或 ARB 控制高血压与降低肾脏不良事件相关[42]。

妊娠和大血管并发症

糖尿病性胃病、神经病变和心血管疾病是与糖尿病相关的常见大血管并发症。它们的发病率随着糖尿病的持续时间和患者年龄的增加而增加。

神经病变是糖尿病的一种未被充分认识和诊断的并发症,尽管它经常发生,并且对患者的生活质量和寿命有负面影响[43]。与自主神经病变相关的症状在妊娠期间尤为突出,因为自主神经系统纤维受损可引起心血管系统、泌尿生殖系统和胃肠道的问题。表现为恶心、呕吐和食欲缺乏的胃轻瘫是自主神经病变的一种症状。在患有 T_1DM 的妇女中,判断这种症状是因为单纯妊娠、糖尿病性胃轻瘫,还是两者皆有是困难的,这已经在第十三章讨论了。对妊娠前患有糖尿病的妊娠妇女,如果出现长时间、严重呕吐和代谢调节障碍应予以怀疑糖尿病性胃轻瘫,尤其是患妊娠剧吐但在常规推荐的治疗方法无效的情况下。

GDM 被发现是在妊娠 9 年内发生心血管疾病的独立危险因素,但仅限于超重妇女。在同一份报道中,妊娠后出现明显糖尿病是心血管疾病的一个主要独立危险因素,并在 GDM 后轻微降低了心血管疾病的调整优势比[44]。高血糖促进高凝、血小板功能障碍和内皮功能障碍。高血糖也会引起氧化应激,这可能导致一氧化氮的产生减少和随之引起的血管舒张的受限[45]。诱发 CVD 的因素(即炎症、低 HDL 和胰岛素抵抗)可能是 GDM 和未来患 CVD 之间的联系[46]。

糖尿病和癌症

与没有糖尿病的人相比,患有 T_1DM[47]和 T_2DM[48]的女性患多种癌症的风险增加。含有致癌基因物质的正常细胞必须受到刺激才能进行恶性转化和生长。在糖尿病中,促进这种转化的机制包括高胰岛素血症、胰岛素抵抗、高血糖、脂肪因子的变化和炎症[49, 50]。

妊娠、妊娠糖尿病与 T_2DM 有常见的胰岛素抵抗和高胰岛素血症。在 T_1DM 中,尽管胰岛素缺乏是主要的发病机制,但由于长期使用外源性胰岛素,常会出现胰岛素过量。因此,这也可能导致短暂的高胰岛素血症和随后增加的胰岛素抵抗。妊娠期间，类固醇激素、人胎盘催乳素和一些脂肪细胞因子的生成增加可能导致胰岛素抵抗和随后的高胰岛素血症。这在发展为 GDM 的患者中尤为严重。因此，妊娠期 T_1DM 和 T_2DM 患者的高胰岛素血症导致的胰岛素增加的一个后果是胰岛素样生长因子结合蛋白（IGFBP1 和 IGFBP2）的减少。胰岛素与胰岛素样生长因子-1（IGF1）分别激活胰岛素和 IGF1 跨膜细胞受体。而这两种受体在恶性细胞中的表达水平都增加了。这些受体的激活导致细胞内胰岛素受体底物-1（IRS1）的激活。丝裂原激活蛋白激酶（MAPK）、磷酸肌醇激酶 Akt（PI3K/Akt）和 Janus 激酶信号传感器与激活器（JAK/STAT）启动了通路的下游激活。这些通路的激活导致蛋白合成、细胞增殖、细胞凋亡保护和癌细胞增殖[49-51]。此外，慢性炎症和高浓度的白细胞介素如白细胞介素 6 或者肿瘤坏死因子-α（TNF-α）促进了肿瘤的发展、存活和侵袭。T_2DM 患者特有的脂肪因子浓度的变化也会影响肿瘤的生长和存活。瘦素的增加与癌细胞的增殖、迁移和侵袭有关。脂联素在 T_2DM 中降低。在正常浓度下，这种脂肪因子可能通过降低可用的胰岛素和葡萄糖及激活 AMPK（AMP 激活蛋白激酶）来降低肿瘤发生，而 AMPK 又会增加一种肿瘤抑制因子 PP2A，该因子在乳腺癌中减少或缺失[49]。脂联素的降低导致 AMPK 活性的降低。

很明显，在患有 T_1DM[47]和 T_2DM[48]的患者中，某些类型的癌症（乳腺癌、胃癌、胰腺癌、结肠癌、直肠、子宫内膜癌和膀胱癌）的发生率增加。目前还不清楚这种同时发生是否是由共同的危险因素（如年龄和肥胖）造成的。考虑到糖尿病妇女中糖尿病和癌症的风险均可以通过健康的饮食、体育活动和体重控制而降低，这三种行为都应该得到鼓励[51]。

糖尿病患者的社会心理问题

女性过渡到母亲

T_1DM 女性在转变为母亲的过程中经历了各种各样的社会心理问题：焦虑程度增加，糖尿病相关的压力、内疚，与卫生专业人员的疏离感，以及对妊娠期间医疗化的关注而不是积极地过渡到母亲[52]。此外，她们可能经历母乳喂养，需要亲戚的帮助。这种依赖可能会导致自我怜悯和与其他母亲相比的无法胜任感[53]。不能处理低血糖的发作会导致她们行为的改变，并对她们的健康有害，如让她们的血糖水平上升到异常高的水平[54]。糖尿病母亲对低血糖的恐惧会造成不安全感，并让人觉得母乳喂养可能有风险。考虑到母乳喂养的好处，这些妇女分娩后在产科病房住院期间和出院后的前数个月应得到特别支持与帮助。妇女应该也确实感到有必要对她们产后的血糖水平负责，这也是她们的伴侣可以做出贡献的目标[54, 55]。

总结

预防 T_1DM 和 T_2DM 的长期不良后果应从产后立即开始。几乎没有证据表明仅仅妊娠就会导致或加重糖尿病的并发症。母乳喂养有助于减轻母亲的体重并加以保持，改善血糖和脂质调节。母乳喂养和减肥对血糖调节有明显的协同作用。妊娠后，正常摄入饮食蛋白和使用血管紧张素转换酶抑制剂可能减缓糖尿病肾病的进展。最后，体重正常化和血糖控制及健康生活方式的改变与定期体育锻炼对患有糖尿病的妇女具有普遍益处，并可能降低她们患心血管疾病和恶性肿瘤的倾向。

选择题

1. 一例 T_1DM 患者在过去 2 年中发生进行性肾衰竭。她还没有接受透析。体格检查没有异常。血红蛋白浓度 9g/dl，血细胞比容 28%，常规控制血压 150/100mmHg，蛋白尿超过 0.7g/d，糖化血红蛋白 5.7%。她打算妊娠。她在妊娠期间会有什么后果（　　）（选择所有适用项）

　　A. 子痫前期　　　　　　B. 肾病的进展
　　C. 胎儿先天畸形　　　　D. 巨大胎儿
　　E. 没有并发症　　　　　F. 早产
正确答案是 A、B、F。

2. 一名 25 岁患有 T_1DM 10 年的女性来到你的办公室寻求妊娠建议。虽然她目前没有妊娠，也从未妊娠过，但她和她的配偶正计划要第一个孩子。她在此之前通过控制饮食、锻炼和每天两次基础胰岛素治疗糖尿病,偶尔在饭前应用短效胰岛素。约 4 个月前,她开始更有规律地监测血糖,她注意到她的空腹血糖水平一直高于 8.3mmol/L。当时她的 HbA1c 水平为 9%。她今天没有什么特别的症状,她的身体检查也没什么特别的。她想知道她应该如何调整她的糖尿病药物来生产一个健康的婴儿,并且没有糖尿病并发症的进展。以下哪一种治疗方法是帮助实现这些目标最合适的方法( )

  A. 她可以继续目前这种治疗,因为在目前的 HbA1c 平下,她有望生下一个健康的宝宝,并且不会出现糖尿病并发症

  B. 在目前胰岛素基础上加用每天两次二甲双胍,以更好地控制血糖

  C. 开始强化胰岛素治疗,努力达到血糖控制目标,如果 HbA1c 低于 8%,她可以尝试妊娠并避免并发症

  D. 开始强化胰岛素治疗,努力达到血糖控制目标,如果 HbA1c 低于 6.5%,她可以尝试妊娠并避免并发症

  E. 因为她没有有效地治疗她的糖尿病,即使她现在改善了血糖控制,她也没有机会生一个健康的孩子,而且并发症的进展风险非常高

  正确答案是 D。

3. 一名 28 岁的 1 型糖尿病患者妊娠了,她接受胰岛素泵治疗(HbA1c 为 6.3%),因轻度高血压服用 ACEI。在妊娠早期,她的蛋白尿为 0.3g/24h;在妊娠的早期和中期,她的平均血压保持在 130/85mmHg 以下;但在妊娠晚期,血压上升到 160/100mmHg,蛋白尿上升到 0.9g/24h。由于胎儿窘迫,她在妊娠第 35 周分娩。

  以下答案正确的是( )

  A. 所有这些肾功能的变化在分娩后仍会存在,因为每次妊娠都会永久地恶化肾功能

  B. 患者有机会恢复到妊娠前血管疾病的状态,因为大多数证据表明妊娠本身并不会导致或促进糖尿病血管疾病的发展

  C. 肾功能在妊娠后常发展为严重的肾病,但高血压可能会回到正常值

D. 妊娠期出现的子痫常导致产后肾功能不全
E. 患者没有机会恢复到妊娠前血管疾病的状态，因为大多数证据表明妊娠导致或有助于糖尿病血管疾病的进展

正确答案是 B。

（刘长春 译，王 冰 校）

参 考 文 献

1. Coton SJ, Nazareth I, & Petersen I. A cohort study of trends in the prevalence of pregestational diabetes in pregnancy recorded in UK general practice between 1995 and 2012. BMJ Open 2016;6(1):e009494. Epub 2016/01/27.
2. Achong N, Duncan EL, McIntyre HD, & Callaway L. Peripartum management of glycemia in women with type 1 diabetes. Diabetes Care 2014;37(2):364–371. Epub 2013/10/17.
3. Roeder HA, Moore TR, & Ramos GA. Changes in postpartum insulin requirements for patients with well-controlled type 1 diabetes. Am J Perinatol 2016;33(7):683–687. Epub 2016/02/11.
4. Quiros C, Patrascioiu I, Perea V, Bellart J, Conget I, & Vinagre I. Postpartum metabolic control in a cohort of women with type 1 diabetes. Endocrinologia y nutricion 2015;62(3):125–129. Epub 2014/12/30.
5. Achong N, McIntyre HD, Callaway L, & Duncan EL. Glycaemic behaviour during breastfeeding in women with Type 1 diabetes. Diabet Med 2016;33(7):947–955. Epub 2015/10/20.
6. Mattila TK & de Boer A. Influence of intensive versus conventional glucose control on microvascular and macrovascular complications in type 1 and 2 diabetes mellitus. Drugs 2010;70(17):2229–2245. Epub 2010/11/18.
7. Huang T, Brown FM, Curran A, & James-Todd T. Association of pre-pregnancy BMI and postpartum weight retention with postpartum HbA1c among women with Type 1 diabetes. Diabet Med 2015;32(2):181–188. Epub 2014/10/28.
8. Park S & Kim SH. Women with rigorously managed overt diabetes during pregnancy do not experience adverse infant outcomes but do remain at serious risk of postpartum diabetes. Endocr J 2015;62(4):319–327. Epub 2015/03/05.
9. Kjos SL, Henry O, Lee RM, Buchanan TA, & Mishell DR Jr. The effect of lactation on glucose and lipid metabolism in women with recent gestational diabetes. Obstet Gynecol 1993;82(3):451–455. Epub 1993/09/01.
10. Gunderson EP, Kim C, Quesenberry CP, Jr., Marcovina S, Walton D, Azevedo RA, et al. Lactation intensity and fasting plasma lipids, lipoproteins, non-esterified free fatty acids, leptin and adiponectin in postpartum women with recent gestational diabetes mellitus: the SWIFT cohort. Metabolism 2014;63(7):941–950. Epub 2014/06/17.
11. Ehrlich SF, Hedderson MM, Quesenberry CP Jr, Feng J, Brown SD, Crites Y, et al. Post-partum weight loss and glucose metabolism in women with gestational diabetes: the DEBI Study. Diabet Med 2014;31(7):862–867. Epub 2014/03/07.
12. Feig DS, Briggs GG, Kraemer JM, Ambrose PJ, Moskovitz DN, Nageotte M, et al. Transfer of glyburide and glipizide into breast milk. Diabetes Care 2005;28(8):1851–1855. Epub 2005/07/27.
13. Hale TW, Kristensen JH, Hackett LP, Kohan R, & Ilett KF. Transfer of metformin into human milk. Diabetologia 2002;45(11):1509–1514. Epub 2002/11/19.

14 Briggs GG, Ambrose PJ, Nageotte MP, Padilla G, & Wan S. Excretion of metformin into breast milk and the effect on nursing infants. Obstet Gynecol 2005;105(6):1437–1441. Epub 2005/06/04.
15 Klein R. Hyperglycemia and microvascular and macrovascular disease in diabetes. Diabetes Care 1995;18(2):258–268. Epub 1995/02/01.
16 Chew EY, Davis MD, Danis RP, Lovato JF, Perdue LH, Greven C, et al. The effects of medical management on the progression of diabetic retinopathy in persons with type 2 diabetes: the Action to Control Cardiovascular Risk in Diabetes (ACCORD) Eye Study. Ophthalmology 2014;121(12):2443–2451. Epub 2014/08/31.
17 Leske MC, Wu SY, Hennis A, Hyman L, Nemesure B, Yang L, et al. Hyperglycemia, blood pressure, and the 9-year incidence of diabetic retinopathy: the Barbados Eye Studies. Ophthalmology 2005;112(5):799–805. Epub 2005/05/10.
18 Estacio RO, McFarling E, Biggerstaff S, Jeffers BW, Johnson D, & Schrier RW. Overt albuminuria predicts diabetic retinopathy in Hispanics with NIDDM. Am J Kidney Dis 1998;31(6):947–953. Epub 1998/06/19.
19 Temple RC, Aldridge VA, Sampson MJ, Greenwood RH, Heyburn PJ, & Glenn A. Impact of pregnancy on the progression of diabetic retinopathy in Type 1 diabetes. Diabet Med 2001;18(7):573–577. Epub 2001/09/13.
20 Diabetes Control and Complications Trial Research Group. Effect of pregnancy on microvascular complications in the diabetes control and complications trial. Diabetes Care 2000;23(8):1084–1091. Epub 2000/08/11.
21 Wender-Ozegowska E, Zawiejska A, Pietryga M, Zozulinska D, Wierusz-Wysocka B, Chmaj K, et al. [Effect of pregnancy on diabetic vascular complications]. Ginekol Pol 2004;75(5):342–351. Epub 2004/11/05.
22 Verier-Mine O, Chaturvedi N, Webb D, & Fuller JH. Is pregnancy a risk factor for microvascular complications? The EURODIAB Prospective Complications Study. Diabet Med 2005;22(11):1503–1509. Epub 2005/10/26.
23 Egan AM, McVicker L, Heerey A, Carmody L, Harney F, & Dunne FP. Diabetic retinopathy in pregnancy: a population-based study of women with pregestational diabetes. J Diabetes Res 2015;2015:310239. Epub 2015/05/07.
24 Arun CS & Taylor R. Influence of pregnancy on long-term progression of retinopathy in patients with type 1 diabetes. Diabetologia 2008;51(6):1041–1045. Epub 2008/04/09.
25 Bloomgarden ZT. American Diabetes Association annual meeting, 1997, and the Teczem Consultant Meeting. Diabetic nephropathy. Diabetes Care 1998;21(2):315–319. Epub 1998/04/16.
26 Eknoyan G, Hostetter T, Bakris GL, Hebert L, Levey AS, Parving HH, et al. Proteinuria and other markers of chronic kidney disease: a position statement of the national kidney foundation (NKF) and the national institute of diabetes and digestive and kidney diseases (NIDDK). Am J Kidney Dis 2003;42(4):617–622. Epub 2003/10/02.
27 Levey AS, Coresh J, Balk E, Kausz AT, Levin A, Steffes MW, et al. National Kidney Foundation practice guidelines for chronic kidney disease: evaluation, classification, and stratification. Ann Intern Med 2003;139(2):137–147. Epub 2003/07/16.
28 Johnson DW, Jones GR, Mathew TH, Ludlow MJ, Chadban SJ, Usherwood T, et al. Chronic kidney disease and measurement of albuminuria or proteinuria: a position statement. Med J Aust 2012;197(4):224–225. Epub 2012/08/21.
29 Krolewski AS, Niewczas MA, Skupien J, Gohda T, Smiles A, Eckfeldt JH, et al. Early progressive renal decline precedes the onset of microalbuminuria and its progression to macroalbuminuria. Diabetes Care 2014;37(1):226–234. Epub 2013/08/14.
30 Garg JP & Bakris GL. Microalbuminuria:

marker of vascular dysfunction, risk factor for cardiovascular disease. Vasc Med 2002;7(1):35–43. Epub 2002/06/27.
31 Molitch ME, Steffes M, Sun W, Rutledge B, Cleary P, de Boer IH, et al. Development and progression of renal insufficiency with and without albuminuria in adults with type 1 diabetes in the diabetes control and complications trial and the epidemiology of diabetes interventions and complications study. Diabetes Care 2010;33(7):1536–1543. Epub 2010/04/24.
32 Diabetes Control and Complications (DCCT) Research Group. Effect of intensive therapy on the development and progression of diabetic nephropathy in the Diabetes Control and Complications Trial. Kidney Intl 1995;47(6):1703–1720. Epub 1995/06/01.
33 Microvascular Complications and Foot Care. Diabetes Care 2016;39 Suppl 1:S72–S80. Epub 2015/12/24.
34 Damm JA, Asbjornsdottir B, Callesen NF, Mathiesen JM, Ringholm L, Pedersen BW, et al. Diabetic nephropathy and microalbuminuria in pregnant women with type 1 and type 2 diabetes: prevalence, antihypertensive strategy, and pregnancy outcome. Diabetes Care 2013;36(11):3489–3494. Epub 2013/09/07.
35 Young EC, Pires ML, Marques LP, de Oliveira JE, & Zajdenverg L. Effects of pregnancy on the onset and progression of diabetic nephropathy and of diabetic nephropathy on pregnancy outcomes. Diabetes Metab Synd 2011;5(3):137–142. Epub 2012/07/21.
36 Miodovnik M, Rosenn BM, Khoury JC, Grigsby JL, & Siddiqi TA. Does pregnancy increase the risk for development and progression of diabetic nephropathy? Am J Obstet Gynecol 1996;174(4):1180–1189. Epub 1996/04/01.
37 Gordin D, Forsblom C, Groop PH, Teramo K, & Kaaja R. Risk factors of hypertensive pregnancies in women with diabetes and the influence on their future life. Ann Med 2014;46(7):498–502. Epub 2014/07/22.
38 Ahmed R, Dunford J, Mehran R, Robson S, & Kunadian V. Pre-eclampsia and future cardiovascular risk among women: a review. J Am Coll Cardiol 2014;63(18):1815–1822. Epub 2014/03/13.
39 Brown MC, Best KE, Pearce MS, Waugh J, Robson SC, & Bell R. Cardiovascular disease risk in women with pre-eclampsia: systematic review and meta-analysis. Eur J Epidemiol 2013;28(1):1–19. Epub 2013/02/12.
40 Drost JT, Arpaci G, Ottervanger JP, de Boer MJ, van Eyck J, van der Schouw YT, et al. Cardiovascular risk factors in women 10 years post early preeclampsia: the Preeclampsia Risk EValuation in FEMales study (PREVFEM). Europ J Prev Cardiol 2012;19(5):1138–1144. Epub 2011/08/24.
41 Ismail-Beigi F, Craven T, Banerji MA, Basile J, Calles J, Cohen RM, et al. Effect of intensive treatment of hyperglycaemia on microvascular outcomes in type 2 diabetes: an analysis of the ACCORD randomised trial. Lancet 2010;376(9739):419–430. Epub 2010/07/03.
42 UK Prospective Diabetes Study Group. Tight blood pressure control and risk of macrovascular and microvascular complications in type 2 diabetes: UKPDS 38. BMJ 1998;317(7160):703–713. Epub 1998/09/11.
43 Vinik AI, Maser RE, Mitchell BD, & Freeman R. Diabetic autonomic neuropathy. Diabetes Care 2003;26(5):1553–1579. Epub 2003/04/30.
44 Fadl H, Magnuson A, Ostlund I, Montgomery S, Hanson U, & Schwarcz E. Gestational diabetes mellitus and later cardiovascular disease: a Swedish population based case-control study. BJOG 2014;121(12):1530–1536. Epub 2014/04/26.
45 Jones TB, Savasan ZA, Johnson Q, & Bahado-Singh R. Management of pregnant patients with diabetes with ischemic heart disease. Clin Lab Med 2013;33(2):243–256. Epub 2013/05/25.
46 D'Souza A, Hussain M, Howarth FC, Woods NM, Bidasee K, & Singh J. Pathogenesis and pathophysiology of accelerated atherosclerosis in the diabetic heart. Mol Cell Biochem 2009;331(1–2): 89–116. Epub 2009/05/26.

47 Carstensen B, Read SH, Friis S, Sund R, Keskimaki I, Svensson AM, et al. Cancer incidence in persons with type 1 diabetes: a five-country study of 9,000 cancers in type 1 diabetic individuals. Diabetologia 2016;59(5):980–988. Epub 2016/03/01.

48 Grote VA, Becker S, & Kaaks R. Diabetes mellitus type 2 – an independent risk factor for cancer? Exp Clin Endocrinol Diabetes 2010;118(1):4–8. Epub 2010/02/04.

49 Zelenko Z & Gallagher EJ. Diabetes and cancer. Endocrinol Metab Clin N Am 2014;43(1):167–185. Epub 2014/03/04.

50 Hua F, Yu JJ, & Hu ZW. Diabetes and cancer, common threads and missing links. Cancer Lett 2016. Epub 2016/02/18.

51 Giovannucci E, Harlan DM, Archer MC, Bergenstal RM, Gapstur SM, Habel LA, et al. Diabetes and cancer: a consensus report. Diabetes Care 2010;33(7):1674–1685. Epub 2010/07/01.

52 Rasmussen B, Hendrieckx C, Clarke B, Botti M, Dunning T, Jenkins A, et al. Psychosocial issues of women with type 1 diabetes transitioning to motherhood: a structured literature review. BMC Preg Childbirth 2013;13:218. Epub 2013/11/26.

53 Sparud-Lundin C & Berg M. Extraordinary exposed in early motherhood – a qualitative study exploring experiences of mothers with type 1 diabetes. BMC Women's Health 2011;11:10. Epub 2011/04/09.

54 Berg M & Sparud-Lundin C. Experiences of professional support during pregnancy and childbirth – a qualitative study of women with type 1 diabetes. BMC Preg Childbirth 2009;9:27. Epub 2009/07/07.

55 Heaman M, Gupton A, & Gregory D. Factors influencing pregnant women's perceptions of risk. MCN Am J Matern Child Nurs 2004;29(2):111–116. Epub 2004/03/19.

第二十八章 妊娠糖尿病：对子代的影响

Anne P. Starling 和 *Dana Dabalea*

Department of Epidemiology, University of Colorado School of Public Health, Aurora, Colorado, USA

> **实践要点**
> - 妊娠高血糖可能对后代造成不良的短期结局，包括巨大儿、先天畸形、新生儿低血糖和呼吸窘迫综合征。
> - 妊娠期间暴露于母体糖尿病已经增加了后代的长期不良结局的风险，包括肥胖、糖尿病和心血管疾病。
> - 未诊断妊娠前或妊娠期糖尿病的轻度妊娠高血糖与出生时的后代大小和肥胖有关；轻度高血糖和长期子代结果的关系尚未得到证实。
> - 虽然通过控制母亲血糖可以使短期不良结局最小化，但还不清楚是否也可以预防长期不良结局。

在本章中，我们将讨论暴露于糖尿病宫内环境对后代的影响。宫内高血糖症会给新生儿带来许多不良结局，其中许多可以通过良好的孕产妇血糖控制来预防。值得关注的是越来越多的证据表明，子宫内暴露于母体糖尿病对后代有长期的影响，并可能增加儿童期和成年期患慢性疾病（包括肥胖、代谢综合征和糖尿病）的风险（图 28.1）。

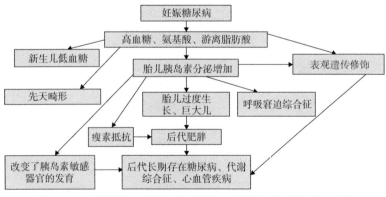

图 28.1 妊娠糖尿病导致后代短期和长期不良结局的潜在路径

新生儿期的风险

巨大儿

妊娠前和妊娠糖尿病妇女较血糖正常妇女更容易有大于胎龄儿（LGA），定义为出生体重在相应胎龄第 90 百分位数以上；或巨大儿，通常定义为出生体重在 4000g 以上[1]。巨大儿与产科并发症有关，包括肩难产和相应的臂丛神经损伤风险，急诊剖宫产的可能性增加[2]。从高血糖和不良妊娠结局（HAPO）的研究结果表明，母亲血糖与 LGA 的概率呈线性关系，妊娠期妇女空腹血糖每增加 1 个标准差，相对风险增加至 1.38 倍[3]。

先天畸形

在妊娠前诊断有糖尿病的妇女，其后代出现先天畸形的风险是一般人群的 2 倍以上，尤其是高风险的神经管缺陷和先天性心脏病[4, 5]。妊娠糖尿病妇女后代的先天异常的主要预测因素是妊娠前的血糖控制情况（如糖化血红蛋白所示）和先前存在的肾病[6, 7]。由于大部分胎儿器官在妊娠早期结束时就已经发育形成，因此妊娠前的备孕阶段就尤为重要（参见第十一章）。

新生儿低血糖

胎儿宫内过度营养和高胰岛素血症的一种可能的短期后果是新生儿低血糖，在严重的情况下可能威胁神经功能甚至生存[8]。HAPO 研究的结果证实了新生儿低血糖与妊娠 24~28 周母体葡萄糖耐量试验及脐带 C 肽浓度呈弱正相关[9]。LGA 婴儿和极早产儿在出生后的最初数小时内发生低血糖的风险更高[8, 9]。

呼吸窘迫综合征

妊娠糖尿病妇女产下的新生儿患呼吸窘迫综合征的风险显著增加[10]。母体高血糖引起的胎儿高胰岛素血症与肺成熟延迟有关[11]。而妊娠前或妊娠期糖尿病的妊娠更容易早产[12]，早产本身是呼吸窘迫综合征的危险因素。妊娠糖尿病是晚期早产（妊娠34~36周）严重呼吸并发症的独立危险因素[13]。

童年和成年风险

2型糖尿病

后代暴露于母亲糖尿病子宫内有更高的慢性疾病的风险，包括肥胖、糖尿病和代谢综合征。亚利桑那州皮马印第安人群中具有很高的2型糖尿病发病率，针对人群的基础性研究发现，患有T_2DM的女性相比血糖正常女性，前者的后代更易出现早发糖尿病[14, 15]。来自芝加哥的民族多元化人口降低T_2DM的背景风险，其中糖耐量受损的患病率较高，在子宫内暴露于母亲妊娠前或妊娠糖尿病的后代在16岁时占20%，患病率是该年龄段的一般人口的10倍[16]。患有T_2DM或糖尿病前期的丹麦妇女的成年后代GDM患病率为21%，而在接受GDM筛查结果为阴性的女性的成年后代中，这一比例为12%[17]。

这些关联并不限于患有T_2DM和GDM的母亲的后代；在妊娠期间患有T_1DM的母亲的成年后代中，也有T_2DM升高和葡萄糖受损的报道。在芝加哥，本节所述的研究表明，多数妊娠前糖尿病的母亲有过胰岛素依赖型糖尿病[16]。在一项奥地利队列研究中，5~15岁没有自身免疫抗体但曾在子宫内暴露于母亲T_1DM的儿童中，与对照组相比有较高的空腹和后负荷血糖、胰岛素和C肽[18]。丹麦人中曾在子宫内暴露于母亲T_1DM的成年后代中T_2DM和糖尿病前期的比例为11%，而对照组为4%[17]。

虽然研究表明T_2DM的宫内环境与子代患糖尿病的风险呈正相关，

但也有一些研究表明，这些结果可能与 T_2DM 的高遗传力相混淆[19, 20]。遗传力估计值为 0.26～0.69，指出高达 69%的 T_2DM 责任可能由遗传因素解释[21, 22]。此外，家庭成员具有可能导致糖尿病相关风险的行为特征；例如，另一方配偶患糖尿病的风险增加 26%[23]。创新的研究设计被用来规避共同的家庭和遗传背景。在一项关于皮马印第安人同胞配对的研究发现，在母亲诊断为 T_2DM 之前出生的婴儿的糖尿病患病率较低，平均 BMI 较诊断后出生的兄弟姐妹低[24]，这表明年幼的同胞患糖尿病的风险很高的原因是接触糖尿病的子宫内环境，而不是遗传易感性或产后家庭环境。其他研究发现过量孕产妇与父亲的糖尿病转移频率[25-28]有关，但这一发现在所有研究中并不一致[29]。

肥胖

妊娠期间暴露于母体糖尿病也与后代肥胖风险增加有关。在患有 T_1DM 的丹麦母亲的后代中，超重（$BMI>25kg/m^2$）的患病率为 41%，而未暴露对照组为 24%[30]。在科罗拉多州人群中，母亲 GDM 暴露与 6～13 岁儿童的 BMI 和腰围增加有关[31]。在皮马印第安人群中，妊娠期间患有 T_2DM 的母亲的后代比血糖正常母亲和糖尿病前期母亲的后代更容易发生肥胖及具有更高的体重[24, 32]。

特别是对于 GDM 和 T_2DM，糖尿病母亲的后代肥胖发病率的增加必须从肥胖的家族聚集中排除。母亲和父亲的 BMI 都与肥胖和后代的腰围呈正相关[33, 34]，这表明共有的遗传因素和共同的出生后环境均有影响。父母肥胖的调整及产后环境因素的调整可能对避免肥胖的长期风险的研究有重要意义[19, 35]。

一些关于轻度母亲高血糖与后代肥胖之间关系的研究已根据父母的肥胖程度进行了调整，但结果并不一致。在贝尔法斯特 HAPO 研究中对女性后代的检查发现，调整母亲 BMI 后，母亲最终高血糖和后代 2 岁[36]和 5～7 岁[37]的肥胖无关联。同样，在英国埃克塞特对非糖尿病高加索妇女进行的一项研究表明，在调整了母亲和父亲的 BMI 后，妊娠期 28 周的母亲空腹血糖与出生后任何时间点的后代体重之间没有正相关[38]。

相比之下，北卡罗来纳州妊娠、感染和营养研究中的一项分析报道显示，妊娠负荷后血糖与后代 3 岁时的 BMI 之间存在显著相关性，而在调整母亲的 BMI 后，这一相关性依然显著[39]。此外，一项对没有妊娠前或妊娠糖尿病的墨西哥裔美国妇女的研究发现，妊娠负荷后血糖浓度与 2~7 岁的子代 BMI 评分呈正相关，这与妊娠期妇女妊娠前肥胖无关[40]。在随后的分层分析中，研究结果仅在没有妊娠前肥胖的女性的后代中显著，这表明母体 BMI 与血糖之间的相互作用与其后代肥胖有关。

这里应该注意调整产妇妊娠前 BMI 可能部分掩盖了胎儿营养过剩的全部影响，因为产妇肥胖也可能有助于宫内葡萄糖升高和能量丰富的环境[41, 42]。另外，筛选 GDM 往往不是普遍的，而且更多可能会提供给女性超重或肥胖，这可能导致正常体重女性的 GDM 漏诊并因此低估调整母亲的 BMI 后产妇 GDM 和后代肥胖/糖尿病之间的真正联系[41]。

干预研究的数据被用来检验妊娠期间降低母亲葡萄糖浓度是否可以阻止后代在以后的生活中肥胖和胰岛素抵抗的风险增加。一项大型观察研究发现，与需要接受治疗（更严重的）GDM 的母亲的后代相比，不需要治疗（更轻微）的 GDM 母亲的后代在 5~7 岁时患肥胖症的风险几乎增加了 1 倍，该研究没有对母亲的 BMI[43]进行调整。相比之下，两项随机对照试验（一项在澳大利亚，一项在加拿大渥太华）表明，患有 GDM 母亲的后代在 4~5 岁或 9 岁时的 BMI 或糖耐量受损与未接受治疗（或最少治疗）的母亲之间没有差别[44, 45]。在一项研究[44]中，作者认为这种影响可能要到童年后期才能被发现，这与一些观察性研究一致，在一些观察研究中，与母亲糖尿病相关的后代体重升高直到上学年龄[46]才明显。第二项研究的样本数量不足以得出关于后代肥胖差异的结论[45]。最后，最近的母胎医学单位多中心试验发现，轻度的 GDM 女性治疗组与未治疗组的后代 5~6 岁或 7~10 岁时，超重或肥胖的频率（BMI 高于第 85 或第 95 百分位数）并无差异[47]。因此，对于患有 GDM 或 T_2DM 的母亲后代，肥胖和 T_2DM 的长期风险是否可以通过控制血糖来降低，目前还没有定论。

心血管疾病

在子宫内暴露于母亲糖尿病的后代可能在以后的生活中会增加罹患

心血管疾病的风险。根据 Carpenter-Coustan 标准，患有 GDM 的母亲的 LGA 后代在 6~11 岁时代谢综合征的患病率高于未接触 GDM 或接触 GDM 但出生时体重适合胎龄的儿童[48]。其他心血管疾病危险因素在儿童暴露于宫外糖尿病或子宫内 GDM 的儿童中升高，包括内皮功能障碍的标志物，更高的 LDL 和更高的收缩压[49, 50]。T_1DM 女性的后代也发现了这些风险因素[51]。丹麦的一项研究报告显示，GDM 女性的后代成年后的代谢综合征风险升高，T_1DM 妇女的后代的风险也升高，但低于前者[30]。然而，一项单独的丹麦登记研究报道发现父亲患有 T_2DM 的后代患心血管和脑血管病的风险也较高[52]，为遗传和产后环境因素的共同影响提供了支持。

长期影响的机制

"燃料"介导的致畸作用

糖尿病妇女妊娠的后代可能在发育的关键窗口暴露于过量的"燃料"（葡萄糖、氨基酸和游离脂肪酸），这可能直接导致整个生命中代谢功能的改变。该途径被称为燃料相关的致畸作用，被认为主要通过胎儿胰岛 B 细胞增生[53, 54]。过量的母体循环葡萄糖穿过胎盘并刺激胎儿胰腺产生胰岛素，而胰岛素反过来会促进增长[55]。胎儿高胰岛素血症可引起胰岛素依赖性器官的改变，包括胰岛素抵抗的发展或胰岛素分泌的下调[56]。在子宫内发生的其他变化可包括脂肪细胞代谢或下丘脑食欲和饱腹感的改变（在文献[57]中综述）。胰岛素长期高水平也可能导致瘦素分泌增加[58]，并且在饮食诱导肥胖的动物模型中观察到中枢对瘦素引起的降低食欲作用产生了抵抗[59]。

葡萄糖可能不是胎儿过量接受的唯一燃料；GDM 还与脂质异常有关。三酰甘油可以水解成游离脂肪酸，其可以穿过胎盘并且可以导致胎儿脂肪细胞的数量和大小增加[60, 61]。在没有诊断为妊娠期或妊娠前糖尿病的女性中，妊娠早期妇女空腹三酰甘油水平和妊娠晚期游离脂肪酸水平与出生 24h 内新生儿体脂百分比显著相关，与母亲的 BMI 无关[62]。子宫内过量母体脂质暴露对长期后代肥胖的相对贡献尚不清楚[53]。

表观遗传学

宫内高血糖可能通过后代 DNA 的表观遗传变化影响后代的健康，导致基因调控持续改变。已经提出了支持这一假设的证据。妊娠期间葡萄糖耐量降低的女性葡萄糖浓度升高与胎盘细胞瘦素和脂联素基因的 DNA 甲基化改变有关[63,64]。在脐带血和女性胎盘细胞中观察到与肥胖有关的 MEST 基因的甲基化水平与 GDM 相比较低[65]。此外，8～12 岁儿童外周血细胞的表观基因组 DNA 甲基化分析揭示与 11 名未暴露儿童相比，暴露于 GDM 子宫内的 11 名儿童存在多个差异甲基化区域（DMR）[66]。尽管没有多重检测对进行校正，但两种 DMR 显示出部分调节暴露于母体 GDM 的后代 VCAM-1 血管内皮功能障碍的标志物之间的关联。据我们所知，尚无对来自胎儿或新生儿细胞中的表观遗传标记的数据进行过这种调控分析，这将更强烈地表明宫内环境的持续影响[20,67]。

总结与未来的方向

妊娠期母体代谢紊乱与后代的短期和长期不良健康结果有关。虽然通过适当的母体血糖控制可以最大限度地减少患糖尿病妇女的新生儿不良结局，但还需要进行更多的研究确定长期不良结局是否也可以预防。GDM 干预研究的长期随访对于解决这个问题非常重要。儿童肥胖和 T_2DM 已成为公共卫生危机，预防是一个高度优先事项。高血糖的宫内环境可能是一个重要的风险因素，可以增强后代代谢疾病的发生风险，加上共同的遗传和行为风险因素，会加剧肥胖和糖尿病的代际循环。

选择题

1. 可以使用以下哪种流行病学研究设计来区分母亲和后代之间共享的遗传易感性的影响，以及暴露于母亲糖尿病宫内对后代的糖尿病风险（　　）

A. 家系研究，比较与母亲糖尿病与父亲糖尿病的后代糖尿病风险

B. 同胞研究，比较母亲诊断糖尿病前出生的后代的糖尿病风险，以及母亲诊断出糖尿病后出生的后代患糖尿病的风险

C. 横断面研究，比较 2 型糖尿病母亲的后代糖尿病患病率与无 T_2DM 母亲的后代糖尿病患病率

D. A 和 B

正确答案是 D。A 和 B 中描述的两种研究设计可能有助于分离[1]来自每个亲代的遗传贡献，以及妊娠期间患有糖尿病的母亲的特定宫内环境对后代患糖尿病风险的影响。

2. 以下哪项不是妊娠期母亲糖尿病可能导致不良后代健康结果的可能机制是（　　）

A. 胎儿细胞的表观遗传修饰

B. 胎儿胰腺过量产生胰岛素

C. 将母体胰岛素转移到胎盘以促进胎儿生长

D. 脂肪细胞代谢的变化，包括脂肪因子的产生

正确答案是 C。母体胰岛素不会穿过胎盘屏障；然而，母体葡萄糖可以穿过胎盘并刺激胎儿胰腺产生胰岛素。

（张　焱　译，朱海清　校）

参 考 文 献

1 Cordero L, Treuer SH, Landon MB, Gabbe SG. Management of infants of diabetic mothers. Arch Pediatr Adolesc Med 1998 Mar;152(3):249–254.

2 Rossi AC, Mullin P, Prefumo F. Prevention, management, and outcomes of macrosomia: a systematic review of literature and meta-analysis. Obstet Gynecol Surv 2013 Oct;68(10):702–709.

3 Metzger BE, Lowe LP, Dyer AR, Trimble ER, Chaovarindr U, Coustan DR, et al. Hyperglycemia and adverse pregnancy outcomes. N Engl J Med 2008 May;358(19):1991–2002.

4 Macintosh MC, Fleming KM, Bailey JA, Doyle P, Modder J, Acolet D, et al. Perinatal mortality and congenital anomalies in babies of women with type 1 or type 2 diabetes in England, Wales, and Northern Ireland: population based study. BMJ 2006 Jul;333(7560):177.

5 Eidem I, Stene LC, Henriksen T, Hanssen KF, Vangen S, Vollset SE, et al. Congenital anomalies in newborns of women with type 1 diabetes: nationwide population-based study in Norway, 1999–2004. Acta Obstetric Gynecolog Scandinav 2010 Nov;89(11):1403–1411.

6 Bell R, Glinianaia SV, Tennant PWG, Bilous RW, Rankin J. Peri-conception hyperglycaemia and nephropathy are associated with risk of congenital anomaly in women with pre-existing diabetes: a

population-based cohort study. Diabetologia 2012 Apr;55(4):936-947.
7. Inkster ME, Fahey TP, Donnan PT, Leese GP, Mires GJ, Murphy DJ. The role of modifiable pre-pregnancy risk factors in preventing adverse fetal outcomes among women with type 1 and type 2 diabetes. Acta Obstetric Gynecolog Scandinav 009;88(10):1153-1157.
8. Mitanchez D. Management of infants born to mothers with gestational diabetes. Paediatric environment. Diabetes Metab 2010 Dec;36(6 Pt 2):587-594.
9. Metzger BE, Persson B, Lowe LP, Dyer AR, Cruickshank JK, Deerochanawong C, et al. Hyperglycemia and adverse pregnancy outcome study: neonatal glycemia. Pediatrics 2010 Dec;126(6):e1545-e1552.
10. Robert MF, Neff RK, Hubbell JP, Taeusch HW, Avery ME. Association between maternal diabetes and the respiratory-distress syndrome in the newborn. N Engl J Med 1976 Feb;294(7):357-360.
11. Lock M, McGillick EV, Orgeig S, McMillen IC, Morrison JL. Regulation of fetal lung development in response to maternal overnutrition. Clinical and Experimental Pharmacology and Physiology 2013 Nov;40(11):803-816.
12. Lai FY, Johnson JA, Dover D, Kaul P. Outcomes of singleton and twin pregnancies complicated by preexisting diabetes and gestational diabetes: a population-based study in Alberta, Canada, 2005-2011. J Diabetes 2016;8(1):45-55.
13. Fung GPG, Chan LM, Ho YC, To WK, Chan HB, Lao TT. Does gestational diabetes mellitus affect respiratory outcome in late-preterm infants? Early Human Development 2014 Sep;90(9):527-530.
14. Pettitt DJ, Aleck KA, Baird HR, Carraher MJ, Bennett PH, Knowler WC. Congenital susceptibility to NIDDM. Role of intrauterine environment. Diabetes 1988 May;37(5):622-628.
15. Dabelea D, Knowler WC, Pettitt DJ. Effect of diabetes in pregnancy on offspring: follow-up research in the Pima Indians. J Matern Fetal Med 2000 Jan-Feb;9(1):83-88.
16. Silverman BL, Metzger BE, Cho NH, Loeb CA. Impaired glucose tolerance in adolescent offspring of diabetic mothers. Relationship to fetal hyperinsulinism. Diabetes Care 1995 May;18(5):611-617.
17. Clausen TD, Mathiesen ER, Hansen T, Pedersen O, Jensen DM, Lauenborg J, et al. High prevalence of type 2 diabetes and pre-diabetes in adult offspring of women with gestational diabetes mellitus or type 1 diabetes: the role of intrauterine hyperglycemia. Diabetes Care 2008 Feb;31(2):340-346.
18. Weiss PA, Scholz HS, Haas J, Tamussino KF, Seissler J, Borkenstein MH. Long-term follow-up of infants of mothers with type 1 diabetes: evidence for hereditary and nonhereditary transmission of diabetes and precursors. Diabetes Care 2000 Jul;23(7):905-911.
19. Donovan LE, Cundy T. Does exposure to hyperglycaemia in utero increase the risk of obesity and diabetes in the offspring? A critical reappraisal. Diabet Med 2015;32(3):295-304.
20. Fraser A, Lawlor DA. Long-term health outcomes in offspring born to women with diabetes in pregnancy. Curr Diab Rep 2014;14(5):489.
21. Almgren P, Lehtovirta M, Isomaa B, Sarelin L, Taskinen MR, Lyssenko V, et al. Heritability and familiality of type 2 diabetes and related quantitative traits in the Botnia Study. Diabetologia 2011 Nov;54(11):2811-2819.
22. Poulsen P, Kyvik KO, Vaag A, Beck-Nielsen H. Heritability of type II (non-insulin-dependent) diabetes mellitus and abnormal glucose tolerance – a population-based twin study. Diabetologia 1999 Feb;42(2):139-145.
23. Leong A, Rahme E, Dasgupta K. Spousal diabetes as a diabetes risk factor: A systematic review and meta-analysis. Bmc Medicine 2014 Jan;12:12.
24. Dabelea D, Hanson RL, Lindsay RS, Pettitt DJ, Imperatore G, Gabir MM, et al. Intrauterine exposure to diabetes conveys risks for type 2 diabetes and obesity: a study of discordant sibships. Diabetes 2000

25 Harder T, Franke K, Kohlhoff R, Plagemann A. Maternal and paternal family history of diabetes in women with gestational diabetes or insulin-dependent diabetes mellitus type I. Gynecol Obstet Invest 2001;51(3):160-164.
26 Dörner G, Mohnike A, Steindel E. On possible genetic and epigenetic modes of diabetes transmission. Endokrinologie 1975 Nov;66(2):225-227.
27 Martin AO, Simpson JL, Ober C, Freinkel N. Frequency of diabetes mellitus in mothers of probands with gestational diabetes: possible maternal influence on the predisposition to gestational diabetes. Am J Obstet Gynecol 1985 Feb;151(4):471-475.
28 McLean M, Chipps D, Cheung NW. Mother to child transmission of diabetes mellitus: does gestational diabetes program Type 2 diabetes in the next generation? Diabet Med 2006 Nov;23(11):1213-1215.
29 Meigs JB, Cupples LA, Wilson PW. Parental transmission of type 2 diabetes: the Framingham Offspring Study. Diabetes 2000 Dec;49(12):2201-2207.
30 Clausen TD, Mathiesen ER, Hansen T, Pedersen O, Jensen DM, Lauenborg J, et al. Overweight and the metabolic syndrome in adult offspring of women with diet-treated gestational diabetes mellitus or type 1 diabetes. J Clin Endocrinol Metab 2009 Jul;94(7):2464-2470.
31 Crume TL, Ogden L, West NA, Vehik KS, Scherzinger A, Daniels S, et al. Association of exposure to diabetes in utero with adiposity and fat distribution in a multiethnic population of youth: the Exploring Perinatal Outcomes among Children (EPOCH) Study. Diabetologia 2011 Jan;54(1):87-92.
32 Pettitt DJ, Knowler WC, Bennett PH, Aleck KA, Baird HR. Obesity in offspring of diabetic Pima Indian women despite normal birth weight. Diabetes Care 1987 1987 Jan-Feb;10(1):76-80.
33 Patel R, Martin RM, Kramer MS, Oken E, Bogdanovich N, Matush L, et al. Familial associations of adiposity: findings from a cross-sectional study of 12,181 parental-offspring trios from Belarus. PLoS One 2011;6(1):e14607.
34 Morandi A, Meyre D, Lobbens S, Kleinman K, Kaakinen M, Rifas-Shiman SL, et al. Estimation of newborn risk for child or adolescent obesity: lessons from longitudinal birth cohorts. PLoS One 2012;7(11):e49919.
35 Wardle J, Guthrie C, Sanderson S, Birch L, Plomin R. Food and activity preferences in children of lean and obese parents. Int J Obes Relat Metab Disord 2001 Jul;25(7):971-977.
36 Pettitt DJ, McKenna S, McLaughlin C, Patterson CC, Hadden DR, McCance DR. Maternal glucose at 28 weeks of gestation is not associated with obesity in 2-year-old offspring: the Belfast Hyperglycemia and Adverse Pregnancy Outcome (HAPO) family study. Diabetes Care 2010 Jun;33(6):1219-1223.
37 Thaware PK, McKenna S, Patterson CC, Hadden DR, Pettitt DJ, McCance DR. Untreated mild hyperglycemia during pregnancy and anthropometric measures of obesity in offspring at age 5-7 years. Diabetes Care 2015 Sep;38(9):1701-1706.
38 Knight B, Shields BM, Hill A, Powell RJ, Wright D, Hattersley AT. The impact of maternal glycemia and obesity on early postnatal growth in a nondiabetic Caucasian population. Diabetes Care 2007 Apr;30(4):777-783.
39 Deierlein AL, Siega-Riz AM, Chantala K, Herring AH. The association between maternal glucose concentration and child BMI at age 3 years. Diabetes Care 2011 Feb;34(2):480-484.
40 Ehrlich SF, Rosas LG, Ferrara A, King JC, Abrams B, Harley KG, et al. Pregnancy glycemia in Mexican-American women without diabetes or gestational diabetes and programming for childhood obesity. American Journal of Epidemiology 2013 Apr;177(8):768-775.
41 Spiegelman D, Israel RG, Bouchard C, Willett WC. Absolute fat mass, percent

body fat, and body-fat distribution: which is the real determinant of blood pressure and serum glucose? Am J Clin Nutr 1992 Jun;55(6):1033–1044.
42 Lawlor DA, Relton C, Sattar N, Nelson SM. Maternal adiposity: a determinant of perinatal and offspring outcomes? Nature Reviews Endocrinology 2012 Nov;8(11):679–688.
43 Hillier TA, Pedula KL, Schmidt MM, Mullen JA, Charles MA, Pettitt DJ. Childhood obesity and metabolic imprinting: the ongoing effects of maternal hyperglycemia. Diabetes Care 2007 Sep;30(9):2287–2292.
44 Gillman MW, Oakey H, Baghurst PA, Volkmer RE, Robinson JS, Crowther CA. Effect of treatment of gestational diabetes mellitus on obesity in the next generation. Diabetes Care 2010 May;33(5):964–968.
45 Malcolm JC, Lawson ML, Gaboury I, Lough G, Keely E. Glucose tolerance of offspring of mother with gestational diabetes mellitus in a low-risk population. Diabet Med 2006 May;23(5):565–570.
46 Silverman BL, Rizzo T, Green OC, Cho NH, Winter RJ, Ogata ES, et al. Long-term prospective evaluation of offspring of diabetic mothers. Diabetes 1991 Dec;40 Suppl 2:121–125.
47 Landon MB, Rice MM, Varner MW, Casey BM, Reddy UM, Wapner RJ, et al. Mild gestational diabetes mellitus and long-term child health. Diabetes Care 2015 Mar;38(3):445–452.
48 Boney CM, Verma A, Tucker R, Vohr BR. Metabolic syndrome in childhood: association with birth weight, maternal obesity, and gestational diabetes mellitus. Pediatrics 2005 Mar;115(3):e290–e296.
49 West NA, Crume TL, Maligie MA, Dabelea D. Cardiovascular risk factors in children exposed to maternal diabetes in utero. Diabetologia 2011 Mar;54(3):504–507.
50 Bunt JC, Tataranni PA, Salbe AD. Intrauterine exposure to diabetes is a determinant of hemoglobin A(1)c and systolic blood pressure in Pima Indian children. J Clin Endocrinol Metab 2005 Jun;90(6):3225–3229.
51 Manderson JG, Mullan B, Patterson CC, Hadden DR, Traub AI, McCance DR. Cardiovascular and metabolic abnormalities in the offspring of diabetic pregnancy. Diabetologia 2002 Jul;45(7):991–996.
52 Wu CS, Nohr EA, Bech BH, Vestergaard M, Olsen J. Long-term health outcomes in children born to mothers with diabetes: a population-based cohort study. PLoS One 2012;7(5):e36727.
53 Whitaker RC, Dietz WH. Role of the prenatal environment in the development of obesity. Journal of Pediatrics 1998 May;132(5):768–776.
54 Heding LG, Persson B, Stangenberg M. B-cell function in newborn infants of diabetic mothers. Diabetologia 1980 Nov;19(5):427–432.
55 PEDERSEN J. Weight and length at birth of infants of diabetic mothers. Acta Endocrinol (Copenh) 1954 Aug;16(4):330–342.
56 Freinkel N. Banting Lecture 1980. Of pregnancy and progeny. Diabetes 1980 Dec;29(12):1023–1035.
57 Taylor PD, Poston L. Developmental programming of obesity in mammals. Exp Physiol 2007 Mar;92(2):287–298.
58 Kolaczynski JW, Nyce MR, Considine RV, Boden G, Nolan JJ, Henry R, et al. Acute and chronic effects of insulin on leptin production in humans: Studies in vivo and in vitro. Diabetes 1996 May;45(5):699–701.
59 Rahmouni K, Morgan DA, Morgan GM, Mark AL, Haynes WG. Role of selective leptin resistance in diet-induced obesity hypertension. Diabetes 2005 Jul;54(7):2012–2018.
60 Knopp RH, Warth MR, Charles D, Childs M, Li JR, Mabuchi H, et al. Lipoprotein metabolism in pregnancy, fat transport to the fetus, and the effects of diabetes. Biol Neonat 1986;50(6):297–317.
61 Tontonoz P, Hu E, Spiegelman BM. Stimulation of adipogenesis in fibroblasts by PPAR gamma 2, a lipid-activated transcription factor. Cell 1994 Dec;79(7):1147–1156.

62 Harmon KA, Gerard L, Jensen DR, Kealey EH, Hernandez TL, Reece MS, *et al.* Continuous glucose profiles in obese and normal-weight pregnant women on a controlled diet: metabolic determinants of fetal growth. Diabetes Care 2011 Oct;34(10):2198–2204.
63 Bouchard L, Thibault S, Guay SP, Santure M, Monpetit A, St-Pierre J, *et al.* Leptin gene epigenetic adaptation to impaired glucose metabolism during pregnancy. Diabetes Care 2010 Nov;33(11):2436–2441.
64 Bouchard L, Hivert MF, Guay SP, St-Pierre J, Perron P, Brisson D. Placental adiponectin gene DNA methylation levels are associated with mothers' blood glucose concentration. Diabetes 2012 May;61(5):1272–1280.
65 El Hajj N, Pliushch G, Schneider E, Dittrich M, Müller T, Korenkov M, *et al.* Metabolic programming of MEST DNA methylation by intrauterine exposure to gestational diabetes mellitus. Diabetes 2013 Apr;62(4):1320–1328.
66 West NA, Kechris K, Dabelea D. Exposure to Maternal Diabetes in Utero and DNA Methylation Patterns in the Offspring. Immunometabolism 2013 Mar;1:1–9.
67 El Hajj N, Schneider E, Lehnen H, Haaf T. Epigenetics and life-long consequences of an adverse nutritional and diabetic intrauterine environment. Reproduction 2014;148(6):R111–R120.

第二十九章 从试验到临床：潜在的未来治疗妊娠糖尿病的方法——改善妊娠期间 B 细胞的质量和功能

David J. Hill

Lawson Health Research Institute, St. Joseph's Health Care, London, Ontario, Canada

概述

GDM 的患病率正在增加，美国最新报道的患病率高达 18%；这与越来越多的肥胖妊娠妇女有关[1]，而且 GDM 的国际诊断标准也发生了变化。GDM 不仅对母亲产生直接的健康风险，而且是患 T_2DM 的危险因素，并且它会增加后代儿童期肥胖和将来患 T_2DM 的风险[2]。虽然已证实 GDM 具有遗传易感性，大多数基因多态性和 T_2DM 相似，但是鉴定单基因谱的遗传风险对个体也有用处[3]。用药物干预来预防 GDM 需要考虑到药物会经胎盘传递给胎儿，目前仅证实二甲双胍在多囊卵巢综合征的妊娠妇女中可不同程度地预防 GDM[4]。因此，重点应放在生活方式的干预上，通过饮食调整，增加运动或两者兼而有之的方式来帮助有 GDM 风险的女性。最近的三项研究结果不一[5-7]，只有一项证实可以降低 GDM 发病率[5]，其中一项证实了母体血糖有所改善[6]。妊娠期胰岛素抵抗会生理性加重，与之伴随的是相应的胰岛 B 细胞数量和分泌胰岛素的增加，未能进行这种功能调整会增加 GDM 的发生风险。展望未来，增强妊娠期自然发生的 B 细胞群的生理性增加可能有助于预防处于危险中的 GDM 女性。然而，这些策略需要将详细了解妊娠期 B 细胞适应性改变的机制作为第一步（图 29.1）。

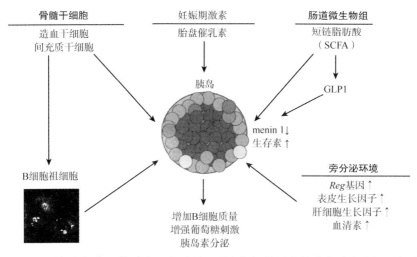

图 29.1　增加妊娠期母体胰岛 B 细胞量以预防妊娠糖尿病的潜在治疗途径和介质

妊娠期 B 细胞的适应性

在所有测试的哺乳动物物种（包括人类）中，母体的 B 细胞在妊娠期间发生适应性扩增（图 29.2）。接下来是分娩后 B 细胞量的消退，主要是通过 B 细胞的靶向凋亡来实现。在妊娠的小鼠中，B 细胞有丝分裂发生率的增加可导致 B 细胞的数量增加 2~3 倍，在妊娠期第 13~15d 附近达到峰值（期限 19d）[8]。Van Assche 等[9]的报道显示，与年龄匹配的非妊娠对照组相比，女性在妊娠晚期或分娩时 B 细胞可增加 1 倍。之后，Butler 等[10]测量了妊娠期间死亡女性胰腺中 B 细胞的面积变化分数，发现妊娠期间增加了 1.4 倍，该数据集还包括妊娠早期死亡的女性。重要的是，B 细胞在妊娠前 3 个月后适应性改变失败与 GDM 有关[11]。扭转 GDM 的未来战略可能包括有针对性地增加产妇 B 细胞的质量，特别是如果它未能进行最佳的适应性扩增。这可以通过以下方式实现：①操纵通常与 B 细胞扩增相关的激素；②用小分子有针对性地操纵胰岛内细胞的分泌环境；③基于细胞的疗法；④营养调节。

B细胞质量的调节变化

- 在成年期间B细胞团先前被认为是有丝分裂的静止状态

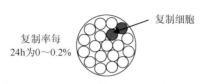

现在可以理解胰岛B细胞质量可以随着生理/病理代谢应激物而改变

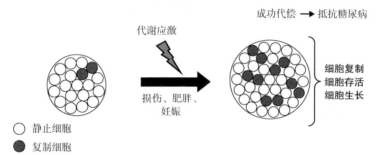

图 29.2　B 细胞团的生理和病理调节变化

尽管 B 细胞在成年期通常处于静止状态，但它们可通过增生、肥大和存活率增加来应对损伤、肥胖或妊娠的代谢应激。引自 Rieck & Kaestner 2010[29]，经 Elsevier 允许使用

B 细胞团的激素控制

妊娠期间增加的 B 细胞量和由此导致的胰岛素分泌能力增加对于抵消增加的母体外周胰岛素抵抗是必要的。造成后者的原因是由于部分母体血液循环中增加的胎盘分泌的生长激素（GH-V）[12]，抑制垂体生长激素释放。胎盘催乳素（PL）和 GH-V 的组合还促进肝脏糖异生和脂解，以支持向胎儿的营养转移。然而，PL 扩大 B 细胞量的能力抵消了母体高血糖的风险。啮齿类动物在妊娠期间的母体 B 细胞量的增加与 PL 的出现和上升相关[13]。通过在 B 细胞中有针对性地促进 PL 的过度表达而扩散[14]。

虽然 PL 的存在可以解释在妊娠期间发生的 B 细胞量的补偿，但它似乎不会直接增强葡萄糖刺激的胰岛素分泌（GSIS）。这可以通过 Kisspeptin 来实现。Kisspeptin 是一种由 *kiss-1* 基因编码的蛋白质，其中酰胺化的 Kisspeptin-54（也称为 metastin）是最丰富的[15]。Kisspeptin 的受体是G蛋白偶联受体（GPCR），GPR54通过偶联G蛋白$G\alpha_q$亚基发出信号，导致磷脂酶C-β（PLC-β）的活化和随后细胞内Ca^{2+}的增加；以及激活蛋白激酶C（PKC）[16, 17]。已显示PKC异构体调节新合成的胰岛素原从内质网的转运，以及胰岛素原转化为胰岛素（图29.3）。Kisspeptin和GPR54由胎盘滋养细胞表达，Kisspeptin-10（能够激活GPR54受体的最短序列）释放到母体循环中[15, 18]。KISS1和GPR54的胎盘信使RNA（mRNA）表达发生在妊娠早期，与滋养细胞侵袭性峰值一致[18]，在妊娠期，上述表达水平降低与早产儿、先兆子痫或1型糖尿病[19, 20]相关。虽然Kisspeptin的循环水平通常在人体中较低，但它们在妊娠期间会增加，在妊娠晚期可以观察到峰值，浓度为20nmol/L或更高[19, 21]。在啮齿类动物中，静脉注射Kisspeptin会导致血浆胰岛素迅速增加4倍，可持续90min[22]。在恒河猴中也有类似的发现[23]。在人类中，患有GDM的女性中Kisspeptin的循环水平降低[24]，表明调节胎盘衍生的PL和Kisspeptin可能增加细胞质量和GSIS。目前尚未测试使用Kisspeptin增加胰岛素释放和预防GDM。

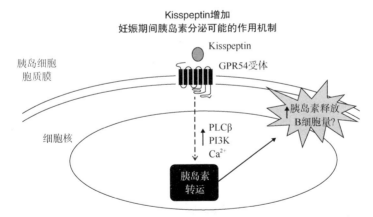

图29.3 Kisspeptin对B细胞的作用机制可能是在妊娠期间增加胰岛素释放。与GPR54受体结合的Kisspeptin导致细胞内活化磷脂酶C（PLC）、磷酸肌醇3激酶（PI3K）水平升高，增加细胞内钙水平，触发胰岛素释放

妊娠期B细胞可塑性的细胞机制

在成人中，胰岛B细胞通常是静止的，具有非常低的增殖周转率。

然而，在啮齿动物妊娠期间，母体 B 细胞发生有丝分裂，导致小鼠在妊娠第 15 天后 B 细胞量至少翻倍，到出生后退化[8]。PL 驱动 B 细胞有丝分裂的再激活，克服了 B 细胞静止并通过催乳素受体的结合和活化诱导增殖。催乳素受体的转基因缺失导致 B 细胞代偿性生长失败，胰岛素释放受损和葡萄糖耐受不良[25, 26]。相反，催乳素受体的表达导致 B 细胞过度生长[26]。在下游，催乳素受体通过与 Jak2 的结合激活许多细胞内第二信使通路，导致激活 Stat5[27]，丝裂原活化蛋白激酶（MAPK）、PI3K 和 Akt[28]（图 29.4）。妊娠啮齿动物 B 细胞内 PL 或催乳素对 Stat5 的激活可以诱导 B 细胞淋巴瘤 6（*Bcl6*）基因表达，这是肿瘤抑制基因的转录抑制因子——menin 1。妊娠期间，催乳素受体缺失的胰岛表现出增加 menin 1 的表达[28]。相反，妊娠期间胰岛内的 menin 1 下调导致了抑制细胞周期调节蛋白 P18 和 P27，以及 B 细胞从细胞周期停滞中释放[29]。

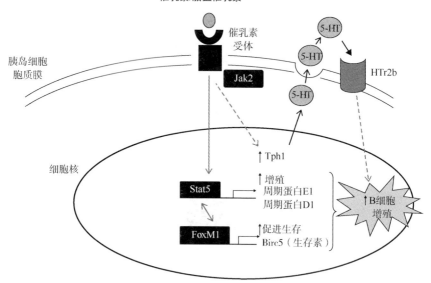

图 29.4 妊娠期间 B 细胞量增加的机制

催乳素或胎盘催乳素与催乳素受体结合。Jak2 和 Stat5 的磷酸化导致细胞循环进展基因的表达增加，如细胞周期蛋白 D1 和 E1，导致 B 细胞复制。Stat5 还可以增加 FoxM1 的表达，导致保存活基因 Birc5 的表达增加。催乳素受体的激活还可以增加色氨酸羟化酶 1（Tph1）的表达，引起血清素（5-HT）的产生和释放。血清素可通过 HTr2b 信号传导后激活 B 细胞增殖受体因此，对于补偿性胰岛生长，下调 menin 1 尤为重要，因为在小鼠母体 B 细胞内靶向过表达 menin 1 会阻止其增殖并导致葡萄糖耐受不良[29]。然而，尚不清楚 Stat5 激活是否是导致 B 细胞中 menin 1 下调的唯一途径，因为单独的葡萄糖可以抑制体外培养 menin 1[30]。葡萄糖的作用依赖于通过 PI3K-Akt 途径的信号传导，表明这可能是调节 menin 1 的整体上游步骤。催乳素增加小鼠 B 细胞量的能力也取决于生存素（Birc5）的表达，小鼠 B 细胞中存活蛋白基因的靶向缺失阻止了妊娠期间的任何适应性改变[31]。menin 1 的小分子拮抗剂或存活蛋白的激动剂理论上可以促进母体 B 细胞量的增加。

妊娠期间，B 细胞量的适应性增加可能不仅是由于静止细胞重新进入细胞增殖周期，而且还来自胰腺祖细胞分化成 B 细胞。在小鼠和人胰腺中均确认有能够成为 B 细胞的多系潜在的祖细胞，特别是存在比胰岛小得多的小内分泌簇中，以及胰管周围[32]。Smukler 等[33]报道这种细胞可以少量表达胰岛素，但是显示葡萄糖转运蛋白 Glut2 的极低表达。因此，这些祖细胞对葡萄糖的胰岛素释放响应性差，但是在代谢应激下可以分化成为成熟的功能性 B 细胞。

这种常驻祖细胞的激活可能有助于妊娠期间 B 细胞的增加。当小鼠模型中的 B 细胞祖细胞被遗传标记时，在妊娠期间观察到稀释的谱系标记细胞，表明从祖细胞产生了一些新的 B 细胞[34]。

类似的机制是否能解释人类妊娠 B 细胞团的适应性变化尚未得到证实。Butler 等[10]使用尸体样本发现妊娠妇女和非妊娠受试者的 B 细胞有丝分裂指数或每个胰岛 B 细胞的相对面积没有变化，但他们观察到分散在整个腺泡组织中并与胰管并列的胰岛素分泌细胞数量的增加。这表明来自祖细胞的 B 细胞的新生可以在人类妊娠期间发生，以及现有 B 细胞的有丝分裂激活。妊娠期间 C 肽的再次出现支持这种机制，其中 90 名妊娠妇女存在 T_1DM，平均病程为 17 年，预计残留的 B 细胞很少[35]。

转录因子表达的变化也是激活妊娠代偿性 B 细胞生长所必需的，这些也可能通过改变信号发出信号 menin1。例如，肝细胞核因子-4α（HNF4α）激活 Ras-Erk1/2 在 PI3K 信号通路下游激活的激酶促有丝分裂途径[36]和叉头框蛋白 M1（FoxM1）抑制 menin1 水平，并激活凋亡抑制因子如生存素[37, 38]。

妊娠期间胰岛旁分泌环境的变化

妊娠期胰岛营养环境的变化远远超过 PL 的增加，需要了解更详细的微环境以选择候选分子靶标而增加 B 细胞量。在妊娠期间，多种旁分泌因子在母体胰腺中大量改变。大鼠胰岛适应妊娠的基因组研究发现，再生蛋白基因-3a（Reg3a）的表达增加了 2.5 倍，表皮生长因子（EGF）表达增加了 3 倍[39]。Reg 基因通过 PI3K 介导的激活转录因子-2（ATF2）的磷酸化激活细胞周期蛋白 D1 表达和 B 细胞增殖。用小鼠或人 Reg3 肽处理正常成年小鼠导致小胰岛平均大小增加，这是由于细胞增殖和出现大量的胰岛素表达细胞[40]。类似的，喂食高脂肪饮食或在妊娠后表达突变 EGF 受体的小鼠未能经历适应性 B 细胞的生长，证明 EGF 信号是成年动物 B 细胞可塑性所必需的[41]。

带有靶向缺失肝细胞生长因子（HGF）受体 c-Met 的成年小鼠在用选择性毒素，如链脲佐菌素（STZ）或部分胰腺切除术治疗后不能再生 B 细胞。而在野生型动物中可以再生，B 细胞上的内源性 c-Met 水平升高[42]。HGF 作用对于妊娠小鼠中的 B 细胞扩增是必需的，因为靶向胰腺缺失 c-Met 导致适应性 B 细胞增殖失败和凋亡率增加[43]。缺失 c-Met 与胰岛中催乳素受体 mRNA 水平降低、Stat5 活化减少、FoxM1 表达降低、p27 抑制失败有关，所有这些都表明 HGF 是 B 细胞 PL 启动的促有丝分裂反应所必需的。缺乏 c-Met 表达的妊娠小鼠发生 GDM，伴有高血糖症和葡萄糖耐量受损。已知刺激 B 细胞增殖的生长因子的变化抑制细胞凋亡也发生在人类母体循环中，包括 HGF[44]和胰岛素样生长因子-1（IGF1）[45]。然而，目前尚不清楚这是否反映出内部存在旁分泌增加小岛。由于肽激素不会穿过胎盘，因此 C 肽激动剂 Met 可能用于增加 B 细胞的质量。

在朗格汉斯小岛内局部产生的 5-HT 也与 B 细胞质量增加和 GSIS 增加相关，并且通过激活催乳素受体发生作用。在妊娠期间，是通过增加表达来调节血清素合成酶、色氨酸羟化酶 1 和 2，从而导致血清素的胰岛含量增加（图 29.4）[46]。5-HT 通过激活 5-HT 调节 GSIS3a 和 3b 受体，而血清素增加 B 细胞质量的能力是由 HTr2b 介导的中期妊娠小鼠和妊娠晚期的 HTr1d[47]。所以，在妊娠期间，尽管经历了 B 细胞团的适应，HTr3a 无效的动物表现出葡萄糖耐受不良[48]。

细胞治疗预防妊娠糖尿病

至少在啮齿动物中，B 细胞的再生需要胰岛微脉管系统的平行扩张，可以通过内皮祖细胞的移植诱导，有助于血管生成。在整个妊娠过程中，在人类母体循环中内源性祖细胞增加与血清雌二醇水平升高有关[49,50]。在小鼠中，雌二醇增强了骨髓造血干细胞（其中一部分发育成内皮细胞）的增殖速度[51]。相应的，患有妊娠糖尿病或葡萄糖耐量降低的女性在妊娠期间，循环内皮祖细胞数量减少[52]。在妊娠期间内皮祖细胞是否存在为了适应性改变而刺激人体 B 细胞的数量改变的情况仍有待证实。然而，来自脐带血或脂肪组织的人间充质干细胞的移植已被证明可增加 C 肽和减少 T_1DM 或 T_2DM 患者的自身调节性 T 细胞[53,54]，提示干细胞诱导的 B 细胞扩增的概念对于妊娠糖尿病也是可行的。

我们和其他人的研究表明，给实验动物进行骨髓干细胞移植可导致糖尿病的逆转[55,56]。骨髓细胞直接转化为胰岛素表达细胞是可能的，但这种情况发生的频率很少，无法解释血糖的快速正常化和胰岛素释放的增加。更有可能的是，B 细胞再生是由骨髓来源的血管祖细胞分化为内皮祖细胞，以渗透胰岛和（或）胰管的分离细胞形式存在，或者是在新血管形成过程中直接掺入微血管系统[55]。新生血管之后是内源性 B 细胞复制的增加，或来自胰管的新胰岛的新生[55,57]。

进一步改进这种临床方法需要了解哪种方法可以使骨髓干细胞更好地诱导内源性 B 细胞扩增。骨髓含有促血管发生的造血祖细胞[（造血细胞）骨髓/单核细胞谱系的干细胞（HSC）]，真正的内皮祖细胞是间充质细胞系（间充质细胞）干细胞（MSC）[58]。HSC 可作为血管生成的旁分泌支持细胞，或者正如我们已经证明的那样，可以直接分化为功能性内皮细胞[55]。我们利用在 Vav 基因启动子控制下表达遗传报道基因的小鼠来标记 HSC。Vav 基因普遍由所有造血谱系细胞表达并且对分化的细胞后代保持活性，包括 T 细胞、B 细胞和巨噬细胞[59]。标记的细胞位于所有年龄的胰腺内，排列在胰腺导管上皮及胰岛周围和内部[60]。

来自导管上皮的小胰岛被造血谱系细胞包围。在用 STZ 诱导糖尿病后，HSC 衍生细胞的丰度在胰岛内和管道周围显著增加，B 细胞的量也相应扩增。虽然这些细胞不表达胰岛素，但约 30%与内皮细胞标志物

CD31 共染色，并且这在 STZ 处理后显著增加，强烈暗示内源性 HSC 衍生的内皮祖细胞参与 B 细胞量的扩增。骨髓的 MSC 成分可通过诱导内源性 B 细胞再生来逆转实验性 T_1DM 中的高血糖症[61]，但 MSC 可能另外转分化为胰岛和导管内的胰岛素表达细胞，后者可能代表胰岛新生[62, 63]。骨髓来源的 MSC 具有趋化因子受体，使它们能够在胰岛细胞提取物中趋化因子的作用下，快速到达糖尿病胰腺[64]，以改善胰岛血管形成[65]并维持胰岛形态[66]。

我们发现，通过 CD44 定位鉴定的 MSC 在 STZ 损伤后在胰腺中更丰富，但其分散在外分泌组织内而不是胰岛内[67]。我们直接比较了骨髓来源的 MSC 或 HSC 在移植到糖尿病小鼠胰腺后诱导 B 细胞再生的能力和机制，以及供体动物年龄的重要性[67]。与对照组相比，用年轻供体的 HSC 或 MSC 移植后 21~40d，糖尿病小鼠的高血糖和血浆胰岛素得到改善，MSC 在 7d 内、HSC 在 14d 内干细胞移植后葡萄糖耐量得到改善。HSC 处理导致胰岛内残留的 B 细胞增殖增加，而 MSC 处理引起胰岛外小分泌细胞团内 B 细胞祖细胞的增殖和分化。HSC 和 MSC 促进 B 细胞再生的能力随着供体年龄的增长而降低，但 MSC 可以通过在移植前体外诱导缺氧来"修复"[68]。因此，MSC 和 HSC 在胰腺 B 细胞丢失后动员，并且可以通过可能互补的不同机制诱导 B 细胞再生。这些研究应在轻度糖尿病的妊娠动物中重复进行，以检查 HSC 或 MSC 增加 B 细胞量对妊娠的适应能力。

微生物群和短链脂肪酸

人体内存在 5000 多种细菌，其中 95%属于拟杆菌属、厚壁菌门和放线菌门三大类[69]。这些细菌比例存在的差异与肥胖有关，就人类而言，其在生活方式干预期间实现的体重减轻与微生物组的初始构成有关[70]。在妊娠期间，与正常体重的女性相比，拟杆菌和葡萄球菌的比例增加，并且在第 2 个月和第 3 个月肠道微生物组成发生了实质性变化[71]。当将人类妊娠晚期的微生物组移植到无菌小鼠时，肥胖和胰岛素抵抗的出现增加，表明人类微生物组的变化可能导致妊娠期胰岛素抵抗[72]。与非妊娠受试者相比，GDM 患者的肠道微生物组多样性进一步改变[72]。

那么，通过益生菌治疗修改微生物组可以防止 GDM 的发展吗？最近的两项试验研究了这种可能性。

芬兰的一项研究检查了 256 名有妊娠糖尿病风险的妊娠妇女，她们在妊娠早期被随机分配到益生菌饮食干预组或对照组中，有或没有强化饮食和生活方式咨询[73]。接受益生菌的妇女在妊娠期间母体血糖降低，GDM 的比率降至 13%，而对照组的女性接受生活方式咨询的比例为 36%。接受益生菌治疗的女性胰岛素敏感指数改善，循环胰岛素水平升高，糖耐量改善。第二项试验的重点是妊娠 24~28 周的 138 名肥胖女性，这些女性有患 GDM 的高风险[74]。接受益生菌的女性在发生 GDM 或葡萄糖耐量方面的百分比没有差异。第三项随机对照试验目前正在进行 SPRING 研究，研究益生菌对大肠杆菌的影响，预防超重和肥胖女性的 GDM[75]。

益生菌的作用机制还可能改善有 GDM 风险女性的血糖控制，其可能与肠道微生物组对能量可用性和新陈代谢的影响有关。肠道微生物组促进厌氧发酵，而且难以消化的多糖产生短链脂肪酸（SCFA），如丁酸盐、丙酸盐和乙酸盐。当把来自常规小鼠的肠道微生物组转移至无菌小鼠时，10d 内脂肪量增加，胰岛素敏感性降低[76]。SCFA 能快速且主动地穿过小肠上皮细胞。丁酸盐可以作为结肠上皮的能量来源；醋酸盐，用于通过肌肉脂肪生成和抑制脂肪分解活性产生能量，它和丙酸盐一起可增强肝脏糖异生[77]。妊娠与母体循环中 SCFA 的产生与外观的变化有关，可能反映了妊娠微生物组的改变[78]。血清乙酸盐水平与妊娠期母体体重增加和母体脂联素水平呈正相关，而丙酸盐与母体瘦素水平和后代出生体重呈负相关。因此，SCFA 的产生可能会影响母体的代谢控制。此外，微生物组的基因组分析显示了与 T_2DM 相关的变化，包括减少了与丁酸盐生产有关的物种[79]，尽管这方面还缺乏妊娠糖尿病的数据。那么，改变 SCFA 产生的从微生物组引起的母体代谢控制的变化与 GDM 的风险有关吗？SCFA 通过与 GPCR 游离脂肪酸受体-3（FFAR3，也称为 Gpr41）和 FFAR2 或 Gpr43[80]的相互作用激活细胞内信号传导途径，如肠上皮细胞、脂肪细胞和胰腺 B 细胞的肠内分泌细胞[81]。在脂肪组织中，已显示活化的 FFAR3 刺激脂肪释放瘦素的产生和增加脂质代谢，同时减少导致胰岛素抵抗的慢性炎症调节剂，如 TNF-α 和 IL-12[82]。缺乏 *Ffar2* 基因的小鼠比野生型小鼠更肥胖，过表达 *Ffar2* 的小鼠在正常饮食条件下，脂肪组织过度消瘦[83]。如果将小鼠维持在无菌环境中则没有发现差异，表明 FFAR2 通过源自肠道微生物组的 SCFA 调节脂肪胰岛素信号传导。因此，FFAR2 激活可以抑制脂肪堆积。在类似的研究中，缺乏 *Ffar3* 基因的小鼠表现出体脂增加和能源消耗减少[84]。

最近，在肠内分泌 L 细胞中发现了 FFAR2 和 FFAR3，其中 SCFA 的刺激介导食欲减少激素、肽-YY（PYY）[85]的下游释放，以及肠降血糖素、胰高血糖素样肽-1（GLP1）的释放[86]。GLP1 可增强 GSIS，抑制 B 细胞凋亡，并改善胰岛素敏感性[87]。然而，SCFA 也可以直接影响胰腺的 GSIS（图 29.5）。MIN6 细胞暴露于 SCFA 导致细胞内 Ca^{2+} 立即增加。此外，灌注分离的小鼠胰岛与 SCFA 导致 GSIS 增加，由 FFAR2 和 FFAR3 介导，而与野生型动物相比，来自 *ffar2*$^{-/-}$ 小鼠的胰岛灌注显示 GSIS 减少[88]。类似的，用针对 FFAR2 的 SCFA 激动剂治疗人胰岛可增加胰岛素的释放[89]。因此，改变微生物组相关联的 SCFA 有效性的变化，特别是在妊娠期间 GLP1 释放水平，B 细胞胰岛素释放和脂肪细胞脂肪因子

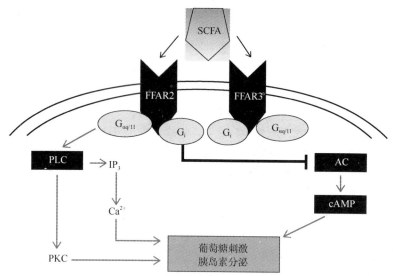

图 29.5 短链脂肪酸（SCFA）可增加葡萄糖刺激的胰岛素 B 细胞释放的可能机制。SCFA 与游离脂肪酸受体 FFAR2 和 FFAR3 结合，引起 G 蛋白亚基 $G_{\alpha q/11}$ 或 G_i 的活化。$G_{\alpha q/11}$ 活化引起磷脂酶 C（PLC）的活化，进一步激活蛋白激酶 C（PKC）并产生肌醇三磷酸（IP3）。IP3 引起细胞内钙的增加，导致胰岛素释放。相反，G_i 的激活可以阻断腺苷酸环化酶（AC）的作用，降低环腺苷—磷酸（cAMP）的水平，从而减少胰岛素释放。适应 SCFA 的这两种途径平衡后的净变化可导致胰岛素分泌的增加

分泌水平而改变对血糖的控制。有趣的是，通过引起 PPARγ 从脂肪生成转变为脂质氧化的依赖性，可以证明膳食补充 SCFA 可以预防高脂饮食对小鼠的致糖尿病作用[90]。

尚未报道用特异性补充 SCFA 预防人类 GDM 的研究。但在动物研究中，丁酸盐的补充改善了肥胖，以及妊娠小鼠的血糖水平及胰岛素水平的增加和 B 细胞的增殖率[91]。总之，妊娠期间母体 B 细胞量和（或）生理适应功能的失败可导致 GDM，目前并无有效预防策略。未来的治疗策略可以通过操纵营养，以及旁分泌和母体内分泌胰腺细胞环境来增加功能性 B 细胞量。

由于母体 B 细胞量通常不包括分娩后的非妊娠 B 细胞量，从理论上来看，如果出生后停止这种疗法不会导致长期病理情况。

选择题

1. 正常妊娠期间胰腺 B 细胞的数量是（　　）
   A. 增加　　　　　　　　B. 减少
   C. 保持不变
   正确答案是 A。
2. 胎盘在妊娠期间直接在母体循环中产生，变异生长激素和胎盘催乳素。哪种激素驱动妊娠的胰岛素抵抗（　　）
   A. 变异生长激素　　　　B. 胎盘催乳素
   正确答案是 A。
3. 妊娠期间补充益生菌会增加产量的是（　　）
   A. 肠道中的长链脂肪酸　B. 短链脂肪酸
   正确答案是 B。

致谢

对于作者发表的被引研究，他感谢西方大学医学系实验医学项目 Alan Thicke 青少年糖尿病研究中心的研究资助，以及欧盟第七框架计划。

（杨　芳　译，朱海清　校）

参 考 文 献

1. The HAPO Study Cooperative Research Group. Hyperglycemia and adverse pregnancy outcomes. N England J Med 2008;358:1991-2002.
2. Kubo A, Ferrara A, Windham GC, Greenspan LC, Deardorff J, Hiatt RA, et al. Maternal hyperglycemia during pregnancy predicts adiposity of the offspring. Diabetes Care 2014;37:2996-3002.
3. Angueira A, Ludvik, AE, Reddy TE, Wicksteed B, Lowe WL, Layden BT. New insights into gestational glucose metabolism: lessons learned from 21st century approaches. Diabetes 2005;64:327-334.
4. Jayasena C, Franks S. The management of patients with polycystic ovary syndrome. Nat Rev Endocrinol 2014;10:624-636.
5. Koivusalo SB, Rönö K, Klemetti MM, Roine RP, Lindström J, Erkkola M, et al. Gestational diabetes mellitus can be prevented by lifestyle intervention: the Finnish Gestational Diabetes Prevention Study (RADIEL): a randomized controlled trial. Diabetes Care 2016;39(1):24-30.
6. Simmons D, Jelsma JG, Galjaard S, Devlieger R, van Assche A, Jans G, et al. Results from a European multicenter randomized trial of physical activity and/or healthy eating to reduce the risk of gestational diabetes mellitus: the DALI Lifestyle Pilot. Diabetes Care 2015;38(9):1650-1656.
7. Poston L, Bell R, Croker H, on behalf of the UPBEAT Trial Consortium. Effect of a behavioural intervention in obese pregnant women (the UPBEAT study): a multicentre, randomised controlled trial. Lancet Diabetes Endocrinol 2015;3(10):767-777.
8. Sorenson RL, Brelje TC. Adaptation of islets of Langerhans to pregnancy: beta-cell growth, enhanced insulin secretion and the role of lactogenic hormones. Horm Metab Res 1997;29:301-307.
9. Van Assche FA, Aerts L, De Prins F. A morphological study of the endocrine pancreas in human pregnancy. Br J Obstet Gynaecol 1978;85:818-820.
10. Butler AE, Cao-Minh L, Galasso R, Rizza RA, Corradin A, Cobelli C, et al. Adaptive changes in pancreatic beta cell fractional area and beta cell turnover in human pregnancy. Diabetologia 2010;53:2167-2176.
11. Xiang A, Takayanagi M, Black MH, Trigo E, Lawrence JM, Watanabe RM, et al. Longitudinal changes in insulin sensitivity and beta-cell function between women with and without a history of gestational diabetes mellitus. Diabetologia 2013;56:2753-2760.
12. Newbern D, Freemark M. Placental hormones and the control of maternal metabolism and fetal growth. Curr Opin Endocrinol Diabetes Obes 2011;18:409-416.
13. Parsons JA, Brelje TC, Sorenson RL. Adaptation of islets of Langerhans to pregnancy: increased islet cell proliferation and insulin secretion correlates with the onset of placental lactogen secretion. Endocrinology 1992;130:1459-1466.
14. Vasavada RC, Garcia-Ocaña A, Zawalich WS, Sorenson RL, Dann P, Syed M, et al. Targeted expression of placental lactogen in the beta cells of transgenic mice results in beta cell proliferation, islet mass augmentation, and hypoglycemia. J Biol Chem 2000;275:15399-15406.
15. Kotani M, Detheux M, Vandenbogaerde A, Communi D, Vanderwinden JM, Le Poul E, et al. The metastasis suppressor gene KiSS-1 encodes kisspeptins, the natural ligands of the orphan G protein-coupled receptor GPR54. J Biol Chem 2001;276:34631-34636.
16. Mizuno N, Itoh H. Functions and regulatory mechanisms of Gq-signaling pathways. Neurosignals 2009;17:42-54.
17. Stafford LJ, Xia C, Ma W, Cai Y, Liu, M. Identification and characterization of mouse metastasis-suppressor KiSS1 and its G-protein-coupled receptor. Cancer Res 2002;62:5399-5404.
18. Hiden U, Bilban M, Knöfler M, Desoye G.

Kisspeptins and the placenta: regulation of trophoblast invasion. Rev Endocr Metab Disord 2007;8:31-39.
19 Smets E, Deurloo KL, Go AT, van Vugt JM, Blankenstein MA, et al. Decreased plasma levels of metastin in early pregnancy are associated with small for gestational age neonates. Prenat Diagn 2008;28:299-303.
20 Cetković A, Miljic D, Ljubić A, Patterson M, Ghatei M, Stamenković J, et al. Plasma kisspeptin levels in pregnancies with diabetes and hypertensive disease as a potential marker of placental dysfunction and adverse perinatal outcome. Endocr Res 2012;37:78-88.
21 Horikoshi Y, Matsumoto H, Takatsu Y, Ohtaki T, Kitada C, Usuki S, et al. Dramatic elevation of plasma metastin concentrations in human pregnancy: metastin as a novel placenta-derived hormone in humans. J. Clin Endocrinol Metab 2003;88:914-919.
22 Bowe JE, King AJ, Kinsey-Jones JS, Foot VL, Li XF, O'Byrne KT, et al. Kisspeptin stimulation of insulin secretion: mechanisms of action in mouse islets and rats. Diabetologia 2009;52:855-862.
23 Wahab F, Riaz T, Shahab M. Study on the effect of peripheral kisspeptin administration on basal and glucose-induced insulin secretion under fed and fasting conditions in the adult male rhesus monkey (Macaca mulatta). Horm Metab Res 2011;43:37-42.
24 Bowe JE, Hill TG, Persaud SJ, Jones PM. A role for kisspeptin in regulating beta cell mass during pregnancy. Diabetic Med 2015;32(Suppl 1):33.
25 Freemark M, Avril I, Fleenor D, Driscoll P, Petro A, Opara E, et al. Targeted deletion of the PRL receptor: effects on islet development, insulin production, and glucose tolerance. Endocrinology 2002;43:1378-1385.
26 Huang C, Snider F, Cross JC. Prolactin receptor is required for normal glucose homeostasis and modulation of β-cell mass during pregnancy. Endocrinology 2009;150:1618-1626.

27 Brelje TC, Stout LE, Bhagroo NV, Sorenson RL. Distinctive roles for prolactin and growth hormone in the activation of signal transducer and activator of transcription 5 in pancreatic islets of Langerhans. Endocrinology 2004;145:4162-4175.
28 Hughes E, Huang C. Participation of Akt, menin, and p21 in pregnancy-induced β-cell proliferation. Endocrinology 2011;152:847-855.
29 Karnik SK, Chen H, McLean GW, Heit JJ, Gu X, Zhang AY, et al. Menin controls growth of pancreatic beta-cells in pregnant mice and promotes gestational diabetes mellitus. Science 2007;318:806-809.
30 Zhang H, Li W, Wang Q, Wang X, Li F, Zhang C, et al. Glucose-mediated repression of menin promotes pancreatic β-cell proliferation. Endocrinology 2012;153:602-611.
31 Xu Y, Wang X, Gao L, Zhu J, Zhang H, Shi H, et al. Prolactin-stimulated surviving induction is required for beta cell mass expansion during pregnancy in mice. Diabetologia 2015;58:2064-2073.
32 Seaberg RM, Smukler SR, Kieffer TJ, Enikolopov G, Asghar Z, Wheeler MB, et al. Clonal identification of multipotent precursors from adult mouse pancreas that generate neural and pancreatic lineages. Nature Biotech 2004;22:1115-1124.
33 Smukler SR, Arntfield ME, Razavi R, Bikopoulos G, Karpowicz P, Seaberg R, et al. The adult mouse and human pancreas contain rare multipotent stem cells that express insulin. Cell Stem Cell 2011;8:281-293.
34 Abouna S, Old RW, Pelengaris S, Epstein D, Ifandi V, Sweeney I, et al. Non-β-cell progenitors of β-cells in pregnant mice. Organogenesis 2010;6:125-133.
35 Nielsen LR, Rehfeld JF, Pedersen-Bjergaard U, Damm P, Mathiesen ER. Pregnancy-induced rise in serum C-peptide concentration in women with type 1 diabetes. Diabetes Care 2009;32:1052-1057.
36 Gupta RK, Gao N, Gorski RK, White P, Hardy OT, Rafiq K, et al. Expansion of adult

beta-cell mass in response to increased metabolic demand is dependent on HNF-4alpha. Genes Dev 2007;21:756–769.
37 Bernado AS, Hay CW, Docherty K. Pancreatic transcription factors and their role in the birth, life and survival of the pancreatic beta cell. Mol Cell Endocrinol 2008;294:1–9.
38 Huang C. Wild-type offspring of heterozygous prolactin receptor-null female mice have maladaptive responses during pregnancy. J Physiol 2013;591:1325–1328.
39 Xue Y, Liu C, Xu Y, Yuan Q, Xu K, Mao X, et al. Study on pancreatic islet adaptation and gene expression during pregnancy in rats. Endocrine 2010;37:83–97.
40 Bonner-Weir S, Taneja M, Weir GC, Tatarkiewicz K, Song KH, Sharma A, et al. In vitro cultivation of human islets from expanded ductal tissue. Proc Natl Acad Sci USA 2000;97:7999–8004.
41 Hakonen E, Ustinov J, Mathijs I, Palgi J, Bouwens L, Miettinen PJ, et al. Epidermal growth factor (EGF)-receptor signaling is needed for murine beta cell mass expansion in response to high fat diet and pregnancy but not after pancreatic duct ligation. Diabetologia 2011;54:1735–1743.
42 Alvarez-Perez JC, Ernst S, Demirci C, Casinelli GP, Mellado-Gil JM, Rausell-Palamos F, et al. Hepatocyte growth factor/c-Met signaling is required for β-cell regeneration. Diabetes 2014;63:216–223.
43 Demirco C, Ernst S, Alvarez-Perez JC, Rosa T, Valle S, Shridhar V, et al. Loss of HGF/c-Met signaling in pancreatic β-cells leads to incomplete maternal β-cell adaptation and gestational diabetes mellitus. Diabetes 2012;61:1143–1152.
44 Horibe N, Okamoto T, Itakura A, Nakanishi T, Suzuki T, Kazeto S, et al. Levels of hepatocyte growth factor in maternal serum and amniotic fluid. Am J Obstet Gynecol 1995;173:937–942.
45 Whittaker PG, Stewart MO, Taylor A, Howell RJ, Lind T. Insulin-like growth factor 1 and its binding protein 1 during normal and diabetic pregnancies. Obstet Gynecol 1990;76:223–229.
46 Schraenen A, Lemaire K, de Faudeur G, Hendrickx N, Granvik M, Van Lommel L, et al. Placental lactogens induce serotonin biosynthesis in a subset of mouse beta cells during pregnancy. Diabetologia 2010;53:2589–2599.
47 Kim H, Toyofuku Y, Lynn FC, Chak E, Uchida T, Mizukami H, et al. Serotonin regulates pancreatic beta cell mass during pregnancy. Nature Med 2010;16:804–808.
48 Ohara-Imaizumi M, Kim H, Yoshida M, Fujiwara, T, Aoyagi K, Toyofuku Y, et al. Serotonin regulates glucose-stimulated insulin secretion from pancreatic β cells during pregnancy. Proc Natl Acad Sci USA 2013;110:19420–19425.
49 Gussin HA, Sharma AK, Elias S. Culture of endothelial cells isolated from maternal blood using anti-CD105 and CD133. Prenat Diagn 2004;24:189–193.
50 Sugawara J, Mitsui-Saito M, Hoshiai T, Hayashi C, Kimura Y, Okamura K. Circulating endothelial progenitor cells during human pregnancy. J Clin Endocrinol Metab 2005;90:1845–1848.
51 Nakada D, Oguro H, Levi BP, Ryan N, Kitano A, Saitoh Y, et al. Oestrogen increases haematopoietic stem-cell self-renewal in females and during pregnancy. Nature 2014;505:555–558.
52 Penno G, Pucci L, Lucchesi D, Lencioni C, Iorio MC, Vanacore R, et al. Circulating endothelial progenitor cells in women with gestational alterations of glucose tolerance. Diab Vasc Dis Res 2014;8:202–210.
53 Thakkar UG, Trevedi HL, Vanikar AV, Dave SD. Insulin-secreting adipose-derived mesenchymal stromal cells with bone marrow-derived hematopoietic stem cells from autologous and allogenic sources for type 1 diabetes mellitus. Cytotherapy 2015;7:940–947.
54 Kong D, Zhuang X, Wang D, Qu H, Jiang Y, Li X, et al. Umbilical cord mesenchymal

cell transfusion ameliorated hyperglycemia in patients with type 2 diabetes mellitus. Clin Lab 2014;60:1969–1976.
55 Hess D, Li L, Martin M, Sakano S, Hill D, Strutt B, et al. Bone marrow derived stem cells rescue hyperglycemia by regeneration of recipient islets. Nature Biotech 2003;21:763–770.
56 Sordi V, Piemonti L. The contribution of hematopoietic stem cells to beta-cell replacement. Curr Diab Rep 2009;9:119–124.
57 Hasegawa Y, Ogihara T, Yamada T, Ishigaki Y, Imai J, Uno K, et al. Bone marrow (BM) transplantation promotes ß-cell regeneration after acute injury through BM cell mobilization. Endocrinology 2007;148:2006–2015.
58 Yoder MC, Mead LE, Prater D, Krier TR, Mroueh KN, Li F, et al. Redefining endothelial progenitor cells via clonal analysis and hematopoietic stem/progenitor cell principals. Blood 2007;109:1801–1809.
59 de Boer J, Williams A, Skavdis G, Harker N, Coles M, Tolaini M, et al. Transgenic mice with hematopoietic and lymphoid specific expression of Cre. Eur J Immunol 2003;33:314–325.
60 Chamson-Reig A, Arany EJ, Hill DJ. Lineage tracing and resulting phenotype of hematopoietic-derived cells in the pancreas during beta cell regeneration. Diabetologia 2010;53:2188–2197.
61 Urban VS, Kiss J, Kovács J, Gócza E, Vas V, Monostori E, et al. Mesenchymal stem cells cooperate with bone marrow cells in therapy of diabetes. Stem Cells 2008;26:244–253
62 Kadam SS, Blonde RR. Islet neogenesis from the constitutively nestin expressing human umbilical cord matrix derived mesenchymal stem cells. Islets 2010;2:112–120.
63 Karaoz E, Ayhan S, Okçu A, Aksoy A, Bayazıt G, Osman Gürol A, et al. Bone marrow-derived mesenchymal stem cells co-cultured with pancreatic islets display β cell plasticity. J Tissue Eng Regen Med 2010;5:491–500.
64 Sordi V, Malosio ML, Marchesi F, Mercalli A, Melzi R, Giordano T, et al. Bone marrow mesenchymal stem cells express a restricted set of functionally active chemokine receptors capable of promoting migration to pancreatic islets. Blood 2005;106:419–427.
65 Johansson U, Rasmusson I, Niclou SP, Forslund N. Gustavsson L, Nilsson B, et al. Formation of composite endothelial cell–mesenchymal stem cell islets: a novel approach to promote islet revascularization. Diabetes 2008;57:2393–2401.
66 Rackham CL, Chagastelles PC, Nardi NB, Hauge-Evans AC, Jones PM, King AJ. Co-transplantation of mesenchymal stem cells maintains islet organisation and morphology in mice. Diabetologia 2011;54:1127–1135.
67 Waseem M, Arany EJ, Strutt B, Hill DJ. Comparison and effect of age on the beta cell regenerative potential of bone marrow-derived mesenchymal (MSC) and haematopoietic stem cells (HSC) in mice. Diabetic Med 2015;32(Suppl 1):33.
68 Waseem M, Strutt B, Rahman Salim A, Hill DJ. Hypoxic preconditioning of adult bone marrow mesenchymal stem cells enhances their ability to reverse diabetes in streptozotocin (STZ) diabetic mice. American Diabetes Association 2015, Abstr 183–OR.
69 Barrett HL, Callaway LK, Nitert MD. Probiotics: a potential role in the prevention of gestational diabetes. Act Diabetol 2012;49(Suppl 1):S1–S13.
70 Santacruz A, Marcos A, Warnberg J, Marti A, Martin-Matillas M, Campoy C, et al. Interplay between weight loss and gut microbiota composition in overweight adolescents. Obesity 2009;17:1906–1915.
71 Collado MC, Isolauri E, Laitinen K, Salminen S. Distinct composition of gut microbiota during pregnancy in overweight and normal-weight women. Am J Clin Nutr

72 Koren O, Goodrich JK, Cullender TC, Spor A, Laitinen K, Bäckhed HK, et al. Host remodeling of the gut microbiome and metabolic changes during pregnancy. Cell 2012;150:470-480.
73 Luoto R, Laitinen K, Nermes M, Isolauri E. Impact of maternal probiotic-supplemented dietary counselling on pregnancy outcome and prenatal and postnatal growth: a double-blind, placebo-controlled study. Br J Nutr 2010;103:1792-1799.
74 Lindsay KL, Kennelly M, Culliton M, Smith T, Maguire OC, Shanahan F, et al. Probiotics in obese pregnancy do not reduce maternal fasting glucose: a double-blind, placebo-controlled, randomized trial (Probiotics in Pregnancy Study). Am J Clin Nutr 2014;99:1432-1439.
75 Nitert MD, Barrett HL, Foxcroft K, Tremellen A, Wilkinson S, Lingwood B, et al. SPRING: an RCT study of probiotics in the prevention of gestational diabetes mellitus in overweight and obese women. BMC Pregnancy Childbirth 2013;13:50.
76 Backhed F, Ding H, Wang T, Hooper LV, Koh GY, Nagy A, et al. The gut microbiota as an environmental factor that regulates fat storage. Proc Natl Acad Sci USA 2004;101:15718-15723.
77 Li D, Kirsop J, Tang WH. Listening to our gut: contribution of gut microbiota and cardiovascular risk in diabetes pathogenesis. Curr Diab Rep 2015;15:634. doi:10.1007/s11892-015-0634-1
78 Priyadarshini M, Thomas A, Reisetter AC, Scholtens DM, Wolever TM, Josefson JL, et al. Maternal short-chain fatty acids are associated with metabolic parameters in mothers and newborns. Transl Res 2014;164:153-157.
79 Qin J, Li Y, Cai Z, Li S, Zhu J, Zhang F, et al. A metagenomewide association study of gut microbiota in type 2 diabetes. Nature 2012;490:55-60.
80 Hara T, Kimura I, Inoue D, Ichimura A, Hirasawa A. Free fatty acid receptors and their role in regulation of energy metabolism. Rev Physiol Biochem Pharmacol 2013;164:77-116.
81 Offermanns S. Free fatty acid (FFA) and hydroxy carboxylic acid (HCA) receptors. Ann Rev Pharmacol Toxicol 2014;54:407-434.
82 Xiong, Y, Miyamoto N, Shibata K, Valasek MA, Motoike T, Kedzierski RM, et al. (2004) Short-chain fatty acids stimulate leptin production in adipocytes through the G protein-coupled receptor GPR41. Proc Natl Acad Sci USA 2004;101:1045-1050.
83 Kimura I, Ozawa K, Inoue D, Imamura T, Kimura K, Maeda T, et al. The gut microbiota suppresses insulin-mediated fat accumulation via the short-chain fatty acid receptor GPR43. Nat Commun 2013;4:1829.
84 Bellahcene M, O'Dowd JF, Wargent ET, Zaibi MS, Hislop DC, Ngala RA, et al. Male mice that lack the G-protein-coupled receptor GPR41 have low energy expenditure and increased body fat content. Br J Nutr 2013;109:1755-1764.
85 Psichas A, Sleeth ML, Murphy KG, Brooks L, Bewick GA, Hanyaloglu AC, et al. The short chain fatty acid propionate stimulates GLP-1 and PYY secretion via free fatty acid receptor 2 in rodents. Int J Obes 2015;39:424-429.
86 Kaji I, Karaki S, Kuwahara A. Short-chain fatty acid receptor and its contribution to glucagon-like peptide-1 release. Digestion 2014;89:31-36.
87 Ma X, Guan Y, Hua X. Glucagon-like peptide 1-potentiated insulin secretion and proliferation of pancreatic β-cells. J Diabetes 2014;6:394-402.
88 Hill TG, Pingitore A, Bowe JE, Bewick GA, Persaud SJ. Direct stimulatory effects of short-chain free fatty acids on insulin secretion from isolated islets. Diabetic Med 2015;32(Suppl 1):39.
89 McNelis JC, Lee YS, Mayoral R, van der Kant R, Johnson AM, Wollam J, et al. GPR43 potentiates beta cell function in obesity. Diabetes 2015;64(9):3203-3217.
90 den Basten G, Bleeker A, Gerding A, van Eunen K, Havinga R, van Dijk TH, et al.

Short chain fatty acids protect against high-fat diet-induced obesity via a PPARγ-dependent switch from lipogenesis to fat oxidation. Diabetes 2015;64:2398-2408.

91 Li HP, Chen X, Li MQ. Butyrate alleviates metabolic impairments and protects pancreatic β cell function in pregnant mice with obesity. Int J Clin Exp Pathol 2013;6:1574-1584.

其他参考文献

92 Rieck S, Kaestner KH. Expansion of beta-cell mass in response to pregnancy. Trends Endocrinol Metab 2010;21:151-158.